The Treatment of Bipolar Disorder
Integrative clinical strategies & future directions

The Treatment of Bipolar Disorder

Integrative clinical strategies & future directions

Edited by

André F. Carvalho

Associate Professor, Department of Clinical Medicine,
Head, Translational Psychiatry Research Group, Faculty of
Medicine, Federal University of Ceará, Fortaleza, Brazil

Eduard Vieta

Chair, Department of Psychiatry and Psychology, Hospital
Clinic, Institute of Neuroscience, IDIBAPS, CIBERSAM,
University of Barcelona, Catalonia, Spain

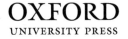

OXFORD
UNIVERSITY PRESS

OXFORD
UNIVERSITY PRESS

Great Clarendon Street, Oxford, OX2 6DP,
United Kingdom

Oxford University Press is a department of the University of Oxford.
It furthers the University's objective of excellence in research, scholarship,
and education by publishing worldwide. Oxford is a registered trade mark of
Oxford University Press in the UK and in certain other countries

Published in the United States of America by Oxford University Press
198 Madison Avenue, New York, NY 10016, United States of America

British Library Cataloguing in Publication Data

Data available

Library of Congress Control Number: 2016955729

ISBN 978–0–19–880103–0

Printed and bound by CPI Group (UK) Ltd, Croydon, CR0 4YY

Foreword

This excellent new book on bipolar disorder is written by leading international experts who have advanced our understanding of the field in recent decades. It starts with modern diagnostic classification, reviews comprehensively and critically the complex field of available treatment methods, and concludes with highlights of current research and discussion of future developments.

Bipolar disorder is a common mental illness, affecting approximately 2.4% of the general population worldwide, although this is arguably a significant underestimation of its true prevalence. One particular feature of the disorder, namely the subjective experience of hypomania as simple well-being or as a return to health after severe depression, leads to substantial under-reporting and under-diagnosis.

On the fundamental issue of classification, the contributors trace the extension of the simple dichotomy of unipolar depression vs bipolar disorder into several subtypes including diverse sub-threshold bipolar and mixed syndromes and discuss the relative merits and appropriateness of categorical and dimensional approaches to the illness. But for treatment decisions a refined categorical classification remains indispensable and should not neglect the patient's comorbid psychiatric and somatic syndromes and diagnoses.

The course of bipolar disorder is characterised by an early onset (often in childhood or adolescence), multiple recurrences of episodes, frequently incomplete inter-episode remission, and substantial consequences in terms of social and cognitive impairment and reduced quality of life. It is furthermore associated with significant morbidity and elevated mortality rates due to comorbidities and suicide.

The volume's main focus is treatment. It provides a masterly description of the evidence-based, effective treatments available for the integrative management of the different stages of this complex and debilitating disorder. These range from early interventions, where a staging model can be helpful, to the numerous acute and long-term maintenance prophylactic therapies, pharmacological and psychotherapeutic. There is ample evidence that specific psychological and psychotherapeutic interventions are valuable adjuncts to pharmacological treatment. A key role is played by psychoeducation (illness awareness, adherence, habits, identification of warning signs) and the involvement of the family (especially in children, adolescents and the elderly). ECT still proves useful in treating some patients, and cognitive dysfunction in bipolar disorder is a new target for evidence-based psychological treatment. But, the authors point out that despite decades of investigation there is still a shortage of clinical trials on bipolar mixed states, rapid cycling bipolar disorder and cyclothymic disorder.

Special chapters deal with differentiated treatments for children/adolescents, the elderly, and women with bipolar disorder.

This volume is an invaluable source of current expertise, a concise guide to the integrative management of bipolar disorder. It provides sound evidence that an appropriate combination of treatments can profoundly improve patients' lives.

Jules Angst

Contents

Abbreviations

ω-3FAs	omega-3 fatty acids	CANMAT	Canadian Network for Mood and Anxiety Treatments
A	amperes		
AA	arachidonic acid		
ACC	anterior cingulate cortex	CBT	cognitive behaviour therapy
ACE	angiotensin-converting enzyme		
		CBT-R	CBT-Regulation
ADHD	attention deficit hyper-activity disorder	CCT	controlled clinical trial
		CD	conduct disorder
ADRs	adverse drug reactions	CGI	Clinical Global Impression
AEDs	antiepileptic drugs		
AIM	antidepressant-induced mania	CIA	clozapine-induced agranulocytosis
AIWG	antipsychotic-induced weight gain	CNR1	cannabinoid receptor 1
		CNS	central nervous system
AMPA	α-amino-3-hydroxyl-5-methyl-4-isoxazoleproprionic acid	COBRA	Cognitive Complaints in Bipolar Disorder Rating Assessment
AN	anorexia nervosa	ConLiGen	Consortium on Lithium Genetics
APA	American Psychiatric Association		
		CONSORT	Consolidated Standards for Reporting Trials
ATP	adenosine triphosphate		
BAD	bipolar affective disorder	COPD	chronic obstructive pulmonary disease
BAP	British Association for Psychopharmacology	COX	cyclooxygenase
		CPS1	carbamoyl phosphate synthase 1
BAR	bipolar at-risk		
BD	bipolar disorder	CR	cognitive remediation
BDNF	brain-derived neurotrophic factor	CRF	corticotropin releasing factor
BED	binge eating disorder	CS	case series
BF	bi-frontal	DALY	disability-adjusted life years
BLT	bright light therapy		
BMI	body mass index	DASS	Depression, Anxiety, and Stress Scale
BN	bulimia nervosa		
BPRS	Brief Psychiatric Rating Scale	DBS	deep brain stimulation
		DHA	docosahexaenoic acid
BT	bi-temporal	DHEA	dehydroepiandrosterone
C	coulombs	DLPFC	dorsolateral prefrontal cortex
CAM	complementary and alternative medicine		
		DPP	depressive predominant polarity

DRD1	dopamine receptor D1
DRD2	dopamine receptor 2
DRD3	dopamine 3 receptor
DRESS	drug-related rash with eosinophilia and systemic symptoms
DSM-5	*Diagnostic and Statistical Manual of Mental Disorders* (5th edition)
DSPD	delayed sleep phase disorder
DTI	diffusion tensor imaging
dTMS	deep repetitive transcranial magnetic stimulation
ECG	electrocardiograph
ECT	electroconvulsive therapy
EDs	eating disorders
EEG	electroencephalography
ELRs	excellent lithium responders
EM	extensive metabolizer
EMBLEM	European Mania in Bipolar Longitudinal Evaluation of Medication
EMDR	eye movement desensitization and reprocessing
EMP +	EM Power Plus
EMRs	electronic medical records
EPA	ethyl-eicosapentanoate/ eicosapentaenoic acid
EPO	erythropoietin
EPS	extrapyramidal side effects
ER	extended release/endoplasmic reticulum
ES	effect size
FAAH	fatty acid amide hydrolase
FAST	Functioning Assessment Short Test
FDA	Food and Drug Administration

FEWP	Free and Easy Wanderer Plus
FFT	family focused treatment/therapy
FGAs	first-generation antipsychotics
FGF2	fibroblast growth factor
FR	functional remediation
FTD	frontotemporal dementia
GABA	central gamma-aminobutyric acid
GAF	global activity
GI	gastrointestinal
GP	general practitioner
GSK-3	glycogen synthase kinase-3
GSK3B	glycogen synthase kinase 3 beta
GWAS	genome-wide association studies
HAM-D	Hamilton Rating Scale for Depression
HCV	hepatitis C virus
HDRS	Hamilton Depression Rating Scale
HIV	human immunodeficiency virus
HLA	human leukocyte antigen
HPA	hypothalamic pituitary adrenal
HR	hazard ratio
hsCRP	high-sensitivity C-reactive protein
Hz	hertz
ICD-10	*International Classification of Diseases* (10th revision)
IGF-1	insulin-growth factor 1
IGF-1-R alpha	insulin-like growth factor 1 receptor alpha subunit
IGFBP5	IGF-binding protein 5
IL	interleukin
IMs	intermediate metabolizers

IPF1	insulin promoter factor 1
IPSRT	interpersonal and social rhythm therapy
ISBD	International Society for Bipolar Disorders
ITT	intention to treat
lDLPFC	left dorsal lateral prefrontal cortex
KA	kainate
KMAP-BP	Korean Medication Algorithm Project for Bipolar Disorder
LCLs	lymphoblastoid cell lines
LD	linkage disequilibrium
LDX	lisdexamphetamine
LOCF	last observation carried forward
LTD	long-term depression
LTP	long-term potentiation
MADRS	Montgomery-Åsberg Depression Rating Scale
MAO	monoamine oxidase
MAS	Mania Assessment Scale
MBCBT	mindfulness-based CBT
mC	millicoulombs
MC4R	melanocortin receptor 4
MCCB	MATRICS Consensus Cognitive Battery
MDD	major depressive disorder
MDQ	mood disorders questionnaire
mECT	maintenance ECT
MetS	Metabolic Syndrome
MF-PEP	multi-family psychoeducational psychotherapy
Mg	magnesium
mGluRs	metabotropic glutamate receptors
MHC	major histocompatibility complex
MMP16	matrix metalloproteinase 16
MPH	methylphenidate
MPP	manic predominant polarity

MRI	magnetic resonance imaging
MRS	Mania Rating Scale/ magnetic resonance spectroscopy
ms	milliseconds
MS	mood stabilizer
MST	magnetic seizure therapy
MT	motor threshold
NAC	N-acetyl cysteine
NESARC	National Epidemiologic Survey on Alcohol and Related Conditions
NICE	National Institute for Health and Care Excellence
NIMH	National Institute of Mental Health
NMDA	N-methyl-D-aspartate
NNH	numbers needed to harm
NNT	number(s) needed to treat
NOS	not otherwise specified
NTRK2	neurotrophic tyrosine kinase receptor type 2
OABD	older-age bipolar disorder
OCD	obsessive–compulsive disorder
OCPs	oral contraceptives
OFC	olanzapine/fluoxetine combination
PCr	phosphocreatine
PED	psychoeducation
PET	positron emission tomography
PI	polarity index/phosphatidyl inositol
PLP1	proteolipid protein 1
PM	poor metabolizer
PMDD	premenstrual dysphoric disorder
POS	polycystic ovarian syndrome
PP	predominant polarity
PTSD	post-traumatic stress disorder

QoL	quality of life	sTNFRSF1A	tumour necrosis factor receptor superfamily, member 1A
RCT	randomized controlled trial		
RDC	research diagnostic criteria	SUD	substance use disorder
		SZA	schizoaffective disorder
rDLPFC	right dorsal lateral prefrontal cortex	TAU	treatment as usual
		TCAs	tricyclic antidepressants
RDoC	Research Domain Criteria	TD	tardive dyskinesia
		tDCS	transcranial direct current stimulation
RfCBT	rumination-focused CBT		
		TEAS	treatment-emerging affective switches
RLAI	risperidone long-acting injectable		
		TEMPS-A	Temperament Evaluation of the Memphis, Pisa, Paris, and San Diego Autoquestionnaire
rTMS	repetitive transcranial magnetic stimulation		
RUL	right unilateral		
SAD	seasonal affective disorder	TEN	toxic epidermal necrolysis
SCIP	Screen for Cognitive Impairment in Psychiatry	TIMA	Texas Implementation of Medication Algorithms
SCN	suprachiasmatic nucleus/nuclei	TMAP	Texas Medication Algorithm Project
SGAs	second-generation antipsychotics	TMS	transcranial magnetic stimulation
SIADH	secretion of antidiuretic hormone	TNF	tumour necrosis factor
		TSD	total sleep deprivation
SJS	Stevens–Johnson syndrome	UD	unipolar disorder
SJW	St John's Wort	UK	United Kingdom
sl-MFB	superolateral medial forebrain bundle	UM	ultrarapid metabolizer
		US	United States
SMR	standardized mortality ratio	VNS	vagus nerve stimulation
		VNTR	variable number of tandem repeats
SNPs	single nucleotide polymorphisms		
		WBT	well-being therapy
SNRIs	serotonin-noradrenaline reuptake inhibitors	WHO	World Health Organization
		WFSBP	World Federation of Societies of Biological Psychiatry
SPECT	single-photon emission computed tomography		
SSC	specialist supportive care	XBP1	X-box binding protein 1
		XR	extended release
SSRIs	selective serotonin reuptake inhibitors	YMRS	Young Mania Rating Scale
STEP-BD	Systematic Treatment Enhancement Program for Bipolar Disorder	ZFPM2	zinc finger protein multitype 2

Contributors

Danilo Arnone
Centre for Affective Disorders,
Department of Psychological Medicine,
Institute of Psychiatry, Psychology and
Neuroscience, King's College London,
London, UK

Vicent Balanzá-Martínez
Teaching Unit of Psychiatry, La Fe
University and Polytechnic Hospital,
Valencia, Spain; Department of
Medicine, University of Valencia,
Valencia, Spain; Centro de Investigación
Biomédica en Red de Salud Mental
(CIBERSAM), Madrid, Spain

Ross J. Baldessarini
International Consortium for Bipolar
and Psychotic Disorders Research,
Mailman Research Center, McLean
Hospital, Belmont, Massachusetts,
USA; Department of Psychiatry,
Harvard Medical School, Boston,
Massachusetts, USA

Danielle Balzafiore
Department of Psychiatry and
Behavioral Sciences, Stanford
University, Stanford, USA; Pacific
Graduate School of Professional
Psychology, Palo Alto University, USA

Michael Berk
IMPACT SRC, School of Medicine,
Deakin University, Geelong, Victoria,
Australia

William V. Bobo
Mayo Clinic Depression Center,
Department of Psychiatry &
Psychology, Mayo Clinic College of
Medicine, Rochester, USA

Sarah Borish
Department of Psychiatry and
Behavioral Sciences, Stanford
University, Stanford, USA; Pacific
Graduate School of Professional
Psychology, Palo Alto University, USA

Sofia Brissos
Lisbon's Psychiatric Hospital Centre,
Lisbon, Portugal

Andre Russowsky Brunoni
Center for Clinical and Epidemiological
Research & Interdisciplinary Center
for Applied Neuromodulation (CINA),
University Hospital, University of São
Paulo, São Paulo, Brazil; Service of
Interdisciplinary Neuromodulation
(SIN), Department and Institute of
Psychiatry, Faculty of Medicine of
University of São Paulo,
São Paulo, Brazil

Vena Budhan
Department of Psychiatry and
Behavioral Sciences, Stanford
University School of Medicine; Pacific
Graduate School of Professional
Psychology, Palo Alto University, USA

Yulisha Byrow
CADE Clinic, Department of
Psychiatry, Royal North Shore Hospital,
St Leonards, NSW, Australia

Edward Callaly
IMPACT SRC, School of Medicine,
Deakin University, Geelong, Victoria,
Australia

Sebastián Camino
Department of Neuroscience, Palermo University, Buenos Aires, Argentina; Braulio Moyano Hospital, Buenos Aires, Argentina

André F. Carvalho
Associate Professor, Department of Clinical MedicineHead, Translational Psychiatry Research Group, Faculty of Medicine, Federal University of Ceará, Fortaleza, Brazil

Francesc Colom
Mental Health Group, IMIM-Hospital del Mar-CIBERSAM, Barcelona, Catalonia, Spain

Paul E. Croarkin
Mayo Clinic Depression Center, Department of Psychiatry & Psychology, Mayo Clinic College of Medicine, Rochester, USA

Sabrina C. da Costa
Department of Psychiatry and Behavioral Sciences, McGovern Medical School, University of Texas Health Science Center at Houston, Texas, USA

Tricia L. da Silva
Institute of Medical Sciences, Faculty of Medicine and Division of Mood and Anxiety Disorders, Centre for Addiction and Mental Health, Toronto, Ontario, Canada

Joao L. de Quevedo
UT Center of Excellence on Mood Disorder, Department of Psychiatry and Behavioral Sciences, The University of Texas Science Center at Houston, Houston, Texas, USA; Center for Translational Psychiatry, Department of Psychiatry and Behavioral Sciences, The University of Texas Medical School at Houston, Houston, Texas, USA

Bernardo de Sampaio Pereira Júnior
Center for Clinical and Epidemiological Research & Interdisciplinary Center for Applied Neuromodulation (CINA), University Hospital, University of São Paulo, São Paulo, Brazil; Service of Interdisciplinary Neuromodulation (SIN), Department and Institute of Psychiatry, Faculty of Medicine of University of São Paulo, São Paulo, Brazil

Caterina del Mar Bonnin
Bipolar Disorders Unit, Institute of Neuroscience, Hospital Clinic, IDIBAPS, CIBERSAM, University of Barcelona, Barcelona, Spain

Dimos Dimellis
Department of Psychiatry, Division of Neurosciences School of Medicine, Aristotle University of Thessaloniki, Greece

Péter Döme
Department of Clinical and Theoretical Mental Health, Semmelweis University, Faculty of Medicine, Budapest, Hungary; National Institute of Psychiatry and Addictions, Laboratory for Suicide Research and Prevention, Budapest, Hungary

Harris A. Eyre
IMPACT SRC, School of Medicine, Deakin University, Geelong, Victoria, Australia; Discipline of Psychiatry, University of Adelaide, Adelaide, Australia

Chiara Fabbri
Department of Biomedical and NeuroMotor Sciences, University of Bologna, Italy

Alberto Forte
International Consortium for Bipolar and Psychotic Disorders Research, Mailman Research Center, McLean Hospital, Massachusetts, USA

Konstantinos N. Fountoulakis
Associate Professor of Psychiatry, Department of Psychiatry, Division of Neurosciences; School of Medicine, Aristotle University of Thessaloniki, Greece

Mark A. Frye
Mayo Clinic Depression Center, Department of Psychiatry & Psychology, Mayo Clinic College of Medicine, Rochester, USA

Xénia Gonda
Department of Clinical and Theoretical Mental Health, Semmelweis University, Faculty of Medicine, Budapest, Hungary; National Institute of Psychiatry and Addictions, Laboratory for Suicide Research and Prevention, Budapest, Hungary

Anna I. Guerdjikova
Lindner Center of HOPE, Mason, Ohio, USA; Department of Psychiatry and Behavioral Neuroscience, University of Cincinnati College of Medicine, Cincinnati, Ohio, USA

Philip Hazell
Discipline of Psychiatry, University of Sydney, Sydney, Australia

Ioline D. Henter
Experimental Therapeutics and Pathophysiology Branch, National Institute of Mental Health, National Institutes of Health, Bethesda, Maryland, USA

Flávio Kapczinski
Bipolar Disorder Program, Laboratory of Molecular Psychiatry, Hospital de Clínicas de Porto Alegre (HCPA), Porto Alegre, Brazil; Graduation Program in Psychiatry and Department of Psychiatry, Universidade Federal do Rio Grande do Sul (UFRGS), Porto Alegre, Brazil

Paul E. Keck
Lindner Center of HOPE, Mason, Ohio, USA; Department of Psychiatry and Behavioral Neuroscience, University of Cincinnati College of Medicine, Cincinnati, Ohio, USA

Muralidharan Kesavan
Additional Professor of Psychiatry, National Institute of Mental Health and Neuro Sciences, Bangalore, India

Lars V. Kessing
Copenhagen Affective Disorders Research Centre (CADIC), Psychiatric Centre Copenhagen, Copenhagen University Hospital, Copenhagen, Denmark; University of Copenhagen, Faculty of Health and Medical Sciences, Copenhagen, Denmark

Sarah Kittel-Schneider
Department of Psychiatry, Psychosomatics and Psychotherapy, University Hospital of Frankfurt, Frankfurt, Germany

Izio Klein
Center for Clinical and Epidemiological
Research & Interdisciplinary Center
for Applied Neuromodulation (CINA),
University Hospital, University of São
Paulo, São Paulo, Brazil; Service of
Interdisciplinary Neuromodulation
(SIN), Department and Institute of
Psychiatry, Faculty of Medicine of
University of São Paulo, São Paulo, Brazil;
Laboratory of Neuroscience (LIM27),
Department and Institute of Psychiatry,
University of São Paulo, São Paulo, Brazil

Simon Kung
Mayo Clinic Depression Center,
Department of Psychiatry &
Psychology, Mayo Clinic College of
Medicine, Rochester, USA

Maria Lacruz
Hospital Francesc de Borja, Gandía,
Valencia, Spain

Rodrigo Machado-Vieira
Experimental Therapeutics and
Pathophysiology Branch, National
Institute of Mental Health, National
Institutes of Health, Bethesda,
Maryland, USA

Gin S. Malhi
Discipline of Psychiatry, Kolling
Institute, Sydney Medical School,
University of Sydney, Sydney, Australia;
CADE Clinic, Department of
Psychiatry, Royal North Shore Hospital,
St Leonards, Australia

Anabel Martinez-Arán
Bipolar Disorders Unit, Institute
of Neuroscience, Hospital Clinic,
IDIBAPS, CIBERSAM, University of
Barcelona, Barcelona, Spain

Lorenzo Mazzarini
cNESMOS Department, Sapienza
University, Sant'Andrea Hospital,
Rome, Italy

Susan L. McElroy
Lindner Center of HOPE, Mason, Ohio,
USA; Department of Psychiatry and
Behavioral Neuroscience, University
of Cincinnati College of Medicine,
Cincinnati, Ohio, USA

Roumen Milev
Mood Disorders Research and
Treatment Service, Providence Care
Hospital; Departments of Psychiatry
and Psychology, Queen's University,
Kingston, Ontario, Canada

Kamilla W. Miskowiak
Copenhagen Affective Disorders
Research Centre (CADIC), Psychiatric
Centre Copenhagen, Copenhagen
University Hospital, Copenhagen,
Denmark, and University of
Copenhagen, Faculty of Health and
Medical Sciences, Denmark

Katherine M. Moore
Mayo Clinic Depression Center,
Department of Psychiatry &
Psychology, Mayo Clinic College of
Medicine, Rochester, USA

Malik M. Nassan
Mayo Clinic Depression Center,
Department of Psychiatry &
Psychology, Mayo Clinic College of
Medicine, Rochester, USA

Bernardo Ng
Assistant Professor of Psychiatry,
University of California, San
Diego, USA

Johannes Pantel
Institute of General Medicine, Goethe
University, Frankfurt/Main, Germany

Gordon Parker
School of Psychiatry, University of New
South Wales, Sydney, Australia; Black
Dog Institute, Sydney, Australia

Ives Cavalcante Passos
UT Center of Excellence on Mood
Disorder, Department of Psychiatry
and Behavioral Sciences, The University
of Texas Science Center at Houston,
Houston, TX, USA; Bipolar Disorder
Program, Laboratory of Molecular
Psychiatry, Hospital de Clínicas de
Porto Alegre (HCPA), Porto Alegre,
RS, Brazil; Graduation Program in
Psychiatry and Laboratory of Molecular
Psychiatry, Federal University of Rio
Grande do Sul, Porto Alegre, RS, Brazil

Amelia Paterson
School of Psychiatry, University of New
South Wales, Sydney, Australia; Black
Dog Institute, Sydney, Australia

Giulio Perugi
Department of Psychiatry, University of
Pisa, Pisa, Italy; Institute of Behavioral
Science G De Lisio, Pisa, Italy

Dina Popovic
Bipolar Disorders Program, Hospital
Clinic, Institute of Neuroscience,
University of Barcelona, IDIBAPS,
CIBERSAM, Barcelona, Spain;
Department of Psychiatry, Sheba
Medical Center, Tel Hashomer, Ramat
Gan, Israel

Natalie Rasgon
Department of Psychiatry and
Behavioral Sciences, Stanford
University, Stanford, USA

Arun V. Ravindran
Department of Psychiatry, Faculty
of Medicine, and Division of Mood
and Anxiety Disorders, Centre for
Addiction and Mental Health, Toronto,
Ontario, Canada

María Reinares
Bipolar Disorders Program, Institute
of Neurosciences, Hospital Clínic,
University of Barcelona, IDIBAPS,
CIBERSAM, Barcelona, Spain

Zoltán Rihmer
Department of Clinical and Theoretical
Mental Health, Semmelweis University,
Faculty of Medicine, Budapest,
Hungary; National Institute of
Psychiatry and Addictions, Laboratory
for Suicide Research and Prevention,
Budapest, Hungary

Thalia Robakis
Department of Psychiatry and
Behavioral Sciences, Stanford
University, Stanford USA

Jan Scott
Professor of Psychological Medicine
at the Institute of Neuroscience at
Newcastle University & the Centre
for Affective Disorders, Institute of
Psychiatry, London, UK

Salih Selek
Associate Professor, Psychiatry
Department, McGovern Medical
School, University of Texas Health
Science Center at Houston, Texas, USA

Alessandro Serretti
Department of Biomedical and
NeuroMotor Sciences, University of
Bologna, Italy

Ajeet B. Singh
IMPACT SRC, School of Medicine,
Deakin University, Geelong, Victoria,
Australia

Jair C. Soares
Psychiatry Department, McGovern
Medical School, University of Texas
Health Science Center at Houston, USA

Gilberto Sousa Alves
Institute of General Medicine, Goethe
University, Frankfurt, Germany;
Translational Psychiatry Research
Group and Department of Clinical
Medicine, Federal University of Ceará,
Fortaleza, Brazil

Felipe Kenji Sudo
Federal University of Rio de Janeiro,
Rio de Janeiro, Brazil

Rafael Tabarés-Seisdedos
Department of Medicine, University
of Valencia, Valencia, Spain; Centro
de Investigación Biomédica en Red
de Salud Mental (CIBERSAM),
Madrid, Spain; Fundación para la
Investigación del Hospital Clínico de
la Comunidad Valenciana (INCLIVA),
Valencia, Spain

Mauricio Tohen
Tenured Professor and Chairman,
Department of Psychiatry and
Behavioral Sciences, University of
New Mexico Health Sciences Center,
Albuquerque, New Mexico, USA

Leonardo Tondo
International Consortium for
Bipolar and Psychotic Disorders
Research, Mailman Research
Center, McLean Hospital,
elmont, Massachusetts, USA;
Department of Psychiatry,
Harvard Medical School, Boston,
Massachusetts, USA

Carla Torrent
Bipolar Disorders Unit, Institute
of Neuroscience, Hospital Clinic,
IDIBAPS, CIBERSAM, University of
Barcelona, Barcelona, Spain

Susannah J. Tye
Mayo Clinic Depression Center,
Department of Psychiatry &
Psychology, Mayo Clinic College of
Medicine, Rochester, USA

Jennifer L. Vande Voort
Mayo Clinic Depression Center,
Department of Psychiatry &
Psychology, Mayo Clinic College of
Medicine, Rochester, USA

Giulia Vannucchi
Department of Psychiatry, University of
Pisa, Pisa, Italy

Gustavo H. Vázquez
International Consortium for Bipolar
and Psychotic Disorders Research,
Mailman Research Center, McLean
Hospital, Belmont, Massachusetts, USA;
Department of Neuroscience, Palermo
University, Buenos Aires, Argentina

Marin Veldic
Mayo Clinic Depression Center,
Department of Psychiatry &
Psychology, Mayo Clinic College of
Medicine, Rochester, USA

Eduard Vieta
Chair, Department of Psychiatry
and Psychology, Hospital Clinic,
Institute of Neuroscience, IDIBAPS,
CIBERSAM, University of Barcelona,
Barcelona, Spain

Nefize Yalin
Centre for Affective Disorders,
Department of Psychological Medicine,
Institute of Psychiatry, Psychology
and Neuroscience, King's College of
London, London, UK

Lakshmi N. Yatham
Professor of Psychiatry, University
of British Columbia, Regional Head,
Department of Psychiatry, Vancouver;
Coastal Health and Providence
Healthcare, Regional Program
Medical Director, Mental Health and
Addictions, Vancouver Coastal Health,
Vancouver, Canada

Allan Y. Young
Director, Centre for Affective Disorders,
Department of Psychological Medicine,
Institute of Psychiatry, Psychology and
Neuroscience, King's College London,
London, UK

Chapter 1

The current classification of bipolar disorders

Gin S. Malhi and Yulisha Byrow

The classification of bipolar disorders in DSM-5 and ICD-10/11

Emotions define humans perhaps even more so than the ability to reason, and drive all forms of experiences—namely, art, music, and literature. This is possible because of the sheer variety and range of emotions that we are able to experience, and this complexity has meant that defining emotional normality and separating aberrations has proven difficult.

In psychiatry, bipolar and related disorders refer to affective disorders that typically consist of fluctuations in mood ranging from depression to mania in varying degrees. Clinically, the first and most pressing problem facing clinicians is the diagnosis of bipolar disorder and its accurate identification and classification. Research findings suggest that approximately 1.25% of patients with major depressive disorder transmute to a diagnosis of bipolar disorder per year.[1] Ruggero and colleagues,[2] who periodically assessed individuals with a bipolar diagnosis, found that the misdiagnosis of bipolar disorder is remarkably common and that 49.7% of individuals were assigned an incorrect non-bipolar diagnosis over a ten-year follow-up period. Part of the complexity of bipolar disorder stems from its natural course, because the illness usually first manifests with depression but bipolar disorder cannot be diagnosed until the occurrence of a manic episode. Consequently, patients experiencing depression, who have never had a manic episode, are understandably and quite appropriately diagnosed with major depressive disorder (MDD), and treated with antidepressants. This is problematic for those patients that have an underlying bipolar illness because antidepressants alone are often ineffective and instead may precipitate mood instability and even a manic episode.[3] This is a major concern because in clinical practice diagnosis determines treatment and provides the necessary shorthand for communication between doctors, health professionals, and patients.

A lack of diagnostic specificity is also a critical issue for research. In order to advance the treatment and prevention of bipolar disorder, findings from clinical research trials need to be satisfactorily mapped onto clinical practice. But the translation of research into practice remains difficult, in both psychiatry and psychology, because of the variable definition of bipolar disorder within extant psychiatric classificatory systems.

Therefore, in this chapter we first describe the diagnosis of bipolar disorders in relation to the most widely used taxonomies; namely, the *Diagnostic and Statistical Manual of Mental Disorders* (5th edition) (DSM-5) and the *International Classification of Diseases* (10th revision) (ICD-10).[4,5] We then compare and contrast the framework and approach used by these classification systems alongside the yet to be released ICD-11, and critically discuss the clinical and research implications of important discrepancies.

Historical perspective

When considering the history of the classification of psychiatric illness it is important to remember that the present-day bipolar disorder nosology is the cumulative product of a wide range of early philosophers and physicians. In this section we selectively describe contributions made by a few influential physicians in the nineteenth and twentieth centuries.

During a time when psychiatry was still taking shape and clinical symptoms were thought to represent different stages of one universal type of insanity, Karl Kahlbaum and his associate Ewald Hecker introduced the complicated concept of *time* into psychiatric nosology. Essentially, they recognized that symptoms and behaviours of patients differ in relation to the age of onset of an illness and accordingly change with time, thus underscoring the clinical significance of the course of an illness.[6] Furthermore, they described and defined psychiatric illnesses such as dysthymia, cyclothymia, and paranoia—terms that remarkably remain relevant and in use today.

Following on from Kahlbaum and Hecker's seminal work, Emil Kraepelin coined the fitting and descriptive term manic-depressive illness, which eventually spawned the modern-day term—bipolar disorder. Kraepelin's model of 'manic depression' was derived purely from clinical observations and thus still applies and influences our modern-day understanding of bipolar disorder. His key achievement in this regard was to separate manic-depression from schizophrenia (dementia praecox) and position mania and depression at opposite poles of a continuum.[7] Following Kraeplin's work, Karl Leonhard in 1957 added to the definition of manic-depressive illness incorporating both unipolarity and bipolarity as separate entities. Notably, he maintained Kraepelin's emphasis on the *cyclical* and *recurrent* nature of these disorders.[8]

Current classification systems

The length of time that has lapsed since the last revision of both DSM and ICD is quite extraordinary. DSM-5 was published 19 years after DSM-IV, and ICD-11, the long-awaited successor to ICD-10 (1992), is yet to be published, with a proposed date of 2018. One of the principal reasons for this delay was the expectation that research would provide a neurobiological basis to psychiatric disorders and that the taxonomy of neuropsychiatric disorders would finally be based on an understanding of aetiology and pathogenesis. But despite valiant efforts no meaningful biomarkers for psychiatric disorders have emerged. Consequently, DSM-5 remains a largely descriptive and phenomenology-based classificatory system that clusters symptoms into syndromes and defines disorders categorically. DSM was developed primarily by American psychiatrists, psychologists, and other health professionals and is therefore widely used in the United States (US). Clinically, it is used to code psychiatric disorders and for investigative purposes and clinical studies. DSM is also utilized by the American legal system to determine medical healthcare rebates governed by insurance schemes. However, outside the US, DSM-5 is principally used for research purposes.

The major alternative classification system is the International Classification of Diseases developed by the World Health Organization (WHO), which published its 10th revision in 1992. It is widely used internationally in health systems including, for example, the United Kingdom (UK) and Australia. The 11th revision of ICD (ICD-11) is underway and is due to be released in 2018. The current chapter, therefore, discusses some of the proposed diagnostic criteria for bipolar disorder set out in the currently available beta version.*

ICD-10 was developed in consultation with many health professionals from different countries and it encompasses all health-related illness and disease in addition to mental disorders. In terms of classifying mental health disorders there are two versions of ICD-10—one that adopts a more clinical focus and the other more oriented towards research. However, in practice, ICD is mostly utilized by medical professionals, particularly in European countries, to measure the use of services.

Importance of diagnosis relevant to research and clinical practice

Given the resources spent developing and implementing classification systems it is imperative to consider why diagnosis is an important concept, and more specifically the usefulness of diagnoses in different contexts. From a research perspective, diagnosis is typically used to select samples for investigative purposes such as aetiology and treatment. The use of a common language facilitates communication between researchers and research groups, and while a categorical approach ensures diagnostic reliability, it often compromises diagnostic validity—a long-standing concern. Robins and Guze were among the first to recognize the importance of developing a structured framework to clarify psychiatric disorders with a view to underpinning diagnosis with neurobiological substrates.[9] Contemporaneously, an influential body of work by Spitzer et al. established the Research Diagnostic Criteria,[10] a classification system using definitive criteria to describe psychiatric illness with the aim of improving the diagnostic reliability of mental illnesses. Today, with the release of the National Institute of Mental Health (NIMH) Research Domain Criteria (RDoC), the importance of biologically derived evidence in diagnosing mental illness is once again in the limelight, with emphasis returning to evidence that draws on neurobiology, as well as the aetiology of mental illnesses.

---

* It is important to note that there are likely to be changes made in the final version of ICD-11.

Importantly, research examining treatment outcomes uses categorical classificatory systems to recruit clinical samples and therefore clinical treatment strategies are based on these findings. There are inherent disadvantages in this approach, because in clinical drug trials patients with comorbidities or particularly complex presentations are routinely excluded and samples that undergo testing tend to be 'over-selected'. For example, many clinical drug trials recruiting a depressed population exclude patients with active suicidal ideation, a common clinical symptom that has key significance for immediate and longer-term management. Therefore, it is unclear whether the samples recruited in such trials are truly representative of the clinical population that they are thought to reflect. Thus, an inevitable tension emerges between competing demands—because it is best to categorize individuals into homogenous samples in order to determine treatment effects for specific populations, but by using a categorical approach and limiting complexity that occurs in the clinical context, the translation of research into practice is invariably constrained.

When adopting a clinical perspective clinicians use diagnoses such as bipolar disorder as a guide for case formulation and to facilitate communication between patients and clinicians, as well as between mental health professionals. While diagnoses offer a significant input into the treatment plan developed for patients with bipolar disorder it is important to remember that bipolar symptoms occur within the context of a broader set of experiences. Thus, it is important to consider aspects of an individual's life that may have contributed to the development of the disorder, such as, adverse life events, dysfunctional personality style, lifestyle issues (eg, smoking and substance misuse), and genetic vulnerability, along with other contextual factors that may facilitate resilience in patients, such as, positive emotions, secure attachment styles, and a supportive social environment, to formulate a comprehensive and individualized treatment plan.[3,11] These contextual factors are not captured by existing diagnostic classification systems.

Limitations of current taxonomy

Successive iterations of DSM culminating in DSM-5 have gradually shifted the classification of bipolar disorders away from Kraepelinian concepts, by placing greater emphasis on polarity than the longitudinal pattern of mood disorders (cyclicity and recurrence). But in reality, the nature of bipolar disorder is only evident when its course is mapped longitudinally and, over time, initial depressive symptoms gradually give way to (hypo)manic episodes. The cross-sectional approach of current classification systems fails to capture the evolution of bipolar disorder and instead views the diagnosis as a 'state' rather than a 'trait'. This is at odds with the true nature of bipolar disorder, which is a relapsing and remitting illness that evolves over the lifetime of an individual.

Another inherent limitation of both DSM and ICD classification systems is the 'equal' weighting of all bipolar disorder symptoms. For example, equal significance is attached to recurrent thoughts of suicide, guilt, and fatigue when determining a diagnosis of a major depressive episode. However, clinically, suicidal thoughts and guilt confer different connotations and are arguably more important and possibly more characteristic of severe presentations of depression than fatigue. Thus, grouping individuals meeting criteria for a broad diagnostic category such as a 'depressive episode' is likely to generate heterogeneous groups with significant variation in illness severity and clinical symptomology.

Brief overview of DSM-5 bipolar and related disorder sections

In DSM-5, bipolar and related disorders are situated between schizophrenia spectrum and other disorders and depressive disorders. For an overview of all the diagnostic categories see Figure 1.1 and for a summary of diagnostic criteria see Table 1.1.

Bipolar I disorder is the modern derivative of manic-depressive illness, and while there is no requirement to have experienced a major depressive episode or psychosis to fulfil criteria, most individuals with this disorder will experience a major depressive episode at some point during their lifetime. The defining feature of bipolar I disorder is mania and the classic features of a manic episode include persistent elevated and expansive, or irritable, mood, and persistently increased activity or energy lasting a period of at least one week. These symptoms must also cause marked impairment in functioning and/or require hospitalization.

Bipolar II disorder requires an individual to have experienced at least one hypomanic and depressive episode with a clinical course defined by recurring mood episodes. Hypomania is similar to mania with elevated mood or euphoria, but these symptoms typically do not cause marked impairment in functioning even though they last at least four consecutive days.

Individuals with *cyclothymic disorder* typically experience chronic fluctuations in mood from hypomania-like symptoms to depressive symptoms for at least two years. However, the changes in mood symptoms would not meet criteria for a hypomanic or depressive episode as they are, by definition, less severe and of shorter duration.

Brief overview of ICD-10 bipolar disorder section

In ICD-10, single manic episodes are distinguished from recurrent manic and/or depressive episodes. For an overview of all the diagnostic categories see Figure 1.2 and for a summary of diagnostic criteria see Table 1.2. Individuals experiencing a single manic episode can potentially receive a diagnosis, ranging in increasing severity, from hypomania to mania with psychotic symptoms. However, note that a single mixed affective episode is considered separately and classed under 'Other single mood disorder'.

Recurrent manic and depressive episodes are classified under 'Bipolar affective disorder' (BAD) (see Figure 1.2). The severity of manic episodes is judged based on the presence of psychotic symptoms and the severity of depressive episodes is captured as mild, moderate, or severe with or without psychosis. The characteristic feature for all BAD diagnoses is the presence of *at least one other affective episode* (from the opposite pole of the mood spectrum) or remission of symptoms.

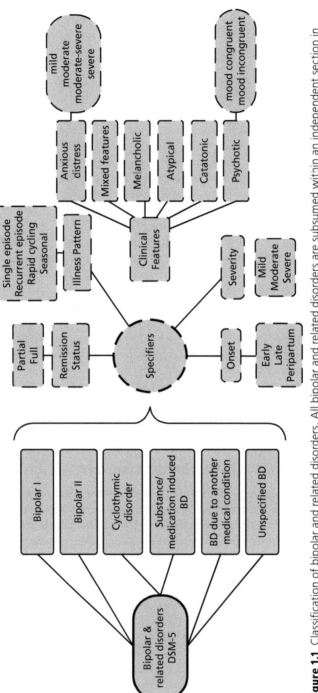

Figure 1.1 Classification of bipolar and related disorders. All bipolar and related disorders are subsumed within an independent section in DSM-5. For each of these diagnoses (solid border) any number of specifiers (dashed border) can be applied.
Data from *Diagnostic and statistical manual of mental disorder*, 5th ed., 2013, American Psychiatric Association.

Table 1.1 Summary of DSM-5 diagnostic criteria for bipolar and related disorders

DSM-5

	BD I	BD II	Cyclothymia
Main Symptom Criteria (Mania)			
Elevated or irritable mood	+	+ (Often irritable)	+
Increased activity or energy	+ (goal directed)	+	+
Increased self-esteem	+	+	+
Decreased need for sleep	+	+	+
Pressured speech	+	+	+
Distractibility	+	+	+
Increased risk taking	+	+	+
Increased sociability/ over-familiarity			
Increased sexual energy			
Delusions/ hallucinations			
Main symptom criteria for major depressive episode (same as MDD)		+	

Severity and duration of episodes

	Mania	Hypomania	Sub-threshold mania
Number of symptoms	≥ 3/≥ 4 if the mood is irritable	≥ 3/≥ 4 if the mood is irritable	≤ 3 symptoms
Duration of episode	≥ 7 days (or any duration if hospitalized)	≥ 4 days	–
Impact on functioning	Disrupts social & occupational functioning or hospitalization or psychotic features	Not severe enough to disrupt functioning or result in hospitalization	Hypomania/depression symptoms cause significant distress or impairment in functioning

Depression

Number of symptoms		≥ 5 symptoms	< 5 symptoms
Duration		2 weeks	< 2 weeks
Frequency of episodes		≥ 1 hypomanic + ≥ 1 depressive episode	Fluctuating between hypomanic and depressive symptoms for ≥ 2 years (1 year for children/ adolescents). Never been without symptoms for > 2 months at a time.

Data from *Diagnostic and statistical manual of mental disorder*, 5th ed., 2013, American Psychiatric Association.

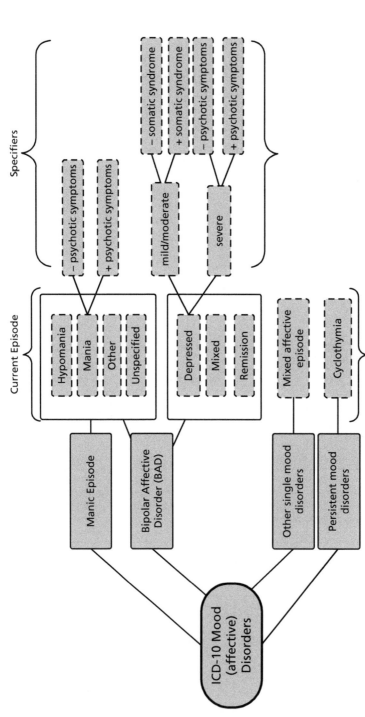

Figure 1.2 The ICD-10 classification system. A parsimonious approach to diagnosis using ICD-10 is to first consider whether the affective episodes are single or multiple present (solid border): a period of mania/hypomania falls under 'manic episode' whereas a single mixed episode falls under 'other single mood disorders'. At least two episodes are necessary to qualify for bipolar affective disorder (BAD). The specifiers are relevant to clinical features and severity of manic and depressive episodes.
Data from *International Classification of Diseases (ICD)*, version 10. Copyright (1992) World Health Organization.

Table 1.2 Summary of ICD-10 diagnostic criteria for bipolar and related disorders

ICD-10

Main symptom criteria	Hypomania	Mania		Cyclothymia
		Mania w/ out psychotic symptoms	Mania with psychotic symptoms	
Elevated or irritable mood	+	+	+	
Increased activity or energy	+	+	+	+
Increased self-esteem	+	+	+	+
Decreased need for sleep	+	+	+	+
Pressured speech	+	+	+	
Distractibility	+	+	+	
Increased risk taking	+	+	+	
Increased sociability/ over-familiarity	+	+ (loss of normal social inhibitions)	+ (loss of normal social inhibitions)	+ (gregariousness)
Increased sexual energy	+	+ (sexual indiscretions)	+ (sexual indiscretions)	+
Delusions/ hallucinations			+ [a]	
Sharpened or atypically creative thinking				+
Increased talkativeness				+
Over-optimism				+

Severity and duration of episodes			
	Mania		
	Hypomania	Mania	Cyclothymia
Number of symptoms	≥ 3 symptoms	≥ 3/≥ 4 irritable mood only	≥ 3 depressive & ≥ 3 elevated mood symptoms
Duration of episode	≥ 4 days (several days)	≥ 7 days (or any duration if hospitalized)	≥ 2 years of mood instability

(continued)

Table 1.2 Continued

ICD-10			
	Depression		
	Mild	**Moderate**	**Severe**
Number of symptoms	≥ 4 symptoms in total	≥ 6 symptoms in total	≥ 8 symptoms in total
Duration of episode	≥ 2 weeks	≥ 2 weeks	≥ 2 weeks

ᵃ Cannot be culturally inappropriate, impossible, third person, or running commentary

Data from *International Classification of Diseases (ICD)*, version 10. Copyright (1992) World Health Organization.

Cyclothymia is classified under 'Persistent mood disorders' and is defined as a persistent course of fluctuating mild depression and mild elation. These 'episodes' are not severe enough to meet criteria for BAD or recurrent depressive disorder.

Summary of major differences in ICD-10, ICD-11, and DSM-5 and their implications

A future aim for both the American Psychiatric Association and World Health Organization has been to harmonize the diagnostic criteria outlined by both DSM-5 and ICD-11, so as to create complementary classification systems. This has not yet been achieved and so this section provides a succinct overview of the more fundamental differences between DSM-5, ICD-10, and the beta version of ICD-11. For a summary of the differences and similarities between these classification systems see Table 1.3.

Structural differences

Perhaps the most conspicuous difference between DSM-5 and ICD-10 is that, in the former, bipolar disorders are placed in a separate section between schizophrenia (and other related disorders) and depressive disorders. This shift reflects the emerging neurobiological links between these disorders, especially in terms of genetics. However, given that phenomenologically bipolar disorder consists of both mania and depression with predominance in fact of the latter, separating depressive and bipolar disorders as distinct entities lacks face validity and may not be meaningful. In contrast, ICD-10 captures both depressive and bipolar disorders within a single mood disorders section. ICD-11 beta version maintains this grouping, which is then divided into depressive and bipolar sections.[12]

Mania

Another key distinction is the diagnosis of bipolar II disorder in DSM-5, which is absent from ICD-10. A second equally significant point of difference is that ICD-10 does not recognize the occurrence of a 'single manic episode' as a criterion sufficient for diagnosing bipolar I disorder whereas DSM-5 does and predicates the diagnosis wholly on mania. Furthermore, DSM-5 distinguishes between mania and more

Table 1.3 Differences and emerging similarities between DSM-5, ICD-10, and ICD-11

	DSM-5	ICD-10	ICD-11 (beta version)
Differences			
Structural grouping	BD and related disorders and depressive disorders defined in two separate but adjacent sections.	BAD and MDD included in mood disorders section.	As ICD-10.
Cyclothymia	Will not satisfy criteria if mood is stabilized for more than 2 months at a time.	Allows for stability of mood for months at a time.	Mood symptoms present more often than not over a 2-year period.
Mixed episodes	Included as a specifier for depressive, manic, & hypomanic episodes in both bipolar disorder and MDD.	Mixed episodes are a separate diagnosis within the BAD section. A separate diagnosis is given for a single mixed episode.	Remains a potentially separate diagnosis (a diagnostic subtype for BD I with equivalence to mania). Can be a single or multiple episode
Points of potential convergence			
Bipolar II disorder	Includes BD I disorder (relevant to manic episodes) and BD II disorder (relevant to hypomanic episodes).	No BD II diagnosis. Hypomanic, manic, and mixed episodes subsumed under BAD diagnosis.	Includes BD I disorder (relevant to manic episodes) and BD II disorder (relevant to hypomanic episodes).
Bipolar I disorder, single manic episode	Requires at least one manic episode to meet criteria for BD I.	Cannot meet criteria for BAD with a single manic episode.	Requires at least one manic episode to meet criteria for BD I.
Increased activity or energy	Included as one of the two key essential criteria for a (hypo)manic episode (criterion A). Thus, is specifically required to meet diagnostic criteria for a (hypo)manic episode and BD I and II.	Not specifically required to meet diagnostic criteria for a (hypo)manic episode; however, included in criterion B.	Included as essential for meeting BD criteria.

Data from *Diagnostic and statistical manual of mental disorder*, 5th ed., 2013, American Psychiatric Association; data from International Classification of Diseases (ICD), version 10. Copyright (1992) World Health Organization.

modest presentations such as hypomania, which in conjunction with depressive episodes define bipolar disorder I and II respectively. In comparison, ICD-10 is less granular and simply subsumes recurrent hypomanic, manic, or mixed episodes within the broader diagnosis of BAD. These fundamental differences in classification can lead to significant discrepancies in clinical, research, and epidemiological data. Fortunately, the soon-to-be-released ICD-11 is likely to partly rectify these problems. The beta version suggests that ICD-11 will distinguish bipolar disorder I and II, as well as redefine bipolar I disorder criteria to include 'one or more manic or mixed episodes'.

Increased activity or energy in mania

An important development in DSM-5 is the addition of 'abnormally and persistently increased goal-directed activity or energy' in combination with the mood elevation (or irritability) criterion. This is specifically required to meet diagnostic criteria for a (hypo)manic episode and bipolar I/II disorder. This refinement better reflects real-world presentations and improves the specificity of diagnosis but there is a risk that it broadens the category and compromises sensitivity. While ICD-10 does include increased energy and activity as a symptom in bipolar disorder, it attracts less emphasis than in DSM-5 (eg, a diagnosis of (hypo)mania does not necessitate an increase in energy or activity). However, the beta version of ICD-11 follows the example of DSM-5 and includes 'increased energy and activity' as an essential criterion for the diagnosis of bipolar disorder.

Another significant development in DSM-5 is that mania persisting beyond the effect of an antidepressant or electroconvulsive therapy is now regarded as equivalent to a manic episode and, in an attempt to recognize variants of mania such as those triggered by treatment, ICD-11 alludes to shortening of the duration criteria in relation to treatment for mania.

Cyclothymia

In DSM-5, cyclothymic disorder essentially describes an individual with abnormal but subsyndromal vicissitudes of mood present for at least half the time during a two-year period. It is relatively unchanged since the time of Kahlbaum and Hecker.[13] Specifically, it stipulates that the individual cannot be without hypomanic or depressive symptoms for longer than two months at a time whereas, interestingly, ICD-10 allows for stability of mood for months at a time. This requirement by DSM-5 for mood stability to last no more than two months at a time has been criticized for being somewhat arbitrary because there is no evidence supporting this particular duration (or indeed any length of time) between episodes. Furthermore, it detracts from the core features of cyclothymia; namely, the persistence of subsyndromal symptoms over a period of years.[14] Thus, the ICD-11 (beta version) definition of cyclothymic disorder does not include this caveat and instead specifies that symptoms should be present for 'more of the time than not' during a period of at least two years.

Mixed episodes

In a dramatic change, DSM-5 has eliminated DSM-IV mixed episodes, effectively negating their status as a separate diagnosis. Instead, mixed presentations are now captured through specifiers attached to either depressive or (hypo)manic episodes and this can be applied to both bipolar disorder and unipolar depression. The 'mixed features' specifier requires that at least three symptoms from the opposite affective pole are present. This relaxation of the previously more stringent requirements in DSM-IV—namely, fulfilment of complete criteria for both a manic and depressive episode for one week—means that mixed presentations will be diagnosed more widely. This reflects reality because, in practice, patients with mixed or subsyndromal features are relatively common but were not coded or captured by DSM-IV criteria.[15,16,17] Thus, including mixed features as a specifier in DSM-5 affords the opportunity to describe patients with greater accuracy and specificity. However, apart from simply increasing the number of individuals who will receive a diagnosis of bipolar disorder, the mixed features specifier, as currently defined, will also generate new problems because of its exclusion of those features that are common to both depression and mania.[18,17] The selection of some features over others has been criticized because exclusion of psychomotor agitation, irritability, and distractibility removes the core features of mixed states. Based on clinical experience and research evidence, mixed presentations often feature distractibility, irritable mood, and psychomotor agitation.[3,19,20,21] Currently, ICD-10 accommodates mixed episodes within BADs, and the diagnosis requires at least two affective episodes that are both prominent for the greater part of the current episode of illness, lasting for at least two weeks. For a single mixed episode, an entirely separate diagnosis exists within the 'other mood disorders' section, which stipulates an affective episode lasting for at least two weeks characterized by either a mixture or rapid alternation (usually within a few hours) of hypomanic, manic, and depressive symptoms. In line with proposals from some researchers, the current beta version of ICD-11 retains mixed features as a separate diagnosis subsumed within bipolar I disorder only.[22] The inclusion of mixed features as a specifier relevant to any bipolar or related disorder diagnosis, as in DSM-5, emulates more of a dimensional rather than categorical approach to defining clinical features, as in ICD-10/11. However, there may be disadvantages associated with including mixed episodes as a specifier rather than a separate diagnosis; for example, it may decrease the specific research focus on mixed states and could potentially lead to ineffective treatment of mixed states with antidepressant monotherapy.[18,21,22]

Conclusion

This chapter has described the nature of the diagnostic classification of bipolar disorders in DSM-5, and ICD-10 and -11. In doing so, it is apparent that while both the American Psychiatric Association and WHO are attempting to harmonize the diagnostic criteria in both DSM-5 and ICD-11, many subtle differences remain. These are important because they will impact both clinicians and researchers and generate differing epidemiological data.

Current psychiatric nosology remains dependent on phenomenology and cannot advance significantly until reliable neurobiological markers are discovered. Therefore, clinicians need to rely on careful clinical assessment, ideally longitudinally, to arrive at diagnoses and this is especially important for an illness such as bipolar disorder—a chronic recurrent illness that remains challenging to define and treat.

References

1. **Angst, J** et al. Diagnostic conversion from depression to bipolar disorders: results of a long-term prospective study of hospital admissions, *Journal of Affective Disorders* 2005;**84**(2–3):149–57.
2. **Ruggero, CJ** et al. 10-Year diagnostic consistency of bipolar disorder in a first-admission sample, *Bipolar Disorders* 2010;**12**(1):21–31.
3. **Malhi, GS** et al. Royal Australian and New Zealand College of Pcyhiatrists clinical practice guidelines for mood disorders, *Australian and New Zealand Journal of Psychiatry* 2015;**49**(12):1087–1206.
4. **American Psychiatric Association**. *Diagnostic and Statistical Manual of Mental Disorders* (5th edn), 2013.
5. **World Health Organization**. *ICD-10 Classifications of Mental Health and Behavioural Disorder: Clinical Descriptions and Diagnostic Guidelines*, Geneva, 1992.
6. **Berrios, GE**. 'The clinico-diagnostic perspective in psychopathology' by K Kahlbaum, *History of Psychiatry* 2007;**18**(2):231–45.
7. **Kraepelin, E**. *Psychiatrie* 5th edn (Leipzig: Barth, 1896).
8. **Leonhard, K**. *The Classification of Endogenous Psychoses* (New York, NY: Irvington Publishers, 1957).
9. **Robins, E** and **Guze, S**. Establishment of diagnostic validity in psychiatric illness: Its application to schizophrenia, *American Journal of Psychiatry* 1970;**126**(107–11):461–2.
10. **Spitzer, RL, Endicott, J**, and **Robins, E**. Research diagnostic criteria: Rationale and reliability, *Archives of General Psychiatry* 1978;**35**:773–82.
11. **Rutten, BPF** et al. Resilience in mental health: linking psychological and neurobiological perspectives, *Acta Psychiatrica Scandinavica* 2013;**128**(1):3–20.
12. **De Dios, C** et al. Bipolar disorders in the new DSM-5 and ICD-11 classifications, *Revista de psiquiatría y salud mental* 2014;**7**(4):179–85.
13. **Malhi, GS, Allwang, C**, and **Keshavan, MS**. Kahlbaum's katatonie and Hecker's hebephrenia, *Acta Neuropsychiatrica* 2007;**19**:314–15.
14. **Phillips, MR**. Dysthymia and cyclothymia in ICD-11, *World Psychiatry* 2012;**11**(Supplement 1):53–8.
15. **Nusslock, R** and **Frank, E**. Subthreshold bipolarity: Diagnostic issues and challenges, *Bipolar Disorders* 2011;**13**:587–603.
16. **Pacchiarotti, I, Mazzarini, L**, et al. Mania and depression. Mixed, not stirred, *Journal of Affective Disorders*,2011;**133**(1–2):105–13.
17. **Vieta, E** and **Valentí, M**. Mixed states in DSM-5: Implications for clinical care, education, and research, *Journal of Affective Disorders* 2013;**148**(1):28–36.
18. **Malhi, GS**. Diagnosis of bipolar disorder: Who is in a mixed state?, *The Lancet* 2013;**381**(9878):1599–600.
19. **Koukopoulos, A, Sani, G**, and **Ghaemi, SN**. Mixed features of depression: Why DSM-5 is wrong (and so was DSM-IV), *British Journal of Psychiatry* 2013;**203**(1):3–5.
20. **Maj, M** et al. Agitated depression in bipolar I disorder: Prevalence, phenomenology, and outcome, *American Journal of Psychiatry* 2003;**160**:2134–40.

21. **Pacchiarotti, I, Valentí, M**, et al. Differential outcome of bipolar patients receiving antidepressant monotherapy versus combination with an antimanic drug, *Journal of Affective Disorders* 2011;**129**:321–6.

22. **Ostergaard, SD** et al. Rethinking the classification of mixed affective episodes in ICD-11, *Journal of Affective Disorders* 2012;**138**(1–2):170–2.

Chapter 2

Should the bipolar disorders be modelled dimensionally or categorically?

Gordon Parker and Amelia Paterson

Introduction

The modelling of psychiatric illness underpins the way we think about disorders, plan treatment approaches, and educate others about these conditions. As such, the modelling of psychiatric conditions may be deceptively important. Psychiatric disorders are either modelled categorically or dimensionally, with diagnostic manuals usually imposing a categorical model as they seek to classify 'cases'. While the modelling of psychiatric illness is of concern to modern psychiatrists, dimensional versus categorical approaches to modelling have been considered and compared since ancient Greek times. As detailed by Goldberg,[1] Plato championed the categorical approach to classification while Aristotle favoured the dimensional approach and, as such, they are often referred to as the Platonic and Aristotelian approaches, respectively.

Goldberg noted several ascriptions to the categorical 'Platonic' approach,[1] later associated with Kraepelin. Firstly, it assumes that conditions are independent. Second, that individuals can be classified as 'cases' or 'non-cases' in relation to a condition. Goldberg suggested that the contrasting Aristotelian dimensional approach is most closely associated with the work of Adolf Meyer—who effectively proposed a model of 'reaction types', with conditions being defined simply by severity. Meyer judged that it was more important to pay attention to the patient's experience than to their clinical features and diagnosis, especially since, as psychotherapy was the treatment of choice for all conditions, diagnosis was considered of little importance. Goldberg observed that 'diagnoses according to the Aristotelians, are man-made abstractions, liable to be discarded or modified according to their usefulness'.

Returning to the issue of 'caseness', Goldberg observed that the strict Platonic view positions illnesses as akin to the concept of pregnancy—in that you either have the condition or you do not. In essence, you cannot sensibly be a 'little pregnant any more than you can be intensely pregnant'. He noted that this approach creates difficulties for those who have symptoms at the sub-threshold level and that the case/non-case model would simply view them as having a *low probability* of having the condition (rather than a *less severe* condition). Goldberg noted that, in contrast, the Aristotelians have no problem with sub-threshold cases as their model is dimensional and they are able to assimilate the concept of severity within their model.

Goldberg's summary position was that 'categorical and dimensional models are merely alternative ways of looking at the same data; it is not that one is right and the other wrong'. We argue an alternate 'and/or' view—that there are some psychiatric conditions (eg melancholia, bipolar disorder) that are quintessentially categorical and some (eg personality disorders) that are dimensional. The task of psychiatric classification is therefore to determine which is *the* valid model for the particular condition rather than adopt a Procrustean approach of imposing a single umbrella model across all conditions as if it has universal application. A reasonable aspiration but, in light of the lack of validating measures, difficult, if not impossible, to resolve for most conditions.

Theoretically, we might also assume that 'diseases' have categorical status (ie you either have the disease or you do not) whereas 'non-diseases' are more likely to reflect extensions of normal states (eg anxiety, personality style) and are therefore intrinsically dimensional. Such a model, therefore, obliges us to define disease and non-disease states. Taylor provided one model in suggesting three levels of categorization—diseases, illnesses, and predicaments.[2] Predictably, the three levels vary by the putative relevance of biological, social, and cultural factors.

The disease category was conceptualized by him as being a physical reality, based on changes in the structure of tissues but does not necessarily include any physical suffering or 'illness' (ie one can have a disease but not be ill) and with schizophrenia being an example. The illness category weights the subjective experience of the patient and incorporates the social role of being ill, and with anxiety states providing an example. In contrast to the disease category, illness is based on the description of its perceived phenomena rather than any alteration in bodily tissues. Finally, the predicaments category was conceptualized as capturing 'problems of living' conditions (eg dependence on illicit drugs) and is both diverse and changeable, being based on the person's experience of environmental phenomena as well as on social and cultural expectations.

Any aversion to categorical models in psychiatry is not mirrored in clinical practice. Clinical psychiatrists who operate to a categorical model generally seek to diagnose with some precision for two principal reasons—firstly, for communication to the patient and to colleagues, and secondly, because they assume that differing conditions require quite differing therapeutic approaches. In contrast, psychiatrists who operate to a dimensional model will have less interest in diagnosis, and weight dimensional constructs like severity as they judge such constructs to shape the patient's level of distress and help-seeking behaviour, and often the treatment to be provided (eg electroconvulsive therapy (ECT) for severe depression, antidepressant drugs for moderate depression, and psychotherapy for mild depression).

Categorical psychiatric models can be readily challenged for their failure to demonstrate clinical features that define the condition at the 'necessary and sufficient' level and are also specific to that condition (ie are not possessed by any other condition), as well as for failure to demonstrate distinct biological determinants and/or to have a benchmark diagnostic test. Such criteria have not been met for any psychiatric condition, a reality that has led to nihilism about any attempt to delineate psychiatric diseases—and the suggestion that psychiatry is unable to 'carve nature at its joints'.

Such a problem is, however, not unique to psychiatry and is handled in varying ways in other fields. For example, anthropologists use the construct of 'thick description' in allowing definition by 'patterns' and accepting that the patterns (not dimensions) are imprecise. In medicine, however, only a minority of conditions have specific clinical features and/or a confirmatory laboratory test. Neurologists nevertheless position Parkinson's disease as a 'categorical' disease—in that it is either present or absent—although it has variable rather than absolutely specific clinical features. Respecting its prototypic expressions, they make a probabilistic estimate as to whether Parkinson's disease is present or absent on the basis of a number of the variable clinical features. In essence, they assume a categorical model and seek to differentiate Parkinson's disease from other causes of parkinsonism rather than adopt a primary dimensional model which might simply weight severity of the condition or of its components such as gait disturbance or tremor.

The use of such a categorical model has advantages (subject to the condition being quintessentially 'categorical') in being more likely to identify those with or without the condition and in heuristically advancing research into its causes and optimal treatment. Thus, there are many advantages to psychiatry seeking to identify those conditions which are categorical. A dimensional model is appropriate for those states that are truly dimensional and may be appropriate as a default option for conditions whose status remains indeterminate. Such an approach—of allowing both models—assumes that the underlying structure of the condition is respected and categorical or dimensional status is accorded on the basis of supportive validity data rather than simply opinion. Building on criteria proposed by Robins and Guze,[3] we can argue that, if a condition is truly intrinsically categorical, it might be reasonably assumed to have prototypic clinical features, to have a relatively specific primary cause (be it biological, psychological, or social), to have its own intrinsic natural history and to have a preferential response to treatment. In considering the bipolar disorders, we will argue the greater relevance of a categorical rather than a dimensional model by reviewing such criteria.

It is important to note that it is possible to dimensionalize everything and, conversely, to create categories or pseudo-categories from intrinsically dimensional constructs. For instance, most people asked to distinguish between a building and a car would effectively differentiate them as independent categorical entities. However, those holding a dimensional view might simply differentiate them as one being big, the other small, both lying along a dimension of 'size'. Which is likely to be the more valid model? Which the most informative? Conversely, entities may be 'dimensionalized'. For example, in a study by Krueger et al. on dimensionalizing psychiatric conditions,[4] factor analyses of DSM-III-R clinical features for ten disorders (major depression, dysthymia, generalized anxiety, agoraphobia, social phobia, simple phobia, obsessive compulsive disorder, conduct disorders, marijuana dependency, and alcohol dependency) were imposed. The authors concluded that their two-factor solution was the best, being able to simply refine the clinical features into two contrasting 'internalizing' and 'externalizing' dimensions. In essence, quite disparate psychiatric conditions were 'dimensionalized' along internalizing and externalizing domains. The model was empirically derived but how intrinsically valid is it and, more importantly, how useful is it in clinical practice?

Psychiatry's classificatory manuals weight or impute diagnostic 'categories' and, commonly, impose categories on underlying dimensions. Recent *Diagnostic and Statistical Manual of Mental Disorders* (DSM) manuals classify personality disorders in this way, by assigning a diagnosis when a set number of criteria are met. The *International Classification of Diseases* (10th revision) (ICD-10) likewise distinguishes between 'severe', 'moderate', and 'mild' depression, albeit with qualitative descriptions differentiating the three 'categories'. The problem with the imposition of any cut-off score is that it will, of necessity, assign some false positives and some false negatives. There is an additional problem that has emerged from the dimensional approach. The DSM-III criteria for obsessive–compulsive disorder were set at a lower cut-off than previous 'case' definitions and resulted in a substantive increase in the prevalence of the condition. DSM-III introduced a diagnosis of major depression and a set of minor depressive categories. Subsequently, the depressive dimension was extended by many theorists to include sub-clinical or sub-syndromal depression. In the 1950s, clinical depression was thought to have a lifetime risk of less than 5%. Now if such depressive extensions are included, it is a ubiquitous experience. Extending 'caseness' to such a low level rightly risks judgements about psychiatry 'pathologizing' sadness and misery in relation to mood disorders, and similar concerns about several other listed conditions.

In considering the bipolar disorders we can examine the data at several levels. Firstly, do the bipolar disorders differ categorically or dimensionally from the unipolar disorders? Secondly, do constituent bipolar disorders differ categorically or dimensionally from each other?

Distinguishing bipolar disorder from unipolar depression

The bipolar disorders were once effectively viewed as belonging with the unipolar depressive disorders. As detailed by Goodwin and Jamison,[5] 'the French 'alienists', Falret and Baillarger, independently and almost simultaneously formulated the concept that mania and depression could represent different manifestations of a single illness. Griesinger viewed mania as the end stage of a progressively worsening melancholic depression and viewed both as reflecting different stages of a unitary condition.[6] While Kraeplin made the distinctive contribution of separating dementia praecox and manic-depressive insanity, he positioned all of the major affective disorders (including mania) into a single category and, as observed by Goodwin and Jamison, doubted that melancholic depression and the bipolar disorders were really separate illnesses.

It was not until 1957 that Leonhard introduced a bipolar-unipolar distinction, following his observation that, for those who had recurrent affective illnesses, some experienced both depression and mania, while others experienced depressive episodes only. He further noted that those patients with a history of mania had a higher rate of mania in their families compared to those with recurrent depressive episodes only.

The categorical bipolar-unipolar distinction was not introduced into formal classificatory systems until 1980 when it was incorporated into the DSM-III and subsequently into the ICD-10 manuals. Thus, prior to Leonhard's classification, the bipolar disorders were positioned together with the unipolar depressive disorders and, at times, positioned together with schizophrenia. Bleuler,[7] in particular, viewed the relationship between manic-depressive illness and schizophrenia as a continuum without a sharp line of demarcation.[5] However, modern psychiatric manuals now unequivocally position the bipolar disorders as categorically different to the unipolar disorders.

Bipolar II disorder similarly developed gradually from what was previously an undifferentiated domain largely neglected by psychiatry. The concept of hypomania was first defined by Mendel in 1881 in his work 'Die Manie. Eine Monographie' (which translates to 'The Mania. A Monograph'), in terms strikingly similar to the modern definition of hypomania. The symptoms were primarily elevated mood, pressured speech, and increased motor activity consistent with the typical clinical picture of mania but to a lesser degree.[8] The term cyclothymia was then used by Kahlbaum in 1882 to describe alterations between elation without psychosis and melancholia which did not progress to dementia.[9]

During the early twentieth century, personality-based mood fluctuations—cyclothymia and hypomania—were lumped together as 'the milder forms of the manic depressive psychosis'[10] and among a subset of practitioners, concern as to how to diagnose and treat such conditions was evident. However, from the 1930s to 1970s, the concept of hypomania or 'milder forms' of bipolar disorder seems to all but have disappeared from the literature. It was not until 1969, when Dunner began work at the National Institute of Mental Health, that research on anything resembling a bipolar II category began. His seminal work looked at a category of bipolar I participants, a category of unipolar participants and a category he describes as 'in between'—who experienced hypomania but not mania (Dunner, personal communication). He reported that the bipolar II participants had manic symptoms similar to the bipolar I sample but to a less severe degree. He also found that the bipolar II group were similar to a bipolar I group in the likelihood of having relatives with bipolar disorder and that the bipolar II group was at higher risk of suicide compared with both bipolar I and unipolar groups.[11]

With the 1980 release of the DSM-III, the concept of hypomania was for the first time officially defined as 'a clinical syndrome that is similar to, but not as severe as, that described by the term "mania" or "manic episode"'. However, bipolar II disorder was still considered an 'atypical bipolar disorder' and considered only briefly in that edition of the manual, without any formal diagnostic guidelines provided. This meant that, although bipolar II began to be used as a category in research studies, without formal diagnostic criteria it was left to each independent research to decide what 'similar to, but not as severe as' mania might mean. Consequently, research studies varied in their classifications and terminology with some referring to 'bipolar other', 'unclassified', or 'UP+' when referring to what we would now consider bipolar II disorder (Dunner, personal communication). Rifkin (a member of the DSM-III Work Group) is quoted as saying that 'a diagnostic scheme must do a lot of lumping, and I doubt if it's worth making a separate category for an episode of hypomania'.[12] Dunner noted that as mania was uncommonly diagnosed in America at the time, supporting both a unipolar/bipolar distinction and bipolar I/bipolar II distinction was an unpopular position (personal communication).

Dunner and Tay[13] eventually established that bipolar II (with a hypomanic episode of three or more days) could be reliably diagnosed by experienced clinicians, a finding which was largely responsible for the inclusion of a bipolar II disorder in the DSM-IV in 1994. However, the ICD-10 had meanwhile defined hypomania as being four or more days and, as a consequence, a minimum period of four or more days was imposed as a DSM-IV criterion for hypomania in order to maintain consistency.[14]

Dimensional modelling of the bipolar disorders

While there are some theorists who position the bipolar disorders (bipolar I and bipolar II) as lying along a dimension that ranges through to the unipolar disorders, dimensional models tend to focus on the extent to which there may be a continuum within the bipolar conditions. The most accepted bipolar disorders are bipolar I and bipolar II and they define the territory for consideration of the extent of which these two conditions are best differentiated. Some consideration should also be given to bipolar III states (which are generally viewed as states of mania or hypomania induced in response to the initiation of an antidepressant or its rapid increase in dose). However, the bipolar dimension has been extended beyond this by many theorists.

Akiskal has been a strong proponent of a 'spectrum' or dimensional model for the bipolar disorders. His bipolar spectrum theory arose from findings that there are some patients lacking documented highs but who have a hyperthymic temperament (a personality style marked by being consistently happier than the average). These hyperthymic unipolar patients are similar to bipolar patients in terms of a family history of bipolar disorder and the percentage of male cases.[15] In one paper,[16] bipolar I is positioned as quintessential manic depression, bipolar II captures those with depressive and hypomanic mood swings, bipolar III is hypomania associated with antidepressant medication, bipolar IV is depression superimposed on a 'hyperthymic temperament', and bipolar V is 'cyclic mixed depressions'.[17,18] In another paper, Akiskal further developed the spectrum model to include both a bipolar VI category defined by cognitive decline and mood instability with an onset in older age[18] and a bipolar II ½ category defined by cyclothymia with depression.[19] Akiskal has further argued[20] for a set of behavioural signs that identify bipolar II disorders being declared in behavioural ways rather than by mood disturbances (a 'soft spectrum'). Such behaviours or traits include polyglotism (the ability to master many languages), eminence, creative achievement, professional instability, multiple marriages, a broad repertoire of sexual behaviour, impulse control problems, as well as ornamentation and flamboyance (principally involving red and other bright colours). Akiskal has proposed the 'rule of three' hinting at soft bipolarity. Exemplars include three failed marriages, three failed antidepressants, three simultaneous jobs, proficiency in three languages, flamboyance expressed in a triad of bright colours, three impulse control behaviours, and simultaneous dating of three individuals.

Such a model is quintessentially dimensional in assuming a gradation of severity. It is—as for diagnostic manuals—categorical in that grades (one to six) are assigned as if diagnostic differentiation can be accorded at each level.

Angst et al.[21] also proposed a categorical broadening of the bipolar disorder domain by use of a bipolar specifier. Their bipolar specifier was designed for use with a DSM-IV-TR diagnosis of a Major Depressive Episode in those with some symptoms of bipolarity. The bipolar specifier broadens bipolar diagnosis to those who are excluded from DSM diagnoses by including those with only three symptoms of bipolar disorder when irritable, those who only experience highs when taking an antidepressant, and those who only experience highs shorter than four days. Use of the bipolar specifier compared to DSM-IV-TR criteria increased the likelihood of bipolar diagnosis in a depressed sample by almost three times. They suggest this indicates that a large number of patients diagnosed with a unipolar condition could be more meaningfully be conceptualized as sub-threshold bipolar disorder.

A strong proponent of a dimensional model is Phelps whose detailed argument[22] will now be summarized. He argues that patients with mood disorders occupy a 'continuum between major depression and bipolar disorder (as extremes) but without any natural dividing points to separate the two', allowing that varying degrees of bipolarity are possible. He is not alone in such an opinion, with the diagnostic guidelines for bipolar disorder issued by the International Society for Bipolar Disorders suggesting that bipolar II disorder is best characterized as part of a spectrum of bipolar illness.[23] Phelps then argued against the categorical model on the basis that if two illnesses present similarly but are truly independent conditions then there should be 'zones of rarity' between them, or points on a continuum where no patients can be placed. Thus, between unipolar and bipolar depression all patients with the unipolar expression should be on one side of the gap and all patients with bipolar disorder on the other side. Phelps refers to two studies which compared the number of hypo/manic symptoms experienced by those with depression and those with bipolar disorder. If a zone of rarity exists then the depressed participants should have few hypo/manic symptoms while the bipolar participants should have many and there should be nobody in between. Such a zone of rarity was not found.[24,25]

Next he reviewed a study by Ghaemi et al.[26] which identified a number of bipolar 'soft signs'. Such features include repeated episodes of major depression, early age of onset of major depression, a first-degree relative with a bipolar disorder, a hyperthymic personality, atypical symptoms when depressed, brief episodes of major depression, a psychotic episode of depression, post-partum depression, hypo/mania while taking an antidepressant medication, loss of response to an antidepressant medication, and seasonal mood shifts. In essence, those authors argued for bipolar status being able to be predicted on the basis of such soft signs rather than on the basis of formal hypo/manic features. The logical problem here is that it risks allocating a bipolar diagnosis to an individual who has never had any hypo/manic symptoms.

Phelps advocated consideration of both soft signs and individual bipolar symptoms when considering where a person may lie on the bipolar spectrum and utilizing a Bipolar Spectrum Diagnostic Scale to examine all of the necessary components in a structured manner. He proposed that using the scale allows the clinician to establish whether the patient shows *any* indication of bipolarity and from there recommends a collaborative approach where the patient is encouraged to investigate their own symptoms. He indicates that a collaborative approach allows the patient to be the expert in their own condition and will so produce a more ecologically valid model of their experiences on which to base treatment.

However, the consideration is then, as conceded by Phelps, how much bipolarity is enough to change a unipolar treatment strategy for a bipolar treatment strategy? Phelps does not provide a pristine answer, instead raising issues important for consideration. Treatment risk is the primary concern, with risks coming in many forms. The risk of treating a patient with underlying bipolarity (who does not meet criteria for bipolar disorder) with an antidepressant has not been established. Phelps extrapolates from the bipolar literature to assume that, as antidepressant treatments have risks in bipolar disorder (in causing switching, mixed states, or a worse illness course), it may be reasonable to assume a level of risk in sub-threshold bipolarity. Inversely treating those with a truly unipolar condition with a mood stabilizer invokes the risk of side effects associated with those medications, which may be greater than the side effects associated with antidepressants. The issue here is how much the patient requires antimanic efficacy in their medication compared to how much they require antidepressant efficacy. Where there is a question of 'how much' bipolarity a patient has, Phelps raises the possibility of an antidepressant treatment which is not an antidepressant and details nine treatments with known antidepressant efficacy which are not antidepressants. These include exercise, psychotherapy, light therapy, lithium, omega 3, thyroid hormones, lamotrigine, quetiapine, and olanzapine. If the patient is aware of their own condition and an active participant in investigating their own symptomatology, then a discussion of the risks and benefits of such treatments may be the most robust solution.

Rather than adopt a spectrum approach entirely, Phelps advocates the use of a spectrum model alongside the traditional categorical model. For example, for a patient with a clear-cut bipolar I condition the inclusion of a spectrum model in psychoeducation may only be confusing. However, when there is some question of bipolarity, a spectrum approach may be an informative conceptualization for both the patient and clinician.

Categorical modelling of the bipolar disorders

Recent DSM manuals (including DSM-5) define mania and hypomania (and thus bipolar I and bipolar II disorders) categorically but, paradoxically, with very similar criteria sets. In essence, DSM symptoms are identical for both mania and hypomania—as is the cut-off score for their presence—so that the two conditions are essentially only differentiated across duration, severity, and hospitalization parameters. Each is limited in application. Duration is problematic as the DSM imposition of four days for hypomania and seven days for mania were generated by expert opinion and consensus rather than empiricism. In one of our studies,[27] the imposition of those minimum duration criteria would have denied a bipolar I diagnosis in 46% of the relevant patients and some 60% of the bipolar II subjects. 'Severity' is extremely difficult to judge, and especially the simple DSM-5 barrier of mania and hypomania being associated with and without 'marked impairment' respectively, and when those in hypomanic states may actually have improved functioning. Hospitalization is theoretically problematic, in that there is no medical condition defined by hospitalization, a criterion which also assumes such an option as being available to all those with the condition.

Categorical models have essentially been developed theoretically rather than from any primary empirical approach. We now overview two empirical studies that we undertook. Firstly, in essence, after examining for differences between bipolar I and bipolar II participants[27] an 'isomer' model for distinguishing between the two groups was proposed. The study used an extension of the DSM-IV diagnosis for mania, where bipolar I participants were required to experience either (i) distinct impairment, (ii) psychotic features at any time, or (iii) hospitalization during a high but were not required to be manic for any particular duration. A bipolar II diagnosis was assigned to those who met DSM-IV criteria for hypomania (again ignoring any duration criterion) but did not experience any of the three noted specific bipolar I features. Of the 157 participants recruited, 49 were assigned to a bipolar I group and 52 to a bipolar II group. Psychotic features were relatively common in the bipolar I group (being experienced by two-thirds) while one-third had required hospitalization. Importantly, 41% of the bipolar I participants had experienced psychotic features when *depressed* compared with 0% of the bipolar II participants. Further, there were no significant differences between the bipolar I and II groups in the severity of manic or hypomanic symptoms, suggesting the 'core' mood and energy constructs to bipolar disorder was not likely to differentiate between the conditions.

A follow-up study was conducted in a larger sample to examine the validity of such a model.[28] Using a clinically diagnosed sample of 632 bipolar participants, those with psychotic symptoms when high were assigned to a bipolar I category while those without such symptoms were assigned to a bipolar II category. Comparable with the previous research, a large number of the bipolar I participants also experienced psychotic symptoms when depressed (57.4%) while only a small number of bipolar II participants experienced psychotic depression (8.1%). The psychosis-weighted diagnostic model also provided greater differentiation between bipolar I and II groups (compared with DSM diagnosis) on employment status, family history of bipolar disorder, and (contrary to expectation) (hypo)manic symptom scores. The differential between bipolar I and bipolar II groups when diagnosed according to this model suggests it is truly separating groups at an intrinsic 'joint' in their natural presentation.

We therefore argue for a categorical 'isomer' or 'mirror image' model. The isomer model posits a core mood and energy component for both mania/hypomania and depression, which is dimensionally but not categorically more severe in bipolar

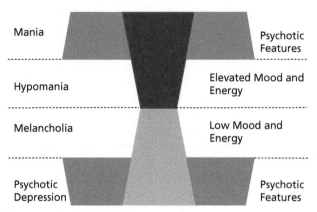

Mania

Psychotic
Features

Hypomania

Elevated Mood and
Energy

Melancholia

Low Mood and
Energy

Psychotic
Depression

Psychotic
Features

Figure 2.1 The core and mantle model

I than in bipolar II. The model then includes a psychotic 'mantle' where, during elevated mood and energy phases the bipolar I patients have experienced categorical psychotic features at some stage of their life during manic episodes (and often during depressive episodes) while the bipolar II patients have never experienced psychotic features when 'high' or when depressed. Thus, the model contains both dimensional and categorical components. The core mood and energy construct is dimensional (and not incisive in differentiating bipolar I and II states) while the presence or absence of psychotic features when high is categorical and provides the point of differentiation between bipolar I and II states (see Figure 2.1).

Less categorical but of some clinical importance is that our findings also indicated that bipolar I depression is likely to be psychotic depression or melancholic depression in its nature, while bipolar II depression is virtually never psychotic in nature but likely to be melancholic in its type.

More recently, in a second study, we[29] conducted a mixture analysis on 1,081 clinically diagnosed bipolar I and II outpatients using scores on hypomanic severity to determine whether there was evidence of bimodality. Our results suggested the presence of a two sub-population solution (thus, indicating bimodality), arguing for a categorical distinction of the bipolar disorders and with the presence/absence of psychotic features when 'high' as the most substantive feature in determining subtype differentiation.

In conclusion, while there are many different ways to conceptualize the bipolar disorders, the choice of a categorical or a dimensional model is based on multiple factors. First and foremost, the model has to respect the underlying nature of the disorders and therefore be a valid reflection of natural conditions. While both dimensional and categorical models have some support from empirical studies, neither is irrefutable and as such it is, as yet, up to the individual clinician to determine which model reflects the clinical population. Secondly, from a utility perspective, it is important to consider which model allows for useful treatment decisions to benefit the patient. While a categorical model allows for simplified treatment decisions and psychoeducation, a spectrum model allows for more variability in presentation which may be of benefit to some patients. It is the opinion of the authors that considering both the underlying nature of the bipolar disorders and the utility of the models in clinical practice, a categorical model would be most appropriate. In particular, hypomanic and manic features show specificity to bipolar I and II disorders respectively, while those conditions appear to show differential response to differing mood-stabilizer medications, with lithium appearing more appropriate for bipolar I and lamotrigine for bipolar II disorder.[30] Additionally, the respective presence or absence of psychotic features distinguishes bipolar I disorder from bipolar II disorder. Thus, a categorical model appears the more appropriate model for conceptualizing differences between the bipolar I and II states.

References

1. **Goldberg, D.** Plato versus Aristotle: categorical and dimensional models for common mental disorders, *Comprehensive Psychiatry* 2000;**41**(2):8–13.

2. **Taylor, D.** The components of sickness: diseases, illnesses, and predicaments, *The Lancet* 1979;**314**(8150):1008–10.

3. **Robins, E** and **Guze, SB.** Establishment of diagnostic validity in psychiatric illness: its application to schizophrenia, *American Journal of Psychiatry* 1970;**126**(7):983–7.

4. **Krueger, RF, Caspi, A, Moffitt, TE,** and **Silva, PA.** The structure and stability of common mental disorders (DSM-III-R): a longitudinal-epidemiological study, *Journal of Abnormal Psychology* 1998;**107**(2):216.

5. **Goodwin, FK** and **Jamison, KR.** *Manic-depressive Illness: Bipolar Disorders and Recurrent Depression* (Oxford: Oxford University Press, 2007).

6. **Jackson, SW.** *Melancholia and Depression: From Hippocratic Times to Modern Times* (New Haven, CT: Yale University Press, 1986).

7. **Bleuler, E.** *Textbook of Psychiatry* (4th German edn). English edited by **AA Brill** (New York, NY: Macmillan, 1924).

8. **Shorter, E.** *A Historical Dictionary of Psychiatry* (US: Oxford University Press, 2005).

9. **Shorter, E.** Bipolar disorder in historical perspective. In **Parker, G** (ed), *Bipolar II Disorder: Modelling, Measuring and Managing* (Cambridge: Cambridge University Press, 2012).

10. **Buzzard, EF, Miller, HE, Riddoch, G, Yellowlees, H, Reynell, WR, Boyle, H,** and **Strauss, EB.** Discussion on the diagnosis and treatment of the milder forms of the manic-depressive psychosis, *Proceedings of the Royal Society of Medicine* 1930;**23**:881–95.

11. **Dunner, DL, Gershon, ES,** and **Goodwin, FK.** Heritable factors in the severity of affective illness, *Biological Psychiatry* 1976;**11**(1):31–42.

12. **Shorter, E.** *What Psychiatry Left out of the DSM-5: Historical Mental Disorders Today* (New York, NY: Routledge, 2015).

13. **Dunner, DL** and **Tay, LK.** Diagnostic reliability of the history of hypomania in bipolar II patients and patients with major depression, *Comprehensive Psychiatry* 1993;**34**(5):303–7.

14. **Dunner, DL.** A review of the diagnostic status of 'bipolar II' for the DSM-IV work group on mood disorders, *Depression* 1993;1:2–10.

15. **Cassano, GB, Akiskal, HS, Savino, M, Musetti, L,** and **Perugi, G.** Proposed subtypes of bipolar II and related disorders: with hypomanic episodes (or cyclothymia) and with hyperthymic temperament, *Journal of Affective Disorders* 1992;**26**(2):127–40.

16. **Akiskal, HS.** The dark side of bipolarity: detecting bipolar depression in its pleomorphic expressions, *Journal of Affective Disorders* 2005a;**84**(2):107–15.

17. **Akiskal, HS** and **Pinto, O.** The evolving bipolar spectrum: prototypes I, II, III, and IV, *Psychiatric Clinics of North America* 1999;**22**(3):517–34.

18. **Ng, B, Camacho, A, Lara, DR, Brunstein, MG, Pinto, OC,** and **Akiskal, HS.** A case series on the hypothesized connection between dementia and bipolar spectrum disorders: Bipolar type VI?, *Journal of Affective Disorders* 2008;**107**(1):307–15.

19. **Akiskal, HS, Akiskal, KK, Lancrenon, S,** and **Hantouche, E.** Validating the soft bipolar spectrum in the French National EPIDEP Study: the prominence of BP-II 1/2, *Journal of Affective Disorders* 2006;**96**(3):207–13.

20. **Akiskal, HS.** Searching for behavioral indicators of bipolar II in patients presenting with major depressive episodes: the 'red sign,' the 'rule of three' and other biographic signs of temperamental extravagance, activation and hypomania, *Journal of Affective Disorders* 2005b;**84**(2):279–90.

21. **Angst, J, Azorin, JM, Bowden, CL, Perugi, G, Vieta, E, Gamma, A,** and **BRIDGE Study Group.** Prevalence and characteristics of undiagnosed bipolar disorders in patients with a major depressive episode: the BRIDGE study, *Archives of General Psychiatry* 2011;**68**(8):791–9.

22. **Phelps, J.** The bipolar spectrum. In: **Parker, G** (ed), *Bipolar II Disorder: Modelling, Measuring and Managing* (Cambridge: Cambridge University Press, 2012).

23. **Ghaemi, SN, Bauer, M, Cassidy, F, Malhi, GS, Mitchell, P, Phelps, J, Vieta, E,** and **Youngstrom, E.** Diagnostic guidelines for bipolar disorder: a summary of the international society for bipolar disorders diagnostic guidelines task force report, *Bipolar Disorders* 2008;**10**(1p2):117–28.

24. **Benazzi, F.** Bipolar II disorder and major depressive disorder: continuity or discontinuity?, *World Journal of Biological Psychiatry* 2003;**4**:166–71.

25. **Akiskal, HS** and **Benazzi, F.** Recurrent major depressive disorder and bipolar II: evidence that they lie on a dimensional spectrum, *Journal of Affective Disorders* 2006;**92**:45–54.

26. **Ghaemi, SN, Ko, JY,** and **Goodwin, FK.** 'Cade's disease' and beyond: misdiagnosis, antidepressant use, and a proposed definition for bipolar spectrum disorder, *Canadian Journal of Psychiatry [Revue canadienne de psychiatrie]* 2002;**47**(2):125–34.

27. **Parker, G, Hadzi-Pavlovic, D,** and **Tully, L.** Distinguishing bipolar and unipolar disorders: an isomer model, *Journal of Affective Disorders* 2006;**96**(1):67–73.

28. **Parker, G, Graham, R, Hadzi-Pavlovic, D, McCraw, S, Hong, M,** and **Friend, P.** Differentiation of bipolar I and II disorders by examining for differences in severity of manic/hypomanic symptoms and the presence or absence of psychosis during that phase, *Journal of Affective Disorders* 2013;**150**(3):941–7.

29. **Parker, GB, Graham, RK,** and **Hadzi-Pavlovic, D.** Are the bipolar disorders best modelled categorically or dimensionally? *Acta Psychiatrica Scandinavica* 2016;**134**(2):104–10.

30. **Parker, G.** Rounding up and tying down, *Bipolar II Disorder: Modelling, Measuring and Managing* 2012:266.

Chapter 3

The treatment of bipolar disorder in its early stages: current techniques, challenges, and future outlook

Ajeet B. Singh, Harris A. Eyre, Edward Callaly and Michael Berk

Introduction

In recent years in psychiatry, a renewed focus on prevention and early intervention across various illness domains has arisen.[1] This is in part related to the simple logic that if a condition can be prevented or illness trajectory optimized, improved prognosis and reduced burden of disease (for the individual and society) may follow. More recently, the increasingly unsustainable costs of healthcare have led to prevention and early intervention becoming even higher health policy and research priorities.[1] For these important reasons, prevention and early intervention are of central importance in the optimal management of bipolar disorders.[1]

Bipolar disorder tends to begin with symptoms of depression rather than mania, which is what is required for diagnosis, and the prodrome of the disorder is even more non-specific, with symptoms of anxiety, sleep disturbance, attention and behavioural symptoms common, as is substance abuse. There is also a lack of robust (sensitive and specific) clinical and biomarker predictors of onset of bipolar disorders.[1] This has made the task of prevention and early intervention more challenging. Nonetheless, given the clear importance of this pursuit, renewed efforts at biomarker discovery have included emphasis on prevention. 'P4 medicine', characterized by predictive, preventative, personalized, and participatory approaches,[2] has become the framework for novel technologies such as genomics and digital healthcare. It is important for clinicians at the frontline of care to remember that new medical technologies need to be housed within the public health wisdom of this P4 model of healthcare.

Early intervention (also known as secondary prevention) has been pioneered in psychiatry over the past two decades, with novel early intervention for psychosis programs gaining global traction since emerging in the mid-1990s in Australia. While the literature and clinical services for early intervention in bipolar disorders are considerably less developed than those for schizophrenia and psychosis, early intervention in bipolar disorders has also been an emergent focus of research over the past decade in particular.[1] This chapter seeks to provide readers with an overview of the current state of the art in early intervention in bipolar, challenges in the field, and promising areas of research which may translate to enhanced clinical care in years to come. Indeed, for early intervention in bipolar disorders there may be even greater opportunity to retard neuroprogression, the progressive damage occurring to the brain with subsequent episodes of illness, than in schizophreniform psychosis, given there seems be less structural brain changes at incident episodes than for schizophreniform psychotic illnesses.[3] The emergence of nutraceutical and lifestyle-based therapeutics acting on inflammatory and neuroprotective pathways offers an interesting opportunity for low-hazard therapeutic trials in the non-specific prodrome of illness.[1] Should the body of evidence for such reach a tipping point, it is plausible that one day there will be active neuroprotective interventions suitable for those in prodrome.[1] As initial studies in this frontier move to larger comparative cohort studies, the utility of this latter approach may eventually be established, but at this stage this area remains an important research front.

Illness staging and minimizing the impact of neuroprogression

Staging bipolar disorder

In several sub-disciplines of medicine, the concept of stage of illness is employed to better tailor care and optimize outcomes. Oncology with its 'Tumour Node Metastasis' system, and cardiology with its American Heart Association 'Classes of Heart Failure' system are prime examples. For most psychiatric conditions—bipolar disorders included—there is a lack of clarity of the underling pathophysiology. This clearly makes application of the staging approach used elsewhere in medicine more difficult. Nonetheless, there do appear to be multiple threads of both clinical and biological empirical data suggesting that a staging model may have real-world utility in bipolar disorders.[1,4]

Historically, in psychiatry many conditions have presented late—after many years of symptoms and untreated illness. With reduced levels of stigma and better community awareness of mental illness, along with generally greater access to psychiatric services, there is much opportunity in the modern era to both engage patients early in their course of bipolar disorder and study differential outcomes based on earlier interventions.[1] These important social factors have enabled greater study of, and care for, those in the early phases of their illness during the past two decades.[1]

Staging models have been proposed (see for reviews[1,4] and see Table 3.1 for an overview of a recent proposal). The earliest stage is stage 0—this stage reflecting individuals who have risk factors, but as yet have not manifested any clinical features of illness. Risk factors include genetic diathesis, perinatal complications, adverse lifestyle risks, childhood maltreatment, psychological stressors, and substance abuse. The non-specific nature of these risk factors makes specific indicated preventative

Table 3.1 A potential clinical staging model for bipolar disorder

Clinical stage	Definition	Potential interventions
0	Increased risk of severe mood disorder (eg, family history, abuse, substance use) No specific current symptoms	Mental health literacy Self-help
1a	Mild or non-specific symptoms of mood disorder	Formal mental health literacy Family psychoeducation Substance abuse reduction Cognitive behavioural therapy, supportive counselling
1b	Prodromal features: ultra-high risk	*1a* plus therapy for episode: phase specific or mood stabilizer
2	First episode threshold mood disorder	*1b* and case management, vocational rehabilitation, specific psychotherapy
3a	Recurrence of sub-threshold mood symptoms	*2* and emphasis on maintenance medication and psychosocial strategies for full remission
3b	First threshold relapse	*2a* and relapse prevention strategies
3c	Multiple relapses	*3b* and combination mood stabilizers
4	Persistent unremitting illness	*3c* and clozapine and other tertiary therapies, social participation despite disability

Data from Bipolar Disorder, 9.7, 2007, Berk M et al., 'Setting the stage: from prodrome to treatment resistance in bipolar disorder', pp. 671–8; data from *Journal of Affective Disorders*, 100.1, 2007, Berk M et al., 'The potential utility of a staging model as a course specifier: a bipolar disorder perspective', pp. 279–81.

interventions problematic due to a large false positive rate—only a fraction of those with risk factors converting to illness over time. But notwithstanding this, among those with generic and non-disorder specific at-risk profiles, there is value in reinforcing general health steps including healthy lifestyles, self-help strategies, psychological counselling, safer use of substances, and mental health literacy. This is salient as risk factors for mental health disorders overlap with those for other common non-communicable disorders.

In particular, greater awareness of the symptoms of bipolar disorders and when to seek help for them is an important element of mental health literacy—something increasingly accessible in the digital age (see, for example, http://www.bipolarcaregivers.org). Stage 1 describes the prodromal stage—a stage where there remains a paucity of evidence to predict the course of illness. For this reason only general measures as outlined earlier are appropriate, with a particular emphasis on awareness of illness symptoms, when to seek help, and where possible serial review by a clinician to monitor at-risk mental state. Developing a therapeutic alliance, engagement, and trust with a clinician early on can be key determinates of subsequent success in care should illness manifest. There is insufficient evidence to argue for specific treatments of the prodrome at present, but fostering a culture of psychoeducation and awareness of how to access services should symptoms emerge is a sensible approach.

Stage 2 is defined as the first episode of illness and since mania is mandatory for a *Diagnostic and Statistical Manual of Mental Disorders* (5th edition) (DSM-5) and *International Classification of Diseases* (10th revision) (ICD-10) diagnosis of bipolar I—stage 2 in bipolar I is the first episode of mania, and in bipolar II disorder the first hypomania. It is at this stage that opportunities for early intervention in bipolar arise. This creates some problems with optimal early interventions, as for many cases the first pole to manifest of the illness is the depressive one, but given the need for elevated states to confirm the diagnosis there is no alternative—early intervention approaches to depression notwithstanding. For some cases, their index mood episodes will be an elevated state without any previous depressive episodes; this group potentially having opportunity for earliest possible intervention in their illness, and potentially best prognosis.

Stage 3 of bipolar is recurrence of mood episodes, and is the stage where most research into bipolar disorder has traditionally been conducted. By stage 4, there is by definition a persistent unremitting nature of the illness. It is hoped that early intervention in stage 2 will improve long-term prognosis, but empirical evidence to establish this has not yet been confirmed. Nonetheless, as with early intervention in psychosis (as in cancer and cardiovascular disease), there is a strong argument that engaging people early in their illness course will be linked to better treatment outcomes, help foster adherence with care, and hopefully translate to better long-term outcomes. This is the basic premise behind early intervention in bipolar disorder. Long-term differential outcomes studies stratified by early intervention versus no early intervention are lacking, leading to a need for some caution in the area. This is particularly important at a policy level where if heath resources are diverted from later-stage sufferers to early stage sufferers of bipolar, there is need to be mindful of the empirical limitations of the evidence. Beyond the psychosocial and putative compliance benefits for early engagement, the early intervention model is also predicated on the importance of neuroprotection as a key goal of treatment.[5] Neuroprotection mitigating against volume change in key brain regions, pathways that promote neuronal growth, proliferation, or survival, and protect against neuronal or glial insults forms a putative biological theoretical underpinning for early stage treatment to improved prognosis.[5] Both neuroimaging and neuropsychological studies suggest the neuroprogression model of bipolar has validity, and in turn helps validate the notion of prioritizing early intervention in the illness.[1,5]

Neuroimaging in the neuroprogression of bipolar disorder

Neuroimaging and cognitive evidence suggest that there may be a neuroprogressive aspect to bipolar disorder.[1] Various brain regions have been implicated, including the anterior cingulate cortex, amygdala, hippocampus, basal-ganglia, dorsolateral-prefrontal cortex, and orbitofrontal cortex.[6,7] Importantly, the volumetric abnormalities appear to be dependent on stage of illness—consistent with the neuroprogression hypothesis.[5] But only a handful of studies have examined patients early in their course of illness. Adler and colleagues[8] identified increased grey matter volumes in a caudal region of the anterior cingulate cortex (ACC). It also appears the pituitary is increased in size in young adults with bipolar disorder,[9] as well as previously published data regarding volumetric increases in the amygdala and pituitary occurring prior to, and shortly after, a first episode of affective psychosis.[3] Collectively, these findings—mindful that there are negative studies—suggest hypertrophy of brain regions involved with elevated stress response around the time of illness onset, ultimately leading to volumetric loss in later stages. Early intervention might be beneficial to inhibit the deleterious downstream biochemical changes associated with bipolar disorder, especially oxidative stress and inflammation, while also exerting neuroprotective effects.[5] These effects may help to mitigate broader neuroprogressive structural changes. For example, the postulated neuroprotective role of lithium is supported in the literature[10] and neuroimaging studies suggest adolescents with bipolar disorder on mood stabilizers—like lithium—may be protected from volumetric brain loss.[11] Additionally, atypical antipsychotics used clinically as mood stabilizers may have neurotrophic or neuroprotective effects,[12] although this literature is inconsistent, and there have been suggestions in preclinical studies that the converse may be true.

Neuropsychology in the neuroprogression of bipolar disorder

Data from neuropsychological studies also helps support the neuroprogressive hypothesis of bipolar disorder, and further underpins the rationale for early intervention. Early studies of cognitive impairments in children at risk of bipolar (due to one or both parents being diagnosed) shows a trend to slowed reaction times on visual tasks,[13] and significant differences between visual and performance IQ.[14] El-Badri and colleagues[15] demonstrated that a greater number of affective episodes were associated with poorer executive functioning and visual task performance in euthymic young adults with varying numbers of previous mood episodes. This finding was supported by a review[16] of 11 studies conducted on the impact of increasing numbers of episodes on neurocognition, concluding there were increasing deficits over increasing numbers of episodes in some papers, while other papers included in the review found no relationship. If the number of previous affective episodes is associated with cognitive impairment, it follows that prophylaxis against affective episodes could slow neuroprogression and improve the prognosis of bipolar disorder in the long term.[1] The literature here is lacking; however, one study found that delay to first treatment was associated with more frequent and more severe episodes of depression and more time spent in rapid cycling states.[17]

Clinical factors in the neuroprogression of bipolar disorder

There is also some evidence that age and illness progression may influence response to treatment. A meta-analysis of 12 double-blinded randomized controlled trials investigating olanzapine (an atypical antipsychotic) use in bipolar disorder found that fewer previous manic episodes was associated with significantly higher response rates to treatment for both mania and depression, and also a lower chance to relapse into manic or depressive episodes.[18] Another study examined 4,714 Danish bipolar disorder sufferers who were prescribed lithium and found that early prophylactic use of lithium was also associated with significantly improved response to treatment.[19] Furthermore, lithium has been found to be effective in adolescents where it is proposed to be more effective in preventing affective episodes than in adults.[20] It has also been suggested that young adults with bipolar disorder may benefit more from group psychoeducation than older adults.[21] However, another study following 764 bipolar disorder patients found that bipolar disorder morbidity during lithium treatment was unrelated to numbers of previous episodes.[22]

Collectively, both neuroimaging and neuropsychological studies suggest that bipolar disorders may have a staged nature, which could be ameliorated by early intervention, but results have been mixed. It may be the case that certain subgroups of patients are more prone to neuroprogression. Delineating a neuroprotective genetic profile and inflammatory load stratification of diathesis to such neuroprogression may be a useful future strategy.[23] It is also possible that some people are predisposed to go on to 'malignant' or 'benign' courses from the outset, and that the scope for intervention may be smaller than conceptualized. In the interim, the progressive nature of bipolar (in at least some sufferers) helps support the case for early intervention being a priority, with potential to improve the long-term prognosis of the condition. Indeed, on average there is a large delay between the onset of bipolar disorder symptoms and correct diagnosis and treatment which represents a large opportunity for improved care.

Influence of neuroprotective pharmacological therapies in bipolar disorder

Mood-stabilizing agents appear to have neuroprotective effects. Their potential to be disease modifying, to alter the course of illness, is a function of their ability to prevent or impede the cascade of cellular loss underpinning the structural, cognitive and clinical changes in bipolar disorder.[5] The putative mechanisms of action of the mood stabilizers, principally lithium and valproate, but increasingly atypical antipsychotics, include actions that reduce apoptosis and oxidative stress.[5] Treatment with either lithium or valproate increases levels of bcl-2 (an anti-apoptotic protein) in animal studies.[24,25] and atypical antipsychotics also appear to increase bcl-2 levels.[26] Glycogen synthase kinase-3 (GSK-3), is another protein involved in regulating apoptosis and cellular resilience, and has cytoprotective effects.[27] It appears to be inhibited by lithium, and this mechanism may be a key element of lithium's mechanism of action.[28] Lithium also appears to help protect cells from excitotoxic apoptosis, a process that contributes to hippocampal atrophy, and has been shown to increase N-acetyl aspartate—a marker of neuronal viability[29] and to increase grey matter in bipolar patients.[30] Markers of oxidative stress appear to be elevated in bipolar disorder, and both lithium and valproate appear to reduce oxidative stress in preclinical models.[31] Neurotrophic factors such as BDNF (brain-derived neurotrophic factor) have also been implicated in the underlying pathophysiology of bipolar disorder, and again both lithium and valproate, as well as some atypical antipsychotics such as quetiapine, appear to increase BDNF in animal models.[32]

Taken collectively, the neuroimaging and neuropsychological evidence for neuro-progression in bipolar, along with putative neuroprotective mechanisms of mood stabilizers used in bipolar, help to support the case for prioritizing early intervention; the simple aim being to minimize neuroprogression and optimize prognosis for sufferers.

Developmental stage and psychosocial impact minimization

Beyond the case for early intervention to potentially attenuate the neuroprogressive aspects of bipolar and enhance long-term prognosis, there is a pressing argument for the value of early intervention to limit the psychosocial developmental impacts of the condition. Bipolar disorders typically have onset during late adolescence and early adulthood. These are key phases of maturation into adulthood, with establishment of both work and personal life foundations for later adulthood.[1] Developmental impacts during these stages of life stand to disproportionally produce psychosocial adjustment handicaps compared with illness that has onset in later life when many developmental milestones have been attained. Furthermore, the total life burden of disease from a health economic perspective stands to be greater for conditions with onset in early adulthood. For these reasons there is a strong case to optimize early treatments in hopes of minimizing impediment or derailment of normal development in early adulthood.[33,34] Tohen and colleagues[34] noted that when functional recovery from bipolar is not achieved early in the course of illness, it is rarely attained later. The early stages of the disorder provide an opportunity to support normal adolescent development and prevent the development of secondary morbidities, such as financial difficulties, employment difficulties, and poor self-esteem, which may accumulate with multiple affective episodes over time. Conus and McGorry[35] also highlighted the protective impact of interventions assisting young bipolar adults to develop and secure their social networks. Such considerations make a compelling case for early intervention in bipolar disorder.

Engagement and adherence

Early intervention in bipolar is an opportunity to optimize both engagement with care and adherence to treatments. Engagement and adherence with treatment are key factors for long-term prognosis, and mould expectations of treatment and long-term attitudes to treatment. Despite the importance of engagement and adherence, there is relatively little empirical data to guide practice. This may in part reflect difficulties in recruiting at times poorly adherent/motivated subjects into longitudinal studies. Nonetheless, there is merit in considering aspects of engagement and adherence in early stage bipolar.

Several factors have been associated with medication and treatment adherence.[36] Psychological factors include: an external locus of control, cognitive dysfunction, fear of side effects, and negative attitudes towards treatment—which can be exacerbated by depressive-phase cognitions. Lack of social support, stigma and family dysfunction appear to also impact engagement and compliance with care. Insight—characteristically poor during manic states—can be a particularly important factor influencing adherence and engagement. A diagnosis of bipolar disorder can enhance insight only if young people identify as mentally ill, which fosters positive attitudes towards pharmacotherapy, while a diagnosis discordant with self-assessment might drive disengagement. This highlghts the importance of cautious information sharing and psychoeducation, tracking the person's level of acceptance.[37] However, this has the potential to be outweighed by stigma stress, which is negatively associated with help-seeking behaviour and service use as well as attitudes towards pharmacotherapy and psychotherapy.[37] Early stage illness is an opportunity for patients to develop secure working relationships with their treating clinician or clinicians. Goodwill and trust in the working relationship between clinician and patient can underpin engagement and adherence—even at times where motivation and insight to do so is impaired or limited. Psychoeducation of the illness and treatment options fosters engagement with care, reducing risk of relapse.[38] Group support and psychoeducation interventions may have specific advantages.[38] More recently, studies suggest that online self-management tools and psychoeducation may assist.[39] Such digital approaches offer an extra layer of accessible care for patients to augment the clinician and group-based measures, potentially enabling even greater engagement and adherence. Clearly, one of the key foci of early intervention in bipolar disorder is fostering engagement with care—doctor–patient and clinician–patient relationships along with peer support and family support all key elements to optimally establish early in the course of illness.

Therapeutic trials and diagnostic stability

One of the great clinical dilemmas in bipolar disorders is diagnosis. Often it requires the passage of years after an index depressive episode before clear elevated episodes confirm the diagnosis of a bipolar disorder.[33] This reality limits optimal early intervention for patients where their index affective episode is depressive rather than manic or hypomanic. Nonetheless, even among the many cases where depressive episodes precede an index manic/hypomanic episode, there may be features of family history and aspects of the depressive symptomatology which might increase one's index of suspicion for bipolarity—enabling closer monitoring.

Firstly, symptoms of bipolar disorders—more usually depressive phases of the illness—characteristically emerge during adolescence. In fact, the mean age of onset for such symptoms is approximately 17 years of age.[40] There are substantial delays to diagnosis given the need for longitudinal clinical manifestations of elevated states and the highly non-specific nature of dysphoric symptoms in adolescence. The mean delay to diagnosis was over 12 years in one study, with the delay greatest in those with the earliest onset.[41] This poses significant challenges to early identification and intervention measures. As the illness progresses, it is normative for it to be expressed by evolving syndromal patterns—the Dutch Bipolar Offspring study showed that offspring of people with bipolar disorder met criteria for many other diagnoses prior to the onset of mania.[42]

Among the earlier age of onset, subgroup depressive episodes predominate, with mania more commonly seen in the later onset patient group.[43] Thus, many cases of bipolar will invariably have delays to treatment, being initially viewed as unipolar depressive states. This situation can also place such patients at risk of monotherapy with antidepressants, possibly exacerbating mood instability. For this reason, any young adult being trialled on antidepressants merits careful mental state monitoring for affective switching and mixed states—potentially manifesting as agitation with risk ideations. In addition, some authors have argued that the 'signature' phenomenology of bipolar depression differs subtly from unipolar depression, expressing features such as more psychomotor retardation atypical patterns, and psychotic symptoms.[44] This may aid early diagnosis/index of suspicion for bipolar diathesis.

While the most common initial misdiagnosis (in clinical course retrospect) is unipolar depression, other diagnoses such as borderline personality and co-morbid conditions such as anxiety and substance misuse are also common—delaying definitive bipolar diagnosis and appropriate intervention. Both borderline personality disorder and anxiety disorders can have a similar age of onset and have symptoms that overlap with mixed mood states characteristic of adolescent bipolar disorder.[45] In some cases a combination of bipolar disorder and borderline personality will exist, such cases meriting tailored expert care—usually in the context of a multidisciplinary team. It is equally true (from clinical experience) that many people with prominent mood instability over time can appear to have predominant personality rather than mood disorders—diagnostic openness and longitudinal follow-up are key to avoid misdiagnosis and associated suboptimal care.

As mentioned earlier—and to emphasize again—beyond the delay in optimal treatment through not considering a differential diagnosis of bipolar in a young adult presenting with depressive symptoms, there are risks associated with inappropriate therapy, particularly manic switching and cycle acceleration with antidepressant monotherapy. Misdiagnosis of bipolar disorder as depression and subsequent inappropriate therapy might result in more psychiatric hospitalizations and psychiatric emergency room visits compared with correctly diagnosed bipolar disorder patients, and thus produce higher per-patient treatment costs.[46] For clinicians, the key is to keep the differential diagnosis in mind, properly educate patients and their families regarding mood switching, and offer frequent mental state review appointments during the initial weeks on an antidepressant medication.

Further complicating accurate initial diagnosis is the observation that mania in young people is more likely to have dysphoric/mixed features leading to diagnosis of bipolar potentially being missed.[47] Clinicians need to be cautious of such 'agitated depression' (depression with mixed features) in young adults—especially if they seem to be exacerbated by antidepressant monotherapy. These concerns are reflected in the 2013 update of DSM-5, which focused on mixed features and may allow more diagnoses to be made in younger patients while maintaining diagnostic flexibility over time.[48] Differentiating features of bipolar depression which may assist with earlier diagnosis of bipolar diathesis include hypersomnia, other 'atypical' depressive symptoms such as 'leaden paralysis' and hyperphagia, psychotic features including pathological guilt, psychomotor slowing, 'flatness' of mood, an abrupt onset or offset of episodes, postpartum onset, a prodrome of cyclothymia or hyperthymia (trait mildly elevated mood), a seasonal pattern of symptoms, lability of mood, irritability, sub-threshold manic symptoms and a family history of bipolar disorder.[41]

There are great clinical challenges in early diagnosis of bipolar disorder, and this in turns impacts the ability for clinicians to intervene early and appropriately. For cases where elevated states present early there is greater opportunity to apply appropriate therapies. For any unipolar depressive presentation early in adulthood, there needs to be an index of suspicion for latent bipolarity, and careful monitoring of the impacts of antidepressants if they are used. There have been attempts to identify criteria of the bipolar disorder prodrome but the data is scarce. The early symptoms of bipolar disorder are non-specific while illness trajectories are difficult to predict and currently a firm diagnosis cannot be made before the onset of manic features. Given the dearth of literature, it remains possible that further research could elucidate characteristics of the bipolar disorder prodrome and aid early diagnosis—this remains to be seen, but promising technological innovations are touched on later in the chapter.

Role of co-morbidities in bipolar disorder

Patients with bipolar disorder are at high risk for a range of co-morbidities that might obscure diagnosis, including childhood anxiety, conduct and attention deficit disorders, as well as migraine, enuresis and substance abuse. These co-morbidities are not only more likely in people with bipolar disorder but also more prevalent before its formal onset. Substance abuse is commonly associated with bipolar disorders, which can be diagnostically problematic and potentially alter the course of illness.

Alcohol is the most commonly used substance with the lifetime prevalence of abuse or dependence as high as 46.2% for bipolar I and 39.2% for bipolar II patients, compared with 13.8% for the general population.[49] Drug use can mimic the signs of psychosis while stimulant use can present similarly to mania, and stimulant withdrawal to depression, and these can be mistaken for signs of bipolar disorder. Bipolar patients with co-morbid drug abuse are less likely to be adherent to medication, with robust data in the case of marijuana misuse.[50] For bipolar disorder patients, substance abuse has been postulated to increase hospitalization rates through treatment non-adherence or potentially destabilize mood in the case of stimulants, but the literature is lacking in these areas. Co-morbidity with alcohol or other substance use disorders is also associated with higher rates of suicide attempts in bipolar disorder patients and co-morbidity could indicate poor coping skills or lack of social support. Together, these factors make the treatment of substance abuse an important goal for clinicians to improve bipolar disorder outcomes.

Anxiety disorders are also frequently comorbid with bipolar disorder and typically presents during childhood or adolescence. Clinically, co-morbid anxiety predicts poorer functioning and quality of life, less time euthymic, increased risk of suicide, and poorer response to treatment.[51] Co-morbid anxiety warrants more intensive treatment and those with lifetime anxiety may benefit from more intensive psychotherapy. Given that anxiety can present before bipolar mania, children and adolescents treated with antidepressants could be at risk of mood destabilization.

Clinical trials in bipolar disorder often exclude patients with co-morbid conditions. This limits the applicability of such trial data to real-world clinical populations where co-morbidity is the norm. Clinicians need to be mindful of this fact, and apply the evidence-based guidelines that exist with a focus on mitigating the impacts of co-morbidities as a priority in care. Clinical experience dictates that patients with marked co-morbidities from the outset of care may have a poorer prognosis and less diagnostic clarity—much impeding optimal outcomes. Rather than such co-morbidities being seen as side issues, aggressively tackling substance abuse and refractory anxiety symptoms can be an essential step to optimize engagement and outcomes.

Future directions

The '4P concept' (prediction, prevention, precision, participation) in modern healthcare holds much promise as a useful framework in the development of early interventions for bipolar disorders. There are a range of promising research techniques supporting these 4Ps. The first is the full leverage of smartphone-based technologies to track, monitor, and motivate patients and those at risk. One company, Monsenso, already has a study underway to investigate via a randomized controlled single-blind parallel-group trial for use of such technology in bipolar disorder (NCT02221336). It is investigating the role of a smartphone-based monitoring system, which includes an integrated feedback loop on both subjective and automatically generated behavioural data on measures of illness activity (phone usage, social activity, physical activity, and mobility). Outcome measures include depressive and manic symptoms, the rate of depressive and manic episodes, the total number of days hospitalized, psychosocial function, perceived stress, quality of life, self-rated depressive symptoms, self-rated manic symptoms, recovery, self-rated sense of empowerment, and medication adherence versus the standard treatment as usual in adult patients with bipolar disorder. Another company, Ginger.IO, also has a study underway using similar technology (NCT02491307). Such proprietary innovations are welcome, but will require independent replication of findings for wide clinical uptake should initial study results be promising. Nonetheless, investment by industry should be welcome—evidence-backed technologies to improve patient outcomes a common goal.

Multimodal longitudinal assessments may be useful in predicting transition from high-risk states to psychosis. A study by Clark et al.[52] explored the risk of individual progression from clinical high risk for psychosis to First Episode Psychosis with multimodal diagnostics from clinical interview, structural magnetic resonance imaging, neuropsychological testing, and electroencephalography. Data from published studies were explored, and predictive models were used based on the odds-ratio form of Bayes' rule. In brief, several modalities of investigation were seen to be necessary to arrive at clinically meaningful risk predictions for conversion to illness. This was particularly true for a group of patients whose initial test results (eg clinical and cognitive) were equivocal. For such individuals, at least four tests were required to determine the actual risk profile. Again, these promising early data will require replication and adequate effect size for clinical utility and broad translation to routine care.

Finally, another key area of technology is precision medicine—genetically guided healthcare. This area has recently generated a global groundswell of interest in potentially helping predict illness risk and optimal preventative and therapeutic options. This entire field—given its great potential—is the subject of a dedicated chapter later in this book.

Conclusion

The burden of bipolar disorders is a pressing public health issue. Prevention, early intervention, optimal application of existing treatments, and development of novel therapies are all keys to progress the field of care. To date, there have been numerous promising lines of enquiry aiming to intervene earlier in bipolar disorder's development, potentially enhancing preventative efforts even before illness formally clinically presents. Such examples include developing staging tools using various biomarkers (genetic, neuroimaging, serum), neuropsychological markers, lifestyle measures, neuroprotective agents, as well as digital health tools to improve biological and psychosocial course and management of illness. Further work is required to enhance the evidence base, but signs are promising that a convergence of technologies and methods will serve to improve patient outcomes in years to come.

References

1. **Berk, M** et al. Stage managing bipolar disorder, Bipolar Disord 2014;**16**(5):471–7.
2. **Hood, L** and **M Flores**. A personal view on systems medicine and the emergence of proactive P4 medicine: predictive, preventive, personalized and participatory, N Biotechnol 2012;**29**(6):613–24.
3. **Velakoulis, D** et al. Hippocampal and amygdala volumes according to psychosis stage and diagnosis: a magnetic resonance imaging study of chronic schizophrenia, first-episode psychosis, and ultra-high-risk individuals, Arch Gen Psychiatry 2006;**63**(2):139–49.
4. **McGorry, PD** et al. Clinical staging of psychiatric disorders: a heuristic framework for choosing earlier, safer and more effective interventions, Aust NZJ Psychiatry 2006;**40**(8):616–22.
5. **Berk, M** et al. Pathways underlying neuroprogression in bipolar disorder: focus on inflammation, oxidative stress and neurotrophic factors, Neurosci Biobehav Rev 2011;**35**(3):804–17.
6. **Monkul, ES, GS Malhi,** and **JC Soares**. Anatomical MRI abnormalities in bipolar disorder: do they exist and do they progress?, Aust NZJ Psychiatry 2005;**39**(4):222–6.
7. **Stork, C** and **PF Renshaw**. Mitochondrial dysfunction in bipolar disorder: evidence from magnetic resonance spectroscopy research, Mol Psychiatry 2005;**10**(10):900–19.
8. **Adler, CM** et al. Voxel-based study of structural changes in first-episode patients with bipolar disorder, Biol Psychiatry 2007;**61**(6):776–81.

9. **MacMaster, FP** et al. Pituitary gland volume in adolescent and young adult bipolar and unipolar depression, Bipolar Disord 2008;**10**(1):101–4.

10. **Silva, R** et al. Lithium blocks stress-induced changes in depressive-like behavior and hippocampal cell fate: the role of glycogen-synthase-kinase-3beta, *Neuroscience* 2008;**152**(3):656–69.

11. **Chang, K** et al. Reduced amygdalar gray matter volume in familial pediatric bipolar disorder, J Am Acad Child Adolesc Psychiatry 2005;**44**(6):565–73.

12. **Kusumi, I, S Boku, and Y. Takahashi**. Psychopharmacology of atypical antipsychotic drugs: From the receptor binding profile to neuroprotection and neurogenesis, Psychiatry Clin Neurosci 2015;**69**(5):243–58.

13. **Winters, KC** et al. Cognitive and attentional deficits in children vulnerable to psychopathology, J Abnorm Child Psychol 1981;**9**(4):435–53.

14. **Decina, P** et al. Clinical and psychological assessment of children of bipolar probands, Am J Psychiatry 1983;**140**(5):548–53.

15. **El-Badri, SM** et al. Electrophysiological and cognitive function in young euthymic patients with bipolar affective disorder, Bipolar Disord 2001;**3**(2):79–87.

16. **Robinson, LJ and IN Ferrier**. Evolution of cognitive impairment in bipolar disorder: a systematic review of cross-sectional evidence, Bipolar Disord 2006;**8**(2):103–16.

17. **Post, RM** et al. Early onset bipolar disorder and treatment delay are risk factors for poor outcome in adulthood, J Clin Psychiatry 2010;**71**(7):864–72.

18. **Berk, M** et al. Does stage of illness impact treatment response in bipolar disorder? Empirical treatment data and their implication for the staging model and early intervention, Bipolar Disord 2011;**13**(1):87–98.

19. **Kessing, LV, E Vradi, and PK Andersen**. Starting lithium prophylaxis early v late in bipolar disorder, Br J Psychiatry 2014;**205**(3):214–20.

20. **Macneil, CA** et al. Psychological needs of adolescents in the early phase of bipolar disorder: implications for early intervention, Early Interv Psychiatry 2011;**5**(2):100–7.

21. **Kessing, LV** et al. Do young adults with bipolar disorder benefit from early intervention?, J Affect Disord 2014;152–4:403–8.

22. **Baldessarini, RJ** et al. Effects of treatment latency on response to maintenance treatment in manic-depressive disorders, Bipolar Disord 2007;**9**(4):386–93.

23. **Fabbri, C and A Serretti**. Genetics of long-term treatment outcome in bipolar disorder, Prog Neuropsychopharmacol Biol Psychiatry 2015;**65**:17–24.

24. **Chen, G** et al. The mood-stabilizing agent valproate inhibits the activity of glycogen synthase kinase-3, J Neurochem 1999;**72**(3):1327–30.

25. **Manji, HK, GJ Moore, and G Chen**. Bipolar disorder: leads from the molecular and cellular mechanisms of action of mood stabilisers, Br J Psychiatry 2001;**178**(Suppl 41):S107–19.

26. **Bai, O, H Zhang, and XM Li**. Antipsychotic drugs clozapine and olanzapine upregulate bcl-2 mRNA and protein in rat frontal cortex and hippocampus, Brain Res 2004;**1010**(1–2):81–6.

27. **Gould, TD and HK Manji**. Glycogen synthase kinase-3: a putative molecular target for lithium mimetic drugs, *Neuropsychopharmacology* 2005;**30**(7):1223–37.

28. **Klein, PS and DA Melton**. A molecular mechanism for the effect of lithium on development, Proc Natl Acad Sci USA 1996;**93**(16):8455–9.

29. **Malhi, GS** et al. Magnetic resonance spectroscopy and its applications in psychiatry, Aust NZJ Psychiatry 2002;**36**(1):31–43.

30. **Moore, GJ** et al. Lithium-induced increase in human brain grey matter, Lancet 2000;**356**(9237):1241–2.

31. **Ng, F** et al. Oxidative stress in psychiatric disorders: evidence base and therapeutic implications, Int J Neuropsychopharmacol 2008;**11**(6):851–76.

32. **Bai, O** et al. Expression of brain-derived neurotrophic factor mRNA in rat hippocampus after treatment with antipsychotic drugs, J Neurosci Res 2003;**71**(1):127–31.

33. **Conus, P** et al. Symptomatic and functional outcome 12 months after a first episode of psychotic mania: barriers to recovery in a catchment area sample, Bipolar Disord 2006;**8**(3):221–31.

34. **Tohen, M** et al. Two-year syndromal and functional recovery in 219 cases of first-episode major affective disorder with psychotic features, Am J Psychiatry 2000;**157**(2):220–8.

35. **Conus, P** and **PD McGorry**. First-episode mania: a neglected priority for early intervention, Aust NZJ Psychiatry, 2002;**36**(2):158–72.

36. **Leclerc, E, RB Mansur**, and **E Brietzke**. Determinants of adherence to treatment in bipolar disorder: a comprehensive review, J Affect Disord 2013;**149**(1–3):247–52.

37. **Theodoridou, A** et al. Early recognition of high risk of bipolar disorder and psychosis: an overview of the ZInEP 'Early Recognition' Study, *Front Public Health* 2014;**2**:166.

38. **Bond, K** and **IM Anderson**. Psychoeducation for relapse prevention in bipolar disorder: a systematic review of efficacy in randomized controlled trials, Bipolar Disord 2015;**17**(4):349–362.

39. **Lauder, S** et al. A randomized head to head trial of MoodSwings.net.au: an Internet based self-help program for bipolar disorder, J Affect Disord 2015;**171**:13–21.

40. **Schulze, TG** et al. Further evidence for age of onset being an indicator for severity in bipolar disorder, J Affect Disord 2002;**68**(2–3):343–5.

41. **Berk, M** et al. Early intervention in bipolar disorders: opportunities and pitfalls, Med J Aust 2007;**187**(7 Suppl):S11–14.

42. **Mesman, E** et al. The Dutch bipolar offspring study: 12-year follow-up, Am J Psychiatry 2013;**170**(5):542–9.

43. **Perugi, G** et al. Polarity of the first episode, clinical characteristics, and course of manic depressive illness: a systematic retrospective investigation of 320 bipolar I patients, Compr Psychiatry 2000;**41**(1):13–18.

44. **Mitchell, PB** et al. The clinical features of bipolar depression: a comparison with matched major depressive disorder patients, J Clin Psychiatry 2001;**62**(3):212–16; quiz 217.

45. **Ruggero, CJ** et al. Borderline personality disorder and the misdiagnosis of bipolar disorder, J Psychiatr Res 2010;**44**(6):405–8.

46. **Stensland, MD, JF Schultz**, and **JR Frytak**. Diagnosis of unipolar depression following initial identification of bipolar disorder: a common and costly misdiagnosis, J Clin Psychiatry 2008;**69**(5):749–58.

47. **Phillips, ML** and **DJ Kupfer**. Bipolar disorder diagnosis: challenges and future directions, Lancet 2013;**381**(9878):1663–71.

48. **Shim, IH, YS Woo**, and **WM Bahk**. Prevalence rates and clinical implications of bipolar disorder 'with mixed features' as defined by DSM-5, J Affect Disord 2015;**173**:120–5.

49. **Frye, MA** and **IM Salloum**. Bipolar disorder and comorbid alcoholism: prevalence rate and treatment considerations, Bipolar Disord 2006;**8**(6):677–85.

50. **Gonzalez-Pinto, A** et al. Assessment of medication adherence in a cohort of patients with bipolar disorder, *Pharmacopsychiatry* 2010;**43**(7):263–70.

51. **Simon, NM** et al. Anxiety disorder comorbidity in bipolar disorder patients: data from the first 500 participants in the Systematic Treatment Enhancement Program for Bipolar Disorder (STEP-BD), Am J Psychiatry 2004;**161**(12):2222–9.

52. **Clark, SR, KO Schubert**, and **BT Baune**. Towards indicated prevention of psychosis: using probabilistic assessments of transition risk in psychosis prodrome, J Neural Transm 2015;**122**(1):155–69.

Chapter 4

Evidence-based treatment of mania

Bernardo Ng and Mauricio Tohen

Introduction

The pharmaceutical agents with antimanic properties have a variety of pharmacologic properties. In the last two decades the most important progress has been the introduction of atypical antipsychotics as monotherapy and/or combination therapy with lithium or valproate.

This chapter will review the evidence of Food and Drug Administration (FDA)-approved agents, and key aspects of the most recent treatment guidelines of different organizations such as the British Association for Psychopharmacology (BAP), the International Society for Bipolar Disorders (ISBD), the Canadian Network for Mood and Anxiety Treatments (CANMAT), and the National Institute for Health and Care Excellence (NICE)(see Table 4.1).[1,2,3]

Antimanic agents

This chapter includes the review of lithium, antiepileptic drugs, antipsychotics (ie typical and atypical), and a segment of their use during pregnancy and lactation.

Lithium

The first report of its use in mania was in 1949. Lithium was widely used in the United States (US) towards the second half of the 1960s for acute mania and maintenance. In the last decade it has also been studied for its neuroprotective effects with the proposal that it may promote the growth of the hypocampal cortex in patients with chronic bipolar disorder.[4,5]

There is evidence of efficacy of lithium for the acute management of mania since 1973. The response rate is superior to placebo and varies from 60 to 80%. It is considered less efficacious than valproate in rapid cyclers and in patients with dysphoria. The full therapeutic action of lithium can take 1–4 weeks, which may become critical in cases of manic patients with limited compliance and/or judgement, where there is a risk of harm to self or others. This is the reason for the frequent combination with benzodiazepines and/or antipsychotics.[6]

The pharmacokinetic considerations include a full absorption through the gastrointestinal (GI) tract, a lack of protein binding in the bloodstream, and a renal

Table 4.1 FDA-approved drugs for mania and recommended daily dosages

Agent	mg/day
Lithium	300–1,800
Divalproex ER	750–1,500
Carbamazepina XR	200–1,600
Risperidone	1–6
Olanzapine	10–15
Olanzapina (IM)	10–15
Quetiapine	50–800
Quetiapine XR	300–800
Quetiapine (adjunct)	50–800
Aripiprazol	15
Aripiprazol (adjunct)	10–15
Aripiprazol (IM)	9.75–29.25
Ziprasidone	80–160
Asenapine	10–20

Data from Food and Drug Administration, U.S. Department of Health and Human Services.

excretion without having been metabolized. Peak plasma levels are reached within 2–4 hours, and it has a half-life of 18 hours. It is filtered by the proximal tubules, which creates a potentially serious interaction with the excretion and reabsorption of sodium. The therapeutic dose of lithium is variable and ranges from 300 to 1,800 mg/day. Because of its narrow therapeutic index, periodic serum levels have to be monitored in order to establish the right dose for the individual patient. Reported therapeutic serum levels range from 0.5 to 1.5 mEq/L; in the acute phase a range between 0.8 and 1.1 mEq/L is preferred.[7,8,9]

Short-term side effects include tremor, nausea, vomiting, abdominal pain, diarrhoea, increased white blood cells, polyuria, polydipsia, dermatitis, extrapyramidal reactions, fatigue, muscle weakness, and electrocardiograph (ECG) changes (ie T wave inversion, U waves). Long-term side effects include weight gain, hypothyroidism (5–30%), diabetes insipidus, decreased glomerular filtration rate, and hyperparathyroidism.[8,9]

Across most treatment guidelines, the main limitation in the use of lithium is its narrow therapeutic index; however, it continues to be one of the most efficacious treatments and with more published evidence.[1,3,9]

Antiepileptic drugs (AEDs)

The AEDs approved by the FDA for mania include carbamazepine and valproate. Gabapentin and topiramate, which are also used to treat acute mania, have none to very limited evidence and are not approved by the FDA.

Carbamazepine

Originally indicated for epilepsy, carbamazepine has published evidence of its efficacy since 1978. Most of the evidence supports that it has an efficacy superior to placebo, and similar to lithium.

It is quickly absorbed from the GI tract and reaches peak plasma concentration within 4–6 hours, and 75–90% binds to serum proteins. It has a half-life of 13–17 hours and gets metabolized through the P450 CYP3A4 hepatic system. A peculiar property of carbamazepine is its ability to enhance the CYP1A2, CYP2C9, and CYP3A4 enzymatic systems, which in turn causes an induction of its own metabolism, frequently requiring a dose adjustment within two months of starting it. Consequently, an adjustment of concomitant medications that share these enzymatic pathways is needed as well.[9,10]

Due to such property, the serum levels of oral contraceptives, warfarin, theophylline, doxycycline, haloperidol, tricyclic antidepressants, valproate, and other agents are reduced when used concomitantly with carbamazepine. Whereas the concomitant use of drugs that inhibit the P450 system such as fluoxetine, cimetidine, erythromycin, isoniazid, calcium channel blockers, and propoxyphene increase the levels of carbamazepine. Finally, drugs such as phenobarbital, phenytoin, and primidone decrease the levels of carbamazepine.[9,10]

Short-term side effects include lethargy, sedation, nausea, tremor, ataxia, and nystagmus; of concern is the possibility of leukopenia and/or thrombocytopenia which is usually transient but in a few cases can evolve to agranulocitosis or aplastic anaemia. The latter occurs in 2 to 5/100,000 cases, and 80% of them occur within the first three months of treatment; it is therefore recommended that carbamazepine be stopped with a white blood count equal or lower than 3,000 wbc/mm^3. Other side effects, rather infrequent, are hyponatremia due to inappropriate secretion of antidiuretic hormone (SIADH), heart conduction defects (ie atrio-ventricular arrhythmia), hepatitis, hypothyroidism, and serious dermatological reactions such as Stevens-Johnson syndrome.[10,11]

Carbamazepine has a greater potential of side effects and toxicity than the rest of the antimanic agents. Therefore, frequent clinical and laboratory monitoring is required, including periodic serum levels, blood cell counts, and liver and thyroid function tests. Serum levels are more useful to monitor for toxicity, since there does not seem to be a correlation between serum concentration and clinical response. These tests must be done every 4–8 weeks during the first few months of treatment, and then repeated yearly. According to treatment guidelines it is second-line treatment as monotherapy and a third-line agent in combination therapy with lithium and valproate.[8,10,11,12]

Valproate

Valproate is FDA-approved for the treatment of manic episodes related to bipolar disorder. The first published placebo-controlled study was a comparison to lithium, in 179 manic patients. Both valproate and lithium separated from placebo with similar efficacy (p=0.004, p=0.025), and a high rate of early termination in all groups especially with those receiving placebo was reported. Subsequent studies in the following decade increasingly demonstrated benefit in patients who were rapid cyclers and mania relapse prevention.[13,14]

It is available in solution, tablets, capsules, and enteric-coated caplets. One of the most common preparations is sodium divalproate, a 1:1 combination of sodium valproate and valproic acid. Its absorption varies depending on the preparation and presentation and if taken with or without meals. Peak plasma levels are reached within 2–4 hours, with a half-life of 6–16 hours, with 90% binding to serum proteins. Depending on the preparation and patient's tolerability it can be prescribed once or twice a day, as bioavailability permits it. Therapeutic plasma levels range from 45 to 125 mg/mL, and there seems to be a direct linear correlation with clinical response. It is metabolized by the cytochrome P450, and it does not induce its own metabolism. Combination with carbamazepine reduces the serum levels of divalproate, and combination with some selective serotonin reuptake inhibitors (SSRIs) increases its serum concentration.[13,14]

The most common side effects include nausea and gastritis, which is frequent and is less likely to appear with the enteric-coated preparations. There is a potential risk of serious hepatic failure, within the first six months of treatment, that has been reported to be more likely in patients two years old or younger and those with pre-existing hepatic pathology. The presence of the latter is therefore a contraindication to the use of divalproate. A more common and non-serious condition is the transient elevation of liver enzymes in serum, which can be present in up to 44% of cases. However, any symptoms associated to enzymatic abnormalities such as malaise, weakness, lethargy, oedema, anorexia, or vomiting should alert the clinician and discontinue the medication if needed. Less frequent side effects, include weight gain, hair loss, decreased platelet aggregation, and serious dermatologic reactions such as Steven-Johnson Syndrome.[12]

According to treatment guidelines it is a first-line agent for the treatment of mania, and it can be safely combined with antipsychotic agents, enhancing its efficacy.[8,9]

Antipsychotics

The evolution of antipsychotics in the treatment of bipolar disorder is one of the most interesting in psychopharmacology. Antipsychotics were widely utilized prior to the availability of lithium. Once approved, lithium became the first choice agent for patients with mania and bipolar disorder in general. During the ensuing decades, the use of antipsychotics further declined as greater risk to develop tardive dyskinesia (TD) was detected in patients with bipolar disorder compared with patients with schizophrenia. Their use was limited to patients with psychotic mania, until the arrival of atypical antipsychotics that evolved up the current use for mania, bipolar depression, and maintenance. Several antipsychotics have now been approved for monotherapy and some of them also for combination therapy in acute mania.[6,15,16,17,18]

Typical antipsychotics

It is worth mentioning that even though these agents are no longer first line for patients with mania, both haloperidol and chlorpromazine enjoyed wide acceptance and their efficacy was established to be comparable to lithium. A major concern was the risk of TD, at the time detected to be more frequent in patients with mood disorders and those with intermittent rather than continuous use.[15,16,17,18,19,20]

Atypical antipsychotics

One of the most interesting outcomes in the last two decades is the development of clinical evidence supporting the use of antipsychotic in the control of mania with or without psychosis, which eventually led researchers to study them in relapse prevention to either pole, and bipolar depression.

Their use has become very popular, they are easy to start, various presentations are available, dosing is flexible, and efficacy has been proven. Regarding safety issues, the risk of TD is lower than with typical antipsychotics, their therapeutic index is wider than lithium, and the teratogenic risks are considerably lower than those with divalproate and carbamazepine. The greatest safety risk resides in its non-acute use where all atypical antipsychotics are associated to a greater or lesser extent with the development of the Metabolic Syndrome (MetS).[21,22]

A meta-analysis of MetS risk factors identified that severe mental illness (ie schizophrenia, bipolar disorder, major depressive disorder) was a risk factor in itself when compared with the general population (RR=1.58, p=0.003). Even though MetS was detected with all antipsychotics, a greater incidence was found in those receiving clozapine and olanzapine, and a lower incidence in those receiving aripiprazole and amilsupride (p<0.001). The data were also analysed by geographical location, and the highest prevalence of MetS was in Australia (50.2%), the lowest was in Brazil (25.8%), and the median was in the US and Europe (32%). The latter suggests environmental factors related to the geographical location in the development of MetS, as supported by a body mass index (BMI) study in Mexico and Colombia of patients receiving antipsychotics, finding that the further south the lower the BMI (30.0 vs 25.5; p<0.01).[22,23]

The first atypical antipsychotic approved for mania was olanzapine in 2000, since then it has been studied in different placebo-controlled trials, in manic patients with and without psychosis, and in maintenance studies. It was first studied in monotherapy with lithium and divalproate as active comparators. Later it was studied as an add-on agent to lithium and valproate. It has also been studied for acute mania in its intramuscular (IM) formulation, compared to lorazepam and haloperidol. Its efficacy in relapse prevention is comparable to lithium and valproate, including patients who are rapid cyclers.[24,25,26,27,28,29,30,31,32,33]

Risperidone was approved in 2003 for acute mania—its efficacy in monotherapy is established against placebo, lithium, haloperidol, divalproate, and olanzapine. It was also tested and demonstrated efficacy as an add-on agent to established mood stabilizer. In its long-term IM-injectable formulation it is the only FDA-approved agent for maintenance. However, long-term injectable agents have been widely used in patients with bipolar disorder and a recent consensus suggests that these agents can aid to a successful outcome in patients with multiple episodes, poor adherence, persistent residual symptoms, multiple medications, and those that prefer IM rather than oral medication.[34,35,36,37,38,39,40,41]

In 2004, quetiapine was approved for acute mania and maintenance as monotherapy and combination therapy with lithium and divalproate; it consistently showed superiority to placebo.[42,43,44,45,46,47] Subsequently, ziprasidone and aripiprazole were FDA-approved in 2004 for bipolar mania.[15] A meta-analysis compared these five antipsychotics and was unable to detect that either one had significantly greater efficacy.[48] Differences in safety and tolerability have been reported with olanzapine and quetiapine having a higher risk of metabolic syndrome. Finally, asenapine was approved, in 2009, for acute mania.[49] In 2014, the FDA approved lurasidone for bipolar depression in monotherapy and combination with lithium or valproate in 2014 but it has not been approved for the treatment of mania.[50]

Fertility, pregnancy, and lactation

This section is included as bipolar disorder affects fertile women and it is the clinician's responsibility to maintain the balance between symptom control and safety to the patient and the fetus. Do not forget that whenever possible the father of the baby and/or patient's significant other should be included in all treatment plan discussions. Especially because many of the pregnancies occur unplanned in patients with bipolar disorder, non-medication measures such as electroconvulsive therapy (ECT) must be considered in this population.[1]

In regards to fertility, divalproate can reduce fertility due to its association to polycystic ovarian syndrome (POS), which is reversible upon its discontinuation. Antipsychotics can cause hiperprolactinaemia to a greater or a lesser degree (ie aripiprazole is a prolactin-sparing antipsychotic), which in turn reduces fertility. On the other hand, due to carbamazepine's ability to reduce serum levels of contraceptives, it can also affect woman's fertility.[51]

As to the use of medications during pregnancy, one must first keep in mind that the spontaneous risk of congenital malformations is 2–4%, and it is positively correlated with the mother's age. It is therefore important that the physician discusses this relevant topic with all female patients during their fertile age. The discussion must take place before the patient becomes pregnant and, furthermore, before she plans on getting pregnant, since the period of greatest risk is during the first trimester of pregnancy. By the same token, patients must be educated about the fact that pregnancy in itself represents a period of high relapse risk regardless of compliance with treatment, which increases if the decision is made to interrupt pharmacological treatment. In general, the risk of medication-induced congenital malformations must be compared to the risk of spontaneous malformations before making a decision about the use of pharmacological agents during pregnancy.[51,52]

Lithium has been traditionally associated to the cardiac malformation known as Epstein's anomaly; systematized studies have established, however, that its incidence is lower than previously suspected (3–12%) such that its use during pregnancy is debatable. Some authors strongly recommend keeping the pregnant patient on lithium with a very close monitoring in conjunction with the obstetrician. On the other hand, both carbamazepine and divalproate have been associated with fetal anomalies of the neural tube, including spina bifida, microcephaly, and also low birth weight; so they are both contraindicated during pregnancy. Finally, there is limited evidence available on the safety of antipsychotics in this population.[52,53,54,55]

The discussion about lactation should be started as soon as the patient realizes that she is pregnant, and it starts with educating the pregnant patient and her significant other about the risks of breastfeeding while taking medication. The first point is that all the medications as previously discussed get excreted through breast milk, yet the relationship between serum concentration and breast milk concentration is rather variable. The risk of lithium toxicity, hepatic failure from divalproate, leukopenia from carbamazepine and clozapine, and extrapyramidal symptoms from antipsychotics should all be considered and carefully monitored if the patient insists on breastfeeding her infant.[1,9,55,56]

Conclusions

In this chapter we have reviewed the published evidence on FDA-approved antimanic pharmacologic agents. It is outstanding that lithium continues to be a first-line treatment option for acute and maintenance treatment. Divalproate also continues to be a first-line agent for mania, in both monotherapy and combination therapy. Typical

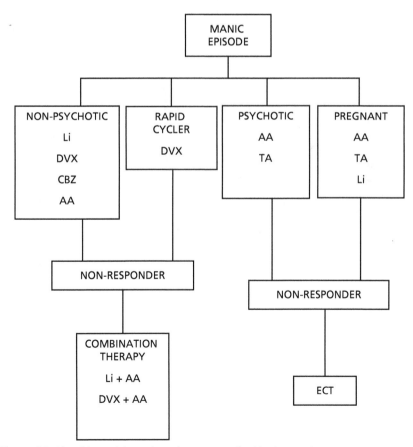

Figure 4.1 Algorithm evidence-based treatments for bipolar mania

Table 4.2 Summary of FDA-approved agents for mania

Family	Agent	Fda label	Short-term side effects	Long-term side effects	Fertility	Pregnancy	Lactation
LITHIUM	lithium	MONOTHERAPY	Nausea, tremor, diarrhoea	Weight gain, hypothyroidism, diabetes insipidus, hypoparathyroidism	No impact	Relative contraindication	All agents are secreted in breast milk
AED	carbamazepine	MONOTHERAPY	Leukopenia, ataxia, sedation	Agranulocytosis, liver failure, Steven-Johnson's syndrome	Decreases effect of oral contraceptives	Absolute contraindication	
	divalproex		Gastritis, tremor		May decrease fertility due to POS		
TA	haloperidol	MONOTHERAPY	Parkinsonism, sedation	Tardive dyskinesia	May decrease fertility due to hyperprolactinaemia	Relative contraindication	
	chlorpromazine						
AA	olanzapine	MONOTHERAPY ADD-ON THERAPY	Sedation, tremor, parkinsonism	Metabolic syndrome tardive dyskinesia	Impact to varying degrees, depending on ability to spare prolactin or not	Limited data, may be safer than lithium and AED	
	risperidone						
	quetiapine						
	ziprasidone						
	aripiprazole						
	asenapine						
	lurasidone						

Data from Food and Drug Administration, U.S. Department of Health and Human Services.

antipsychotics also continue to be used in cases of severe agitation and/or psychosis. Atypical antipsychotics have widened their use to include mania and bipolar depression as well as maintenance treatment (see Figure 4.1).[1,3,9,56]

Regarding safety issues, lithium's main obstacle is its reduced therapeutic index requiring periodic blood tests. Valproate safety risks include weight gain and polycystic ovaries. They are both contraindicated during pregnancy. Typical antipsychotics represent a risk for TD, which appears to be lower with atypical antipsychotics. The main risk with the latter as a group is the risk of MetS, hyperglycaemia, and alterations of the lipid metabolism, especially with clozapine, olanzapine, and quetiapine (see Table 4.2).[1,3,9,56]

Bipolar disorder continues to be a complex psychiatric condition, yet the progress in treatment options for the manic phase has evolved such that we have more options than ever before, allowing the well-informed and sensitive physician to offer precise and appropriate clinical solutions to these patients.

Disclosures

Dr Ng has received honoraria from or consulted for Otsuka, Lundbeck, Takeda, Lilly, GlaxoSmithKline, and AstraZeneca.

Dr Tohen was a full-time employee at Lilly (1997–2008). He has received honoraria from or consulted for Abbott, AstraZeneca, Bristol Myers Squibb, GlaxoSmithKline, Lilly, Johnson & Johnson, Allergan, Otsuka, Merck, Sunovion, Forest, Geodon Richter Plc, Roche, Elan, Alkermes, Lundbeck, Teva, Pamlab, Minerva, Wyeth, and Wiley Publishing.

His spouse was a full-time employee at Lilly (1998–2013).

References

1. **Goodwin GM.** Consensus group of the British Association for Psychopharmacology. Evidence based guidelines for treating bipolar disorder: revised second edition— recommendations from the British Association for Psychopharmacology, J of Psychopharm 2009;**23**(4):346–88.

2. **Young LT, Milev R, Bond DJ, Frey BN, Goldstein BI, Lafer B, Birmaher B, Ha K, Nolen WA,** and **Berk M.** Canadian Network for Mood and Anxiety Treatments (CANMAT) and International Society for Bipolar Disorders (ISBD) collaborative update of CANMAT guidelines for the management of patients with bipolar disorder: update 2013, Bipolar Disord 2013;**15**:1–44.

3. NICE. National Institute for Health and Care Excellence. Bipolar disorder: the assessment and management of bipolar disorder in adults, children, and young people in primary and secondary care. 2014, http://www.guidance.nice.org.uk/cg185.

4. **Cade JFJ:** Lithium salts in the treatment of psychotic excitement, *Medical Journal of Australia* 1949;**2**:349–52.

5. **Giakoumatos CI, Nanda P, Mathew IT, Tandon N, Shah J, Bishop JR, Clementz BA, Pearlson GD, Sweeney JA, Tamminga CA,** and **Keshavan MS.** Effects of lithium on cortical thickness and hippocampal subfield volumes in psychotic bipolar disorder, J Psychiatr Res 2015;**61**:180–7.

6. **Prien RF, Caffey EM, and Klett CJ.** Comparison of lithium carbonate and chlorpromazine in the treatment of mania, Arch Gen Psychiatry 1973;**26**:146–53.

7. **Gelenberg AJ, Kane JM, Keller MB, Lavori P, Rosenbaum JF, Cole K, and Lavelle J.** Comparison of standard and low serum levels of lithium for maintenance treatment of bipolar disorder, N Eng J Med 1989;**321**:1489–93.

8. **Murru A, Popovic D, Pacchiarotti I, Hidalgo D, León-Caballero J, and Vieta E.** Management of adverse effects of mood stabilizers, Curr Psychiatry Rep 2015;**17**(8):603.

9. **Yatham LN, Kennedy SH, Parikh SV, Schaffer A, Beaulieu S, Alda M, O'Donovan C, MacQueen G, McIntyre RS, Sharma V, Ravindran A, Young LT, Milev R, Bond DJ, Frey BN, Goldstein BI, Lafer B, Birmaher B, Ha K, Nolen WA, and Berk M.** Canadian Network for Mood and Anxiety Treatments (CANMAT) and International Society for Bipolar Disorders (ISBD) collaborative update of CANMAT guidelines for the management of patients with bipolar disorder: update 2013, Bipolar Disord 2013;**15**:1–44.

10. **Pichler EM, Hattwich G, Grunze H, and Muehlbacher M.** Safety and tolerability of anticonvulsant medication in bipolar disorder, Expert Opin Drug Saf 2015;**14**(11):1703–24.

11. **Miura T, Noma H, Furukawa TA, Mitsuyasu H, Tanaka S, Stockton S, Salanti G, Motomura K, Shimano-Katsuki S, Leucht S, Cipriani A, Geddes JR, and Kanba S.** Comparative efficacy and tolerability of pharmacological treatments in the maintenance treatment of bipolar disorder: a systematic review and network meta-analysis, *Lancet Psychiatry* 2014;**1**(5):351–9.

12. **Yatham LN, Kusumakar V, Calabrese JR, Rao R, Scarrow G, and Kroeker G.** Third generation anticonvulsants in bipolar disorder: A review of efficacy and summary of clinical recommendations, J Clin Psychiatry 2002;**63**:275–83.

13. **Bowden CL, Brugger AM, Swann AC, Calabrese JR, Janicak PG, Petty F, Dilsaver SC, Davis JM, Rush AJ, Small JG**, et al. Efficacy of divalproex vs lithium and placebo in the treatment of mania. The Depakote Mania Study Group, JAMA 1994;23–30;**271**(12):918–24.

14. **Harrison G Pope Jr**, MD, **Susan L McElroy, E Keck Jr**, MD, and **James I Hudson,** MD. Valproate treatment of acute mania. A placebo-controlled, Arch Gen Psychiatry 1991;**48**(1):62–8.

15. **Gajwani P, Kemp DE, Muzina DJ, Xia G, Gao K, and Calabrese JR.** Acute treatment of mania: an update on new medications, Curr Psychiatry Rep 2006;**8**(6):504–9.

16. **Baastrup PC, Hollnagel P, Sorensen R, and Schou M.** Adverse reactions in treatment with lithium carbonate and haloperidol, JAMA 1976;**236**(23):2645–6.

17. **Tohen M and Zarate CA Jr.** Antipsychotic agents and bipolar disorder. J Clin Psychiatry 1998;**59**(Suppl1):38–48.

18. **Tohen M and Vieta E.** Antipsychotic agents in the treatment of bipolar mania, Bipolar Disord 2009;**11**(Suppl 2):45–54.

19. **Goodwin FK and Zis AP.** Lithium in the treatment of mania: comparisons with neuroleptics, Arch Gen Psychiatry 1979;**20**;36(suppl):840–4.

20. **Shopsin B, Gershon S, Thompson H, and Collins P.** Psychoactive drugs in mania. A controlled comparison of lithium carbonate, chlorpromazine, and haloperidol, Arch Gen Psychiatry 1975;**32**(1):34–42.

21. **Tohen M, Bowden CL, Smulevich AB, Bergstrom R, Quinlan T, Osuntokun O, Wang WV, Oliff HS, Martenyi F, Kryzhanovskaya LA, and Greil W.** Olanzapine plus

carbamazepine v carbamazepine alone in treating manic episodes, Br J Psychiatry 2008;**192**(2):135–43.

22. **Vancampfort D, Stubbs B, Mitchell AJ, De Hert M, Wampers M, Ward PB, Rosenbaum S, and Correll CU.** Risk of metabolic syndrome and its components in people with schizophrenia and related psychotic disorders, bipolar disorder and major depressive disorder: a systematic review and meta-analysis, *World Psychiatry* 2015;**14**(3):339–47.

23. **Ng B, Camacho A, Parra K, DelaEspriella R, Rico V, Villagomez RI, Lozano S, Trancoso M, Castilla-Puentes RC, Cook BL, and Jimenez DE.** Differences in BMI between Mexico and Colombia among patients receiving new generation antipsychotics. Results from the International Study of Latinos on Antipsychotics (ILA). Submitted to publication.

24. **Tohen M, Sanger TM, McElroy SL, Tollefson GD, Chengappa KN, Daniel DG, Petty F, Centorrino F, Wang R, Grundy SL, Greaney MG, Jacobs TG, David SR, and Toma V.** Olanzapine versus placebo in the treatment of acute mania. Olanzapine HGEH Study Group, Am J Psychiatry 1999;**156**(5):702–9.

25. **Tohen M, Chengappa KN, Suppes T, Zarate CA Jr, Calabrese JR, Bowden CL, Sachs GS, Kupfer DJ, Baker RW, Risser RC, Keeter EL, Feldman PD, Tollefson GD, and Breier A.** Efficacy of olanzapine in combination with valproate or lithium in the treatment of mania in patients partially nonresponsive to valproate or lithium monotherapy, Arch Gen Psychiatry 2002a;**59**(1):62–9.

26. **Tohen M, Baker RW, Altshuler LL, Zarate CA, Suppes T, Ketter TA, Milton DR, Risser R, Gilmore JA, Breier A, and Tollefson GA.** Olanzapine versus divalproex in the treatment of acute mania, Am J Psychiatry 2002b;**159**(6):1011–17.

27. **Tohen M, Goldberg JF, Gonzalez-Pinto Arrillaga AM, Azorin JM, Vieta E, Hardy-Bayle MC, Lawson WB, Emsley RA, Zhang F, Baker RW, Risser RC, Namjoshi MA, Evans AR, and Breier A.** A 12-week, double-blind comparison of olanzapine vs haloperidol in the treatment of acute mania, Arch Gen Psychiatry 2003a;**60**(12):1218–26.

28. **Tohen M, Chengappa KN, Suppes T, Baker RW, Zarate CA, Bowden CL, Sachs GS, Kupfer DJ, Ghaemi SN, Feldman PD, Risser RC, Evans AR, and Calabrese JR.** Relapse prevention in bipolar I disorder: 18-month comparison of olanzapine plus mood stabiliser v mood stabiliser alone, Br J Psychiatry 2004;**184**:337–45.

29. **Tohen M, Greil W, Calabrese JR, Sachs GS, Yatham LN, Oerlinghausen BM, Koukopoulos A, Cassano GB, Grunze H, Licht RW, Dell'Osso L, Evans AR, Risser R, Baker RW, Crane H, Dossenbach MR, and Bowden CL.** Olanzapine versus lithium in the maintenance treatment of bipolar disorder: a 12-month, randomized, double-blind, controlled clinical trial, Am J Psychiatry 2005;**162**(7):1281–90.

30. **Tohen M, Vieta E, Goodwin GM, Sun B, Amsterdam JD, Banov M, Shekhar A, Aaronson ST, Bardenstein L, Grecu-Gabos I, Tochilov V, Prelipceanu D, Oliff HS, Kryzhanovskaya L, and Bowden C.** Olanzapine versus divalproex versus placebo in the treatment of mild to moderate mania: a randomized, 12-week, double-blind study, J Clin Psychiatry 2008a;**69**(11):1776–89.

31. **Tohen M, Bowden CL, Smulevich AB, Bergstrom R, Quinlan T, Osuntokun O, Wang WV, Oliff HS, Martenyi F, Kryzhanovskaya LA, and Greil W.** Olanzapine plus carbamazepine v carbamazepine alone in treating manic episodes, Br J Psychiatry 2008b;**192**(2):135–43.

32. **Tohen M, Sutton VK, Calabrese JR, Sachs GS, and Bowden CL.** Maintenance of response following stabilization of mixed index episodes with olanzapine monotherapy

in a randomized, double-blind, placebo-controlled study of bipolar 1 disorder, J Affect Disord 2009;**116**(1–2):43–50.

33. **Meehan K, Zhang F, David S, Tohen M, Janicak P, Small J, Koch M, Rizk R, Walker D, Tran P, and Breier A.** A double-blind, randomized comparison of the efficacy and safety of intramuscular injections of olanzapine, lorazepam, or placebo in treating acutely agitated patients diagnosed with bipolar mania. J Clin Psychopharmacol 2001;**21**(4):389–97.

34. **Sachs GS, Grossman F, Ghaemi SN, Okamoto A, and Bowden CL.** Combination of a mood stabilizer with risperidone or haloperidol for treatment of acute mania: a double-blind, placebo-controlled comparison of efficacy and safety, Am J Psychiatry 2002;**159**(7):1146–54.

35. **Yatham LN, Grossman F, Augustyns I, Vieta E, and Ravindran A.** Mood stabilisers plus risperidone or placebo in the treatment of acute mania. International, double-blind, randomised controlled trial, Br J Psychiatry 2003;**182**:141–7.

36. **Hirschfeld RM, Keck PE Jr, Kramer M, Karcher K, Canuso C, Eerdekens M, and Grossman F.** Rapid antimanic effect of risperidone monotherapy: a 3-week multicenter, double-blind, placebo-controlled trial, Am J Psychiatry 2004;**161**(6):1057–65.

37. **Smulevich AB, Khanna S, Eerdekens M, Karcher K, Kramer M, and Grossman F.** Acute and continuation risperidone monotherapy in bipolar mania: a 3-week placebo-controlled trial followed by a 9-week double-blind trial of risperidone and haloperidol, Eur Neuropsychopharmacol 2005;**15**(1):75–84.

38. **Han C, Lee MS, Pae CU, Ko YH, Patkar AA, and Jung IK.** Usefulness of long-acting injectable risperidone during 12-month maintenance therapy of bipolar disorder. Prog Neuropsychopharmacol Biol Psychiatry 2007;**15**;**31**(6):1219–23.

39. **Bobo WV and Shelton RC.** Risperidone long-acting injectable (Risperdal Consta®) for maintenance treatment in patients with bipolar disorder, Expert Rev Neurother 2010;**10**(11):1637–58.

40. **Chou YH, Chu PC, Wu SW, Lee JC, Lee YH, Sun IW, Chang CL, Huang CL, Liu IC, Tsai CF, and Yen YC.** A systemic review and experts' consensus for long-acting injectable antipsychotics in bipolar disorder. Clin Psychopharmacol Neurosci 2015;**31**;**13**(2):121–8.

41. **Camacho A, Ng B, Galangue B, and Feifel D.** Use of risperidone long-acting injectable in a rural border community clinic in southern California. *Psychiatry* (Edgmont) 2008;**5**(6):43–9.

42. **Bowden CL, Grunze H, Mullen J, Brecher M, Paulsson B, Jones M, Vågerö M, and Svensson K.** A randomized, double-blind, placebo-controlled efficacy and safety study of quetiapine or lithium as monotherapy for mania in bipolar disorder, J Clin Psychiatry 2005;**66**(1):111–21.

43. **Vieta E, Mullen J, Brecher M, Paulsson B, and Jones M.** Quetiapine monotherapy for mania associated with bipolar disorder: combined analysis of two international, double-blind, randomised, placebo-controlled studies. Curr Med Res Opin 2005;**21**(6):923–34.

44. **Ketter TA, Jones M, and Paulsson B.** Rates of remission/euthymia with quetiapine monotherapy compared with placebo in patients with acute mania, J Affect Disord 2007;**100**(Suppl 1):S45–53.

45. **Young AH, McElroy SL, Bauer M, Philips N, Chang W, Olausson B, Paulsson B, Brecher M; and EMBOLDEN I (Trial 001) Investigators.** A double-blind, placebo-controlled study of quetiapine and lithium monotherapy in adults in the acute phase of bipolar depression (EMBOLDEN I), J Clin Psychiatry 2010;**71**(2):150–62.

46. Vieta E, Suppes T, Eggens I, Persson I, Paulsson B, and Brecher M. Efficacy and safety of quetiapine in combination with lithium or divalproex for maintenance of patients with bipolar I disorder (international trial 126), J Affect Disord 2008;109(3):251–63.

47. Vieta E, Suppes T, Ekholm B, Udd M, and Gustafsson U. Long-term efficacy of quetiapine in combination with lithium or divalproex on mixed symptoms in bipolar I disorder, J Affect Disord 2012;15;142(1–3):36–44.

48. Perlis RH, Welge JA, Vornik LA, Hirschfeld RM, and Keck PE Jr. Atypical antipsychotics in the treatment of mania: a meta-analysis of randomized, placebo-controlled trials, J Clin Psychiatry 2006;67(4):509–16.

49. McIntyre RS, Cohen M, Zhao J, Alphs L, Macek TA, and Panagides J. Asenapine in the treatment of acute mania in bipolar I disorder: a randomized, double-blind, placebo-controlled trial, J Affect Disord 2010;122(1–2):27–38.

50. Loebel A, Cucchiaro J, Silva R, Kroger H, Sarma K, Xu J, and Calabrese JR. Lurasidone as adjunctive therapy with lithium or valproate for the treatment of bipolar I depression: a randomized, double-blind, placebo-controlled study, Am J Psychiatry 2014;171(2):169–77.

51. Grunze H, Vieta E, Goodwin GM, Bowden C, Licht RW, Möller HJ, Kasper S; and WFSBP Task Force on Treatment Guidelines for Bipolar Disorders. The World Federation of Societies of Biological Psychiatry (WFSBP) guidelines for the biological treatment of bipolar disorders: update 2012 on the long-term treatment of bipolar disorder, World J Biol Psychiatry 2013 Apr;14(3):154–219.

52. Jacobson SJ, Jones K, Johnson K, Ceolin L, Kaur P, Sahn D, et al. Prospective multicentre study of pregnancy outcome after lithium exposure during first trimester, Lancet 1992;339(8792):530–3.

53. Källen B and Tandberg A. Lithium and pregnancy—a cohort study on manic-depressive women, Acta Psychiatrica Scandinavica 1983;8(2):134–9.

54. Reis M and Kallen B. Maternal use of antipsychotics in early pregnancy and delivery outcome, J Clin Psychopharmacol 2008;28:279–88.

55. Austin MP and Mitchell PB. Use of psychotropic medications in breast-feeding women: acute and prophylactic treatment, Aust NZJ Psychiatry 1998;32:778–84.

56. Jong-Hyun J, Jeong GL, Moon-Doo K, Inki S, Se-Hoon S, Hee RW, Young SW, Duk-In J, Jeong SS, Young-Chul S, Kyung JM, Bo-Hyun Y, and Won-Myong B. Korean Medication Algorithm for Bipolar Disorder 2014: comparisons with other treatment guidelines, Neuropsychiatric Disease and Treatment 2015;11:1561–71.

Chapter 5

The treatment of bipolar mixed states

Sarah Kittel-Schneider

Introduction

Mixed affective states in bipolar disorder (BD) are defined by co-occurrence of manic and depressive symptoms and have also been described as dysphoric mania or depressive mania. Kraepelin was the first one to depict the concept of mixed episodes.[1] Mixed episodes as described in the *Diagnostic and Statistical Manual of Mental Disorders* (4th edition) (DSM-4) text revision (TR) can only be classified in bipolar patients.[2] To diagnose a mixed episode by means of DSM-IV TR symptoms of as well a major depressive episode as a manic or hypomanic episode have to be present simultaneously nearly every day for at least one week. In DSM-5, there is no possibility to diagnose a mixed episode in bipolar disorder anymore. Instead, a 'mixed feature' specifier can be added to manic and hypomanic episodes in BD and to major depressive episode in BD and also to a major depressive episode in patients suffering from major depressive disorder (MDD).[3] This 'mixed features' specifier can be assigned to the patients' diagnosis when at least three depressive symptoms are present in a manic episode or at least three manic symptoms occur during a depressive episode. Patients who fulfil full episode criteria for both major depressive episode and manic episode should be diagnosed as manic episode with mixed features.[3] The prevalence of mixed states in BD patients ranges from 9 to 23% according to the definition used.[4]

Mixed affective states are difficult to treat and the incidence of mixed mania and also mixed depression is associated with a more severe and chronic course of BD as well as a higher rate of suicide (for a review see[5]). Mixed states seem to occur more often in females than males. Moreover, mixed manic episodes have been shown to be associated with increased depression during follow-up and patients suffering from mixed states display a greater risk of rapid cycling course.[5] Furthermore, a higher prevalence of physical co-morbidities is reported in patients with mixed states.[6] Bipolar patients suffering from mixed states also display increased psychiatric comorbidities such as personality disorders, borderline personality disorder (in particular), and substance abuse disorders.[5]

Treatment of mixed states is less investigated than treatment of pure manic or depressive episodes. In most studies, manic and mixed patients are analysed together and the data regarding mixed states are derived from sub-analysis or post hoc analysis of those clinical trials. National German S3 guidelines[7] as well as the Canadian Network for Mood and Anxiety Treatments (CANMAT) guidelines update[8] also do not give special recommendation regarding treatment of mixed episodes as most of the other guidelines (the British Association for Psychopharmacology (BAP), the International Society for Bipolar Disorders (ISBD), the National Institute for Health and Care Excellence (NICE), and Australian and New Zealand clinical practice guidelines for treatment of BDs).

Previous early studies suggested that patients with mixed episodes show poorer lithium response[9] and seem to respond better to valproic acid,[10] but there is no prospective randomized controlled trial to confirm those findings. Since the approval of the so-called atypical antipsychotics or second-generation antipsychotics (SGAs), the majority of the trials were investigating the efficacy of those SGAs or combination therapy with SGAs and mood stabilizers in manic and mixed bipolar patients.

There is some direct and indirect evidence that antidepressant-only treatment is rather worsening mixed-affective states.[11,12] Most guidelines and clinical advice recommend to discontinue antidepressants even as an add-on to mood-stabilizer and/or atypical antipsychotics in bipolar mixed states; however, randomized controlled trials focusing on this question are rare.[11,13]

Treatment

Psychopharmacological treatment

Second-generation antipsychotic monotherapy: acute therapy

The majority of published trials have investigated manic and mixed manic patients together. Therefore, in most studies, only improvement in manic symptoms measured by Young Mania Rating Scale (YMRS) is reported and depressive symptoms are only registered in a few trials. Treatment of mixed states with atypical antipsychotics in all studies was superior to placebo regarding improvement in YMRS. A meta-analysis from Muralidharan et al. which analysed the efficacy of SGAs in monotherapy and as an add-on to mood stabilizers concluded, despite lack of data, that atypical antipsychotic treatment leads to a greater improvement of the manic symptoms than of depressive symptoms in mixed patients.

The efficacy of atypical antipsychotics in treating depressed mixed episodes according to the DSM-5 criteria remains rather unclear due to the lack of specific clinical trials.[14] Ziprasidon, asenapine, and lurasidone might also improve depressed mixed states.[15–17]

Aripiprazole In studies investigating manic and mixed episode patients together, post hoc analysis also found significant improvement in mixed patients due to treatment with aripiprazole; however, only differences in the YMRS were assessed. Studies were conducted in comparison to placebo, lithium, and haloperidol (reviewed in[14]).

Asenapine Asenapine has showed to be effective in comparison to placebo and non-inferior to olanzapine in acute mania and mixed states (reviewed in[14]). Szegedi and colleagues also measured the effect of asenapine treatment on depressive symptoms in a post hoc analysis, which was greater compared with olanzapine.[15]

Lurasidone A post hoc analysis of patients with mixed features in bipolar depression revealed that lurasidone was effective in the treatment of patients with bipolar depression who presented with mixed features as well as in those without mixed features by measuring Montgomery-Åsberg Depression Rating Scale (MADRS) scores.[16]

Olanzapine Placebo-controlled (reviewed in[12,14]) as well as controlled-parallel studies in comparison to active substances (vs haloperidol,[18] vs risperidone,[19] vs lithium,[20] vs valproate[21]) showed evidence for an improvement in mixed episodes in post hoc analysis for the treatment with olanzapine regarding YMRS scores.

Paliperidone Efficacy of paliperidone was tested in placebo-controlled studies and in comparison to quetiapine as an active substance in manic and mixed bipolar patients. Paliperione was superior to placebo in change from baseline YMRS[22] and non-inferior to quetiapine. However, paliperidone led to a higher switch to depression compared with quetiapine after three months of treatment.[23]

Risperidone Risperidone was superior to placebo measured by YMRS scores in the treatment of manic and mixed bipolar patients.[24]

Ziprasidone One placebo-controlled study showed ziprasidone being superior to placebo in reducing manic symptoms in manic and mixed bipolar patients.[25] And there is a trial that included unipolar and bipolar II patients in a depressive mixed state that revealed superiority to placebo—the effect was more pronounced in bipolar II patients.[17]

Second-generation antipsychotic monotherapy: maintenance therapy

Trials specifically investigating if atypical antipsychotics are able to prevent reoccurrence of mixed episodes are sparse.

Clozapine Clozapine has shown to be effective in a small study with therapy-refractory bipolar patients with predominant manic and mixed episodes in maintenance therapy.[26]

Asenapine and olanzapine Asenapine and olanzapine seem to be effective in maintenance treatment; for olanzapine there are two placebo-controlled studies showing a significant reduction in time to symptomatic relapse after 48 weeks in manic and mixed patients (reviewed in[12,14]).

Mood-stabilizer monotherapy: acute therapy

There are noticeable fewer trials studying the effect of mood stabilizers than SGAs regarding treatment of mixed bipolar episodes.

Carbamazepine Carbamazepine seems to be more effective in reducing YMRS scores in manic and mixed patients than placebo. In a post hoc analysis analysing manic and mixed patients separately, Weisler et al. found hints that carbamazepine was also improving Hamilton Depression Rating Scale (HDRS) scores in mixed patients (reviewed in[11]).

Lamotrigine There is no evidence that lamotrigine is effective in treating acute mixed episodes.[27]

Valproate and lithium Most studies compared the effect of valproate versus lithium in groups of manic and mixed patients together. It has been suggested that an increasing number of previous mixed episodes negatively correlates with lithium response in bipolar patients, which is not the case for valproate.[28] Lithium, as well as valproate, significantly improved Mania Rating Scale (MRS) scores compared with placebo in manic and mixed patients.[29] Overall, valproate seems to be more effective than lithium in acute mixed episodes; however, prospective randomized controlled trials to confirm those findings are lacking (for a review see[11]).

Mood-stabilizer monotherapy: maintenance therapy

In patients who experienced a dysphoric manic episode there was no significant difference in terms of the prophylactic effect of lithium vs valproate and both were superior to placebo.[30] Randomized controlled trials investigating the prophylactic effect of mood stabilizers specifically regarding the reoccurrence of mixed episodes are non-existent.

Combination therapy: acute therapy

In general, combination therapy was consistently more effective to treat acute mixed episodes than monotherapy.

Quetiapine and valproate A recent clinical trial investigating manic and mixed patients showed that add-on lithium treatment to quetiapine enhanced the antimanic treatment effect of quetiapine significantly. The mixed patients were not analysed separately post hoc.[31] Add-on quetiapine to valproate medication led to improvement in manic and mixed patients in a previous trial also regarding depressive symptoms.[32]

Olanzapine and lithium/valproate Several studies analysed the effect of adjunctive olanzapine treatment to lithium or valproate in manic, mixed, and dysphoric manic patients. Olanzapine add-on was consistently improving YMRS scores in comparison with placebo (reviewed in[12,14]). One study could also show reduced suicidal ideation in mixed patients due to combination therapy.[33]

Ziprasidone and lithium/valproate Adjunctive ziprasidone treatment failed to separate from mood stabilizer plus placebo (lithium or valproate) treatment on primary (change in YMRS scores) and secondary end points (MADRS, Positive and Negative Syndrome Scale, Clinical Global Impressions Severity of Illness and Improvement scales, and Global Assessment of Functioning) in a trial with manic and mixed bipolar patients.[34]

Oxcarbazepin/carbamazepine and lithium As an add-on treatment to lithium, oxcarbazepine reduced depression rating scale scores more than carbamazepine in a group of partly remitted manic patients with residual symptoms on both the MADRS and on the HDRS.[35] As those patients scored on MADRS and HDRS as well as on YMRS, there were potentially patients in mixed states among them.

Lithium and valproate In a naturalistic study, lithium and valproate combination led to greater improvement in the Clinical Global Impressions–Bipolar Version Scale scores in mixed, anxiety, and psychotic symptoms than in patients receiving lithium as monotherapy.[36]

Fluoxetine and olanzapine One trial evaluated the effect of fluoxetine as adjunctive treatment to olanzapine in comparison to olanzapine monotherapy in bipolar patients. This study was a post hoc analysis of patients with mixed depression and the olanzapine/fluoxetine combination seemed to be effective treatment for bipolar I mixed depression on trend level.[37]

Risperidone/haloperidol and lithium/valproate Risperidone and haloperidol as adjunctive treatments to mood stabilizer (lithium or valproate) were both superior to placebo in reducing YMRS scores in manic or mixed patients.[38]

Combination therapy: maintenance therapy

Regarding maintenance therapy, there are two trials which evaluated the effect of combination therapy in a sample including mixed patients. Time to recurrence of any episode was the primary outcome and quetiapine as add-on treatment to lithium or valproate significantly prolonged the time until relapse/recurrence compared with placebo.[39,40]

Non-pharmacological treatment: electroconvulsive therapy (ECT)

There are only a few studies that include mixed patients but it seems that ECT could prove useful in therapy-refractory cases of bipolar mixed states. In a small study in which lithium-non-responders suffering from mixed episodes were treated with ECT, all of those patients had significant reduction in both manic and depressive symptoms.[41] Similar results could be obtained in another study with a greater number of patients including bipolar patients in depressed or mixed states who had been resistant to pharmacological treatment.[42] A very recent publication from the same group confirmed response and remission rates of approximately 40% and 30% respectively in ECT-treated mixed bipolar patients; the sample described in parts overlapping with the earlier study.[43] There are hints that mixed patients benefit as well as depressed or manic patients from ECT but require a greater number of ECT sessions.[44]

Transcranial magnetic stimulation (TMS)

Deep TMS and other forms of TMS have been investigated primarily in depressed bipolar patients. Pallanti and colleagues suggested from the results of an exploratory study investigating 40 bipolar patients in mixed states that low frequency repetitive TMS on the right dorsolateral prefrontal cortex might improve both depressive and manic symptoms as an add-on treatment to mood stabilizers.[45]

Light therapy and sleep-deprivation therapy

As both treatments are used to treat depressive states and have a known risk of switch into mania, even though it is small, it is unlikely that mixed states will be improved. However, there are no clinical studies investigating the effect of those chronobiological therapies in mixed patients.

Deep brain stimulation (DBS)

Existing studies only evaluated DBS in therapy-resistant depression in unipolar or bipolar patients; in those studies it is not clear whether patients with depressive mixed states were included.[46] DBS in Parkinson's disease has rather been shown to be able to induce manic states.[47]

Psychotherapy

To date there is no study in which the effect of psychotherapy specifically on mixed states, neither acute nor prophylactic, has been investigated. So, it is still unclear if psychotherapy is effective in the acute treatment or the prophylaxis of mixed episodes.

Conclusion

Conolly and Thase reviewed four guidelines for the treatment of bipolar disorder in 2011 (those from Malhi et al. in the framework of an Australian project, those of the BAP, and those produced by the ISBD and the CANMAT and the Texas Implementation of Medication Algorithms project) and concluded from those guidelines that mixed episodes should be treated first-line with valproate or an atypical antipsychotic. Other more recently published reviews came to similar conclusions.[12,48] The best evidence in treating manic and depressive symptoms at the same time exists for monotherapy with aripiprazole, asenapine, carbamazepine, valproate, olanzapine, and ziprasidone. Regarding combination treatment, add-on olanzapine to lithium or valproate has the best evidence. Studies investigating prophylactic treatment are even rarer; monotherapy with valproate, olanzapine, and quetiapine seems to prevent mixed episodes. Adjunctive therapy with valproate or lithium to quetiapine has also shown to be effective in prophylaxis of mixed episodes.

However, there is still a lack of clinical trials addressing the efficacy of psychopharmacological medication on treating mixed affective symptoms and also guidelines do not fully reflect the evidence to hand.[48]

With reference to non-pharmacological treatments, only for ECT is there enough evidence to consider this as an efficacious treatment, specifically in pharmacotherapy-resistant mixed bipolar patients.

Furthermore, more studies are needed to explore treatment options for different groups of patients diagnosed with mixes states according to DSM-5. This is especially with respect to MDD patients with mixed specifier and those bipolar patients suffering from major depressive episode with mixed specifier because there are barely any trials focusing on these groups of patients.

References

1. Kraepelin E, ed. *Manic Depressive Insanity and Paranoia*. Edinburgh: E&S Livingstone; 1921.

2. Association AP. *APA—American Psychiatric Association: Diagnostic and Statistical Manual of Mental Disorders—DSM-IV-TR* 4th edn. Washington DC: American Psychiatric Association; 2000.

3. Association AP, ed. *Diagnostic and Statistical Manual of Mental Disorders*. VA: American Psychiatric Association; 2013 [DSM-5] edn: Arlington 2013.

4. Vieta E and Morralla C. Prevalence of mixed mania using 3 definitions, J Affect Disord 2010 Sep;**125**(1–3):61–73.

5. Vieta E and Valenti M. Mixed states in DSM-5: implications for clinical care, education, and research, J Affect Disord 2013 May 15;**148**(1):28–36.

6. Gonzalez-Pinto A, Aldama A, Mosquera F, and Gonzalez Gomez C. Epidemiology, diagnosis and management of mixed mania, CNS Drugs 2007;**21**(8):611–26.

7. Pfennig A, Bschor T, Baghai T, Braunig P, Brieger P, Falkai P, et al. [S3 guidelines on diagnostics and therapy of bipolar disorders: development process and essential recommendations], Nervenarzt 2012 May;**83**(5):568–86.

8. Yatham LN, Kennedy SH, Parikh SV, Schaffer A, Beaulieu S, Alda M, et al. Canadian Network for Mood and Anxiety Treatments (CANMAT) and International Society for Bipolar Disorders (ISBD) collaborative update of CANMAT guidelines for the management of patients with bipolar disorder: update 2013, Bipolar Disord 2013 Feb;**15**(1):1–44.

9. Prien RF, Himmelhoch JM, and Kupfer DJ. Treatment of mixed mania, J Affect Disord 1988 Jul–Aug;**15**(1):9–15.

10. Swann AC, Bowden CL, Morris D, Calabrese JR, Petty F, Small J, et al. Depression during mania. Treatment response to lithium or divalproex, Arch Gen Psychiatry 1997 Jan;**54**(1):37–42.

11. Fountoulakis KN, Kontis D, Gonda X, Siamouli M, and Yatham LN. Treatment of mixed bipolar states, Int J Neuropsychopharmacol 2012 Aug;**15**(7):1015–26.

12. Fagiolini A, Coluccia A, Maina G, Forgione RN, Goracci A, Cuomo A, et al. Diagnosis, epidemiology and management of mixed states in bipolar disorder, CNS Drugs 2015 Sep 14.

13. Azorin JM, Belzeaux R, Cermolacce M, Kaladjian A, Correard N, Dassa D, et al. [Recommendations for the treatment of mixed episodes in current guidelines], Encephale 2013 Dec;**39**(Suppl 3):S185–7.

14. Muralidharan K, Ali M, Silveira LE, Bond DJ, Fountoulakis KN, Lam RW, et al. Efficacy of second-generation antipsychotics in treating acute mixed episodes in bipolar disorder: a meta-analysis of placebo-controlled trials, J Affect Disord 2013 Sep 5;**150**(2):408–14.

15. Szegedi A, Zhao J, van Williigenburg A, Nations KR, Mackle M, and Panagides J. Effects of asenapine on depressive symptoms in patients with bipolar I disorder experiencing acute manic or mixed episodes: a post hoc analysis of two 3-week clinical trials, BMC Psychiatry 2011;**11**:101.

16. McIntyre RS, Cucchiaro J, Pikalov A, Kroger H, and Loebel A. Lurasidone in the treatment of bipolar depression with mixed (subsyndromal hypomanic) features: post hoc analysis of a randomized placebo-controlled trial, J Clin Psychiatry 2015 Apr;**76**(4):398–405.

17. Patkar A, Gilmer W, Pae CU, Vohringer PA, Ziffra M, Pirok E, et al. A 6-week randomized double-blind placebo-controlled trial of ziprasidone for the acute depressive mixed state, PLoS One 2012;7(4):e34757.

18. Tohen M, Goldberg JF, Gonzalez-Pinto Arrillaga AM, Azorin JM, Vieta E, Hardy-Bayle MC, et al. A 12-week, double-blind comparison of olanzapine vs haloperidol in the treatment of acute mania, Arch Gen Psychiatry 2003 Dec;60(12):1218–26.

19. Perlis RH, Baker RW, Zarate CA, Jr, Brown EB, Schuh LM, Jamal HH, et al. Olanzapine versus risperidone in the treatment of manic or mixed States in bipolar I disorder: a randomized, double-blind trial, J Clin Psychiatry 2006 Nov;67(11):1747–53.

20. Niufan G, Tohen M, Qiuqing A, Fude Y, Pope E, McElroy H, et al. Olanzapine versus lithium in the acute treatment of bipolar mania: a double-blind, randomized, controlled trial, J Affect Disord 2008 Jan;105(1–3):101–8.

21. Tohen M, Baker RW, Altshuler LL, Zarate CA, Suppes T, Ketter TA, et al. Olanzapine versus divalproex in the treatment of acute mania, Am J Psychiatry 2002 Jun;159(6):1011–17.

22. Berwaerts J, Xu H, Nuamah I, Lim P, and Hough D. Evaluation of the efficacy and safety of paliperidone extended-release in the treatment of acute mania: a randomized, double-blind, dose-response study, J Affect Disord 2012 Jan;136(1–2):e51–60.

23. Vieta E, Nuamah IF, Lim P, Yuen EC, Palumbo JM, Hough DW, et al. A randomized, placebo and active-controlled study of paliperidone extended release for the treatment of acute manic and mixed episodes of bipolar I disorder, Bipolar Disord 2010 May;12(3):230–43.

24. Khanna S, Vieta E, Lyons B, Grossman F, Eerdekens M, and Kramer M. Risperidone in the treatment of acute mania: double-blind, placebo-controlled study, Br J Psychiatry 2005 Sep;187:229–34.

25. Keck PE, Jr, Versiani M, Warrington L, Loebel AD, and Horne RL. Long-term safety and efficacy of ziprasidone in subpopulations of patients with bipolar mania, J Clin Psychiatry 2009 Jun;70(6):844–51.

26. Zarate CA, Jr, Tohen M, Banov MD, Weiss MK, and Cole JO. Is clozapine a mood stabilizer?, J Clin Psychiatry 1995 Mar;56(3):108–12.

27. Amann B, Born C, Crespo JM, Pomarol-Clotet E, and McKenna P. Lamotrigine: when and where does it act in affective disorders? A systematic review, J Psychopharmacol 2011 Oct;25(10):1289–94.

28. Swann AC, Bowden CL, Calabrese JR, Dilsaver SC, and Morris DD. Mania: differential effects of previous depressive and manic episodes on response to treatment, Acta Psychiatr Scand 2000 Jun;101(6):444–51.

29. Bowden CL, Brugger AM, Swann AC, Calabrese JR, Janicak PG, Petty F, et al. Efficacy of divalproex vs lithium and placebo in the treatment of mania. The Depakote Mania Study Group, JAMA 1994 Mar 23–30;271(12):918–24.

30. Bowden CL, Collins MA, McElroy SL, Calabrese JR, Swann AC, Weisler RH, et al. Relationship of mania symptomatology to maintenance treatment response with divalproex, lithium, or placebo, Neuropsychopharmacology 2005 Oct;30(10):1932–9.

31. Bourin MS, Severus E, Schronen JP, Gass P, Szamosi J, Eriksson H, et al. Lithium as add-on to quetiapine XR in adult patients with acute mania: a 6-week, multicenter, double-blind, randomized, placebo-controlled study, Int J Bipolar Disord 2014;2:14.

32. Sokolski KN and Denson TF. Adjunctive quetiapine in bipolar patients partially responsive to lithium or valproate, Prog Neuropsychopharmacol Biol Psychiatry 2003 Aug;27(5):863–6.

33. Houston JP, Ahl J, Meyers AL, Kaiser CJ, Tohen M, and Baldessarini RJ. Reduced suicidal ideation in bipolar I disorder mixed-episode patients in a placebo-controlled trial of olanzapine combined with lithium or divalproex, J Clin Psychiatry 2006 Aug;67(8):1246–52.

34. Sachs GS, Vanderburg DG, Karayal ON, Kolluri S, Bachinsky M, and Cavus I. Adjunctive oral ziprasidone in patients with acute mania treated with lithium or divalproex, part 1: results of a randomized, double-blind, placebo-controlled trial, J Clin Psychiatry 2012 Nov;73(11):1412–19.

35. Juruena MF, Ottoni GL, Machado-Vieira R, Carneiro RM, Weingarthner N, Marquardt AR, et al. Bipolar I and II disorder residual symptoms: oxcarbazepine and carbamazepine as add-on treatment to lithium in a double-blind, randomized trial, Prog Neuropsychopharmacol Biol Psychiatry 2009 Feb 1;33(1):94–9.

36. Muti M, Del Grande C, Musetti L, Marazziti D, Pergentini I, Corsi M, et al. Prescribing patterns of lithium or lithium + valproate in manic or mixed episodes: a naturalistic study, Int Clin Psychopharmacol 2013 Nov;28(6):305–11.

37. Benazzi F, Berk M, Frye MA, Wang W, Barraco A, and Tohen M. Olanzapine/fluoxetine combination for the treatment of mixed depression in bipolar I disorder: a post hoc analysis, J Clin Psychiatry 2009 Oct;70(10):1424–31.

38. Sachs GS, Grossman F, Ghaemi SN, Okamoto A, and Bowden CL. Combination of a mood stabilizer with risperidone or haloperidol for treatment of acute mania: a double-blind, placebo-controlled comparison of efficacy and safety, Am J Psychiatry 2002 Jul;159(7):1146–54.

39. Suppes T, Vieta E, Liu S, Brecher M, and Paulsson B. Maintenance treatment for patients with bipolar I disorder: results from a North American study of quetiapine in combination with lithium or divalproex (trial 127), Am J Psychiatry 2009 Apr;166(4):476–88.

40. Vieta E, Suppes T, Eggens I, Persson I, Paulsson B, and Brecher M. Efficacy and safety of quetiapine in combination with lithium or divalproex for maintenance of patients with bipolar I disorder (international trial 126), J Affect Disord 2008 Aug;109(3):251–63.

41. Gruber NP, Dilsaver SC, Shoaib AM, and Swann AC. ECT in mixed affective states: a case series, J ECT 2000 Jun;16(2):183–8.

42. Medda P, Perugi G, Zanello S, Ciuffa M, Rizzato S, and Cassano GB. Comparative response to electroconvulsive therapy in medication-resistant bipolar I patients with depression and mixed state, J ECT 2010 Jun;26(2):82–6.

43. Medda P, Toni C, Mariani MG, De Simone L, Mauri M, and Perugi G. Electroconvulsive therapy in 197 patients with a severe, drug-resistant bipolar mixed state: treatment outcome and predictors of response, J Clin Psychiatry 2015 Apr 14.

44. Devanand DP, Polanco P, Cruz R, Shah S, Paykina N, Singh K, et al. The efficacy of ECT in mixed affective states, J ECT 2000 Mar;16(1):32–7.

45. Pallanti S, Grassi G, Antonini S, Quercioli L, Salvadori E, and Hollander E. rTMS in resistant mixed states: an exploratory study, J Affect Disord 2014 Mar;157:66–71.

46. Holtzheimer PE, Kelley ME, Gross RE, Filkowski MM, Garlow SJ, Barrocas A, et al. Subcallosal cingulate deep brain stimulation for treatment-resistant unipolar and bipolar depression, Arch Gen Psychiatry 2012 Feb;69(2):150–8.

47. Chopra A, Tye SJ, Lee KH, Matsumoto J, Klassen B, Adams AC, et al. Voltage-dependent mania after subthalamic nucleus deep brain stimulation in Parkinson's disease: a case report, Biol Psychiatry 2011 Jul 15;70(2):e5–7.

48. Grunze H and Azorin JM. Clinical decision making in the treatment of mixed states, World J Biol Psychiatry 2014 Jul;15(5):355–68.

Chapter 6

The treatment of rapid cycling bipolar disorder

Konstantinos N. Fountoulakis
and Dimos Dimellis

Introduction

Rapid cycling should not be regarded simply as a course specifier for bipolar disorder (BD). The presence of a rapid cycling pattern has been associated with other clinical phenotypes, mainly with mixed affective features, and it may constitute a source of diagnostic uncertainties. In addition, rapid cycling BD represents a rather complicated clinical situation, which demands clarification, and whose treatment constitutes a challenge.[1]

In the *Diagnostic and Statistical Manual of Mental Disorders* (5th edition) (DSM-5), a rapid cycling course specifier applies for patients with BD who experience at least four affective episodes during a 12-month period. Evidence indicates that a rapid cycling pattern may be a transient phenomenon, which may occur in up to 43% of individuals with BD over a lifetime.[2] Notwithstanding, the precise aetiology of rapid cycling remains unknown, a causal or triggering role for exposure to antidepressants and hypothyroidism (including subclinical) have been implicated.

Evidence indicates that pharmacotherapy may be less effective for rapid cycling BD patients than for non-rapid cycling patients.[2] In addition, a rapid cycling pattern may be associated with several illness characteristics which indicate a worse prognosis in BD, including an earlier age of illness onset, a higher prevalence of co-morbid substance use disorders, more frequent suicidal behaviours, and greater functional disability.[1]

Several strategies have been proposed to treat rapid cycling BD.[3,4] The standard mood stabilizers (lithium, divalproex, and carbamazepine) have been used either as monotherapy or in combination, and also the efficacy of atypical antipsychotics and antidepressants has been studied.[5] The use of other experimental agents, such as levothyroxine or melatonin, has generated mixed results.[6-9] Only a limited number of studies has specifically investigated the pharmacological management of rapid cycling BD. This chapter aims to provide a critical review of available evidence for the management of rapid cycling BD.

Treatment of acute episodes in rapid cycling patients

Several treatment choices have been studied in patients with rapid cycling BD, including: (i) antidepressant monotherapy; (ii) antipsychotic monotherapy; (iii) mood stabilizer-anticonvulsant monotherapy; (iv) mood stabilizer-anticonvulsant combinations; and (v) mood stabilizer-anticonvulsant plus a member of other psychopharmacological class (see Table 6.1).

Antidepressant monotherapy

Randomized trials regarding antidepressant monotherapy exist for two second-generation antidepressants; namely, escitalopram and venlafaxine.[10,11] Escitalopram (10 mg) was studied in a nine-month randomized, double-blind, placebo-controlled, cross-over trial versus placebo. This was a three-phase study of a small sample of ten patients. Parker et al.[11] reported that escitalopram, when compared with placebo, reduced the severity of depressive symptoms and the percentage of days depressed or high, but remission rates for depression were not reported. An interesting but weak trend for reduction in hypomania was also found. The small sample size of this underpowered study limits the generalizability of its results.

Venlafaxine was compared to Lithium for BD-II patients suffering from a depressive episode. Venlafaxine achieved a greater reduction in Hamilton Depression Rating Scale-28 (HDRS-28) scores independently of the cycling status and also achieved higher response (p = 0.021) and remission (p = 0.001) rates in the rapid cycling group. Although this study was not powered to detect treatment-emerging affective switches (TEAS) between groups, venlafaxine did not result in a higher proportion of TEAS when compared to lithium in either rapid cycling or non-rapid cycling patients.[10]

Antipsychotic monotherapy

The efficacy of atypical antipsychotics in the treatment of mania in rapid cyclers is well established.[12] Aripiprazole, olanzapine, and quetiapine have shown efficacy in this subpopulation of BD patients. More specifically, aripiprazole has been assessed in a post hoc analysis of two three-week randomized, controlled trials, regarding its efficacy and safety in subpopulations of patients experiencing an acute bipolar I manic or mixed episode. Patients with a history of rapid cycling during the preceding year demonstrated significantly greater improvements in Young Mania Rating Scale (YMRS) with aripiprazole compared with placebo. In addition, aripiprazole-treated patients presented statistically significantly higher response and remission rates compared with placebo.[13]

Olanzapine was efficacious and well tolerated in reducing symptoms of mania in rapid cycling BD-I patients. This was shown is a post hoc analysis[14] of a data set that was derived from a double-blind, placebo-controlled study of olanzapine in acute mania.[15] Data from this study were pooled with data from a second one which employed a similar design.[16] This analysis indicated that improvement in mania with

Table 6.1 Treatment of acute episodes in rapid cycling (RC) patients

Antidepressant monotherapy

Study	Design	Active Drug	Comparator	Duration	N	Outcome	Comments
Parker et al. 2006	Double-blind, cross-over	Escitalopram (10 mg)	Placebo	9 months	10	Escitalopram reduced the severity of depressive symptoms and the percentage of days depressed or high	Remission rates for depression were not reported Small sample size

Antipsychotic monotherapy

Study	Design	Active Drug	Comparator	Duration	N	Outcome	Comments
Suppes et al.	Post hoc analysis from two RCTs	Aripiprazole	Placebo	3 weeks	516	RC patients: greater reductions in YMRS scores, higher response and remission rates	
Sanger et al.	Post hoc analysis	Olanzapine (5–20 mg)	Placebo	3 weeks	45	Olanzapine was effective in reducing manic symptoms in BD-I patients with RC course	
Vieta et al.	Pooled analysis from 2 RCTs with an open-label extension up to 1 year	Olanzapine (5–20 mg)	Placebo (double-blind phase)	1st RCT: 3 weeks 2nd RCT: 4 weeks	254 in DB phase 164 in open-label extension	Early response to olanzapine favoured RC patients Long-term outcome favoured non-RC patients Fewer RC patients achieved initial symptomatic remission RC patients were more likely to experience recurrence, had more hospitalizations and suicide attempts	

(Continued)

Table 6.1 Continued

Antidepressant monotherapy

Study	Design	Active Drug	Comparator	Duration	N	Outcome	Comments
Suppes et al.	Post hoc analysis of a 47-week RCT	Olanzapine (5–20 mg)	Divalproex (500–2,500 mg)	47 weeks	251	Olanzapine and divalproex were equal in YMRS score reductions Overall, RC patients did less well regardless of treatment	High dropout rates in both treatment arms Cycle frequency was not taken into account
Cutler et al.	RCT	Quetiapine (400–800 mg)	Placebo	3 weeks	308	Quetiapine was not efficacious in RC, acutely manic patients	
Vieta et al.	RCT (sub-analysis of the data set)	Quetiapine (300 or 600 mg)	Placebo	8 weeks	108	Quetiapine was more effective (vs placebo) in reducing total MADRS scores	
Suppes et al.	RCT (sub-analysis of the data set)	Quetiapine (300 mg)	Placebo	8 weeks	270	Quetiapine was more effective (vs placebo) in reducing total MADRS scores	

Mood stabilizer-anticonvulsant monotherapy

Study	Design	Active Drug	Comparator	Duration	N	Outcome	Comments
Suppes et al.	Post hoc analysis of a 47-week RCT	Olanzapine (5–20 mg)	Divalproex (500–2,500mg)	47 weeks	251	Olanzapine and divalproex were equal in YMRS score reductions Overall, RC patients did less well regardless of treatment	High dropout rates in both treatment arms Cycle frequency was not taken into account

Muzina et al.	RCT	Divalproex	Placebo	6 weeks	54 (67% RC)	BD-I (but not BD-II) patients improved significantly regarding MADRS scores	Results for RC patients were not reported separately
Mood stabilizer—anticonvulsant combination							
Wang et al.	RCT	Addition of lamotrigine to lithium plus divalproex	Addition of placebo to lithium plus divalproex	12 weeks	36	No significant differences in favour of lamotrigine	
Mood stabilizer—anticonvulsant plus other class							
Post et al.	RCT	Addition of venlafaxine, sertraline, or bupropion to mood stabilizer	Addition of placebo to mood stabilizer	10 weeks	174 (27% prior RC history)	All antidepressants were associated with similar range of acute response and remission rates. Increased risk of switch for venlafaxine (a strong relationship between RC history and TEAS was reported)	Results for RC patients were not reported separately (regarding response and remission rates)
Keck et al.	RCT	Addition of ethyl-eicosapeptanoate (EPA) to mood stabilizer	Addition of placebo to mood stabilizer	4 months	59	No significant differences in favour of EPA	

RCT: randomized controlled trial, RC: rapid cycling, BD: bipolar disorder, TEAS: treatment-emergent affective switch, TAU: treatment as usual olanzapine was similar for rapid cyclers and non-rapid cyclers, while rapid cyclers presented an earlier response.[17]

A post hoc analysis of a 47-week trial of olanzapine versus divalproex sodium in patients with an index manic or mixed episode has been conducted.[18] Overall, rapid cycling patients did less well during the extended observation period regardless of treatment. Among rapid cycling patients, olanzapine and divalproex appeared equally efficacious in terms of YMRS changes from baseline to endpoint, while no significant differences were also detected in Clinical Global Impression (CGI) Mania or Bipolar Severity (CGI-BP), or in the HDRS.

Quetiapine was not efficacious for the treatment of acute mania in rapid cycling BD patients in one trial.[19] On the other hand, an a priori planned sub-analysis of the data from rapid cycling patients with acute BD-I or BD-II disorder with a major depressive episode found quetiapine monotherapy (300–600 mg/day) to be more effective than placebo in reducing MADRS total scores; quetiapine was also well tolerated.[20] The post hoc analysis of the rapid cycling subsample participants with bipolar disorder from the BOLDER study has confirmed this finding.[21] Finally, the sub-analysis of the data from a small number of depressed rapid cycling BD patients again suggested that 300 mg of quetiapine monotherapy was superior to placebo.[22]

Mood stabilizer-anticonvulsant monotherapy

Lithium was compared to venlafaxine, as previously mentioned.[10] Additionally, lithium and lamotrigine were studied in an open-label study that enrolled participants with BD-II depressed patients.[23] Of the sample, 72% showed rapid cycling features within the previous year and they were treated with either lamotrigine or lithium for 16 weeks. HDRS-17 (primary outcome), MADRS, and YMRS scores improved significantly ($p < 0.001$) in both treatment groups concerning the rapid cycling subgroup of patients, without any significant differences between lamotrigine and lithium. Rapid cyclers also presented significant improvements in overall mood severity according to the CGI scale ($p < 0.001$).[23]

Valproate has been also studied in rapid cycling patients, as aforementioned. Beyond the comparative study versus olanzapine,[18] a second, more recent one explored the efficacy of extended-release divalproex sodium in comparison to placebo and in BD I and II patients suffering from depression within six weeks.[24] Of the patients, 67% that took part in this study met the DSM-4 criteria for rapid cycling. BD-I (but not BD-II) patients achieved significantly superior improvements in MADRS scores on active treatment compared with placebo. Although significantly more patients met the response criteria while on divalproex, no between-group differences were detected for remission rates. A major drawback of this study was that the authors did not report separately the results for the rapid cycling subgroup versus the non-rapid cycling one.

Mood stabilizer-anticonvulsant combinations

Wang et al.[25] studied the efficacy of the addition of lamotrigine to the combination of lithium and valproate in rapid cycling bipolar depressed patients with substance use disorder comorbidity. It was a 12-week, double-blind, placebo-controlled trial. At the endpoint, no significant differences between placebo and lamotrigine were detected on MADRS and YMRS scores. In addition, lamotrigine did not differ from placebo on either response or remission rates.

Mood stabilizer-anticonvulsant plus other class psychotropic combinations

Post et al.[26] investigated the effects of adding a second-generation antidepressant to mood stabilizers in a sample with bipolar depression. More specifically, the authors performed a ten-week, randomized study in in which the efficacy of add-on venlafaxine, sertraline, or bupropion was investigated in a sample under current treatment with mood stabilizers. Of the participants, 27% had a prior history of rapid cycling. Although response and remission rates were not reported separately for rapid cyclers, no differences were detected between the three antidepressants. On the other hand, a strong relationship between a history of rapid cycling and TEAS rates was verified. Burpopion seemed to carry a lower risk than venlafaxine to induce TEAS among rapid cyclers, whereas no significant differences were detected between sertraline and venlafaxine or sertraline and bupropion.

Keck et al.[27] studied the efficacy of adding ethyl-eicosapentanoate (EPA) on top of a mood stabilizer in patients with bipolar depression that also met the criteria for rapid cycling within the previous year. This was a four-month, placebo-controlled, randomized study in which 6 g/day doses of EPA were added to ongoing treatment. At the endpoint, no significant differences between active treatment and placebo were identified, offering no support to the notion that omega-3 fatty acids might have antidepressant efficacy in BD patients with rapid cycling features.

Relapse prevention in rapid cycling patients

Treatment choices that were studied for the prevention of mood episodes in patients with rapid cycling BD include: (i) antipsychotic monotherapy; (ii) mood stabilizer-anticonvulsant monotherapy; (iii) treatment combinations; and (iv) continuation versus discontinuation of antidepressants (see Table 6.2).

Antipsychotic monotherapy

A post hoc analysis of a 100-week, randomized controlled trial reported the effects of aripiprazole in a sample of rapid cycling BD patients who had experienced a recent manic or mixed episode.[28] Notwithstanding the small sample size of this trial (N = 28), aripiprazole significantly extended time to relapse compared with placebo. In addition, aripiprazole was well tolerated.

Vieta et al. reported the acute and long-term effects of olanzapine in both rapid cyclers and non-rapid cyclers in an open-label trial.[17] Olanzapine treatment for one year resulted in fewer symptomatic remissions and more frequent recurrences (especially into depression) among BD patients with rapid cycling. Suicide attempts and hospitalizations were also more frequent in this subgroup. On the other hand, the

Table 6.2 Relapse prevention in rapid cycling (RC) patients

Antipsychotic monotherapy

Muzina et al.	RCT	Aripiprazole	Placebo	100 weeks	28	Aripiprazole increased significantly time to relapse	
Vieta et al.	Pooled analysis from 2 RCTs with an open-label extension up to 1 year	Olanzapine (5–20 mg)	Placebo (double-blind phase)	1st RCT: 3 weeks 2nd RCT: 4 weeks	254 in DB phase 164 in open-label extension	Early response to olanzapine favoured RC patients Long-term outcome favoured non-RC patients Fewer RC patients achieved initial symptomatic remission RC patients were more likely to experience recurrence, had more hospitalizations and suicide attempts	
Suppes et al.	Post hoc analysis of a 47-week RCT	Olanzapine (5–20 mg)	Divalproex (500–2,500 mg)	47 weeks	251	Olanzapine and divalproex were equal in YMRS score reductions Overall, RC patients did less well regardless of treatment	High dropout rates in both treatment arms Cycle frequency was not taken into account

Mood stabilizer-anticonvulsant monotherapy

Denicoff et al.	RCT	Lithium	Carbamazepine or combination	1 year	106 (> 50% RC history)	Prior history of RC was associated with better response to combination	Treatment-specific effects (time to relapse, number of relapses, TEAS) were not reported for RC patients separately

Study	Type	Treatment	Comparator	Duration	N	Outcome	Notes
Calabrese et al.	RCT	Lamotrigine	Placebo	6 months	182	No significant difference between groups regarding time to additional pharmacotherapy for emerging symptoms. Lamotrigine was superior regarding premature discontinuation, and the percentage of patients that remained stable for the whole duration of the study	
Calabrese et al.	RCT	Lithium	Divalproex	20 months		Divalproex was not more effective than lithium	
Findling et al.	RCT	Lithium	Divalproex	76 weeks	139	Divalproex was not more effective than lithium	
Kemp et al.	RCT	Lithium	Lithium and divalproex combination	6 months	149	No significant differences between lithium and combination treatment	Number of relapses and TEAS were not reported
Calabrese et al.	RCT	Lithium	Divalproex	20 months	60	Divalproex was not more effective than lithium in relapse prevention	
Treatment combinations							
Suppes et al.	RCT	Quetiapine in combination with lithium or divalproex	Placebo in combination with lithium or divalproex	Up to 104 weeks	628	Quetiapine was more efficacious than placebo in preventing relapse	
Vieta et al.	RCT	Quetiapine in combination with lithium or divalproex	Placebo in combination with lithium or divalproex	Up to 104 weeks		Quetiapine was more efficacious than placebo in preventing relapse	
Macfadden et al.	RCT	Risperidone long-acting injectable plus TAU	Placebo plus TAU	52 weeks	124	Relative relapse risk 2.3 times higher for adjunctive placebo	

RCT: randomized controlled trial, RC: rapid cycling, BD: bipolar disorder, TEAS: treatment-emergent affective switch, TAU: treatment as usual mean number of the new mood episodes was 1.44 (ie, participants did seem to meet the criteria for rapid cycling by the end of the trial). The aforementioned post hoc analysis performed by Suppes et al. reported that rapid cycling patients did less well had more relapses during the extended observation period than non-rapid cycling ones, regardless of treatment.[18] In addition, olanzapine and divalproex appeared comparable in terms of long-term efficacy.

Finally, quetiapine was compared to sodium valproate in a randomized pilot study, regarding its long-term efficacy and safety.[29] BD patients in full or partial remission and with a history of rapid cycling were treated with either quetiapine or valproate for 12 months. Although patients on antipsychotics had significantly fewer depressive days (according to the Life Chart Method data), no significant differences between the two treatment groups emerged regarding days with manic or hypomanic symptoms, response rates, and reduction in scores of the HDRS, MADRS, and YMRS.

Mood stabilizer-anticonvulsant monotherapy

One prospective study reported the comparative, prophylactic effects of carbamazepine, lithium and their combination in a sample of BD-I patients.[30] More than half of these patients had a prior history of rapid cycling, and this was associated with a better response on the combination (on the CGI), a lower number of episodes (vs lithium), and higher number of days to the first manic episode. Nevertheless, treatment-specific effects on time to relapse, number of relapses, and TEAS rates were not reported for rapid cyclers.

A preliminary report of the potential prophylactic effects of lamotrigine in BD patients with a history of rapid cycling during the year prior to study commencement was published by Walden et al.[31] A small sample of patients was randomized to receive either lithium or lamotrigine monotherapy for 12 months. Six out of seven patients in the lamotrigine group had fewer than four episodes, while this was the case for three out of seven patients allocated to lithium treatment. Time to relapse and rates of TEAS were not reported.

The prophylactic effects of lamotrigine were reported by Calabrese et al. in a double-blind, placebo-controlled study in which mood-stabilized BD patients with a history of rapid cycling during the preceding year were randomized to receive either lamotrigine or placebo monotherapy for six months.[32] Lamotrigine did not differentiate from placebo regarding the primary outcome that was the time to additional pharmacotherapy for emerging symptoms, although it proved to be superior in two secondary outcome measures; namely, time for premature discontinuation for any reason and the percentage of patients that remained stable on monotherapy for the whole duration of the study. A prospective analysis of the same data set, using the prospective Life Chart Method, showed that patients on lamotrigine were 1.8 times more likely to achieve euthymia at least once weekly during the six-month period.[33] Number of relapses and time to relapse were not reported.

For the prevention phase, the data so far suggest that divalproex was not more effective than lithium[4] and also that the combination of lithium plus divalproex was not more efficacious than lithium monotherapy.[34] A small study reported that the combination of lithium plus carbamazepine was more effective than either agent alone.[30] Notwithstanding the data were negative for lamotrigine, some secondary outcome measures provided a signal for efficacy, especially for BD-II patients.[32]. Overall, the widely believed concept, among clinicians, that divalproex is more effective than lithium for the prophylaxis of mood episodes in rapid cycling BD was not supported by a trial involving 139 patients.[35]

Beyond the previously mentioned studies that had compared the mood-stabilizing effects of lithium versus carbamazepine[30] or lamotrigine,[31] Kemp et al. conducted a comparative, double-blind, six-month study of lithium monotherapy and its combination with divalproex in 31 rapid cyclers with co-morbid substance use disorders.[34] Lithium did not produce differential results when compared to the combination therapy; however, the number of relapses and the rate of TEAS were not reported.

Previously, Calabrese et al. conducted a double-blind, parallel-group study that compared lithium versus divalproex monotherapy.[4] The sample of this trial comprised 60 recently manic or hypomanic patients (stratified for BD-I and BD-II) who achieved a persistent response for at least six months on a combination of lithium plus divalproex; trial duration was 20 months. The results failed to support the hypothesis that divalproex was more efficacious than lithium in relapse prevention, although the small sample of patients and the potential effects of lithium discontinuation do not allow the generalizability of these findings.

Treatment combinations

The efficacy of the combination of carbamazepine plus lithium and of the addition of lamotrigine following non-response to lithium plus divalproex combination have been previously discussed.[30,36] Overall, the results seemed inconsistent. Although lithium monotherapy was not found to be inferior in efficacy to the lithium–divalproex combination for relapse prevention, the history of rapid cycling predicted a superior response to the lithium–carbamazepine combination than to either drug in monotherapy.

Two studies have explored the efficacy and safety of quetiapine combined with lithium or divalproex in the prevention of mood episodes in rapid cycling BD-I patients with their most recent episode being either manic/mixed or depressive.[37,38] Both studies had a similar design. Specifically, BD patients who achieved and maintained stability on quetiapine plus lithium or divalproex combination for at least 12 weeks were randomized to remain on this combination or to be switched to placebo plus lithium or divalproex. The patients were treated in this double-blind studies for up to 104 weeks. Both trials have found that maintenance with adjunctive quetiapine was significantly more efficacious than placebo in preventing relapse.

Another large controlled trial evaluated the efficacy of adjunctive maintenance treatment with risperidone long-acting injectable (RLAI) on treatment as usual (TAU) in 240 BD-I patients with at least four mood episodes in the 12 months prior to study entry.[39] Of 240 participants, 124 met stability criteria and were thus randomized to RLAI or placebo for 52 weeks. By the end of the trial, relapse rates were significantly higher for placebo than for RLAI, and relative relapse risk was 2.3 higher for adjunctive placebo ($p = 0.011$).

Another recent trial has randomized adults with rapid cycling type I or type II BD to receive either RLAI plus TAU or TAU alone for 12 months. By the end of this open-label randomized trial, any-cause relapse rates did not significantly differ between RLAI plus TAU and TAU alone.[40]

Continuation of antidepressants versus discontinuation

The effects of continuing *versus* discontinuing antidepressants after acute recovery of bipolar depression on the long-term course of BD were explored within the frames of the Systematic Treatment Enhancement Program for Bipolar Disorder (STEP-BD) trial.[41] It was observed that of the presence of rapid cycling predicted three times more depressive episodes with antidepressant continuation, while patients with rapid cycling BD showed increased number of depressive episodes, shorter episode latency, and consequently fewer weeks in remission. These results should be translated with caution as the number of patients with a rapid cycling course was relatively small (n = 17). This finding was supported by the European Mania in Bipolar Longitudinal Evaluation of Medication (EMBLEM) study, which found that patients who had continued the use of antidepressants in the maintenance phase of the study (14%; n = 341) were more likely to be rapid cyclers compared with those who were not taking antidepressants.

Evidence from meta-analysis

A meta-analysis has suggested that lithium is at least in part efficacious in rapid cycling BD patients,[42] while a second meta-analystic review has found no consistent advantage of any treatment option versus the others for rapid cycling BD.[2] The meta-analysis of 20 studies published in 1974–2002 comparing subjects with rapid and non-rapid cycling BD reported that in contrast to common beliefs, lithium prophylaxis may be efficacious for a considerable number of rapid cyclers, especially when prescription of antidepressants is avoided. Hypothyroidism may be associated with mood destabilization in vulnerable patients.[42]

Conclusion

This chapter has evaluated evidence for treatment options for rapid cycling BD. Accessible evidence is scarce and limited. Only a limited number of trials have been designed to specifically address the question of how to treat effectively bipolar patients with a rapid cycling pattern. On the other hand, the majority of the published data consists of either post hoc analyses or open-label studies. Despite the dearth of bibliographical documentation, some basic recommendations could be made based on the existing data.

The treatment of rapid cycling BD patients is being based on two axons: the treatment of the acute episode and the prevention of relapses. Regarding the management of acute episodes, the strongest and more robust data exist for atypical antipsychotics. Both aripiprazole and olanzapine were found to be efficacious and well tolerated in acutely manic rapid cycling patients, whereas quetiapine reduced, only, the intensity of the depressive symptomatology. The second more extensively studied class of psychotropic medication in the treatment of acutely ill rapid cycling patients is that of mood stabilizers and anticonvulsants, for which the data are even more limited and controversial. Finally, newer antidepressants such as venlafaxine and escitalopram have also been studied with positive results in reducing the severity of depressive symptomatology.

Concerning relapse prevention, both atypical antipsychotics and mood stabilizers and anticonvulsants have also been studied. Aripirpazole and olanzapine increased the time to relapse, whereas quetiapine resulted in fewer depressive days. RLAI, on the other hand, produced mixed results. Regarding mood stabilizers and anticonvulsants, lithium, divalporex, carbamazepine, and lamotrigine have been studied either as monotherapy or in combination. The most interesting finding was about the efficacy of lithium, especially in comparison with divalproex. Despite the common belief that the latter is more effective, lithium was found to be at least as effective as divalporex and also was not inferior to the combination with divalproex.

As aforementioned, the literature regarding both acute and chronic treatment of rapid cycling BD patients is limited and its quality is generally poor. Its supplementation with randomized controlled trials that will recruit patients' samples, adequately powered for rapid cycling BD, is needed in order to clarify the benefits and also the drawbacks of the existing medications.

References

1. **Fountoulakis KN, Kontis D, Gonda X,** and **Yatham LN.** A systematic review of the evidence on the treatment of rapid cycling bipolar disorder, *Bipolar Disorders* 2013;**15**(2):115–37.

2. **Tondo L, Hennen J,** and **Baldessarini RJ.** Rapid-cycling bipolar disorder: effects of long-term treatments, *Acta Psychiatrica Scandinavica* 2003;**108**(1):4–14.

3. **Dunner DL** and **Fieve RR.** Clinical factors in lithium carbonate prophylaxis failure, *Archives of General Psychiatry* 1974;**30**(2):229–33.

4. **Calabrese JR, Shelton MD, Rapport DJ,** et al. A 20-month, double-blind, maintenance trial of lithium versus divalproex in rapid-cycling bipolar disorder, Am J Psychiatry 2005;**162**(11):2152–61.

5. **Schneck CD.** Treatment of rapid-cycling bipolar disorder, *The Journal of Clinical Psychiatry* 2006;**67**(Suppl 11):22–7.

6. **Extein IL.** High doses of levothyroxine for refractory rapid cycling, Am J Psychiatry 2000;**157**(10):1704–5.

7. **Afflelou S, Auriacombe M, Cazenave M, Chartres JP,** and **Tignol J.** [Administration of high dose levothyroxine in treatment of rapid cycling bipolar disorders. Review of the literature and initial therapeutic application apropos of 6 cases], *L'Encephale* 1997;**23**(3):209–17.

8. **Leibenluft E, Feldman-Naim S, Turner EH, Wehr TA,** and **Rosenthal NE.** Effects of exogenous melatonin administration and withdrawal in five patients with rapid-cycling bipolar disorder. *The Journal of Clinical Psychiatry* 1997;**58**(9):383–8.

9. **Bauer MS** and **Whybrow PC.** Rapid cycling bipolar affective disorder II. Treatment of refractory rapid cycling with high-dose levothyroxine: a preliminary study, *Archives of General Psychiatry* 1990;**47**(5):435–40.

10. **Amsterdam JD, Wang CH, Shwarz M,** and **Shults J.** Venlafaxine versus lithium monotherapy of rapid and non-rapid cycling patients with bipolar II major depressive episode: a randomized, parallel group, open-label trial, *Journal of Affective Disorders* 2009;**112**(1–3):219–30.

11. **Parker G, Tully L, Olley A,** and **Hadzi-Pavlovic D.** SSRIs as mood stabilizers for bipolar II disorder? A proof of concept study, *Journal of Affective Disorders* 2006;**92**(2–3):205–14.

12. **Cipriani A, Barbui C, Salanti G,** et al. Comparative efficacy and acceptability of antimanic drugs in acute mania: a multiple-treatments meta-analysis, *Lancet* 2011;**378**(9799):1306–15.

13. **Suppes T, Eudicone J, McQuade R, Pikalov A,** 3rd, and **Carlson B.** Efficacy and safety of aripiprazole in subpopulations with acute manic or mixed episodes of bipolar I disorder, *Journal of Affective Disorders* 2008;**107**(1–3):145–54.

14. **Sanger TM, Tohen M, Vieta E,** et al. Olanzapine in the acute treatment of bipolar I disorder with a history of rapid cycling. *Journal of Affective Disorders* 2003;**73**(1–2):155–61.

15. **Tohen M, Sanger TM, McElroy SL,** et al. Olanzapine versus placebo in the treatment of acute mania. Olanzapine HGEH Study Group, Am J Psychiatry 1999;**156**(5):702–9.

16. **Tohen M, Jacobs TG, Grundy SL,** et al. Efficacy of olanzapine in acute bipolar mania: a double-blind, placebo-controlled study. The Olanzipine HGGW Study Group, *Archives of General Psychiatry* 2000;**57**(9):841–9.

17. **Vieta E, Calabrese JR, Hennen J,** et al. Comparison of rapid-cycling and non-rapid-cycling bipolar I manic patients during treatment with olanzapine: analysis of pooled data, *The Journal of Clinical Psychiatry* 2004;**65**(10):1420–8.

18. **Suppes T, Brown E, Schuh LM, Baker RW,** and **Tohen M.** Rapid versus non-rapid cycling as a predictor of response to olanzapine and divalproex sodium for bipolar mania and maintenance of remission: post hoc analyses of 47-week data, *Journal of Affective Disorders* 2005;**89**(1–3):69–77.

19. **Cutler AJ, Datto C, Nordenhem A, Minkwitz M, Acevedo L,** and **Darko D.** Extended-release quetiapine as monotherapy for the treatment of adults with acute mania: a randomized, double-blind, 3-week trial, Clin Ther 2011;**33**(11):1643–58.

20. **Vieta E, Calabrese JR, Goikolea JM, Raines S,** and **Macfadden W.** Quetiapine monotherapy in the treatment of patients with bipolar I or II depression and a rapid-cycling disease course: a randomized, double-blind, placebo-controlled study, *Bipolar Disorders* 2007;**9**(4):413–25.

21. **Cookson J, Keck PE, Jr, Ketter TA,** and **Macfadden W.** Number needed to treat and time to response/remission for quetiapine monotherapy efficacy in acute bipolar depression: evidence from a large, randomized, placebo-controlled study, Int Clin Psychopharmacol 2007;**22**(2):93–100.

22. **Suppes T, Datto C, Minkwitz M, Nordenhem A, Walker C,** and **Darko D.** Effectiveness of the extended release formulation of quetiapine as monotherapy for the treatment of acute bipolar depression, *Journal of Affective Disorders* 2010;**121**(1–2):106–15.

23. **Suppes T, Marangell LB, Bernstein IH,** et al. A single blind comparison of lithium and lamotrigine for the treatment of bipolar II depression, *Journal of Affective Disorders* 2008;**111**(2–3):334–43.

24. **Muzina DJ, Gao K, Kemp DE,** et al. Acute efficacy of divalproex sodium versus placebo in mood stabilizer-naive bipolar I or II depression: a double-blind, randomized, placebo-controlled trial, *The Journal Of Clinical Psychiatry* 2011;**72**(6): 813–19.

25. **Wang Z, Gao K, Kemp DE**, et al. Lamotrigine adjunctive therapy to lithium and divalproex in depressed patients with rapid cycling bipolar disorder and a recent substance use disorder: a 12-week, double-blind, placebo-controlled pilot study, *Psychopharmacology Bulletin* 2010;**43**(4):5–21.

26. **Post RM, Altshuler LL, Leverich GS**, et al. Mood switch in bipolar depression: comparison of adjunctive venlafaxine, bupropion and sertraline, *The British Journal of Psychiatry: the Journal of Mental Science* 2006;**189**:124–31.

27. **Keck PE, Jr, Mintz J, McElroy SL**, et al. Double-blind, randomized, placebo-controlled trials of ethyl-eicosapentanoate in the treatment of bipolar depression and rapid cycling bipolar disorder, Biol Psychiatry 2006;**60**(9):1020–2.

28. **Muzina DJ, Momah C, Eudicone JM**, et al. Aripiprazole monotherapy in patients with rapid-cycling bipolar I disorder: an analysis from a long-term, double-blind, placebo-controlled study, Int J Clin Pract 2008;**62**(5):679–87.

29. **Langosch JM, Drieling T, Biedermann NC**, et al. Efficacy of quetiapine monotherapy in rapid-cycling bipolar disorder in comparison with sodium valproate, *Journal of Clinical Psychopharmacology* 2008;**28**(5):555–60.

30. **Denicoff KD, Smith-Jackson EE, Disney ER, Ali SO, Leverich GS**, and **Post RM**. Comparative prophylactic efficacy of lithium, carbamazepine, and the combination in bipolar disorder, *The Journal of Clinical Psychiatry* 1997;**58**(11):470–8.

31. **Walden J, Schaerer L, Schloesser S**, and **Grunze H**. An open longitudinal study of patients with bipolar rapid cycling treated with lithium or lamotrigine for mood stabilization, *Bipolar Disorders* 2000;**2**(4):336–9.

32. **Calabrese JR, Suppes T, Bowden CL**, et al. A double-blind, placebo-controlled, prophylaxis study of lamotrigine in rapid-cycling bipolar disorder. Lamictal 614 Study Group, *The Journal of Clinical Psychiatry* 2000;**61**(11):841–50.

33. **Goldberg JF, Bowden CL, Calabrese JR**, et al. Six-month prospective life charting of mood symptoms with lamotrigine monotherapy versus placebo in rapid cycling bipolar disorder, Biol Psychiatry 2008;**63**(1):125–30.

34. **Kemp DE, Gao K, Ganocy SJ**, et al. A 6-month, double-blind, maintenance trial of lithium monotherapy versus the combination of lithium and divalproex for rapid-cycling bipolar disorder and co-occurring substance abuse or dependence, *The Journal of Clinical Psychiatry* 2009;**70**(1):113–21.

35. **Findling RL, McNamara NK, Youngstrom EA**, et al. Double-blind 18-month trial of lithium versus divalproex maintenance treatment in pediatric bipolar disorder, J Am Acad Child Adolesc Psychiatry 2005;**44**(5):409–17.

36. **Kemp DE, Gao K, Fein EB**, et al. Lamotrigine as add-on treatment to lithium and divalproex: lessons learned from a double-blind, placebo-controlled trial in rapid-cycling bipolar disorder, *Bipolar Disorders* 2012;**14**(7):780–9.

37. **Suppes T, Vieta E, Liu S, Brecher M**, and **Paulsson B**. Maintenance treatment for patients with bipolar I disorder: results from a North American study of quetiapine in combination with lithium or divalproex (trial 127), Am J Psychiatry 2009;**166**(4):476–88.

38. **Vieta E, Suppes T, Eggens I, Persson I, Paulsson B**, and **Brecher M**. Efficacy and safety of quetiapine in combination with lithium or divalproex for maintenance of patients with bipolar I disorder (international trial 126), *Journal of Affective Disorders* 2008;**109**(3):251–63.

39. **Macfadden W, Alphs L, Haskins JT**, et al. A randomized, double-blind, placebo-controlled study of maintenance treatment with adjunctive risperidone long-acting

therapy in patients with bipolar I disorder who relapse frequently, *Bipolar Disorders* 2009;**11**(8):827–39.

40. **Bobo WV, Epstein RA, Lynch A, Patton TD, Bossaller NA, and Shelton RC.** A randomized open comparison of long-acting injectable risperidone and treatment as usual for prevention of relapse, rehospitalization, and urgent care referral in community-treated patients with rapid cycling bipolar disorder, *Clinical Neuropharmacology* 2011;**34**(6):224–33.

41. **Ghaemi SN, Ostacher MM, El-Mallakh RS**, et al. Antidepressant discontinuation in bipolar depression: a Systematic Treatment Enhancement Program for Bipolar Disorder (STEP-BD) randomized clinical trial of long-term effectiveness and safety, *The Journal of Clinical Psychiatry* 2010;**71**(4):372–80.

42. **Kupka RW, Luckenbaugh DA, Post RM, Leverich GS, and Nolen WA.** Rapid and non-rapid cycling bipolar disorder: a meta-analysis of clinical studies, *The Journal of Clinical Psychiatry* 2003;**64**(12):1483–94.

Chapter 7

Evidence-based treatment of bipolar depression

Mark A. Frye, Paul E. Croarkin, Marin Veldic, Malik M. Nassan, Katherine M. Moore, Simon Kung, Susannah J. Tye, William V. Bobo, and Jennifer L. Vande Voort

Introduction

It is increasingly recognized that bipolar disorder illness morbidity is driven by depression.[1] Depressive symptoms, whether acute or chronic treatment resistant, often are accompanied by mixed symptoms, suicidality (disease related and treatment emergent), catatonia, and medical co-morbidity further fuelling symptom burden and clinical challenges in successful treatment intervention.[2] Despite the predominant illness burden, the evidence base for acute bipolar depression is significantly less than the evidence bases for acute mania (lithium, divalproex sodium, carbamazepine, typical antipsychotic chlorpromazine, and atypical antipsychotics aripiprazole, asenapine, cariprazine, olanzapine, quetiapine (immediate and extended release), risperidone, and ziprasidone) and maintenance relapse prevention (lithium, lamotrigine, aripiprazole, olanzapine, quetiapine extended release, risperidone intramuscular injection, ziprasidone adjunctive therapy). Most of the drug development for bipolar depression has focused on atypical antipsychotic therapies.

Atypical antipsychotics

Quetiapine, olanzapine/fluoxetine, olanzapine (Japan only), and lurasidone all have regulatory approval for treatment of bipolar depression. The evidence base for quetiapine includes more than 2,500 bipolar I/II depressed subjects who participated in four eight-week, placebo-controlled trials.[3,4,5,6] In comparison to placebo, 300 and 600 mg alike were associated with higher rates of response (50% symptom reduction), remission (Montgomery-Åsberg Depression Rating Scale (MADRS) ≤12), and overall baseline to endpoint symptom reduction utilizing MADRS. Both doses as well outperformed lithium[6] and paroxetine[4] with selective serotonin reuptake inhibitor (SSRI) monotherapy showing a threefold increase in treatment-emergent switch in comparison with quetiapine.

The initial lurasidone evidence base includes two, six-week, randomized, double-blind studies comparing lurasidone monotherapy (low dose—20–60 mg/day, high dose—80–120 mg/day) or lurasidone adjunct (20–120 mg/day) to therapeutic lithium or valproate to placebo in patients (total n=853) with bipolar I depression.[7,8] Compared with placebo, lurasidone, both monotherapy doses (mean low 31.8 mg and mean high dose 82.0 mg) and adjunctive (mean dose 66.3 mg), was associated with higher rates of response, remission, and overall depressive symptom burden (baseline to endpoint change in MADRS). In an exploratory post hoc analysis of the monotherapy study, mixed features (defined as a Young Mania Rating Scale (YMRS) score ≥4 at study baseline) was highly prevalent (>50%) and treatment with lurasidone, in comparison with placebo, was associated with greater depressive (ie MADRS) symptom reduction in both mixed and non-mixed groups.[9] A more recent study in major depression with mixed features (n=209), using pre-*Diagnostic and Statistical Manual of Mental Disorders* (5th edition) (DSM-5) criteria defined as major depression with two or three protocol-defined non-overlap core manic symptoms, lurasidone (mean daily dose 36.2 mg) was more effective than placebo in reducing both depressive and manic symptoms.[10] The latter two studies support the DSM-5 transdiagnostic concept of the mixed specifier.

The evidence base for olanzapine/fluoxetine combination (OFC) was, in essence, an exploratory arm (n=86) of OFC to an eight-week, placebo-controlled randomized trial comparing olanzapine monotherapy (n=370) to placebo (n=377) in bipolar I depression.[11] The combination of olanzapine (mean daily dose 7.4 mg)/fluoxetine (mean daily dose 39.3 mg) was superior to placebo in baseline to eight-week endpoint change in MADRS and both response and remission rates. Olanzapine monotherapy (mean dose 9.7 mg daily) was superior to placebo in improving depression; however, the overall symptoms reduction of depression was significantly greater with OFC versus olanzapine. The evidence base for olanzapine has a second six-week, placebo-controlled study showing olanzapine monotherapy (n=343) for bipolar I depression was more effective than placebo (n=171); this significant difference was in overall symptoms burden (baseline to endpoint change in MADRS rated depression), response, and remission rates, but not recovery.[12]

Early evidence would suggest that cariprazine, a dopamine D3 and D2 receptor partial agonist atypical antipsychotic with regulatory approval for acute mania, may have broader mood stabilization properties. In an eight-week, randomized, double-blind placebo-controlled investigation of patients with bipolar I depression (n=571), cariprazine 1.5 mg daily, in comparison with placebo, was associated with a greater reduction in depressive symptoms as measured by the MADRS at week six (primary outcome) and week eight (completer analysis of 'efficacy persistence'). At week six, there was no significant difference between low-dose cariprazine (0.75 mg) and placebo; higher-dose cariprazine 3.0 mg demonstrated greater symptom reduction than placebo, but did not retain significance for multiple comparison adjustment.[13]

While lurasidone has not been systematically evaluated in acute mania (ie no evidence base nor regulatory approval) and clozapine, despite antimanic evidence, is not Food and Drug Administration (FDA)-approved, atypical antipsychotics as a class, are generally considered to possess antimanic properties. The evidence base, notwithstanding some methodological design issues, however, does not suggest that atypical antipsychotics as a class possess antidepressant properties (ie negative studies with aripiprazole and ziprasidone).[14,15] Major concerns for atypical antipsychotics focus on weight gain, cardiometabolic risk factors, and risk of tardive dyskinesia (TD). These issues become increasingly relevant when shifting from acute treatment to maintenance treatment.

Lithium and mood-stabilizing anticonvulsants

In comparison to a gold standard status as an active comparator in acute mania, the contemporary evidence based for lithium in bipolar depression is limited. One secondary analysis has suggested greater depressive symptom reduction with maintenance therapeutic (>0.8 mmol/L) versus non-therapeutic (</=0.8 mmol/L) lithium levels.[16] Similar data on longer time to episode recurrence (manic or depressive) in bipolar I patients stabilized on a lithium level of 0.6–1.2 mEq/L versus <0.6 mEq/L suggests that higher dosing of mood stabilizers, if tolerated, may reduce symptoms and possibly reduce need complex multimodal treatment.[17]

Lithium-associated changes in thyroid economy may impede therapeutic effectiveness, particularly for depression, and may provide a novel treatment intervention in treatment-resistant cases of bipolar depression. A number of studies have suggested that lower mean serum free T4 and/or higher TSH levels respectively during lithium maintenance are associated with increased depression symptom severity, rapid cycling, and depression recurrence.[18,19] In medication-free patients with depression, a significant inverse correlation between TSH and cerebral blood flow and glucose metabolism has been identified that may represent a neurobiological correlate to this depression relapse risk.[20] Finally, in a novel, placebo-controlled trial design that randomized 62 treatment-resistant bipolar I/II depressed patients (35% on lithium) to high-dose levothyroxine (300 micrograms), a secondary analysis revealed a significant improvement in depressive symptoms in bipolar women (vs men) with a significant association in baseline TSH and subsequent decrease in depressive symptoms.[21]

The evidence base for lamotrigine, FDA-approved for maintenance (ie manic and depressive relapse)[22] is based primarily on meta-analysis. Geddes et al.[23] conducted a meta-analysis on five placebo-controlled trials (n=1072 bipolar I and II patients). While there was variable study duration (7–10 weeks) and dosing strategy (fixed 50 mg and 200 mg, flexible dose 100–400 mg), there was evidence that lamotrigine, in comparison with placebo, was associated with a higher rate of treatment response defined as a 50% or greater decrease in symptoms: MADRS (RR=1.22, 95% CI 1.06–1.41), HDRS (RR=1.27, 95% CI 1.09–1.47); remission rates, however, did not differ by treatment. The evidence base has been further supported by the LamLit study; in an eight-week, randomized, placebo-controlled trial of 124 lithium maintained bipolar I/II depressed outpatients, 200 mg adjunct lamotrigine was associated, in comparison with placebo, with a significantly greater reduction of depressive symptoms and higher response rate.[24] In a considerably smaller meta-analysis of four, short-term (6–8 week), placebo-controlled trials with a total of 142 bipolar I or II depressed patients, divalproex monotherapy, in comparison with placebo, was associated with greater depressive symptom reduction and higher rates of clinical response and remission.[25,26] Furthermore, a secondary analysis of a valproate maintenance study suggests less symptom severity and need for adjunctive antidepressant therapy.[27]

Neuromodulation

While electroconvulsive therapy (ECT) has been an available treatment for depression, arguably the treatment of choice for severe (ie catatonia, psychotic depression) acute depression, there has been little systematic study of ECT for bipolar depression. Schoeyen et al.[28] in a six-week, six-site study randomized 73 bipolar patients to thrice weekly right unilateral ECT versus algorithm-based pharmacological treatment for broadly defined treatment-resistant depression. Baseline to six-week endpoint depressive symptom severity was significantly reduced with ECT in comparison with algorithm pharmacological treatment; in a completer analysis, response rates (73.9% vs 35%) were significantly higher in ECT versus pharmacological treatment but there was no difference in remission rates. While further work needs to evaluate the longer-term benefits of acute intervention, merits of bilateral ECT known to have greater efficacy and side effects than unilateral, and evaluating ECT response rate standardizing treatment resistance to the index (vs lifetime) episode, this study underscores the therapeutic potential of ECT.[29,30]

Repetitive transcranial magnetic stimulation (rTMS) has an evidence base and regulatory approval for major depressive disorder in adults whose index episode of depression has failed to achieve satisfactory improvement prior to antidepressant medication. There is has been great interest in looking at this neuromodulatory treatment for bipolar depression. In the first meta-analysis (19 studies, n=181) of rTMS in bipolar disorder, the clinical response rate (50% symptom reduction) was significantly higher in patients receiving active rTMS versus sham rTMS (McGirr et al., 2016).[31] A limitation of this early meta-analysis for a novel neuromodulatory device is the substantial clinical trial design heterogeneity including stimulation target, laterality, and high (10 Hz) versus low (1 Hz) stimulation parameters. Targeting right dorsal lateral prefrontal cortex (rDLPFC) had the highest rate of clinical response; laterality and stimulation parameters did not statistically separate in secondary analyses. In the largest trial to date, 49 bipolar depressed patients were randomized to bilateral sequential (1 Hz rDLPFC followed by 10 Hz lDLPFC) versus sham rTMS for four weeks.[32] There was no significant difference between groups in baseline to endpoint symptom burden reduction, nor response or remission rates. Further work with adequate sample size is encouraged to further characterize the evidence base for rTMS in bipolar depression.

An early two-year open-label investigation of bilateral subcallosal cingulate white matter deep brain stimulation (DBS) showed a significant decrease in depressive symptoms with similar response and remission rates for both treatment-resistant unipolar (n=10) and bipolar (n=7) depressed patients.[33] There is interest in better understanding the potential role of this neuromodulatory brain stimulation for treatment-resistant bipolar depression[34] recognizing well-established risk for DBS-induced mania in DBS-treated Parkinson's patients (Chopra et al., 2011).[35]

Antidepressants

With the exception of fluoxetine, all regulatory-approved antidepressants have received their indication in major depressive disorder; patients with a history of mania or hypomania in these regulatory development studies were routinely excluded from participation. As such, given the dearth of approved treatments for bipolar depression, there has been widespread use of unimodal antidepressants with little guidance from an evidence base.[36,37] Meta-analysis of 16 acute clinical trials comparing antidepressant therapy to placebo or active control (n=3113) found no significant benefit of antidepressant therapy in rates of response (relative risk RR = 1.17, 95% CI, 0.88–1.57; p=0.28) or remission (RR=1.14, 95% CI, 0.90–1.45; p=0.28).[38,39]

The evidence base for the acute phase or short-term use of antidepressants in bipolar II depression is limited, but may challenge previous meta-analyses. In a 12-week randomized double-blind comparison of venlafaxine versus lithium monotherapy for bipolar II depression (n=129), venlafaxine was associated with a significantly higher rate of response (68% vs 34%) with no difference in hypomanic symptoms.[40] Conversely, 142 bipolar II depressed patients participated in a 16-week randomized, double-blind study of lithium monotherapy, sertraline monotherapy, and lithium/sertraline combination therapy. All three treatments were associated with similar response rates (63%) and switch rates (majority within the first five weeks); the combination group was associated with the higher dropout rate with no added benefit of acceleration of treatment response.[10]

While the Sidor and Macqueen work did not identify a risk of antidepressant-induced mania or treatment-emergent affective switch (TEAS), there is increasing recognition that a subset of clinical factors (mixed symptoms, age, bipolar I subtype, tricyclic antidepressant) and genetic/other biological factors, rarely powered to be studied in clinical trial development programmes, may identify individualized risk.[41,42] While early work focused appropriately on serotonin transporter candidate gene and risk of antidepressant-induced mania (AIM +), genome wide association studies may identify areas of novel investigation.[43]

Psychotherapy

The psychotherapeutic evidence base for bipolar depression is best exemplified by the one-year randomized Systematic Treatment Enhancement Program.[44] 293 bipolar I or II medicated depressed outpatients were randomized to biweekly 30 sessions of intensive psychotherapies (family-focused, interpersonal, or cognitive behaviour therapy) versus general psychoeducation for three sessions. One-year recover rates, defined as no more than one or two moderate symptoms of depression for at least eight weeks, were significantly higher in the intensive psychotherapy groups than with general education (64% vs 52%).

Novel drug development

Some of the early evidence base for novel drug develop in bipolar depression appear promising. The NMDA antagonist ketamine has clearly demonstrated a rapid, non-sustained antidepressant response in both unipolar and bipolar depression;[45] as reviewed by Bobo et al.,[46] the strength of symptom-burden reduction appears to be more robust for unipolar versus bipolar depression. While the unipolar signal may be stronger in this initial review and development programmes go forward with treatment-resistant depression and suicidal ideation, single-dose ketamine treatment followed by glycine co-receptor NMDA antagonist d-cycloserine treatment (eight weeks, 1,000 mg daily) has been associated with remission in 4 out of 7 bipolar depressed patients.[47] Thus, longer-term treatment designs of modulating the NMDA receptor may have therapeutic benefit for bipolar depression. D-cycloserine is also part of a fixed-dose combination alongside lurasidone (marketed as Cyclurad') that is undergoing investigation, after a similar single dose of ketamine, as a treatment for acute suicidality in bipolar depression (http://www.neurorxpharma.com). Early work also appears promising for riluzole,[48,49] dopamine D3 partial agonist pramipexole,[50,51] and based on inflammatory models of illness progression[52] N-acetylcysteine,[53] celecoxib,[54] pioglitazone, an insulin sensitizing agent,[55] and other anti-inflammatory agents.[56]

Despite early positive signals from modafinil[57] and armodafinil,[58] two subsequent studies failed to show significant difference between armodafinil and placebo;[59,60] these negative studies have identified important designs concerns of extensive heterogeneity of study sample attempting to maximize generalizability that ultimately failed. Similarly, early investigation of agomelatine for bipolar depression did not show significant difference from placebo.[61]

Conclusion

While the evidence base for bipolar depression has increased over the last decade, there remains unmet need to develop new interventions that are effective, fast-acting, sustainable, and with low side effect burden. After the evidence base contributes to regulatory approval, there will be increasing interest to develop personalized or precision-guided predictors or biomarkers of response to best optimize interventions for bipolar depression (see Box 7.1).

Box 7.1 Level of evidence base for bipolar depression

Regulatory approval
Olanzapine/fluoxetine combination, quetiapine, lurasidone, and olanzapine (Japan only)
Controlled evidence and or meta-analyses
Cariprazine, lamotrigine, valproate, ECT, intensive psychotherapy
Exploratory
rTMS, pramipexole, ketamine, ketamine/D-cycloserine, anti-inflammatories

References

1. **Frye, MA.** Bipolar disorder—a focus on depression, N Engl J Med 2011;**364**(1):51–9.

2. **Goodwin, FK** and **Jamison, KR.** *Manic-Depressive Illness: Bipolar Disorders and Recurrent Depression* 2nd edn (New York, NY: Oxford University Press, 2007).

3. **Calabrese, JR, Keck, PE, Jr, Macfadden, W, Minkwitz, M, Ketter, TA, Weisler, RH, Cutler, AJ, McCoy, R, Wilson, E, Mullen, J; the BOLDER Study Group.** A randomized, double-blind, placebo-controlled trial of quetiapine in the treatment of bipolar I or II depression, Am J Psychiatry 2005;**162**(7):1351–60.

4. **McElroy, SL, Weisler, RH, Chang, W, Olausson, B, Paulsson, B, Brecher, M, Agambaram, V, Merideth, C, Nordenhem, A,** and **Young, A;** EMBOLDEN II (Trial D1447C00134) Investigators. A double-blind, placebo-controlled study of quetiapine and paroxetine as monotherapy in adults with bipolar depression (EMBOLDEN II), J Clin Psychiatry 2010;**71**(2):163–74.

5. **Thase, ME, Macfadden, W, Weisler, RH, Chang, W, Paulsson, B, Khan, A,** and **Calabrese, JR; BOLDER II Study Group.** Efficacy of quetiapine monotherapy in bipolar I and II depression: a double-blind, placebo-controlled study (the BOLDER II study), J Clin Psychopharmacol 2006;**26**(6):600–9.

6. **Young, AH, McElroy, SL, Bauer, M, Philips, N, Chang, W, Olausson, B, Paulsson, B,** and **Brecher, M; for the EMBOLDEN I (Trial 001) Investigators.** A double-blind, placebo-controlled study of quetiapine and lithium monotherapy in adults in the acute phase of bipolar depression (EMBOLDEN I), J Clin Psychiatry 2010;**71**(2):150–62.

7. **Loebel, A, Cucchiaro, J, Silva, R, Kroger, H, Hsu, J, Sarma, K,** and **Sachs, G.** Lurasidone monotherapy in the treatment of bipolar I depression: a randomized, double-blind, placebo-controlled study, *The American Journal of Psychiatry* 2014a;**171**(2):160–8.

8. **Loebel, A, Cucchiaro, J, Silva, R, Kroger, H, Sarma, K, Xu, J,** and **Calabrese, JR.** Lurasidone as adjunctive therapy with lithium or valproate for the treatment of bipolar I depression: a randomized, double-blind, placebo-controlled study, *The American Journal of Psychiatry* 2014b;**171**(2):169–77.

9. **McIntyre, RS, Cucchiaro, J, Pikalov, A, Kroger, H,** and **Loebel, A.** Lurasidone in the treatment of bipolar depression with mixed (subsyndromal hypomanic) features: post hoc analysis of a randomized placebo-controlled trial, *The Journal of Clinical Psychiatry* 2015;**76**(4):398–405.

10. **Altshuler, LL, Sugar, CA, McElroy, SL, Calimlim, B, Gitlin, M, Keck, PE, Aquino-Elias, A, Martens, BE, Fischer, EG, English, BA, Roach, J,** and **Suppes, T.** Switch rates during lithium monotherapy, sertraline monotherapy, and lithium/sertraline combination therapy for acute treatment of bipolar II depression: a randomized, double-blind comparison, Am J Psychiatry 2016 (in press).

11. **Tohen, M, Vieta, E, Calabrese, J, Ketter, TA, Sachs, G, Bowden, C, Mitchell, PB, Centorrino, F, Risser, R, Baker, RW, Evans, AR, Beymer, K, Dubé, S, Tollefson, GD,** and **Breier, A.** Efficacy of olanzapine and olanzapine-fluoxetine combination in the treatment of bipolar I depression, Arch Gen Psychiatry 2003;**60**(11):1079–88.

12. **Tohen, M, McDonnell, DP, Case, M, Kanba, S, Ha, K, Fang, YR, Katagiri, H,** and **Gomez, JC.** Randomised, double-blind, placebo-controlled study of olanzapine in patients with bipolar I depression, Br J Psychiatry 2012;**201**(5):376–82.

13. **Durgam, S, Earley, W, Lipschitz, A, Guo, H, Laszlovszky, I, Nemeth, G, Vieta, E, Calabrese, JR,** and **Yatham, LN.** An 8-week randomized, double-blind,

placebo-controlled evaluation of the safety and efficacy of cariprazine in patients with bipolar i depression, *The American Journal of Psychiatry* 2016;**173**(3):271–81.

14. Sachs, GS, Ice, KS, Chappell, PB, Schwartz, JH, Gurtovaya, O, Vanderburg, DG, and Kasuba, B. Efficacy and safety of adjunctive oral ziprasidone for acute treatment of depression in patients with bipolar I disorder: a randomized, double-blind, placebo-controlled trial, J Clin Psychiatry 2011;**72**(10):1413–22.

15. Thase, ME, Jonas, A, Khan, A, Bowden, CL, Wu, X, McQuade, RD, Carson, WH, Marcus, RN, and Owen, R. Aripiprazole monotherapy in nonpsychotic bipolar I depression: results of 2 randomized, placebo-controlled studies, J Clin Psychopharmacol 2008;**28**(1):13–20.

16. Nemeroff, CB, Evans, DL, Gyulai, L, Sachs, GS, Bowden, CL, Gergel, IP, Oakes, R, and Pitts, CD. Double-blind, placebo-controlled comparison of imipramine and paroxetine in the treatment of bipolar depression, Am J Psychiatry 2001;**158**(6):906–12.

17. Nolen, WA and Weisler, RH. The association of the effect of lithium in the maintenance treatment of bipolar disorder with lithium plasma levels: a post hoc analysis of a double-blind study comparing switching to lithium or placebo in patients who responded to quetiapine (Trial 144), Bipolar Disord 2013;**15**(1):100–9.

18. Frye, MA, Denicoff, KD, Bryan, AL, Smith-Jackson, EE, Ali, SO, Luckenbaugh, D, Leverich, GS, and Post, RM. Association between lower serum free T4 and greater mood instability and depression in lithium-maintained bipolar patients, Am J Psychiatry 1999;**156**(12):1909–14.

19. Frye, MA, Yatham, L, Ketter, TA, Goldberg, J, Suppes, T, Calabrese, JR, Bowden, CL, Bourne, E, Bahn, RS, Adams, B. Depressive relapse during lithium treatment associated with increased serum thyroid-stimulating hormone: results from two placebo-controlled bipolar I maintenance studies, Acta Psychiatr Scand 2009b;**120**(1):10–13.

20. Marangell, LB, Ketter, TA, George, MS, Pazzaglia, PJ, Callahan, AM, Parekh, P, Andreason, PJ, Horwitz, B, Herscovitch, P, and Post, RM. Inverse relationship of peripheral thyrotropin-stimulating hormone levels to brain activity in mood disorders, Am J Psychiatry 1997;**154**(2):224–30.

21. Stamm, TJ, Lewitzka, U, Sauer, C, Pilhatsch, M, Smolka, MN, Koeberle, U, . . . and Bauer, M. Supraphysiologic doses of levothyroxine as adjunctive therapy in bipolar depression: a randomized, double-blind, placebo-controlled study, *The Journal of Clinical Psychiatry* 2014;**75**(2):162–8.

22. Goodwin, GM, Bowden, CL, Calabrese, JR, Grunze, H, Kasper, S, White, R, Greene, P, and Leadbetter, R. A pooled analysis of 2 placebo-controlled 18-month trials of lamotrigine and lithium maintenance in bipolar I disorder, J Clin Psychiatry 2004;**65**(3):432–41.

23. Geddes, JR, Calabrese, JR, and Goodwin, GM. Lamotrigine for treatment of bipolar depression: independent meta-analysis and meta-regression of individual patient data from five randomised trials, Br J Psychiatry 2009;**194**(1):4–9.

24. van der Loos, ML, Mulder, PG, Hartong, EG, Blom, MB, Vergouwen, AC, de Keyzer, HJ, Notten, PJ, Luteijn, ML, Timmermans, MA, Vieta, E, and Nolen, WA. Efficacy and safety of lamotrigine as add-on treatment to lithium in bipolar depression: a multicenter, double-blind, placebo-controlled trial, J Clin Psychiatry 2009;**70**(2):223–31.

25. Bond, DJ, Lam, RW, and Yatham, LN. Divalproex sodium versus placebo in the treatment of acute bipolar depression: a systematic review and meta-analysis, J Affect Disord 2010;**124**(3):228–34.

26. **Smith, LA, Cornelius, VR, Azorin, JM, Perugi, G, Vieta, E, Young, AH, and Bowden, CL.** Valproate for the treatment of acute bipolar depression: systematic review and meta-analysis, J Affect Disord 2010;**122**(1–2):1–9.

27. **Gyulai, L, Bowden, CL, McElroy, SL, Calabrese, JR, Petty, F, Swann, AC, Chou, JC, Wassef, A, Risch, CS, Hirschfeld, RM, Nemeroff, CB, Keck, PE, Jr, Evans, DL, and Wozniak, PJ.** Maintenance efficacy of divalproex in the prevention of bipolar depression, *Neuropsychopharmacology* 2003;**28**(7):1374–82.

28. **Schoeyen, HK, Kessler, U, Andreassen, OA, Auestad, BH, Bergsholm, P, Malt, UF, Morken, G, Oedegaard, KJ, and Vaaler, A.** Treatment-resistant bipolar depression: a randomized controlled trial of electroconvulsive therapy versus algorithm-based pharmacological treatment, *The American Journal of Psychiatry* 2015;**172**(1):41–51.

29. **Tohen, M and Abbott, CC.** Use of electroconvulsive therapy in bipolar depression, *The American Journal of Psychiatry* 2015;**172**(1):3–5.

30. **Kotzalidis, GD, Pacchiarotti, I, Rapinesi, C, Murru, A, Colom, F, and Vieta, E.** Differential effectiveness of right unilateral versus bilateral electroconvulsive therapy in resistant bipolar depression, Am J Psychiatry 2015;**172**(3):294.

31. **McGirr, A, Karmani, S, Arsappa, R, Berlim, MT, Thirthalli, J, Muralidharan, K, and Yatham, LN.** Clinical efficacy and safety of repetitive transcranial magnetic stimulation in acute bipolar depression, *World Psychiatry: Official Journal of the World Psychiatric Association* 2016;**15**(1):85–6.

32. **Fitzgerald, PB, Hoy, KE, Elliot, D, McQueen, S, Wambeek, LE, and Daskalakis, ZJ.** A negative double-blind controlled trial of sequential bilateral rTMS in the treatment of bipolar depression, *Journal of Affective Disorders* 2016;**198**:158–62.

33. **Holtzheimer, PE, Kelley, M., Gross, RE, Filkowski, MM, Garlow, SJ, Barrocas, A,** . . . and **Mayberg, HS.** Subcallosal cingulate deep brain stimulation for treatment-resistant unipolar and bipolar depression, *Archives of General Psychiatry* 2012;**69**(2):150–8.

34. **Gippert, SM, Switala, C, Bewernick, BH, Kayser, S, Brauer, A, Coenen, VA, and Schlaepfer, TE.** Deep brain stimulation for bipolar disorder-review and outlook. CNS Spectrums 2016;1–4.

35. **Chopra, A, Tye, SJ, Lee, KH, Matsumoto, J, Klassen, B, Adams, AC, and Frye, MA.** Voltage-dependent mania after subthalamic nucleus deep brain stimulation in Parkinson's disease: a case report, *Biological Psychiatry* 2011;**70**(2):e5–7.

36. **Baldessarini, RJ, Leahy, L, Arcona, S, Gause, D, Zhang, W, and Hennen, J.** Patterns of psychotropic drug prescription for US patients with diagnoses of bipolar disorders, Psychiatr Serv 2007;**58**(1):85–91.

37. **Pacchiarotti, I., Bond, DJ, Baldessarini, RJ, Nolen, WA, Grunze, H, Licht, RW,** . . . and **Vieta, E.** The International Society for Bipolar Disorders (ISBD) task force report on antidepressant use in bipolar disorders, *The American Journal of Psychiatry* 2013;**170**(11):1249–62.

38. **Sidor, MM, and Macqueen, GM.** An update on antidepressant use in bipolar depression, Curr Psychiatry Rep 2012;**14**(6):696–704.

39. **Sidor, MM and Macqueen, GM.** Antidepressants for the acute treatment of bipolar depression: a systematic review and meta-analysis, J Clin Psychiatry 2011;**72**(2):156–67.

40. **Amsterdam JD, Lorenzo-Luaces L, Soeller I, Li SQ, Mao JJ, and DeRubeis RJ.** Short-term venlafaxine vs lithium monontherapy for bipolar II major depressive episodes: effectiveness and mood conversion rate, *British Journal of Psychiatry* Feb 2016, DOI: 10.1192/bjp.bp.115.169375.

41. Frye, MA, Helleman, G, McElroy, SL, Altshuler, LL, Black, DO, Keck, PE, Jr, Nolen, WA, Kupka, R, Leverich, GS, Grunze, H, Mintz, J, Post, RM, and Suppes, T. Correlates of treatment-emergent mania associated with antidepressant treatment in bipolar depression, Am J Psychiatry 2009a;**166**(2):164–72.

42. Frye, MA, McElroy, SL, Prieto, ML, Harper, KL, Walker, DL., Kung, S, . . . and Biernacka, JM. Clinical risk factors and serotonin transporter gene variants associated with antidepressant-induced mania, *The Journal of Clinical Psychiatry* 2015b;**76**(2):174–80.

43. Frye MA, McElroy SL, Prieto ML, Kung S, Veldic M, Bobo WV, Cuellar-Barboza AB, Colby CL, Geske J, Bond DJ, Feeder S, Mori N, and Biernacka JM. Genome-wide association study of antidepressant-induced mania. Presented at the Annual Meeting of the International Society of Bipolar Disorder, Amsterdam, the Netherlands, 14 July 2016.

44. Miklowitz, DJ, Otto, MW, Frank, E, Reilly-Harrington, NA, Wisniewski, SR, Kogan, JN, Nierenberg, AA, Calabrese, JR., Marangell, LB, Gyulai, L, Araga, M, Gonzalez, JM, Shirley, ER, Thase, ME, and Sachs, GS. Psychosocial treatments for bipolar depression: a 1-year randomized trial from the Systematic Treatment Enhancement Program, Arch Gen Psychiatry 2007;**64**(4):419–26.

45. Newport, DJ, Carpenter, LL, McDonald, WM, Potash, JB, Tohen, M, and Nemeroff, CB. Ketamine and other NMDA antagonists: early clinical trials and possible mechanisms in depression, *The American Journal of Psychiatry* 2015;**172**(10):950–66.

46. Bobo, WV, Voort, JL, Croarkin, PE, Leung, JG, Tye, SJ, and Frye, MA. Ketamine for treatment-resistant unipolar and bipolar major depression: critical review and implications for clinical practice, *Depression and Anxiety* 2016;**00**:1–13.

47. Kantrowitz, JT, Halberstam, B, and Gangwisch, J. Single-dose ketamine followed by daily D-Cycloserine in treatment-resistant bipolar depression. The Journal of Clinical Psychiatry 2015;**76**(6):737–8.

48. Brennan, BP, Hudson, JI, Jensen, JE, McCarthy, J, Roberts, JL, Prescot, AP, Cohen, BM, Pope, HG, Jr, Renshaw, PF, and Ongur, D. Rapid enhancement of glutamatergic neurotransmission in bipolar depression following treatment with riluzole, *Neuropsychopharmacology* 2010;**35**(3):834–46.

49. Zarate, CA, Jr, Brutsche, NE, Ibrahim, L, Franco-Chaves, J, Diazgranados, N, Cravchik, A, Selter, J, Marquardt, CA, Liberty, V, and Luckenbaugh, DA. Replication of ketamine's antidepressant efficacy in bipolar depression: a randomized controlled add-on trial, Biol Psychiatry 2012;**71**(11):939–46.

50. Goldberg, JF, Burdick, KE, and Endick, CJ. Preliminary randomized, double-blind, placebo-controlled trial of pramipexole added to mood stabilizers for treatment-resistant bipolar depression, Am J Psychiatry 2004;**161**(3):564–6.

51. Zarate, CA, Jr, Payne, JL, Singh, J, Quiroz, JA, Luckenbaugh, DA, Denicoff, KD, Charney, DS, and Manji, HK. Pramipexole for bipolar II depression: a placebo-controlled proof of concept study, Biol Psychiatry 2004;**56**(1):54–60.

52. Leboyer, M, Soreca, I, Scott, J, Frye, M, Henry, C, Tamouza, R, and Kupfer, DJ. Can bipolar disorder be viewed as a multi-system inflammatory disease?, J Affect Disord 2012;**141**(1):1–10.

53. Berk, M, Dean, OM, Cotton, SM, Gama, CS, Kapczinski, F, Fernandes, B, Kohlmann, K, Jeavons, S, Hewitt, K, Moss, K, Allwang, C, Schapkaitz, I, Cobb, H, Bush, AI, Dodd, S, and Malhi, GS. Maintenance N-acetyl cysteine treatment for bipolar disorder: a double-blind randomized placebo controlled trial, BMC Med 2012;**10**:91.

54. **Nery, FG, Monkul, ES, Hatch, JP, Fonseca, M, Zunta-Soares, GB, Frey, BN, Bowden, CL, and Soares, JC,.** Celecoxib as an adjunct in the treatment of depressive or mixed episodes of bipolar disorder: a double-blind, randomized, placebo-controlled study, Hum Psychopharmacol 2008;**23**(2):87–94.

55. **Kemp, DE, Schinagle, M, Gao, K, Conroy, C, Ganocy, SJ, Ismail-Beigi, F, and Calabrese, JR.** PPAR-gamma agonism as a modulator of mood: proof-of-concept for pioglitazone in bipolar depression. CNS Drugs 2014;**28**(6):571–81.

56. **Rosenblat, JD, Kakar, R, et al.** Anti-inflammatory agents in the treatment of bipolar depression: a systematic review and meta-analysis, *Bipolar Disorders* 2016;**18**(2):89–101.

57. **Frye, MA, Grunze, H, Suppes, T, McElroy, SL, Keck, PE, Jr, Walden, J, Leverich, GS, Altshuler, LL, Nakelsky, S, Hwang, S, Mintz, J, and Post, RM.** A placebo-controlled evaluation of adjunctive modafinil in the treatment of bipolar depression, Am J Psychiatry 2007;**164**(8):1242–9.

58. **Calabrese, JR, Frye, MA, Yang, R, and Ketter, TA.** Efficacy and safety of adjunctive armodafinil in adults with major depressive episodes associated with bipolar I disorder: a randomized, double-blind, placebo-controlled, multicenter trial, The Journal of Clinical Psychiatry 2014;**75**(10):1054–61.

59. **Ketter, TA, Yang, R, and Frye, MA.** Adjunctive armodafinil for major depressive episodes associated with bipolar I disorder, *Journal of Affective Disorders* 2015;**181**:87–91.

60. **Frye, MA, Amchin, J, Bauer, M, Adler, C, Yang, R, and Ketter, TA.** Randomized, placebo-controlled, adjunctive study of armodafinil for bipolar I depression: implications of novel drug design and heterogeneity of concurrent bipolar maintenance treatments, *International Journal of Bipolar Disorders* 2015a;**3**(1):34.

61. **Yatham, LN, Vieta, E, Goodwin, GM, Bourin, M, de Bodinat, C, Laredo, J, and Calabrese, JR.** Agomelatine or placebo as adjunctive therapy to a mood stabiliser in bipolar I depression: randomised double-blind placebo-controlled trial, *The British Journal of Psychiatry: the Journal of Mental Science* 2016;**208**(1):78–86.

Calabrese, JR, Ketter, TA, Youakim, JM, Tiller, JM, Yang, R, and Frye, MA. Adjunctive armodafinil for major depressive episodes associated with bipolar I disorder: a randomized, multicenter, double-blind, placebo-controlled, proof-of-concept study, *The Journal of Clinical Psychiatry* 2010;**71**(10):1363–70.

Chapter 8

Evidence-based maintenance treatment of bipolar disorder

Dina Popovic and Eduard Vieta

Introduction

The ongoing research on bipolar disorder (BD) has highlighted its pervasive and debilitating nature, characterized by lifelong recurrent episodes and residual intra-episodic symptomatology.[1] Almost half of all treated patients experience a recurrence within two years and 70–90% within five years,[2] while the lifetime recurrence rate is 95%.[3]

Management of BD after acute treatment of mood episodes entails first continuation therapy aiming to prevent relapses, followed by maintenance therapy focusing on prevention of recurrences.[4] Although the main aim of long-term treatment is the prevention of future mood episodes, the more realistic key goal is to reduce inter-episode symptomatology alongside with a reduction in the frequency and severity of episodes.

The maintenance treatment of BD represents a major clinical challenge. The current first-line treatment strategies for long-term treatment of BD are represented by lithium, lamotrigine, valproate, olanzapine, quetiapine in monotherapy and as adjunctive therapy, aripiprazole for the prevention of manic events, risperidone long-acting injection monotherapy and as adjunctive therapy, and adjunctive ziprasidone for the prevention of mood events.[5]

When several treatment options are available for a specific indication, having a reliable estimate of comparative efficacy (prevention of any mood episode, of manic, hypomanic, or mixed episode, and of depressive episode), tolerability, and acceptability is clinically useful.

Another common dilemma that clinicians face is whether they should combine treatments. It is usually recommended to initially attempt to manage patients in monotherapy in order to enhance adherence and minimize side effects, but combination therapy is often necessary.

Monotherapy trials against placebo remain the gold standard design for determining efficacy in BD.[6] A recommended tool for reporting results of clinical trials for bipolar disorder is represented by the number needed to treat (NNT) analysis.[7] NNT summarizes the effect of treatment in terms of the number of patients a clinician needs to treat with a particular therapy to expect to prevent one adverse event. NNT is a measure of effect size, and calculation of the NNT can quantify the clinical relevance of a statistically significant study result.[8] Although NNT has been described as 'the least misleading and most clinically useful measure of treatment effectiveness',[9] it is considered likely to help translate efficacy-driven clinical data to information that will more readily guide clinicians on the benefits of specific interventions in BD.[7]

Polarity index (PI) is a novel metric for bipolar disorders that aims to guide clinicians in choosing optimal management strategy for long-term maintenance treatment. PI is a measure of the relative prophylactic efficacy of drugs used in BD. PI is derived by dividing the number needed to treat (NNT) for the prevention of depressive episodes by the NNT for the prevention of manic episodes.[10] Drugs with a PI superior to one have stronger antimanic versus antidepressant prophylactic properties, whereas those with PI inferior to one are more effective for preventing depressive episodes than the manic ones. Drugs with the PI of one have a comparable antimanic and antidepressive potential.[10]

Drugs for maintenance treatment of bipolar disorder

In general, if a patient has responded satisfactorily to a certain drug during the acute phase, the same treatment should be maintained during maintenance treatment. This was confirmed in two randomized controlled trials (RCTs).[11,12]

Table 8.1 summarizes the characteristics of the placebo-controlled RCTs for all the antipsychotics used for maintenance treatment of BD.

Aripiprazole

Two of three RCTs have found aripiprazole efficacious for maintenance treatment of bipolar I disorder, as monotherapy or as adjunctive treatment. One relapse-prevention study was performed on efficacy of aripiprazole in monotherapy in 161 BD I patients.[13] The results suggested that aripiprazole 15–30 mg/day was significantly superior to placebo in prevention of relapse into any mood episode during a 100-week-long double-blind treatment, with an NNT value of 6.[13] Aripiprazole was significantly superior to placebo in preventing relapse to mania, which translates into an NNT of 7. No difference in prevention of depressive relapses was noted between aripiprazole and placebo. Results have been similar in RCTs involving aripiprazole as adjunctive therapy. This was shown in a 52-week, relapse-prevention RCT (N=337) that assessed the efficacy of aripiprazole as adjunctive treatment to lithium or divalproex in patients with manic/mixed episodes who displayed inadequate response to lithium or divalproex.[14] Results suggested that patients in remission for 12 weeks who were randomized to add-on treatment with aripiprazole had lower rates of relapse to manic (NNT=10) but not depressive episodes (NNT=33.3).[14,10]

According to the pooled data from these two studies,[13,14] the PI of aripiprazole is 4.38, suggesting a higher antimanic versus antidepressive efficacy.

Given that efficacy was shown for the prevention of any mood episode and for mania in particular, aripiprazole represents a first-line option for treatment and prevention of mania in maintenance treatment of bipolar disorder.[15]

Table 8.1 Characteristics of included randomized controlled studies of antipsychotics in maintenance treatment of bipolar disorder

Trial (in order of appearance in text)	Patient inclusion criteria (maintenance phase)	Duration (weeks)	Number randomized	Dosage (mg/day) or plasma levels/ Mean dosage
Keck et al., 2007	Bipolar I ≥ 18 years YMRS ≤ 10 MADRS ≤ 13 No hospitalization in previous 3 months	100	ARI=78 PLA=83	ARI: 15–30mg/day Mean: 23.8 mg/day
Marcus et al., 2011	Bipolar I YMRS ≥ 16 Current or recent manic/mixed episode Inadequate response to lithium or valproate YMRS ≥ 16 and ≤ 35% decrease from baseline at 2 weeks	52	ARI + LI/VPA=168 PLA + LI/VPA=169	ARI: 10–30 mg/day
Tohen et al., 2006	Bipolar I ≥ 18 years YMRS ≤ 12 HAM-D ≤ 8 2 prior mixed or manic episodes in past 6 years	48	OLZ=225 PLA=136	OLZ: 5–20 mg/day
Vieta et al., 2008(a)	Bipolar I ≥ 18 years YMRS ≤ 12 HAM-D ≤ 12	104	QUE + LI/VPA=336 PLA + LI/VPA=367	QUE: 400–800 mg/day Mean: 497 mg/day LI: 0.5–1.2 mEq/L VPA:50–125 μg/mL
Suppes et al., 2009	Bipolar I ≥ 18 years YMRS ≤ 10 MADRS ≤ 13	104	QUE + LI/VPA=310 PLA + LI/VPA=313	QUE: 400–800 mg/day Mean: 519 mg/die LI: 0.5–1.2 mEq/L Mean: 0.71–0.74 mEq/L VPA:50–125 μg/mL Mean: 68.91–71.38 μg/mL
Weisler et al.	Bipolar I YMRS ≤ 12 MADRS ≤ 12 Acute current or recent (past 26 weeks) manic, depressive, or mixed index episode treated with QUE	104	QUE=404 LI=364 PLA=404	QUE: 300–800 mg/day Li: 0.6–1.2 mEq/L

Table 8.1 Continued

Trial (in order of appearance in text)	Patient inclusion criteria (maintenance phase)	Duration (weeks)	Number randomized	Dosage (mg/day) or plasma levels/ Mean dosage
Quiroz et al., 2010	Bipolar I 18–65 years Recent manic/mixed episode or stable patients with ≥ 1 mood episode in past 4 months	96	RLAI=140 PLA=136	RLAI: 12.5–50 mg i.m. Mean: 25 mg
Macfadden et al., 2009	Bipolar I 18–70 years ≥ 4 episodes in the past year	52	RLAI + TAU=65 PLA + TAU=59	RLAT: 25–50 mg / 2 weeks
Bowden et al., 2010	Bipolar I ≥ 18 years Current or recent manic/ mixed episode MRS ≥ 14	24	ZIP + LI/ VPA=127 PLA + LI/ VPA=113	ZIP: 80-160 mg/die LI: 0.6–1.2 mEq/L Mean: 0.7– 0.9 mEq/L VPA:50–125 µg/mL Mean: 67.4–72.8
Berwaerts et al., 2012	Bipolar I Manic or mixed episode YMRS ≥ 20 18–65 years Minimum 2 lifetime episodes	171	PALI:146 PLA: 144 OLZ: 82	PALI: 3–12 mg/day OLZ: 5–20 mg/day
Vieta et al., 2012	Bipolar I ≥ 2 mood episodes in the previous year	52	RLAI: 132 OLZ: 131 PBO: 135	OLZ: 10 mg/day RIS: 25–50 mg i.m.

* NNT analyses refer to 12-month period

PLA=placebo, ARI=aripiprazole, OLZ=olanzapine, QUE=quetiapine, RLAI=risperidone long-acting injection, TAU=treatment as usual, ZIP=ziprasidone, PALI=paliperidone ER

Aripiprazole is usually started at a dose of 10 or 15 mg per day, and may be increased to 15 or 30mg per day. Lower starting doses of 2 or 5 mg per day may help prevent side effects. Common side effects include tremor, akathisia and other extrapiramidal symptoms, headache, agitation, anxiety, nausea, and xerostomia. The incidence of extrapyramidal symptoms may be higher in subjects taking aripiprazole compared with other second-generation antipsychotics such as quetiapine and olanzapine.[16]

Olanzapine

Two placebo-controlled studies with maintenance treatment phases of 12 and 18 months have assessed the efficacy of olanzapine as maintenance treatment of BD,[17,18] and two additional RCTs where olanzapine was included as control arm.[19,20]

When comparing olanzapine to placebo over 12 months,[17] the NNT was 3 for prevention of symptomatic relapse to any mood episode, indicating a large clinical maintenance effect size difference between olanzapine and placebo. When olanzapine plus lithium or valproate was compared with placebo plus lithium or valproate over an 18-month period, the NNT for the prevention of any episode was not significant.

Furthermore, olanzapine showed a significant difference in the risk of relapse into manic episodes over placebo for up to 12 months,[17] corresponding to an NNT of 5; however, no significant differences emerged from the study comparing olanzapine combined with lithium or valproate with placebo combined with lithium or valproate over 18 months.[18] Olanzapine in monotherapy or combined with lithium or divalproex was not significantly superior to placebo in preventing relapse into depressive episodes.[17]

Olanzapine was included as an active control arm in two additional RCTs.[19,20] In both studies, patients receiving olanzapine had a significantly longer time to a recurrence of mood episode than either risperidone long-acting injection (RLAI)[19] and paliperidone extended release (ER).[20]

Overall, olanzapine in monotherapy has proven efficacy for prevention of any mood episode as well as manic episodes. The PI of olanzapine, based on the weighted mean of three RCTs[18,17,19] is 2.98.[10]

Notwithstanding olanzapine's proven efficacy, it has a number of potentially serious metabolic side effects, such as increased weight gain and increased risk of developing diabetes mellitus type II. Other side effects include increased cholesterol and triglycerids, dyspepsia, constipation, xerostomia, somnolence, fatigue, insomnia, and extrapyramidal symptoms.[16] The recommended dose is 5–20 mg at bedtime.

Quetiapine

Three placebo-controlled randomized double-blind studies assessed the efficacy of quetiapine in long-term treatment of BD I.[21,22,23,24] Two studies[21,23] assessing effectiveness of quetiapine as add-on therapy during continuation treatment for up to 104 weeks demonstrated that quetiapine in combination with lithium or divalproex was significantly more effective than lithium or divalproex alone in the prevention of mood episodes, which translates into an NNT of 4. In a study by Weisler et al.,[24] evaluating quetiapine as monotherapy for up to 104 weeks, quetiapine was found effective in the prevention of any mood episode, with an NNT of 3.

Quetiapine in combination with lithium or divalproex was significantly more effective than the placebo in combination with lithium or divalproex in preventing recurrence of mania, assuming an NNT value of 7 in the study by Vieta et al.[21] and 9 in the study by Suppes et al.[23] Likewise, quetiapine in monotherapy[24] was significantly more effective than placebo in the prevention of mania, with an NNT of 3.

NNTs were significant for quetiapine plus lithium or divalproex in preventing depressive relapses in the two studies evaluating quetiapine as adjunctive therapy, with values of 7[21] and 6.[23]

Quetiapine in monotherapy assumed an NNT value of 4 in the prevention of depressive episodes.[24]

Taken together, these data indicate that quetiapine alone and combined with lithium or valproate was effective in preventing any mood episode.[15] Quetiapine seems to have a similar efficacy for prevention of mania and depression, with polarity index of 1.14.[10]

Generally the starting dose is 100–200 mg/die, with typical dose of 400–800 mg/die in both acute and maintenance treatment. Quetiapine can cause clinically meaningful increase in insulin resistance. Other common side effects include dizziness, dry mouth, headache, and somnolence.[16]

Risperidone long-acting injection

Although the long-term efficacy of oral risperidone has not been assessed,[5] four RCTs have examined the efficacy of RLAI for maintenance treatment in BD.[25,26,19]

The first study, by Quiroz et al.,[25] examined the long-term efficacy of RLAI[25] in patients with recent manic or mixed episode followed up for up to 24 months. RLAI monotherapy was shown to be superior to placebo in preventing any mood episode with an NNT of 4. A study conducted by Macfadden et al.[26] assessed RLAI as an adjunct to treatment as usual for 52 weeks in 139 patients who had frequently relapsing BD. Significantly fewer patients in the adjunctive RLAI group relapsed into any mood episode compared with those in the placebo group, corresponding to an NNT of 5.

When comparing RLAI to placebo over 24 months,[25] NNT was 4 for the prevention of manic recurrences and 8 in the 52-week follow-up trial conducted by Macfadden et al.[26]

The third randomized controlled trial assessing efficacy and safety of RLAI monotherapy for recurrence prevention in patients with bipolar I disorder.[19] Time to recurrence of any mood episode was significantly longer with RLAI versus placebo; the difference was significant for time to recurrence of elevated mood episodes but not depressive episodes.

Overall, RLAI has proven efficacy for the prevention of any kind of mood episodes, as well as for the prevention of mania (NNT=5) while it did not result effective for the prevention of depressive episodes (NNT=54). PI of RLAI, based on the results of the three studies, is 12.09, depicting its predominantly antimanic action.[10]

The usual starting dose of RLAI is 12.5–25 mg every two weeks, with lower dosage recommended in patients with lower body mass index or increased sensitivity to side effects. The dose may be increased to 37.5 or 50 mg every two weeks. A minimum of four weeks should pass between dose adjustments.[16]

Ziprasidone

The efficacy of adjunctive ziprasidone for maintenance treatment of bipolar mania was demonstrated in a recent six-month-long RCT in 239 patients with BD I.[27] When comparing ziprasidone to placebo, NNT assumed the value of 8 for the prevention of any mood episode while it was not significant for the prevention of manic (NNT=15) or depressive episodes (NNT=56). Thus, the PI of ziprasidone is 3.91. No maintenance studies have examined the efficacy of ziprasidone in monotherapy. The recommended starting dose of ziprasidone—in adjunct to lithium or ziprasidone—is 40 mg twice per day, but may be increased to 160 mg/day based on tolerability and efficacy. Common side effects (>10%) are somnolence and headache. Less common side effects include extrapyramidal symptoms.[27,16]

Paliperidone ER

One recent RCT assessed the efficacy of paliperidone ER in maintenance treatment of BD.[20] In this two-year-long RCT, paliperidone ER was compared to placebo in 290 patients who remitted from acute manic or mixed episode, and to olanzapine in 82 patients who remitted with olanzapine and where maintained on it (non-randomized arm). The median time to recurrence was longer in patients who received paliperidone than placebo, but olanzapine was found to be more effective in prevention of mood episodes than paliperidone. Other RCTs are necessary to assess the efficacy and tolerability of paliperidone.

Paliperidone can be initiated at dose of 6 mg/day and the dose can be titrated up by 3 mg every 2–3 days within the range of 2–12 mg per day. Common side effects are akathisia, headache, somnolence, dizziness, and nausea.[16]

Table 8.2 summarizes all the RCTs of mood stabilizers in the maintenance treatment of BD.

Lamotrigine

Two RCTs compared lamotrigine, lithium, and placebo in maintenance treatment of recently manic[28] and depressed[29] bipolar I patients. Since the studies were prospectively designed for combined analyses, a pooled analysis from the two discussed studies,[30] allowing greater power with respect to the original studies, was available for NNT analysis and therefore included in the present chapter. An additional double-blind, placebo-controlled study examining lamotrigine as maintenance monotherapy for rapid cycling bipolar patients was available for NNT analysis exclusively for prevention of any mood episode.[31]

Compared to placebo, lamotrigine in monotherapy was found to be effective in the prevention of any mood episode in recently manic patients[28] with an NNT of 5, and showed no significant difference in recently depressed patients.[29,10] Data emerging from the pooled analyses[30] evidenced an NNT of 11 for prevention of any mood episode.

Lamotrigine was not significantly superior to placebo in the prevention of mania in any of the studies discussed.[28,29,30]

Lamotrigine was found to be superior to placebo in preventing depressive episodes in recently manic patients,[28] with an NNT value of 7. In contrast, lamotrigine was not significantly superior to placebo in the prevention of depressive episode neither in recently depressed patients[29] nor in the pooled analyses.[30]

Lamotrigine in monotherapy was found effective in preventing any kind of mood episode. Its effectiveness was also demonstrated for the prevention of depressive episodes in recently manic patients (NNT=21). The PI of lamotrigine, indicative of its predominantly antidepressive properties, is 0.40.

Table 8.2 Characteristics of included randomized controlled studies of mood stabilizers in maintenance treatment of bipolar disorder

Trial (in order of appearance in text)	Patient inclusion criteria (maintenance phase)	Duration (weeks)	Number randomized	Dosage (mg/day) or plasma levels / Mean dosage
Tohen et al., 2004	Bipolar I 18–70 years YMRS ≤ 12 HRSD-21 ≤ 8	72	LI/VPA + PLA=48 LI/VPA + OLZ=51	OLZ: 5–20 mg/day Mean: 12.5 mg/day LI: 0.66–0.86 mEq/l VPA: 60.1–73.8 μg/mL
Bowden et al., 2003	Bipolar I ≥ 18 years Current or recent (hypo)mania ≥ 1 additional (hypo)manic and 1 depressive episode in the past 3 years	76	LAM: 59 LI: 46 PLA:70	LAM: 100–400 mg/die LI: 0.8–1.1 mEq/L
Calabrese et al., 2003	Bipolar I ≥ 18 years Current or recent MDE ≥1 additional (hypo)manic and 1 depressive episode in the past 3 years	72	LAM: 221 LI: 121 PLA: 121	LAM: 50–400 mg/die Mean: 200 mg/die LI: 0.8–1.1 mEq/L Mean: 0.8 ± 0.3 mEq/L
Calabrese et al., 2000	Bipolar I and II rapid cycling ≥ 18 years ≤ 14 HAM-D ≤ 12 MRS < 3 on item 3 HAM-D stable for 4 weeks	26	LAM: 90 PLA: 87	LAM: 100–300 mg/day
Prien et al., 1973	Manic-depressive, manic type	24*	LI:101 PLA: 104	LI: 0.5–1.4 mEq/L
Bowden et al., 2000	Bipolar I 18–70 years Manic episode ≤ 3 months before randomization MRS ≤ 11 DSS ≤ 13 GAS > 60 No serious suicidal risk	52	VPA: 187 LI: 90 PLA: 92	VPA: 71–125 μg/mL LI: 0.8–1.2 mmol/L
Vieta et al., 2008(b)	Bipolar I or II ≥ 18 years YMRS ≤ 12 MADRS ≤ 20 No acute episodes in 6 months	52	OXC + LI=26 PLA + LI=29	OXC: 1,200 mg/day LI: 0.6 mEq/l

* NNT analyses refer to 12-month period

PLA=placebo, LI=lithium, VPA=valproate, TAU=treatment as usual, LAM=lamotrigine, OXC=oxcarbazepine

Treatment guidelines recommend a starting dose of 25 mg per day for the first two weeks, which can be increased then to 50mg/die, taken in two separate doses. Following this, the dose may be increased by 25–50mg/day, one week at a time for each increase. The slow titration reduces the risk of serious and potentially life-threatening skin rash (0.1% risk of toxic epidermal necrolysis—Stevens-Johnson syndrome). The target dose generally ranges from 50 to 200 mg per day. An ER formulation is available for once-per-day dosing. Common side effects include nausea, dyspepsia, pain, insomnia, and benign cutaneous reactions.[16]

Lithium

Lithium has long been considered the gold standard of BD maintenance treatment. The first double-blind trial by Prien et al.[32] assessed the efficacy of lithium over a two-year period. NNT analyses relevant to a one-year period evidenced effectiveness of lithium in preventing any mood episode, translating to an NNT of 4.[10] Since the mid 1970s until 2000, no RCTs assessing lithium efficacy were published. From 2000 on, four double-blind studies examined the efficacy of lithium as a maintenance treatment.[33,28,29,24] In the study by Bowden et al.,[33] neither lithium nor valproate were significantly superior to placebo in preventing mood episodes over one year in a cohort of 372 patients with BD I. In two studies,[28,29] lithium was studied as an active comparator medication compared to a lamotrigine-enriched sample of patients with BD I. In the study by Bowden et al.,[28] lithium was found to be significantly more effective than placebo in preventing any mood episode, with an NNT of 4 while in recently depressed BD I patients the difference was not significant. In a pooled analysis of the two studies,[30] lithium was significantly more effective than placebo in preventing any mood episode, with an NNT value of 7. In a RCT conducted by Weisler et al.[24] where bipolar I patients were followed up for up to 104 weeks, lithium, assessed as active comparator, has proven its effectiveness in preventing any kind of mood episode, with an NNT of 3.

Regarding the prevention of manic episodes, in the study by Prien et al.[32] lithium was effective in the prevention of manic episodes, with an NNT of 4. Lithium was also found to be significantly more effective than placebo in preventing mania in recently manic patients,[28] with an NNT of 2, as well as in pooled analyses of the two studies.[30]

Likewise, in the study by Weisler et al.,[24] lithium assumed an NNT value of 3 for mania prevention; however, lithium was not significantly superior to placebo in preventing manic recurrences in the remaining two studies.[33,29]

Lithium was found significantly superior to placebo in preventing depressive episodes, with an NNT of 4, only in the study by Weisler et al.[24] while it resulted not significantly superior to placebo in preventing depression in any other of the studies as discussed previously.[32,33,28,29,30]

In conclusion, since the efficacy of lithium was largely demonstrated for the prevention of any mood episode, in particular for mania, lithium continues to represent a first-line maintenance treatment for bipolar disorder for the treatment and prevention of mania.

Pooled results of the previously discussed five studies suggest an NNT of 4.4 for prevention of manic episodes, and NNT of 6.1 for the prevention of depressive episodes, with PI of 1.39, suggesting that lithium may be the only predominantly antimanic mood stabilizer.[15]

Lithium was also shown to reduce suicide risk in patients with bipolar disorder I. A meta-analysis on 33 RCTs by Baldessarini et al.[34] yielded 13-fold lower rates of suicide and reported suicide attempts.

The initial dose of lithium is 300 mg once a day. It is then titrated to achieve serum levels of 0.5mEq/L- 1.2 mEq/L. The efficacy of lithium is dose-dependent and reliably correlates with serum concentrations. Lower levels are considered to be non-effective, and serum level above this range would lead to side effects and toxicity.

Common side effects include weight gain, tremor, gastrointestinal distress, impaired concentration, thirst, polyuria, and hypothyiroidism.[35]

If lithium needs to be discontinued it needs to be done very gradually, since abrupt discontinuation is associated with higher rate of recurrence, even after a good response and long illness-free period.[36]

Valproate

There is only one published study assessing valproate in maintenance treatment of BD. A randomized, double-blind, parallel-group multicentre study of treatment outcomes was conducted over a 52-week maintenance period.[33] Patients with a previous manic episode were randomized to maintenance treatment with divalproex, lithium, or placebo. Although the authors concluded that the treatment arms did not differ significantly on time to recurrence of any mood episode during maintenance therapy, the NNT for prevention of any mood episode was 7; however, valproate did not result superior to placebo in preventing neither manic (NNT=22) nor depressive episodes (NNT=11).[15,10]

Other randomized not placebo-controlled trials showed that valproate may be as effective as lithium or olanzapine in the prevention of recurrences, in particular depressive recurrences.[37]

Valproate is initiated at a dose of 300–500 mg once a day, and titrated to achieve a target serum level of 50–125 mcg/mL. Long-acting preparations are available that can be prescribed once per day.[16]

Carbamazepine

Although carbamazepine was the first agent after lithium to be advocated for long-term treatment of BD and two lithium-controlled studies indicate the drug's efficacy in relapse prevention,[38,39] currently there are no available long-term placebo-controlled trials. There is also evidence that carbamazepine may be more effective in preventing recurrences in subjects affected by bipolar II disorder compared with those with BD I.[40]

A meta-analysis of four RCTs, with a total of 464 patients, supports that carbamazepine has similar efficacy to lithium regarding rates of relapse, but higher withdrawal rate due to side effects. Due to the absence of placebo-controlled studies, tolerability issues, and the fact that carbamazepine is inducer of cytochrome p450 (and thus induces the metabolism of various other agents, as well as its own metabolism, which requires adjustment of dose of carbamazepine), treatment guidelines recommend carbamazepine as second-line maintenance option for BD.[16]

Carbamazepine is initially prescribed at a dose of 200 mg twice per day and can be incremented by 200 mg/die. The maximum daily dose is 800 mg twice per day. Common side effects include dizziness, somnolence, ataxia, gastrointestinal distress, and benign elevation of transaminases. Slow titration reduces the occurrence of these side effects. Serious side effects include blood dyscrasias and rashes.[16]

Oxcarbazepine

One RCT assessed the efficacy of oxcarbazepine compared to placebo as adjuncts to ongoing treatment with lithium in 55 patients with BD I and BD II for a period of 52 weeks.[22] The results evidenced a lower risk of recurrence to any mood episode with oxcarbazepine, corresponding to an NNT of 5, but this difference was not significant since the confidence interval crossed infinity. The same was true for the prevention of manic and depressive episodes, with NNT values of 9 and 6, respectively, neither statistically significant.[15] The lack of significant difference could be due to lack of power for the small sample size in the study.

The initial dose of oxcarbazepine is 300 mg twice daily, which can be titrated to a target dose of up to 1,200–2,400 mg/day, taken twice daily. Common side effects include dizziness, ocular disturbances, gastrointestinal distress, and somnolence. Serum levels of sodium should be monitored because oxcarbazepine can cause hyponatraemia, especially early in treatment.[16]

Other drugs

Asenapine is an atypical antipsychotic that has positive data in acute and mixed mania,[41,42,43] but no trials have been carried out so far in bipolar depression and in maintenance. For both acute studies[41,42] an extension study of nine and 40 weeks was performed.[44,45]

Cariprazine has positive data in mania[46,47,48] and bipolar depression[49] but not yet on maintenance. Clozapine has only been tested in open-label studies.[16] No placebo-controlled maintenance trials are available with antidepressants. Maintenance electroconvulsive therapy (ECT) may be advised in treatment-resistant patients who responded to acute ECT.[50,51]

Issues with bipolar maintenance treatment trials

Unlike the acute treatment trials, with more than 50 trials for only acute bipolar mania, there are surprisingly few maintenance studies. In a recent review by Popovic et al.,[15] which included all the RCTs assessing the effectiveness of drugs in the prophylactic treatment of BD compared to placebo, only 15 trials were found (inclusion criteria was: a minimal duration of six months; patients over 18; while exclusion criteria was: small sample sizes (ie, fewer than 17 subjects per arm); a study sample not exclusively composed of bipolar patients; those using rating scales not validated in patients with bipolar disorder . . .). Since then, a further two trials satisfying the same inclusion criteria have been published.[20,14] It is noteworthy that some trials (eg, McIntyre et al.)[42] were excluded because they did not have a long-term placebo group. The studies were not homogeneous with respect to clinical characteristics of the sample (rapid cycling course, manic/mixed states or depression, refractory patients, or unbiased samples), sample size, and rates of study completion. In that regard, as discussed by Popovic et al.,[10] most studies enrolled enriched populations of patients who were currently or recently manic or mixed. Missing from most study designs was the recruitment of patients with index depressive episodes. Exclusion of depressed patients at enrolment may affect the polarity of mood episodes during the blinded relapse prevention phase since the study design was primarily configured to demonstrate efficacy in the delay or prevention of manic recurrence. The absence of depressive index episodes in a compound whose primary spectrum of efficacy is in depression biases outcome against the drug, or vice versa. However, the main reason why some compounds have been studied only in the context of index mania is their failure to separate from placebo in acute bipolar depression trials indicating a stronger antimanic action, which makes it more suitable for the treatment of mania and the prevention of subsequent manic episodes.[10]

Conclusion

BD is an episodic and chronic psychiatric disorder which requires maintenance treatment. The goals of maintenance treatment include preventing or delaying recurrences of new mood episodes, reducing subsyndromal symptoms, preventing cognitive decline and suicidal risk, and enhancing patients' psychosocial functioning. It is necessary to educate patients about the chronic nature of BD and the need for ongoing maintenance treatment.

References

1. Keck Jr, PE, Calabrese, JR, McIntyre, RS, McQuade, RD, Carson, WH, Eudicone, JM, Carlson, BX, Marcus, RN, and Sanchez, R. Aripiprazole monotherapy for maintenance therapy in bipolar I disorder: a 100-week, double-blind study versus placebo, J Clin Psychiatry 2007;**68**(10):1480–91.

2. Perlis, RH, Delbello, MP, Miyahara, S, Wisniewski, SR, Sachs, GS, Nierenberg, AA, and STEP-BD investigators. Revisiting depressive-prone bipolar disorder: polarity of initial mood episode and disease course among bipolar I systematic treatment enhancement program for bipolar disorder participants, Biol Psychiatry 2005;**58**(7):549–53.

3. Goodwin, FK and Jamison, K. Manic-depressive illness. In: *Bipolar Disorders and Recurrent Depression* 2nd edn (Cambridge: Oxford Press, 2007).

4. Calabrese, JR, Goldberg, JF, Ketter, TA, Suppes, T, Frye, M, White, R, DeVeaugh-Geiss, A, and Thompson, TR. Recurrence in bipolar I disorder: a post hoc analysis excluding relapses in two double blind maintenance studies, Biol Psychiatry 2006;**59**:1061–4.

5. Yatham, LN, Kennedy, SH, Schaffer, A, Parikh, SV, Beaulieu, S, O'Donovan, C, MacQueen, G, McIntyre, RS, Sharma, V, Ravindran, A, Young, LT, Young, AH, Alda, M, Milev, R, Vieta, E, Calabrese, JR, Berk, M, Ha, K, and Kapczinski, F.

Canadian Network for Mood and Anxiety Treatments (CANMAT) and International Society for Bipolar Disorders (ISBD) collaborative update of CANMAT guidelines for the management of patients with bipolar disorder: update 2009, Bipolar Disord 2009;**11**(3):225–55.

6. **Goodwin, GM, Anderson, I, Arango, C, Bowden, CL, Henry, C, Mitchell, PB, Nolen, WA, Vieta, E,** and **Wittchen, HU.** ECNP consensus meeting. Bipolar depression. Nice, March (2007), Eur Neuropsychopharmacol 2008;**18**:535–49.

7. **Martinez-Aran, A, Vieta, E, Chengappa, KN, Gershon, S, Mullen, J,** and **Paulsson, B.** Reporting outcomes in clinical trials for bipolar disorder: a commentary and suggestions for change, Bipolar Disord 2008;**10**(5):566–79.

8. **Citrome, L.** Compelling or irrelevant? Using number needed to treat can help decide, Acta Psychiatr Scand 2008;**117**:412–19.

9. **Gray, G.** *Concise Guide to Evidence-based Psychiatry* (Washington, DC: American Psychiatric Publishing Inc, 2004), 67–76.

10. **Popovic, D, Reinares, M, Goikolea, JM, Bonnin, CM, Gonzalez-Pinto, A,** and **Vieta, E.** Polarity index of pharmacological agents used for maintenance treatment of bipolar disorder, Eur Neuropsychopharmacol 2012;**22**:339–46.

11. **McElroy, SL, Bowden, CL, Collins, MA, Wozniak, PJ, Keck, PE,** Jr, and **Calabrese, JR.** Relationship of open acute mania treatment to blinded maintenance outcome in bipolar I disorder, J Affect Disord 2008 Apr;**107**(1–3):127–33.

12. **Weisler, RH, Nolen, WA, Neijber, A, Hellqvist, A, Paulsson, B;** Trial 144 Study Investigators. Continuation of quetiapine versus switching to placebo or lithium for maintenance treatment of bipolar I disorder (Trial 144: a randomized controlled study), J Clin Psychiatry 2011 Nov;**72**(11):1452–64.

13. **Keck Jr, PE, Calabrese, JR, McIntyre, RS, McQuade, RD, Carson, WH, Eudicone, JM, Carlson, BX, Marcus, RN,** and **Sanchez, R.** Aripiprazole monotherapy for maintenance therapy in bipolar I disorder: a 100-week, double-blind study versus placebo, J Clin Psychiatry 2007;**68**(10):1480–91.

14. **Marcus, R, Khan, A, Rollin, L,** et al. Efficacy of aripiprazole adjunctive to lithium or valproate in the long-term treatment of patients with bipolar I disorder with an inadequate response to lithium or valproate monotherapy: a multicenter, double-blind, randomized study, Bipolar Disord 2011;**13**:133–44.

15. **Popovic, D, Reinares, M, Amann, B, Salamero, M,** and **Vieta, E.** Number needed to treat analyses of drugs used for maintenance treatment of bipolar disorder. *Psychopharmacology* 2011;**213**:657–67.

16. **Kudlow, PA, Cha, DS, McIntyre, RS,** and **Suppes, T.** Maintenance treatments in bipolar disorder. In: *The Bipolar Book* (New York, NY: Oxford University Press, 2015), 299–318.

17. **Tohen, M, Calabrese, JR, Sachs, GS,** et al. Randomized, placebo-controlled trial of olanzapine as maintenance therapy in patients with bipolar I disorder responding to acute treatment with olanzapine, Am J Psychiatry 2006;**163**:247–56.

18. **Tohen, M, Chengappa, KN, Suppes, T, Baker, RW, Zarate, CA, Bowden, CL, Sachs, GS, Kupfer, DJ, Ghaemi, SN, Feldman, PD, Risser, RC, Evans, AR,** and **Calabrese, JR.** Relapse prevention in bipolar I disorder: 18-month comparison of olanzapine plus mood stabiliser v mood stabiliser alone, Br J Psychiatry 2004;**184**:337–45.

19. **Vieta, E, Montgomery, S, Sulaiman, AH, Cordoba, R, Huberlant, B, Martinez, L,** and **Schreiner, A.** A randomized, double-blind, placebo-controlled trial to assess prevention

of mood episodes with risperidone long-acting injectable in patients with bipolar I disorder, Eur Neuropsychopharmacol 2012 Nov;**22**(11):825–35.

20. **Berwaerts, J, Melkote, R, Nuamah, I**, and **Lim, P.** A randomized, placebo- and active-controlled study of paliperidone extended-release as maintenance treatment in patients with bipolar I disorder after an acute manic or mixed episode, J Affect Disord 2012 May;**138**(3):247–58.

21. **Vieta, E, Cruz N, García-Campayo, J, de Arce, R, Manuel Crespo, J, Vallès, V, Pérez-Blanco, J, Roca, E, Manuel Olivares, J, Moríñigo, A, Fernández-Villamor, R**, and **Comes, M.** A double-blind, randomized, placebo-controlled prophylaxis trial of oxcarbazepine as adjunctive treatment to lithium in the long-term treatment of bipolar I and II disorder, Int J Neuropsychopharmacol 2008a;**11**:445–52.

22. **Vieta, E, Suppes, T, Eggens, I, Persson, I, Paulsson, B**, and **Brecher, M.** Efficacy and safety of quetiapine in combination with lithium or divalproex for maintenance of patients with bipolar I disorder (international trial 126), J Affect Disord 2008b;**109**:251–63.

23. **Suppes, T, Vieta, E, Liu, S, Brecher, M**, and **Paulsson, B.** Maintenance treatment for patients with bipolar I disorder: results from a North American study of quetiapine in combination with lithium or divalproex (trial 127), Am J Psychiatry 2009;**166**:476–88.

24. **Weisler, RH, Nolen, WA, Neijber, A, Hellqvist, A**, and **Paulsson, B.** Quetiapine or lithium versus placebo for maintenance treatment of bipolar I disorder after stabilization on quetiapine. Presented at the 60th Institute on Psychiatric Services Congress, **Chicago, IL**, 2–5 October 2008.

25. **Quiroz, JA, Yatham, LN, Palumbo, JM, Karcher, K, Kushner, S**, and **Kusumakar, V.** Risperidone long-acting injectable monotherapy in the maintenance treatment of bipolar I disorder, Biol Psychiatry 2010;**68**(2):156–62.

26. **Macfadden, W, Alphs, L, Haskins, JT, Turner, N, Turkoz, I, Bossie, C, Kujawa, M**, and **Mahmoud, R.** A randomized, double-blind, placebo-controlled study of maintenance treatment with adjunctive risperidone long-acting therapy in patients with bipolar I disorder who relapse frequently, Bipolar Disord 2009;**11**(8):827–39.

27. **Bowden, CL, Vieta, E, Ice, KS, Schwartz, JH, Wang, PP**, and **Versavel, M.** Ziprasidone plus a mood stabilizer in subjects with bipolar I disorder: a 6-month, randomized, placebo-controlled, double-blind trial, J Clin Psychiatry 2010;**71**(2):130–7.

28. **Bowden, CL, Calabrese, JR, Sachs, G, Yatham, LN, Asghar, SA, Hompland, M, Montgomery, P, Earl, N, Smoot, TM, DeVeaugh-Geiss, J; Lamictal 606 Study Group.** A placebo-controlled 18-month trial of lamotrigine and lithium maintenance treatment in recently manic or hypomanic patients with bipolar I disorder, Arch Gen Psychiatry 2003;**60**(4):392–400.

29. **Calabrese, JR, Bowden, CL, Sachs, G, Yatham, LN, Behnke, K, Mehtonen, OP, Montgomery, P, Ascher, J, Paska, W, Earl, N, DeVeaugh-Geiss, J; Lamictal 605 Study Group.** A placebo controlled 18-month trial of lamotrigine and lithium maintenance treatment in recently depressed patients with bipolar I disorder, J Clin Psychiatry 2003;**64**(9):1013–24.

30. **Goodwin, GM, Bowden, CL, Calabrese, JR, Grunze, H, Kasper, S, White, R, Greene, P**, and **Leadbetter, R.** A pooled analysis of 2 placebo-controlled 18-month trials of lamotrigine and lithium maintenance in bipolar I disorder, J Clin Psychiatry 2004;**65**:432–41.

31. Calabrese, JR, Suppes, T, Bowden, CL, Sachs, GS, Swann, AC, McElroy, SL, Kusumakar, V, Ascher, JA, Earl, NL, Greene, PL, Monaghan, ET; Lamictal 614 Study Group. A double-blind, placebo-controlled, prophylaxis study of lamotrigine in rapid-cycling bipolar disorder, J Clin Psychiatry 2000;**61**:841–50.

32. Prien RF, Klett J, and Caffey Jr EF. Lithium carbonate and imipramine in prevention of affective episodes, Arch Gen Psychiatry 1973;**29**:420–5.

33. Bowden, CL, Calabrese, JR, McElroy, SL, Gyulai, L, Wassef, A, Petty, F, Pope, HG, Jr, Chou, JC, Keck, PE, Jr, Rhodes, LJ, Swann, AC, Hirschfeld, RM, and Wozniak, PJ. A randomized, placebo-controlled 12-month trial of divalproex and lithium in treatment of outpatients with bipolar I disorder. Divalproex Maintenance Study Group, Arch Gen Psychiatry 2000;**57**:481–9.

34. Baldessarini, RJ, Tondo, L, and Hennen, J. Treating the suicidal patient with bipolar disorder. Reducing suicide risk with lithium, Ann NY Acad Sci 2001 Apr;**932**:24–38.

35. Frye, MA, Yatham, L, Ketter, TA, Goldberg, J, Suppes, T, Calabrese, JR, Bowden, CL, Bourne, E, Bahn, RS, and Adams, B. Depressive relapse during lithium treatment associated with increased serum thyroid-stimulating hormone: results from two placebo-controlled bipolar I maintenance studies, Acta Psychiatr Scand 2009 Jul;**120**(1):10–13.

36. Suppes, T, Baldessarini, RJ, Faedda, GL, and Tohen, M. Risk of recurrence following discontinuation of lithium treatment in bipolar disorder, Arch Gen Psychiatry 1991 Dec;**48**(12):1082–8.

37. Tohen, M, Ketter, TA, Zarate, CA, Suppes, T, Frye, M, Altshuler, L, Zajecka, J, Schuh, LM, Risser, RC, Brown, E, and Baker, RW. Olanzapine versus divalproex sodium for the treatment of acute mania and maintenance of remission: a 47-week study, Am J Psychiatry 2003 Jul;**160**(7):1263–71.

38. Greil, W, Ludwig-Mayerhofer, W, Erazo, N, Engel, RR, Czernik, A, Giedke, H, Muller-Oerlinghausen, B, Osterheider, M, Rudolf, GA, Sauer, H, Tegeler, J, and Wetterling, T. Lithium vs carbamazepine in the maintenance treatment of schizoaffective disorder: a randomised study, Eur Arch Psychiatry Clin Neurosci 1997;**247**(1):42–50.

39. Hartong EG, Moleman P, Hoogduin CA, Broekman TG, and Nolen WA; LitCar Group. Prophylactic efficacy of lithium versus carbamazepine in treatment-naive bipolar patients, J Clin Psychiatry 2003 Feb;**64**(2):144–51.

40. Greil, W, Kleindienst, N, Erazo, N, and Müller-Oerlinghausen, B. Differential response to lithium and carbamazepine in the prophylaxis of bipolar disorder, J Clin Psychopharmacol 1998 Dec;**18**(6):455–60.

41. McIntyre, RS, Cohen, M, Zhao, J, Alphs, L, Macek, TA, and Panagides, J. A 3-week, randomized, placebo-controlled trial of asenapine in the treatment of acute mania in bipolar mania and mixed states, Bipolar Disord 2009a Nov;**11**(7):673–686.

42. McIntyre, RS, Cohen, M, Zhao, J, Alphs, L, Macek, TA, and Panagides, J. Asenapine in the treatment of acute mania in bipolar I disorder: a randomized, double-blind, placebo-controlled trial, J Affect Disord 2010a Apr;**122**(1–2):27–38.

43. Landbloom, RL, Mackle, M, Wu, X, Kelly, L, Snow-Adami, L, McIntyre, RS, Mathews, M, and Hundt, C. Asenapine: efficacy and safety of 5 and 10 mg bid in a 3-week, randomized, double-blind, placebo-controlled trial in adults with a manic or mixed episode associated with bipolar I disorder, J Affect Disord 2015.

44. McIntyre, RS, Cohen, M, Zhao, J, Alphs, L, Macek, TA, and Panagides, J. Asenapine versus olanzapine in acute mania: a double-blind extension study, Bipolar Disord 2009b Dec;**11**(8):815–26.

45. McIntyre, RS, Cohen, M, Zhao, J, Alphs, L, Macek, TA, and **Panagides, J**. Asenapine in the treatment of acute mania in bipolar I disorder: a randomized, double-blind, placebo-controlled trial, J Affect Disord 2010b Apr;**122**(1–2):27–38.

46. **Calabrese, JR, Keck, PE, Jr, Starace, A, Lu, K, Ruth, A, Laszlovszky, I, Németh, G**, and **Durgam, S**. Efficacy and safety of low- and high-dose cariprazine in acute and mixed mania associated with bipolar I disorder: a double-blind, placebo-controlled study, J Clin Psychiatry 2015 Mar;**76**(3):284–92.

47. **Sachs, GS, Greenberg, WM, Starace, A, Lu, K, Ruth, A, Laszlovszky, I, Németh, G**, and **Durgam, S**. Cariprazine in the treatment of acute mania in bipolar I disorder: a double-blind, placebo-controlled, phase III trial, J Affect Disord 2015 Mar 15;**174**:296–302.

48. **Durgam, S, Starace, A, Li, D, Migliore, R, Ruth, A, Németh, G**, and **Laszlovszky, I**. The efficacy and tolerability of cariprazine in acute mania associated with bipolar I disorder: a phase II trial, Bipolar Disord 2015a Feb;**17**(1):63–75.

49. **Durgam, S, Earley, W, Lipschitz, A, Guo, H, Laszlovszky, I, Németh, G, Vieta, E, Calabrese, JR**, and **Yatham, LN**. An 8-week randomized, double-blind, placebo-controlled evaluation of the safety and efficacy of cariprazine in patients with bipolar I depression, Am J Psychiatry 2015b Nov (ahead of print).

50. **Santos Pina, L, Bouckaert, F, Obbels, J, Wampers, M, Simons, W, Wyckaert, S**, and **Sienaert, P**. Maintenance electroconvulsive therapy in severe bipolar disorder: a retrospective chart review, J ECT 2015 Jul (Epub ahead of print).

51. **Minnai, GP, Salis, PG, Oppo, R, Loche, AP, Scano, F**, and **Tondo, L**. Effectiveness of maintenance electroconvulsive therapy in rapid-cycling bipolar disorder, J ECT 2011 Jun;**27**(2):123–6.

Chapter 9

The treatment of bipolar II disorder

Lakshmi N. Yatham and Muralidharan Kesavan

Introduction

Bipolar II disorder (BD II) was first described by Dunner, Gershon, and Goodwin in 1976.[1] As per the *Diagnostic and Statistical Manual of Mental Disorders* (5th edition) (DSM-5), a diagnosis of BD II is made if the patient has experienced at least one major depressive episode and one or more hypomanic episodes, in the absence of any lifetime manic episodes.[2] Hypomanic symptoms are essentially the same as manic symptoms, but of lesser severity and no psychotic features. Further, hypomanic patients do not require hospitalization and symptoms lasting for a minimum of four days is sufficient for a diagnosis of a hypomanic episode as per DSM-5.[2] The prevalence of BD II varies from 0.5 to 6.4% in the general population, depending on the criteria used.[3,4] BD II is recognized in DSM-5 but not in the *International Classification of Diseases* (10th revision) (ICD-10).

BD II has been considered a milder variant of BD by some while a more accepted conceptualization places it on a continuum between bipolar I disorder (BD I) and unipolar depression.[5] Hypomania tends to be missed often, leading to a misdiagnosis of unipolar depression.[6] While the hypomanic symptoms are less severe than the manic symptoms, the course of BD II tends to be more chronic than BD I[7] and is characterized by more depressive episodes, more time spent in depression, more frequent episodes, suicidality, and co-morbidity.[8] The predominant polarity in BD II is depression, with patients spending most of their illness in depression than hypomania. Dunner et al. reported that over a ten-year period, BD II patients experienced depression 39 times more than hypomania (50.3% vs 1.3%).[9] Similar rates were reported by Judd et al. in a study that had followed BD patients up to 20 years in which depression was experienced for 59.1% of the weeks during the study period compared to 1.9% of the weeks for hypomania.[8] It has been suggested that more suicidality in BD II might be related to BD II patients spending more time in depression.[10]

BD II tends to have high diagnostic stability as borne out by a ten-year follow-up study which reported that only 7.2% of the sample of 96 BD II patients experienced a full-blown manic episode during this period compared with 66% of patients with BD I.[11] Despite the lifetime prevalence rates of BD II being high and a course as chronic as BD I, there is little consensus on how to optimally manage this condition.

Foundations of management

Diagnose early

Since patients with BD II tend to typically seek help during a depressive episode, and not during hypomania, the diagnosis of BD II are often missed by clinicians.[6] We suggest a step-wise approach (Figure 9.1) to improve the diagnosis of BD II.

Clinicians should be vigilant for a diagnosis of BD II in any patient presenting for help with a depressive episode. As a first step, clinicians should examine the phenomenology and course of the depressive episodes to identify any indicators of bipolarity. Depression tends to typically have a younger age at onset in BD II patients compared with those with a major depressive disorder (MDD). Most individuals with BD II will describe a symptom pattern dominated by 'melancholic symptoms' (eg a profound non-reactive and anhedonic mood, impaired concentration, diurnal variation of mood and energy), although they are less likely to report the more characteristic melancholic features of early morning wakening, and appetite and weight loss—and more likely (especially in younger patients) to report converse features of hypersomnia and hyperphagia that are considered to be associated with 'atypical depression'.[12] Presence of psychotic symptoms during depression is more likely indicative of BD I than BD II. If previous treatment for depression resulted in 'mild highs' or 'irritability and dysphoria' that is more likely indicative of a BD II depression. Switching from a depressive episode to a hypomanic episode may occur either spontaneously or with treatment during the course of the disorder. About 5–15% of the patients may go on to develop a full-blown manic episode which then changes the diagnosis to BD I, irrespective of whether they experience another manic episode in their lifetime or

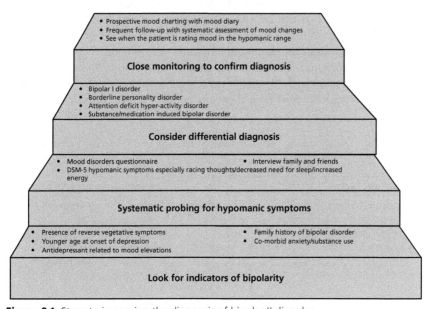

Figure 9.1 Steps to improving the diagnosis of bipolar II disorder

not. Presence of co-morbid anxiety and substance use as well as a family history of BD is more common in BD II than in those with MDD. For instance, recent evidence points towards a clustering of BD II in families, with more relatives having BD II and unipolar depression and fewer relatives with BD I.[13] Genetic factors may influence the onset of BD II, which reportedly has a slightly earlier onset than BD I, though this has not been formally investigated.

In addition, patients must be systematically probed for history of hypomanic symptoms/episodes. We recommend that all patients presenting with depressive episodes should be asked to complete a mood disorders questionnaire (MDQ).[14] This tends to help trigger patients' memory about their previous hypomanic behaviours. Those that answered yes to one or more symptoms on the checklist should be further questioned in greater detail using the DSM-5 checklist for hypomanic symptoms. As well, interviewing family members or those that live with the patient to obtain longitudinal information is often very helpful.

It is important to rule out other conditions that present with overlapping symptoms before confirming a diagnosis of BD II (see Tables 9.1–9.3).

The majority of patients with BD II will have a prior diagnosis of MDD, either because the hypomania has not yet presented or has not been formally assessed. A careful assessment as described previously, including the clinical features of depression, will help in determining a diagnosis of BD II. Borderline personality disorder also shares some components of BD II including mood swings and impulsivity, but they differ in the quality, degree, and duration of mood alterations, the degree of mood lability, and the pattern of troublesome behaviours including instability in relationships, onset, and family history.[15] Attention deficit hyperactivity disorder (ADHD) also needs to be excluded. ADHD is usually marked by ongoing concentration, attention, and academic problems in childhood (with or without hyperactivity), while those with a BD II will have either not shown such behaviours or have only experienced periods of inattention and concentration problems (along with some features of highs such as insomnia) intermittently in childhood, if at all.[16] In addition, specific cyclothymic or hyperthymic temperaments and cyclothymic disorder may cluster in families with BD and in some cases are antecedents of a frank BD I or BD II.[17] These chronic conditions more often mimic the symptoms of hypomania

Table 9.1 Differential diagnosis between bipolar disorder and borderline personality disorder

Bipolar II disorder	Borderline personality disorder
• Biphasic mood dysregulation • Mood symptoms meet threshold criteria for major depressive disorder (MDD) • Reasonable functioning during euthymic periods • Family history of bipolar II disorder or MDD	• Mood dysregulation in the depressive spectrum • Mood symptoms often do not reach threshold for MDD • Dysfunction persists even in euthymic periods • Family history of deprivation and abuse

Table 9.2 Differential diagnosis of bipolar disorder and ADHD

Bipolar II disorder	ADHD
• Onset of clear-cut symptoms typically after age 12 years	• Onset of clear-cut symptoms before age 12 years
• Onset with dysthymia or depression	• Onset of hyper or disruptive behaviours
• Episodicity	• Continuous
• Family history of mood disorders	• Family history of disruptive disorders
• Variable or negative response to stimulants	• Response to stimulants
• Response to mood stabilizers/some atypical antipsychotics	• Variable or no response to mood stabilizers/atypical antipsychotics

Table 9.3 Differential diagnosis between bipolar disorder and substance-induced mood lability

Bipolar II disorder	Substance-induced mood lability
• Alcohol, cocaine, and amphetamine use	• Polysubstance use
• Episodicity	• Continuous
• Mood problems in the absence of substance use	• Substance use without any mood problems
• Hypomania present	• Hypomania usually absent
• Family history of bipolar or other mood disorders	• Family history of externalizing and anxiety disorders

and, often, atypical episode of MDD, similar to those in BD II but of milder degree and without obvious dysfunction. Patients who abuse substances can also experience mood problems but typically those with primary substance abuse tend to abuse multiple substances, and the mood problems tend to be temporally associated with substance use.

DSM-5 requires the presence of hypomania for at least four-days to make a diagnosis. Empirical studies have often discounted this criterion as sometimes hypomania tends to last only for up to two days or less and applying the DSM criteria could result in a rejection of the diagnosis of BD II. This is particularly so in patients who may have ultra-rapid or ultradian cycling.

Communicating the diagnosis to the patient

This is probably the most difficult part in clinically managing BD II. Many patients are overwhelmed by the diagnosis and find BD II more stigmatizing. Most are concerned about the implications it may have for their work and other responsibilities. 'Denial' is a commonly encountered response. A few patients may be relieved that they finally have a diagnosis and a management plan to go with it.

It is important to emphasize that BD II is a lifetime condition and that both pharmacotherapy and psychological treatments are helpful. Psychoeducation could include information about illness, potential destabilizing factors, the role of medications and their side effects, and the impact of co-morbidities on outcome. The key message is that while the condition cannot be 'cured', as is the case with most chronic medical illnesses like diabetes and hypertension, it can be brought under sufficient 'control' for the patient to continue with their life in a constructive manner.

Management

A comprehensive management plan needs to be developed, keeping in mind both the psychological and pharmacological interventions, in discussion with the patients and their families. The evidence for these interventions in BD II is summarized as follows.

Role of psychological interventions

Psychological interventions seem to have a role in the treatment of BD II disorder, though the evidence for its use is limited. Further, the policy of one glove fits all cannot be used as far as psychotherapy goes in BD II. Many clinicians recommend cognitive behaviour therapy (CBT) or some other form of psychotherapy for all patients with BD II, even though it may not be required. Patient selection is important to decide if therapy would be useful or not. The role of psychotherapy in the treatment of BD II depression has been understudied. Nonetheless, the predominance of depressive symptoms in patients with BD II and the fact that BD II depression shares many clinical characteristics with MDD suggest that psychotherapy may improve outcomes in these patients.

Psychotherapy for BD II depression

A small (n = 17), 12-week feasibility study demonstrating that 41% of patients with BD II depression achieved a response ($\geq$ 50% reduction in depression scores) with interpersonal and social rhythm therapy (IPSRT), without an increase in mania scores, suggests that IPSRT may be useful in the acute management of BD II depression.[18] A randomized study of IPSRT (n = 14) versus quetiapine (n = 11) for acute BD II depression showed significant differences in depression scores over time but no difference between the two groups in response rates (29% for IPSRT vs 27% for quetiapine).[19]

Psychotherapy for maintenance treatment of BD II

A post hoc analysis of 20 patients with BD II who participated in a single-blind randomized controlled trial (RCT) demonstrated the benefits of adjunctive group psychoeducation (21 sessions over six months) compared with unstructured support groups, with lasting benefits for up to five years. Significantly fewer patients in the psychoeducation group experienced any mood, depressive, or hypomanic relapse during follow-up, and had significantly better psychosocial functioning at both two- and five-year follow-up.[20]

A recent meta-analysis examined the role of psychoeducation in preventing relapses in patients with BD and concluded that psychoeducation was effective in preventing any relapses (odds ratio, OR: 1.98–2.75) and manic/hypomanic relapses (1.68–2.52) but not depressive relapses. Group psychoeducation was more effective than individual psychoeducation. Very few studies in the meta-analysis included patients with BD II and, furthermore, the results were not presented separately for BD II patients.[21]

A recent review identified 18 trials of psychotherapy for BD, which included 481 subjects with BD II (> 10% of the total sample in each study). In all studies except one,[18] patients received pharmacotherapy in addition to psychotherapy. Despite the lack of empirical evidence for the use of psychotherapy in BD II, it has been suggested by the authors that psychotherapy can be employed to develop strategies for recognizing cycling mood states, addressing illness related traumas, and managing psychosocial consequences of the illness.[22] IPSRT is being increasingly viewed as a good treatment option for patients with BD II.[22]

Pharmacological treatment options

Hypomania

Since depressive episodes predominate the course of BD II, treatments for hypomania are not well studied. Most studies that have evaluated acute treatments for BD have included mixed samples of BD I and BD II and do not present the results separately for hypomania. Though most guidelines do not recommend the use of antidepressants for bipolar depression, they are still commonly prescribed. If a patient develops hypomania while on antidepressants, they should be discontinued immediately. Treatment approaches for hypomania have generally followed that of manic episodes.[23] The available evidence is summarized as follows.

Anticonvulsants

An eight-week double-blind placebo-controlled trial (n = 60) showed significantly greater reduction of Young Mania Rating Scale (YMRS) scores in patients with hypomania/mild mania with oral divalproex extended release (ER) (maximum dose 30 mg/kg body weight), in addition to showing more improvement in depressive symptoms.[24]

Atypical antipsychotics

One of the first studies evaluated the role of risperidone in the management of hypomania. 34 patients with DSM-4 BD II completed the trial and showed good improvement within one week of starting treatment at a mean dose of 2.8 mg/day of risperidone compared to placebo. 32% of these patients received risperidone monotherapy while the rest were also on a mood stabilizer.[25] One eight-week RCT showed that quetiapine (n = 39; mean dose 232 mg/day) was marginally more effective than placebo in treating hypomania/mild mania.[26]

Guidelines for clinical management

BD II patients with persistent or new hypomanic symptoms should be treated with an antimanic agent to rapidly alleviate hypomanic symptoms. Prior history of treatment response, adverse effects of medications, and patient preferences are important considerations in treatment selection. If a patient had been taking a prophylactic antimanic agent, an increase in the dose of that medication may be sufficient in some cases. Medications that could potentially be contributing to hypomanic symptoms such as antidepressants should be discontinued.

The Canadian Network for Mood and Anxiety Treatments (CANMAT) guidelines 2013 update has the following recommendation. Due to the lack of systematic studies of the commonly used mood-stabilizing medications in hypomania, it is difficult to formulate evidence-based treatment recommendations. However, clinical practice suggests that medications that are effective in mania are also efficacious in treating hypomanic symptoms. In patients with persistent and/or impairing symptoms of hypomania, clinicians should treat according to their clinical judgement, using lithium, divalproex, or atypical antipsychotic agents and tapering and discontinuing potentially contributory medications such as antidepressants.[23]

Bipolar II depression

Acute management of BD II depression remains a challenge. Most studies have evaluated antipsychotics, antidepressants, and anticonvulsants for the management of bipolar I depression and some of these studies had included BD II depressed patients. However, studies examining treatments specifically for BD II depression are sparse. The available evidence for treating BD II depression is presented as follows.

Lithium

The EMBOLDEN I trial included a lithium comparator arm (36% of the total n = 136 in the lithium group) at doses of 600–1,800 mg per day along with two separate arms of quetiapine 300 mg and 600 mg, and is the only placebo-controlled, parallel-group RCT data for lithium in acute BD II depression.[27] In this trial, neither lithium nor quetiapine were superior to placebo in improving depression scores in BD II. However, the mean lithium levels were < 0.8 mEq/L, which could have had an influence on the treatment outcome, as some previous studies suggest that higher serum lithium levels are required for antidepressant effect of lithium.

Anticonvulsants

Divalproex A meta-analysis of four small studies (total n = 142) in patients with BD I or BD II depression found that the RR of response was double (RR = 2.01), and of remission (risk ratio, RR = 1.61) almost two-thirds greater, with divalproex monotherapy compared with placebo but did not have sufficient data to present results separately for BD II.[28] One RCT of divalproex monotherapy in mood stabilizer naïve bipolar depression reported results separately for BD I and BD II (n = 34), and outcomes for the BD II group showed no separation from placebo.[29] A seven-week open-label trial of divalproex ER in acute BD II depression reported significant improvement in Montgomery-Åsberg Depression Rating Scale (MADRS) scores from baseline to endpoint and 54% response rates.[30] Further studies are clearly warranted to fully understand the role of divalproex in BD II depression.

Lamotrigine The results of two previously unpublished RCTs of lamotrigine have been published in a review article. In the first study, 221 patients with BD II received lamotrigine 200 mg/day or placebo for eight weeks, while in the second 206 patients with BD I or BD II depression were randomized to lamotrigine 100–400 mg/day or placebo. In neither trial was lamotrigine superior to placebo. The negative results may be related to the slow titration of lamotrigine and high placebo response rates.[31] Further, a meta-analysis of lamotrigine trials in BD I or BD II depression showed greater response rates with lamotrigine than placebo, although the effect size was very modest, but the discontinuation rates were not different for lamotrigine compared to placebo.[32] Further, lamotrigine was more effective in patients with severe depression (Hamilton Depression Rating Scale (HDRS) > 24 at baseline) than placebo.[32]

Atypical antipsychotics

Quetiapine It has the largest evidence base for the treatment of BD depression. It includes five placebo-controlled trials with a total n of more than 3,000.

In BOLDER I study, which was a multisite, randomized, double-blind study, two fixed doses of quetiapine monotherapy (300 mg and 600 mg) were evaluated, but the drug versus placebo effect was not found to be significant in BD II.[33] In BOLDER II study, both doses of quetiapine were found to be efficacious with separation from placebo occurring as early as week one.[34] A pooled analysis of data from the BOLDER I and II and EMBOLDEN I and II studies including 776 patients has demonstrated that quetiapine 300 mg or 600 mg to be superior to placebo in treating core depressive symptoms in BD II, with a rapid onset of action, separating from placebo typically after one week. Furthermore, quetiapine was relatively well tolerated, with sedation and, less commonly, weight gain being the limiting concerns.[35] In two of the studies, quetiapine was superior to lithium and paroxetine monotherapy, respectively.

Other agents

Quetiapine + lamotrigine A 12-week, open-label trial assessed the benefit of adding lamotrigine or quetiapine to pre-existing therapy in a mixed sample of patients with BD (BD I n = 15, BD II n = 22, or BD not otherwise specified (NOS) n = 1) on multiple medications. Adding quetiapine to lamotrigine in patients who had not responded to lamotrigine (n = 17 patients with BD II), and adding lamotrigine to quetiapine in patients who had not responded to quetiapine, was associated with improvements in the overall sample. Data were not reported separately for patients with BD II.[36]

Antidepressant monotherapy

Mood elevation with antidepressants has been a major deterrent of antidepressant monotherapy trials in BD II. A paroxetine comparator arm in the EMBOLDEN II trial represents the largest placebo-controlled sample to evaluate antidepressant monotherapy in BD II depression. Paroxetine was not superior to placebo at 20 mg per day and quetiapine did not separate from placebo in this study. Similar switch rates were reported with paroxetine and placebo.[37]

Two open-label studies have examined antidepressant monotherapy in BD II. In a 14-week, open-label study of fluoxetine monotherapy (n = 148), 60% of patients responded and 58% remitted. Although about 24% experienced hypomania/sub-syndromal hypomania, this did not result in treatment discontinuation.[38] In a post hoc analysis of a previously reported open-label study in 83 patients with BD II, the significantly greater improvements in depression scores with venlafaxine compared with lithium were independent of rapid cycling status, and venlafaxine did not result in a higher proportion of mood conversions (versus lithium) in either the rapid or non-rapid cycling patients. Patients in this study who were unresponsive to lithium therapy (n = 14) and who were subsequently crossed over to venlafaxine experienced significantly greater reductions in depression and overall mood scores, with no differences in mania scores versus prior lithium.[39]

Somatic treatments

Electroconvulsive therapy (ECT): an open-label study of twice weekly bilateral ECT included patients with BD II who were medication refractory (n = 67). They achieved a response rate of 79% and a remission rate of 57%. This response rate was intermediate between patients with MDD (94%) and those with BD I (67%).[40]

Guidelines for clinical management

The CANMAT guidelines for BD, 2013 update makes the following recommendations for the acute treatment of BD II depression. Queitapine and quetiapine extended release (XR) are the only recommended first-line drugs for acute depression in BD II. Lithium, lamotrigine, divalproex, lithium or divalproex + antidepressants, lithium + divalproex, and atypical antipsychotic agents + antidepressants are to be considered as second-line drugs based on the strength of the available evidence. Antidepressant monotherapy (in subjects with infrequent hypomanias), quetiapine + lamotrigine, and ECT are recommended as third-line agents.[23]

Maintenance treatment of bipolar II disorder

As mentioned earlier, patients with BD II spend a greater proportion of their illness in depression than in hypomania. Therefore, maintenance treatments tend to focus more on preventing depressive episodes than hypomania. In most situations, patients are continued on the drug to which they responded well during the acute phase of treatment. Due to a scarcity of trials, most guidelines make recommendations based on available evidence and expert consensus.

Lithium

The prophylactic benefit of lithium in patients with BD II has been replicated in three small RCTs; however, in one trial the prophylactic benefit of lithium was less clear in BD II than in BDI, while in another, only the reduction in depressive episodes was statistically significant.[41] Long-term observational data suggest that lithium maintenance has superior benefits in BD II patients, who experience significantly fewer episodes per year, and significantly less time ill, compared with the time prior to initiation of lithium therapy.

Anticonvulsants

Lamotrigine In a large, six-month RCT, there were no significant differences between lamotrigine and placebo in terms of time to additional therapy for BD I and II rapid cycling patients. However, significantly more patients treated with lamotrigine compared with placebo were stable without recurrence at six months among patients with BD II (46% vs 18%).[42]

Adjunctive lamotrigine In a 52-week, open-label study in 109 patients with treatment-refractory BD II, adjunctive lamotrigine was associated with a significant improvement in depressive symptoms and sustained response. Depressive symptoms continued to improve over a 52-week period.[43] Similarly, a retrospective chart review reported that the majority of 31 patients with treatment-resistant BD II depression who received adjunctive lamotrigine for ≥ 6 months were much or very much improved. The mean dose of lamotrigine was 199 mg/day and the maximum 400 mg/day, suggesting that a substantial number of patients required ≥ 200 mg for maximal benefit.[44]

Divalproex Divalproex has been evaluated as a maintenance therapy in rapid cycling BD II patients and in women with BD II and co-morbid borderline personality disorder. Divalproex did not significantly decrease depressive symptoms compared with placebo in a small RCT involving women with BD II and co-morbid borderline personality disorder. However, attrition was high with only 11 patients remaining in the study at six months.[45] In a small, open trial over three years, divalproex was effective in reducing mood episodes in patients with BD II and rapid cycling. 11 patients with BD II reported sustained mood stabilization during the study period with low doses of divalproex (mean dose = 351 mg; blood level = 32.5 mg/ml) while five patients with BD II did not respond to lower doses but improved substantially with divalproex prescribed at 50–100 mg/ml range.[46]

Carbamazepine/oxcarbazepine In an RCT in BD I (n = 27) or BD II (n = 25) patients who displayed residual manic or depressive symptoms on maintenance lithium treatment, the addition of eight weeks of carbamazepine or oxcarbazepine resulted in significant symptom reduction, with oxcarbazepine being more effective than carbamazepine. Results were not presented separately for patients with BD II.[47]

Atypical antipsychotics

Quetiapine A pooled analysis of maintenance data from the EMBOLDEN I and II trials has been presented in abstract form. Among patients with BD II (n = 231) who achieved remission during acute-phase treatment with quetiapine, those who continued quetiapine monotherapy for up to 52 weeks were significantly less likely to experience relapse into any mood episode (hazard ratio (HR) 0.47 for 300 mg and 0.18 for 600 mg) or depressive mood episode (HR 0.35 and 0.21) compared with those who switched to placebo. Rates of hypomania were low and were similar for quetiapine and placebo.[35]

Adjunctive quetiapine Naturalistic studies in combined populations of patients with BD I and BD II demonstrated high rates of sustained euthymia with adjunctive quetiapine, in spite of the fact that the quetiapine doses used in clinical practice were substantially lower than those used in clinical trials. Neither of these studies reported separate results for patients with BD II.[23]

Other agents

Fluoxetine monotherapy Two small RCT extension studies examined the efficacy of fluoxetine in the maintenance treatment of BD II. The first was a six-month RCT in patients with BD II and BD NOS who had responded to fluoxetine, in which relapse rates were 43% with continued fluoxetine versus 100% with placebo.[48]

The second was a one-year RCT in patients with BD II depression (n = 81) who had responded to fluoxetine. It reported that patients were significantly more likely to remain well if they continued on fluoxetine than if they switched to lithium. However, neither fluoxetine nor lithium was significantly better than placebo in mean time to relapse (fluoxetine 249.9 days, lithium 156.4 days, placebo 186.9 days).[49]

Somatic treatments

Electroconvulsive therapy: In one small case series of 14 patients with rapid-cycling BD (nine with BD II) who received maintenance ECT for a mean of 21 months, all patients experienced significant improvement and a resolution of rapid-cycling status.[50]

Guidelines for clinical management

The CANMAT guidelines for BD 2013 update makes the following recommendations. Lithium, lamotrigine, and quetiapine are recommended first-line maintenance treatments for BD II. Divalproex, lithium, or divalproex or atypical antipsychotic + antidepressant are recommended second-line agents along with adjunctive quetiapine and adjunctive lamotrigine. The rest, including ECT, are third-line agents.[23]

There are no studies that have evaluated the role of repetitive transcranial magnetic stimulation or transcranial direct current stimulation in the acute or maintenance treatments for BD II.

Conclusion

Diagnosis of BD II is often missed as patients typically do not seek help when they are hypomanic. Therefore, all patients presenting with a depressive episode must be routinely screened for previous hypomanic episodes. While this might improve detection and early diagnosis of BD II, treating BD II continues to remain a challenge for clinicians in the absence of controlled studies to guide clinical management. Treatment recommendations in guidelines are often based on the available evidence, extrapolation of data from BD I studies, and expert consensus. Since the clinical presentations, course, and outcome and treatment response of BD II are often significantly different from BD I, it can be argued that the results of BD I treatment studies cannot and should not be extrapolated to BD II. While we recommend that clinicians follow the evidence and guidelines as articulated in this chapter to treat BD II, further trials investigating newer agents are urgently required to better understand the efficacy of treatments and provide optimal treatments for the acute and maintenance phases of BD II.

References

1. **Dunner DL, Gershon ES, and Goodwin FK.** Heritable factors in the severity of affective illness, Biol Psychiatry 1976 Feb;**11**(1):31–42.

2. **American Psychiatric Association.** *Diagnostic and Statistical Manual of Mental Disorders* 5th edn (Washington, DC: author, 2013).

3. **Merikangas KR, Akiskal HS, Angst J, Greenberg PE, Hirschfeld RM, Petukhova M, and Kessler RC.** Lifetime and 12-month prevalence of bipolar spectrum disorder in the National Comorbidity Survey replication, Arch Gen Psychiatry 2007 May;**64**(5):543–52. Erratum in: Arch Gen Psychiatry 2007 Sep;64(9):1039.

4. **Benazzi F.** Testing predictors of bipolar-II disorder with a 2-day minimum duration of hypomania, Psychiatry Res 2007 Oct 31;**153**(2):153–62. Epub 16 Jul 2007.

5. **Benazzi F.** Is there a continuity between bipolar and depressive disorders?, Psychother Psychosom 2007;**76**:70–6.

6. **Piver A, Yatham L, and Lam R.** Bipolar spectrum disorders. New perspectives, Can Fam Physician 2002;**48**:896–904.

7. **Maina G, Albert U, Bellodi L, Colombo C, Faravelli C, Monteleone P, Bogetto F, Cassano GB, and Maj M.** Health-related quality of life in euthymic bipolar disorder patients: differences between bipolar I and II subtypes, J Clin Psychiatry 2007 Feb;**68**(2):207–12.

8. **Judd LL, Akiskal HS, Schettler PJ, Coryell W, Endicott J, Maser JD, Solomon DA, Leon AC, and Keller MB.** A prospective investigation of the natural history of the long-term weekly symptomatic status of bipolar II disorder, Arch Gen Psychiatry 2003 Mar;**60**(3):261–9.

9. **Feinman JA and Dunner DL.** The effect of alcohol and substance abuse on the course of bipolar affective disorder, J Affect Disord 1996 Feb;**37**(1):43–9.

10. **Valtonen HM, Suominen K, Haukka J, Mantere O, Leppämäki S, Arvilommi P, and Isometsä ET.** Differences in incidence of suicide attempts during phases of bipolar I and II disorders, Bipolar Disord 2008 Jul;**10**(5):588–96.

11. **Coryell W, Endicott J, Maser JD, Keller MB, Leon AC, and Akiskal HS.** Long-term stability of polarity distinctions in the affective disorders, Am J Psychiatry 1995 Mar;**152**(3):385–90.

12. **Goodwin FK and Jamison KR.** *Manic-Depressive Illness: Bipolar Disorders and Recurrent Depression* 2nd edn (New York, NY: Oxford University Press, 2007).

13. **Coryell W, Endicott J, Reich T, Andreasen N, and Keller M.** A family study of bipolar II disorder, Br J Psychiatry 1984 Jul;**145**:49–54.

14. **Hirschfeld RM, Williams JB, Spitzer RL, Calabrese JR, Flynn L, Keck PE Jr, Lewis L, McElroy SL, Post RM, Rapport DJ, Russell JM, Sachs GS, and Zajecka J.** Development and validation of a screening instrument for bipolar spectrum disorder: the Mood Disorder Questionnaire, Am J Psychiatry 2000 Nov;**157**(11):1873–5.

15. **Bayes A, Parker G, and Fletcher K.** Clinical differentiation of bipolar II disorder from borderline personality disorder, Curr Opin Psychiatry 2014 Jan;**27**(1):14–20.

16. Karaahmet E, Konuk N, Dalkilic A, Saracli O, Atasoy N, Kurçer MA, and Atik L. The comorbidity of adult attention-deficit/hyperactivity disorder in bipolar disorder patients, Compr Psychiatry 2013 Jul;**54**(5):549–55.

17. Hantouche EG and Akiskal HS. Toward a definition of a cyclothymic behavioral endophenotype: which traits tap the familial 113-22 diathesis for bipolar II disorder?, J Affect Disord 2006;**96**:233–7.

18. Swartz HA, Frank E, Frankel DR, Novick D, and Houck P. Psychotherapy as monotherapy for the treatment of bipolar II depression: a proof of concept study, Bipolar Disord 2009 Feb;**11**(1):89–94.

19. Swartz HA, Frank E, and Cheng Y. A randomized pilot study of psychotherapy and quetiapine for the acute treatment of bipolar II depression, Bipolar Disord 2012 Mar;**14**(2):211–16.

20. Colom F, Vieta E, Sánchez-Moreno J, Goikolea JM, Popova E, Bonnin CM, and Scott J. Psychoeducation for bipolar II disorder: an exploratory, 5-year outcome subanalysis, J Affect Disord 2009 Jan;**112**(1–3):30–5.

21. Bond K and Anderson IM. Psychoeducation for relapse prevention in bipolar disorder: a systematic review of efficacy in randomized controlled trials, Bipolar Disord 2015 Jun;**17**(4):349–62.

22. Swartz HA, Levenson JC, and Frank E. Psychotherapy for bipolar II disorder: the role of interpersonal and social rhythm therapy, Prof Psychol Res Pr 2012 Apr;**43**(2):145–53.

23. Yatham LN, Kennedy SH, Parikh SV, Schaffer A, Beaulieu S, Alda M, O'Donovan C, Macqueen G, McIntyre RS, Sharma V, Ravindran A, Young LT, Milev R, Bond DJ, Frey BN, Goldstein BI, Lafer B, Birmaher B, Ha K, Nolen WA, and Berk M. Canadian Network for Mood and Anxiety Treatments (CANMAT) and International Society for Bipolar Disorders (ISBD) collaborative update of CANMAT guidelines for the management of patients with bipolar disorder: update 2013, Bipolar Disord 2013 Feb;**15**(1):1–44.

24. McElroy SL, Martens BE, Creech RS, Welge JA, Jefferson L, Guerdjikova AI, and Keck PE Jr. Randomized, double-blind, placebo-controlled study of divalproex extended release loading monotherapy in ambulatory bipolar spectrum disorder patients with moderate-to-severe hypomania or mild mania, J Clin Psychiatry 2010 May;**71**(5):557–65.

25. Vieta E, Gastó C, Colom F, Reinares M, Martínez-Arán A, Benabarre A, and Akiskal HS. Role of risperidone in bipolar II: an open 6-month study, J Affect Disord 2001 Dec;**67**(1–3):213–19.

26. McElroy SL, Martens BE, Winstanley EL, Creech R, Malhotra S, and Keck PE Jr. Placebo-controlled study of quetiapine monotherapy in ambulatory bipolar spectrum disorder with moderate-to-severe hypomania or mild mania, J Affect Disord 2010 Jul;**124**(1–2):157–63.

27. Young AH, McElroy SL, Bauer M, Philips N, Chang W, Olausson B, Paulsson B, Brecher M; EMBOLDEN I (Trial 001) Investigators. A double-blind, placebo-controlled study of quetiapine and lithium monotherapy in adults in the acute phase of bipolar depression (EMBOLDEN I), J Clin Psychiatry 2010 Feb;**71**(2):150–62.

28. Bond DJ, Lam RW, and Yatham LN. Divalproex sodium versus placebo in the treatment of acute bipolar depression: a systematic review and meta-analysis, J Affect Disord 2010 Aug;**124**(3):228–34.

29. Muzina DJ, Gao K, Kemp DE, Khalife S, Ganocy SJ, Chan PK, Serrano MB, Conroy CM, and Calabrese JR. Acute efficacy of divalproex sodium versus placebo in mood

stabilizer-naive bipolar I or II depression: a double-blind, randomized, placebo-controlled trial, J Clin Psychiatry 2011 Jun;**72**(6):813–19.

30. **Wang PW, Nowakowska C, Chandler RA, Hill SJ, Nam JY, Culver JL, Keller KL**, and **Ketter TA.** Divalproex extended-release in acute bipolar II depression, J Affect Disord 2010 Jul;**124**(1–2):170–3.

31. **Calabrese JR, Huffman RF, White RL**, et al. Lamotrigine in the acute treatment of bipolar depression: results of five double-blind, placebo-controlled clinical trials, Bipolar Disord 2008;**10**:323–33.

32. **Geddes JR, Calabrese JR**, and **Goodwin GM.** Lamotrigine for treatment of bipolar depression: independent meta-analysis and meta-regression of individual patient data from five randomised trials, Br J Psychiatry 2009;**194**:4–9.

33. **Calabrese JR, Keck PE Jr, Macfadden W, Minkwitz M, Ketter TA, Weisler RH, Cutler AJ, McCoy R, Wilson E**, and **Mullen J.** A randomized, double-blind, placebo-controlled trial of quetiapine in the treatment of bipolar I or II depression, Am J Psychiatry 2005 Jul;**162**(7):1351–60.

34. **Thase ME, Macfadden W, Weisler RH, Chang W, Paulsson B, Khan A, Calabrese JR; BOLDER II Study Group.** Efficacy of quetiapine monotherapy in bipolar I and II depression: a double-blind, placebo-controlled study (the BOLDER II study), J Clin Psychopharmacol 2006 Dec;**26**(6):600–9. Erratum in: J Clin Psychopharmacol 2007 Feb;27(1):51.

35. **Young AH, Calabrese JR, Gustafsson U**, et al. The efficacy of quetiapine monotherapy in bipolar II depression: combined data from the BOLDER and EMBOLDEN studies, Bipolar Disord 2010;**12**(Suppl. 1):58.

36. **Ahn YM, Nam JY, Culver JL, Marsh WK, Bonner JC**, and **Ketter TA.** Lamotrigine plus quetiapine combination therapy in treatment-resistant bipolar depression, Ann Clin Psychiatry 2011;**23**:17–24.

37. **McElroy SL, Weisler RH, Chang W, Olausson B, Paulsson B, Brecher M, Agambaram V, Merideth C, Nordenhem A, Young AH;** EMBOLDEN II (Trial D1447C00134) Investigators. A double-blind, placebo-controlled study of quetiapine and paroxetine as monotherapy in adults with bipolar depression (EMBOLDEN II), J Clin Psychiatry 2010 Feb;**71**(2):163–74.

38. **Amsterdam JD** and **Shults J.** Efficacy and mood conversion rate of short-term fluoxetine monotherapy of bipolar II major depressive episode, J Clin Psychopharmacol 2010;**30**:306–11.

39. **Amsterdam JD, Wang G**, and **Shults J.** Venlafaxine monotherapy in bipolar type II depressed patients unresponsive to prior lithium monotherapy, Acta Psychiatr Scand 2010;**121**:201–8.

40. **Medda P, Perugi G, Zanello S, Ciuffa M**, and **Cassano GB.** Response to ECT in bipolar I, bipolar II and unipolar depression, J Affect Disord 2009;**118**:55–9.

41. **Amsterdam JD, Luo L**, and **Shults J.** Efficacy and mood conversion rate during long-term fluoxetine v lithium monotherapy in rapid- and non-rapid-cycling bipolar II disorder, Br J Psychiatry 2013 Apr;**202**(4):301–6.

42. Calabrese JR, Suppes T, Bowden CL, Sachs GS, Swann AC, McElroy SL, Kusumakar V, Ascher JA, Earl NL, Greene PL, and Monaghan E. A double-blind, placebo-controlled, prophylaxis study of lamotrigine in rapid-cycling bipolar disorder. Lamictal 614 Study Group, J Clin Psychiatry 2000 Nov;**61**(11):841–50.

43. **Chang JS, Moon E, Cha B**, and **Ha K.** Adjunctive lamotrigine therapy for patients with bipolar II depression partially responsive to mood stabilizers, Prog Neuropsychopharmacol Biol Psychiatry 2010 Oct 1;34(7):1322–6.

44. **Sharma V, Khan M**, and **Corpse C.** Role of lamotrigine in the management of treatment-resistant bipolar II depression: a chart review, J Affect Disord 2008;111:100–5.

45. **Frankenburg FR** and **Zanarini MC.** Divalproex sodium treatment of women with borderline personality disorder and bipolar II disorder: a double-blind placebo-controlled pilot study, J Clin Psychiatry 2002 May;63(5):442–6.

46. **Jacobsen FM.** Low-dose valproate: a new treatment for cyclothymia, mild rapid cycling disorders, and premenstrual syndrome, J Clin Psychiatry 1993 Jun;54(6):229–34.

47. **Juruena MF, Ottoni GL, Machado-Vieira R**, et al. Bipolar I and II disorder residual symptoms: oxcarbazepine and carbamazepine as add-on treatment to lithium in a double-blind, randomized trial, Prog Neuro-psychopharmacol Biol Psychiatry 2009;33:94–9.

48. **Amsterdam JD** and **Shults J.** Fluoxetine monotherapy of bipolar type II and bipolar NOS major depression: a double-blind, placebo-substitution, continuation study, Int Clin Psychopharmacol 2005;20:257–64.

49. **Amsterdam JD** and **Shults J.** Efficacy and safety of long-term fluoxetine versus lithium monotherapy of bipolar II disorder: a randomized, double-blind, placebo-substitution study, Am J Psychiatry 2010;167:792–800.

50. **Minnai GP, Salis PG, Oppo R, Loche AP, Scano F**, and **Tondo L.** Effectiveness of maintenance electroconvulsive therapy in rapid-cycling bipolar disorder, J ECT 2011;27:123–6.

Chapter 10

The treatment of cyclothymia

Giulio Perugi, Giulia Vannucchi,
and Lorenzo Mazzarini

Introduction

Cyclothymia is by now the most neglected mood disorder despite its first description dates back to the period when modern psychiatry was born and manic-depressive insanity was conceptualized. Prevalence rates ranging from 0.4% to 2.5% have been reported for cyclothymic disorder in non-clinical populations.[1-3] These rates are even higher among psychiatric patients.[4] The lack of interest in treatment, research, as well as the under-recognition of cyclothymia in clinical settings is probably related to the ambiguity regarding its conceptualization and the common tendency to describe cyclothymia only in terms of mood symptoms.

Current diagnostic classifications as per the *Diagnostic and Statistical Manual of Mental Disorders* (5th edition) and the *International Classification of Diseases* (10th revision) (DSM-5 and ICD-10, respectively) include cyclothymia as a separate category among bipolar disorders (BDs). The categorical approach provides an arbitrary clear-cut separation between cyclothymic and BD II and I disorders. In clinical practice, most cyclothymic patients are referred for major affective episodes, but if a cyclothymic subject experiences a major depressive or a (hypo)manic episode, the diagnosis is dropped and the patient is reclassified as BD I or BD II. In this context, cyclothymia is viewed as a residual category, while its clinical importance and independent profile is left unappreciated. Moreover, a definition based only on the long-lasting alternation of mood symptoms of opposite polarity neglects most of the behavioural and psychological features of the disorder and its continuity with temperamental and personality characteristics. Mood reactivity and affective instability, extreme emotionality, and impulsivity, which should be considered as true core features of cyclothymia, as well as most of their psychological, behavioural, and interpersonal consequences are described from a different perspective among the DSM-5 criteria for dramatic or anxious clusters of personality disorders and the ICD-10 definition of emotionally unstable and histrionic personality disorders. This approach represents a major limitation for understanding not only the relationship between constitutional traits and major episodes in mood-disordered patients, but also the close link between cyclothymia and other anxious and impulse control disorders, with relevant implications for their treatment and clinical management.

Behavioural and psychological aspects of cyclothymia, as well as the associated 'co-morbidity', should be considered major targets for an integrative management strategy. The correct recognition of a putative cyclothymic matrix in these 'complex' clinical presentations constitutes a fundamental step to implement effective and integrative treatment strategies. Thus, despite cyclothymia requires more sophisticated treatments than do classical bipolar I and II disorders, its proper operationalization remains an obscure area in psychiatry research. The evidence on psychological and pharmacological treatments in this area is very sparse so that, even when cyclothymia is correctly identified, there is neither evidence-based treatment, nor consensus on the strategy to treat it.

The purpose of this chapter is to summarize available evidence on both pharmacological and psychological treatments for cyclothymia and to provide specific treatment strategies.

Clinical studies

Psychopharmacological treatment

Pharmacological treatment of cyclothymia is surprisingly under-studied, especially when compared with mania and depression. Mood stabilizers such as lithium, valproate, carbamazepine, and lamotrigine have been studied mainly in bipolar I and, to a lesser extent, in bipolar II patients. Similarly, there are only few controlled studies that have focused on the use of antidepressants in bipolar depression in general, and cyclothymia in particular. The lack of adequate research in this area is even more astonishing when we consider the chronicity and the major impact on functioning of cyclothymic depressive and hypomanic symptoms, as well as related complications, such as substance abuse and suicidality.

There is a paucity of systematic studies and a substantial lack of randomized placebo-controlled studies of psychopharmacological treatments[5] and most information is derived from a small number of open naturalistic studies. Some observational studies support the efficacy of lithium in cyclothymia. The first reports date from the mid-70s and found that patients with classical features of endogenous depression, who had shown previous cyclothymic swings and resistance to antidepressants, responded to lithium.[6] Few studies on non-complicated cases of cyclothymia showed mild to moderate prophylactic properties of lithium for depressive episodes,[7] as well as a successful prevention of severe mood episodes of other polarities (ie, mixed or hypomanic), in 97% of the lithium-treated patients.[8] Similarly, in a comparative naturalistic study, lithium response rates seemed higher in cyclothymic patients than in other psychiatric controls.[9] In the same period, some studies showed that cyclothymic features should have been considered as predictor of good response to lithium (both as monotherapy or as add-on therapy) on a variety of conditions, such as BD,[10] premenstrual tension (which is now included under the label of premenstrual dysphoric disorder in the DSM-5),[11] and cocaine abuse.[12]

Baldessarini and colleagues[13] published the results of a long-term follow-up of bipolar patients treated with lithium. The authors compared the treatment response on the basis of the presence of rapid cycling. As expected, they found that rapid cycling is more common among BD II patients and that 28% of them had premorbid cyclothymia. Notwithstanding the common belief that lithium would be less effective in rapid cycling, in this sample a similar response to lithium was observed for rapid and non-rapid cyclers, except for a doubled risk mainly for depressive recurrences among rapid cyclers. Recently, soft bipolar patients with a cyclothymic temperament treated with lithium showed significantly higher rates of remission than those without lithium treatment.[14]

The reports on lithium response in cyclothymia are not all positive. A study comparing unipolar, bipolar II, and cyclothymic patients found that lithium prophylactic efficacy was less evident in the cyclothymic subgroup.[15] Similarly, in a five-year follow-up study on 71 BD patients, a hyperthymic temperament was associated to a better lithium response in comparison with anxious, cyclothymic, and depressive temperaments.[16]

Data on medications other than lithium are even scarcer. There are two studies on valproate in cyclothymia; in the first one, 70% of 32 patients with mood swings achieved a mood stabilization in term of frequency and/or amplitude of mood fluctuations;[17] in the second study, valproate was employed in the treatment of cyclothymia and BD II with mild rapid cycling. In the five-year follow-up study, 79% of enrolled patients obtained sustained partial or complete mood stabilization with low-dose valproate, while a further 6% required high doses.[18]

Two studies have evaluated the efficacy of valproate in the offspring of bipolar patients at high risk of developing a mood disorder.[19,20] An open-label study showed that 78% of this bipolar offspring, aged 6–18, with mood or behavioural disorders and at least mild affective disorders, were responders to valproate. The second study assessed 56 patients with mood symptoms compatible with the diagnoses of cyclothymia or BD Not Otherwise Specified (NOS).[20] At the end of the study, valproate did not differ from placebo in preventing the onset of a full-blown BD.

Other anticonvulsants commonly used in clinical practice for the treatment of cyclothymic patients are lamotrigine and gabapentin, but evidence pertaining these two drugs is limited and inconsistent. To the best of our knowledge, there are only two studies on lamotrigine in cyclothymia/soft bipolar spectrum or cyclothymic temperament. Montes and colleagues[21] provided the chart reviews of 34 depressive bipolar patients, followed up along an average 30-week period. Lamotrigine, as monotherapy or adjunctive treatment, during an index depressive episode was more effective in patients with a bipolar spectrum condition than in patients with BD I. The drug demonstrated prophylactic properties and one-third of the sample remained euthymic for the entire observation period. Another naturalistic study showed that 23 female patients with cyclothymic temperament and refractory depression achieved sustained remission with lamotrigine augmentation or monotherapy.[22]

Gabapentin, which failed in controlled trials to be proven efficacious in BD, resulted effective in patients with bipolar spectrum disorders in a study conducted in a naturalistic setting, as monotherapy or adjunctive treatment.[23] The authors advocated the utility of this medication in depressive patients mostly due to its efficacy on associated anxiety symptoms and sleep disturbances.

A case series study has shown that a very low dosage of quetiapine (25–75 mg/day) in patients with cyclothymic temperament can lead to a sustained symptom remission by managing anxiety, activation, sleep disturbances, and benzodiazepines abuse.[24] Other typical or atypical antipsychotics have not been systematically studied in cyclothymic patients.

The use of antidepressants in cyclothymic patients is a debated issue. In spite of this, there are few positive reports regarding the efficacy of tricyclic antidepressants like imipramine[25] and amitriptiline alone or associated with perfenazine.[26] On the contrary, in a recent study[14] of cyclothymic or hyperthymic patients with major depressive patients, the treatment with selective serotonin reuptake inhibitors (SSRIs) was associated with lower rates of remission than in patients without such temperamental traits.

On the basis of their clinical experience, several authors[27] reported a worsening of the illness course in soft bipolar patients induced by antidepressant drugs, as demonstrated by the appearance of antidepressant-induced hypomanic and mixed-manic switches and long-term mood instability, chronic course, attenuated mixed features, rapid cycling, and increased suicidality.

Another important phenomenon is represented by the 'wear-off'.[28] The development of tolerance and the emergence of relapses and/or recurrences during a previously effective maintenance treatment with antidepressants have been considered a sign of bipolarity per se among depressive patients.[29] Among patients with resistant depression almost 80% showed evidence of bipolarity, including depressive episodes in patients with underlying cyclothymia.[29] In such patients, a diagnostic reassessment may alter the initial treatment plan (ie the use of mood stabilizers in detriment of antidepressants may be prioritized).

Psychotherapy and psychoeducation

Studies investigating psychotherapy and psychoeducation strategies, specifically addressing cyclothymic patients, are sparse. The few available studies on cyclothymia are heterogeneous, consisting in the application of different techniques, based on different psychopathological models of the disorder.

Shen and colleagues[30] took into account the social zeitgeber theory, and conducted a randomized trial in 71 cyclothymic college students. They found that the more severe was a lifestyle, the more severe were depressive and mood lability symptoms. Although a positive trend emerged, an increase in lifestyle regularity proved insufficient to significantly interfere with cyclothymic mood symptoms.

Cognitive behavioural therapy (CBT) has been explored initially in case reports and series. In a case report treated with nine months of CBT and followed up for 11 weeks, the target of the treatment was to reduce mood variability by enhancing cognitive awareness on changes in mood states. At the end of the study, the authors found a positive effect of CBT especially on depressive symptoms, although the patient remained psychosocially impaired.[31] More recently, Fava and colleagues[32] proposed the association of CBT and well-being therapy (WBT) in a standardized sequential combination of ten sessions for a period of five months. They conducted a randomized trial in 62 cyclothymic patients with three-point follow-up (at the end of the treatment, after one year and after two years). Patients treated with CBT/WBT reported a significant reduction in both depressive and hypomanic symptomatology compared with the control group. In addition, this improvement was maintained after one and two years of follow-up: thus, during the follow-up period, a proportion of treated patients did not continue to meet diagnostic criteria for cyclothymia. Although this study has several limitations in terms of sampling bias, the lack of a control group and a poor definition of outcome measures, it may represent an interesting starting point for further research in this unexplored field.

Most cyclothymic patients do not match with the psychoeducational approach proposed for 'classic' BD forms.[33] When cyclothymic patients are included in BD I groups of psychoeducation, they may feel 'not understood' and may say 'this is not my illness'. Actually, psychoeducation for BD I cannot fit with the main psychological, behavioural and interpersonal features related to cyclothymia.

Hantouche and colleagues in the Anxiety and Mood Centre team (Paris, France)[34] elaborated a psychoeducation group therapy specific for cyclothymia. The format consisted of six weekly two-hour sessions. During the first session, a clinical description of cyclothymia is provided together with a discussion regarding causes and medications. The second session is relative to monitoring of mood swings, assessment of warning signs, strategies to cope with early relapses, and planning of 'positive' routines. Sessions three and four are dedicated to the assessment of psychological vulnerabilities assessed (eg, emotional dependency, sensitivity to rejection, excessive need to please, testing limits, need for control, and compulsive behaviours). During the fifth session, cognitive processes linked to ups-and-downs are examined. Finally, the sixth session is focused on interpersonal conflicts.[35] Systematic long-term follow-up data regarding this psychoeducational approach remain unavailable. However, the authors reported the results of the open follow-up from a minimum of six to a maximum of 42 weeks from several clinical samples. This approach obtained promising preliminary results in terms of better understanding of the nature of the illness, less opposition to medications, and better adherence to treatments in general. Psychoeducation seemed to also improve some psychological, social, and behavioural aspects linked to the illness, such as reduction of uncertainty, shame or despair, attenuation of conflicts in family and workplace, and the formation of small self-help/support groups. The final effect was so positive and motivating that more than half of participants insisted to continue an individual-based psychotherapy.

Clinical management

The clinical picture of cyclothymia is extremely complex, variable, and very rich in terms of clinical features. Emotional deregulation with instability and over-reactivity to external and internal stimuli is associated with fluctuations involving not only mood but also cognition and psychomotricity (eg energy, hedonic pattern, motivation, sleep and circadian rhythms, etc). Intense and rapid mood swings draw major psychological, interpersonal, and behavioural consequences, which usually are the most prominent expression of the disorder (see Figure 10.1).

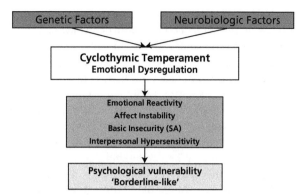

Figure 10.1 Cyclothymia well suited to developmental disorder

In most cases, the first clinical manifestations of cyclothymia appear during adolescence and are frequently misinterpreted as age-related 'problems' and 'physiological' character and personality modifications. Depressive symptoms are frequently attributed to concomitant stressful life events or more or less 'self-perceived' traumatic events, whereas hypomanic and related sub-excitatory symptoms go unrecognized or are considered part of the 'normal adolescence turmoil'. A major cause of distress is represented by the intensity, rapidity, and unpredictability of mood swings, which are invariably associated with a considerable degree of instability in terms of self-esteem, vocational attitudes, and interpersonal relationships.

Depressive and hypomanic phases are extremely variable in terms of duration, severity, and symptomatology.[36] Usually, depression in cyclothymic individuals is of mild to moderate severity and is marked by despair, anguish, fatigue, and atypical features.[37] Feelings of low self-worth and guilt, insecurity and dependence, emotionality, agitation, and extremely high sensitivity have been reported, along with high levels of irritability and anxiety,[38] as well as a tendency to emphasize social and interpersonal difficulties.[4] Typically, during depressive or mixed periods, cyclothymic patients report frequent suicidal thoughts and, quite often, self-injuring or suicidal gestures.[39] Hypomanic phases are often difficult to identify, especially due to their brevity. In addition, the 'dark' side of excitement with irritability, impulsivity, hostility, and risk-taking behaviour seem to predominate.[4] People with cyclothymic disorder tend to be impulsive and unpredictable during hypomanic or mixed states, with irritable mood directed to others, whereas during depressive periods they may be very sensitive, but also tend to experience self-directed irritability consistent with guilt, ruminations, and low self-esteem.

The psychological and behavioural consequences of the underlying emotional instability and reactivity may constitute major complaints in many cases. Hyperreactivity to judgement, criticism, and rejection with consequent interpersonal sensitivity are very common manifestations of cyclothymia. When emotional reactions are particularly intense, a tendency to be interpretative and to develop overvalued

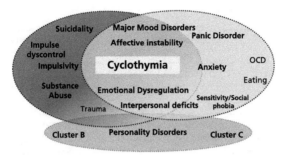

Figure 10.2 Major psychopathological domains of cyclothymia: multidimensionality and complexity

ideas may episodically appear, with destructive consequences on social and interpersonal relationships. Similarly, the fragile self-esteem associated to the fear of being disapproved, rejected, or abandoned may give reason of submissive behaviour and persistent involvement in abusive relationships. A pathological dependence on compliments and emotional reward may be observed in some cases, sometimes in association with inappropriate seductive, provocative, and manipulative behaviours. These manifestations may complicate the patient–doctor relationship.

Cyclothymic mood instability is the common factor underlying a wide range of co-morbidity and complications associated with bipolarity, including anxiety, impulsivity, suicidality, and drug abuse.[40,41] The presence of impulsivity may be associated with sensation seeking and self-stimulating behaviour, which becomes amplified during hypomanic phases.[36] In this perspective, cyclothymia seems to offer a fertile ground for drug abuse and addiction.[41] Both sensation-seeking behaviour and marked reactivity to substances facilitate the approach to and use of any sort of drug, alcohol, stimulant, and cocaine, but also hypnotics and sedatives. Anxious 'comorbidity' is very common and anxiety disorders rather than mood symptoms are in many cases chief complaints when these individuals seek specialized treatment[36,40] (see Figure 10.2).

The complex, multidimensional clinical picture is a major reason for difficulties in treatment management of cyclothymia, but it is not the only one. We already mentioned the difficult patient–doctor relationship, which may negatively influence treatment compliance and long-term outcomes.

In clinical practice, it is common that evidence-based treatment regimens for BD I or II result inadequate or even detrimental for cyclothymic individuals. These patients seem to be extremely sensitive and reactive to medications. Side effects or even 'paradoxical' unexpected reactions are very common and may exceed benefits. Thus, in spite of the general opinion that cyclothymia is a 'minor' mood disorder, it can be a very severe, debilitating condition and requires more sophisticated treatment than other classical bipolar forms. A correct treatment strategy should include a 'sartorial' psychopharmacological approach and a specific psychoeducational intervention. Treatment strategy for cyclothymia is summarized in Table 10.1.

Table 10.1 Treatment strategy for cyclothymia

Acute 0–8 weeks	Continuation 1–6 months	Maintenance Indefinite
Depressive, mixed, or hypomanic states Symptomatic recovery	Psychosocial maladjustment Functional recovery	Stability Coping with psychological faults
Mood-stabilizers (MS) + adjunctive drugs if needed: antidepressant, antipsychotic 'Go slow, stay low'	Mood-stabilizers (MS) Tapering adjunctive drugs	Long-term MS (which should 'stay low'); anticipate hypomania and depression
Psychoeducation	Cognitive reorganization, emotional coaching, changes in behavioural systems, and so on	Optimizing adaptation: goodness of fit

Pharmacological treatment

Though not adequately studied, available data and clinical experience strongly suggest the value of mood-stabilizer agents including lithium and some anticonvulsants, both in the mid- and long term.[5,42] As a general rule, the use of antidepressant or antipsychotic drugs should be considered for short periods of time and only after the failure of mood stabilizers, to manage depressive, anxious, or hypomanic symptoms.

In clinical practice, pharmacological strategies for the treatment of cyclothymia should be based on three fundamental principles: (i) establish the hierarchy of clinical targets and priority on the basis of severity and functional impairment; (ii) draw principal objectives both in mid- and long-term perspectives (in this respect, it is very important to involve in detail and motivate the patient); and (iii) follow the rule of 'go slow and stay low', considering that these patients are abnormally sensitive to the effects of medications.

In the majority of cases the hierarchical approach provides the treatment of the current acute episode, which is mostly represented by non-psychotic mixed depressive states, often chronic and following a history of multiple antidepressants failure. Once the acute phase is managed, emotional reactivity, intensity, and instability should be considered the primary target of the treatment. Co-morbidity (as obsessive–compulsive disorder (OCD), panic, impulsivity, drug/alcohol abuse, and bulimia) may have different hierarchical importance on the basis underlying risks and/or severity. For example, a severe alcohol- or drug-use disorder has to be treated with priority. Similarly, the presence of suicidal risk and self-harm behaviours need prompt intervention.

The principal objectives of treatment include, in the mid-term, the achievement of relative mood stability, meant as the decrease of amplitude and frequency of ups-and-downs, and a greater behavioural control throughout positive routines. As mid-term, we mean a period ranging from six months to one year following treatment initiation. It is very important at the beginning of treatment to explain this term to the patient and to remind throughout the entire treatment period. Improvement and long-lasting results are possible only by avoiding the temptation to prematurely give up medications (especially mood stabilizers) because of the impression of ineffectiveness. Involving and encouraging the patient to be 'patient' may make the difference between the stabilization and 'medication roulette'. After a mood stabilization, in the long term, the aim of a continuous treatment is to enhance functional adjustment and to aid in the correction dysfunctional life schemas.

We use to stratify the pharmacologic intervention on the basis of specific dimensions involved respecting the rule of 'go slow and stay low'. The majority of cyclothymic patients would benefit from a small dose of valproate (if mixicity and mood reactivity are dominant), lamotrigine (when anxious–depressive polarity is dominant), or lithium (if affect intensity is present). Many patients received the combination of a small dose of lithium (200–400 mg/day) plus lamotrigine (25–100 mg/day).[43] Careful attention is required for adverse effects, such as skin reactions, thyroid dysfunction, polycystic ovary syndrome, and weight gain.

Antidepressants should be used with caution, but in real-world practice, almost all cyclothymic patients receive antidepressants and a correct diagnosis is frequently established in recurrent, difficult-to-treat, resistant 'depression'. When possible, a gradual removal of the antidepressant and unnecessary drugs and the introduction of one or more specific mood stabilizers should be attempted. In ideal conditions, antidepressants should be avoided from the beginning and reserved as second- or third-line choices only to long-lasting severe depressive or anxious symptomatology. A possible option is represented by quetiapine, which has been reported to be effective in the treatment of acute bipolar depression and has been recently suggested useful for the control of dysphoria, irritability, anxiety, and sleep symptoms in cyclothymics.[24] Low doses (not exceeding 100 mg/day) are usually utilized because intolerance to quetiapine and even more to other antipsychotic drugs (with high doses most patients will drop these drugs during the first two weeks). The use of antipsychotics should be limited regarding both doses and treatment duration. Cyclothymic patients are likely to develop in a short period psychomotor adverse effects such as motor impairment, blunted affect, loss of motivation, and depression. Because of this heightened sensitivity, cyclothymia is also associated with an increased risk of the early development of tardive neuropsychiatric side effects. In this respect, the use of first-generation antipsychotics or drugs with selective blockade of D2-receptors should be avoided, unless strictly necessary. Other antipsychotics with different receptor profiles should be preferred and used at low doses. For example, 25–50 mg/day of quetiapine as well as 2.5–5 mg/day of olanzapine or 2–6 mg/day of perfenazine may be useful for the management of irritability, impulsivity, and other excitatory phenomena during an acute hypomanic or mixed state.

Another important issue concerns the frequent co-morbidity with anxiety, impulse–control or eating disorders, and attention deficit hyperactivity disorder in youths. Each co-morbid condition requires a selection of treatments, which are mostly based on open clinical experience.[44,45] For example, high anxiety, panic attacks, inner tension (usually observed in mixed depressive state), and ultra-rapid cycling would be a predictor of response to valproate rather than to lithium.

Gabapentin, which has been shown to be effective in panic disorder and social phobia, seems to be helpful when anxiety disorders or an alcohol-use disorder are co-morbid. Topiramate would be indicated when co-morbid binge-eating disorder is present. Less information is available for treating co-morbid social phobia; the same problem applies to co-morbid post-traumatic stress disorder. Co-morbid OCD is probably the most challenging condition to treat. A complex combination of different mood stabilizers with serotonergic drugs and antipsychotics is often applied.[38,40]

Although hypomania and mood reactivity are more likely to determine functional impairment and negative consequences than depression, cyclothymic patients usually perceive greater distress linked to depression and anxiety, rather than hypomanic symptoms or emotional instability. For this reason, most patients seek treatments to manage depressive symptoms or anxious co-morbidity and are treated with antidepressants and sedatives. Although the evidence concerning the efficacy and safety of antidepressants in cyclothymic individuals is substantially lacking, there is broad agreement among clinicians that, in this population, the use of these drugs should be carefully monitored in order to minimize mood switches and long-term destabilization. Exposure to antidepressants, indeed, may be associated with a variety of possible negative consequences, such as increased amplitude of highs and lows and frequency of cycling.[42] In other patients, mood destabilization might assume the aspect of chronic mixed-depressive states, usually resistant to standard treatments and involving the co-occurrence of dysphoric and excitatory symptoms simultaneously present or rapidly fluctuating. This type of symptomatology is frequently associated with an increased risk of suicidal behaviours.[39] Finally, as cyclothymia may be a harbinger of full-blown bipolarity, antidepressants might be responsible for the onset of severe manic or mixed episodes in certain individuals.

Another important phenomenon commonly observed employing antidepressant drugs in cyclothymia is the wear-off. Cyclothymic patients are very likely to show tolerance and decreasing response to antidepressants over time.[46] The wear-off phenomenon is frequently associated to rapid onset of benefits, sometimes in few days or even few hours, after the first exposure to antidepressants.

Mood disorders are accompanied by circadian deregulations, which are particularly common among cyclothymic patients. These latter frequently report abnormalities in sleep/wake cycles and show abnormal oscillating melatonin secretion and frequent delayed sleep phase disorder (DSPD),[47] a circadian rhythm disorder characterized by the inability to fall asleep and wake up until much later than is desired or socially acceptable. Melatonin and agomelatine are known to have chronobiotic properties. In cyclothymic patients, it is possible to hypothesize that the restoration of circadian rhythms, such as the improvement of sleep efficiency together with the reduction of intra-sleep awakening, through MT1 and MT2 agonism, may contribute to improve mood symptomatology, motivational aspects, and psychosocial functioning. The efficacy of melatonin and agomelatine and the importance of a resynchronization of circadian rhythms in the therapy of cyclothymia deserve further investigations.

Finally, cyclothymic patients should be considered at high risk of developing sedative misuse (particularly for benzodiazepines) because of hypersensitivity to all substances and high rates of anxiety disorders, mostly panic. The long-term use of sedatives is a frequent complication in such patients: the most evident effect is the worsening of mood lability, behavioural control, and cognitive functions, over the worsening of sleep disturbances and anxiety itself. Thus, it seems very important to promote a gradual tapering down of sedatives according to adapted but rigid protocols choosing long half-life medications to reduce withdrawal symptoms and craving.

Adapted psychoeducation

A psychoeducational approach is the first step for a correct and effective management of cyclothymia. Differently from bipolar I and II patients, psychoeducation should start from the beginning and would promote acceptance of the illness, confidence in the doctor, adherence to medications, and circumscribe the objectives of the treatment focusing on the behavioural and interpersonal consequences of the illness.

In cyclothymia, the patient has to face attenuated but continuous and deceitful mood shift between depression and excitement, which are strongly related to each other. Over-reactivity and inter-episodic instability are deeply ingrained with the life of the patient; thus, psychological and physical stressors may trigger exaggerated emotional reactions and disproportionate consequences. In some cases, the development of over-valued ideas, interpretations, and distorted perspective, on the basis of a temporary affective state, may complicate the clinical picture and, in these situations, the subject tends to misattribute the cause–effect sequence, reinforcing affective instability and its behavioural consequences. These clinical features have nothing to do with the characteristics of classical BD, characterized by severe, often psychotic, major depressive and mixed-manic episodes separated by periods of remission.

Because of the temperamental nature of the disorder, psychoeducation is endless and should be an integral part of every single follow-up visit. The physician should give the patient a continuous feedback to circumscribe the behavioural and interpersonal consequences of the illness. Assessing periodically the psychological aspects of cyclothymia becomes particularly important, even after months of psychopharmacological treatment and psychoeducation.

In most cases, medications and adapted psychoeducation are sufficient to mitigate psychological dysfunction. For a minority of patients it might be useful to be part of an individual psychotherapy package. Research is not advanced in this field and at the moment there is no rigid or strict format for psychological therapy. The therapist should keep in mind the model in which moods swings and circularity are linked with mood reactivity, affect intensity, emotion sensitivity, interpersonal sensitivity, and basic insecurity, which illustrate the endogenous cyclicity in cyclothymia.

In clinical practice, CBT techniques could be adapted to fit with specific individual objectives such as: (i) recording levels of mood and energy; (ii) helping 'healthy' daily routines to enhance circadian rhythms, especially in those patients with comorbid DSPD; (iii) implementing specific strategies to manage the cognitive aspects related to ups-and-downs (activation and inhibition), especially in ultra-rapid mood-swings—this objective might be obtained throughout the discussion of dysfunctional and overvalued beliefs linked to the mood;[48] (iv) attenuating co-morbid anxiety, such as panic attacks, OCD, social anxiety, or post-traumatic stress disorder, in order to avoid or limit the use of antidepressants; (v) rebuilding self-esteem.

This process should start from the reduction of the affective resonance of the interpersonal events, which is mostly related to uncontrolled mood reactivity rather than the actual importance of the event itself. Indirectly, also a greater affective stability could be achieved.[49] Self-esteem and over-reactivity are linked by means of sensitivity to judgement, criticism, and rejection. As already said, cyclothymic subjects are promptly offended and sensitive to the possibility of being wounded, with feelings of hostility and anger towards those who evocate these reactions and that are considered responsible for their sufferings; (vi) restoring healthy social support by mitigating hostility, over-evaluation of minor disputes, and enhancing rage control—the ultimate goal would be to interrupt the processes which usually lead to destructive consequences on interpersonal life;[35] and (vii) replacing repetitive dysfunctional life schemas linked to cyclothymia with different cognitive style. More specifically cyclothymic individuals have been found to be variously subdued to five schemas: abandonment, self-sacrifice, insufficient self-control, affective dependence, and the need for control.[50] Those schemas tend to create unrelenting standards and determine great personal sufferings and consequences.

Conclusion

Treatment of cyclothymia is an understudied issue despite the evidence that 30–50% of depressives, anxious, impulsive, and borderline patients are affected by this disorder. There are a lot of challenging issues concerning diagnostic delimitation, psychoeducation, and pharmacological treatment. We need to confirm the specificity of the disorder within the bipolar spectrum and to improve its recognition in early phase of the illness, especially in youth. Cyclothymia, indeed, is a topic well suited to a developmental psychopathology approach: it tends to have an onset during childhood and adolescence and it is important that diagnosis and treatment are initiated early. An appropriate approach of cyclothymia will permit to reduce controversy surrounding the over-diagnosis of bipolar spectrum in youths. A therapeutic model combining the focus on cyclothymic presentations of bipolarity with a temperamental perspective represents a clear and precise approach for complex clinical syndromes with mood instability, depression, excitement, anxiety, impulse control, substance use, and so-called 'personality' disorders. Early recognition means establishing a specific treatment and clinical management since the beginning, and avoiding unnecessary complications and risks, especially those related to antidepressants exposure. It is necessary to confirm if early detection and treatment of cyclothymia can guarantee a significant change in the long-term prognosis. Prospective observation in our practice is in favour of persistent significant improvement. This is more visible when specific pharmacotherapy, psychological approach and psychoeducation are applied to young patients never treated before.

References

1. **Perugi G, Toni C, Maremmani I, Tusini G, Ramacciotti S, Madia A**, et al. The influence of affective temperaments and psychopathological traits on the definition of bipolar disorder subtypes: a study on bipolar I Italian national sample, J Affect Disord 2012;**136**(1–2):e41–9.

2. **Van Meter AR, Youngstrom EA**, and **Findling RL**. Cyclothymic disorder: a critical review, Clin Psychol Rev 2012;**32**(4):229–43.

3. **Vazquez GH, Tondo L, Mazzarini L**, and **Gonda X**. Affective temperaments in general population: a review and combined analysis from national studies, J Affect Disord 2012;**139**(1):18–22.

4. **Hantouche EG, Angst J**, and **Akiskal HS**. Factor structure of hypomania: interrelationships with cyclothymia and the soft bipolar spectrum, J Affect Disord 2003;**73**(1–2):39–47.

5. **Baldessarini RJ, Vazquez G**, and **Tondo L**. Treatment of cyclothymic disorder: commentary, Psychother Psychosom 2011;**80**(3):131–5.

6. **Neubauer H** and **Bermingham P**. A depressive syndrome responsive to lithium. An analysis of 20 cases, J Nerv Ment Dis 1976;**163**(4):276–81.

7. **Peselow ED, Dunner DL, Fieve RR**, and **Lautin A**. Prophylactic effect of lithium against depression in cyclothymic patients: a life-table analysis, Compr Psychiatry 1981;**22**(3):257–64.

8. **Rosier YA, Broussolle P**, and **Fontany M**. Lithium gluconate: systematic and factorial analysis of 104 cases which have been studied for 2 and one-half to 3 years in patients regularly observed and showing periodic cyclothymia or dysthymia, Ann Med Psychol (Paris) 1974;**1**(3):389–97.

9. **Akiskal HS, Khani MK**, and **Scott-Strauss A**. Cyclothymic temperamental disorders, Psych Clin North Am 1979;**2**:527–54.

10. **Ananth J, Engelsmann F, Kiriakos R**, and **Kolivakis T**. Prediction of lithium response, Acta Psychiatr Scand 1979;**60**(3):279–86.

11. **Steiner M, Haskett RF, Osmun JN**, and **Carroll BJ**. Treatment of premenstrual tension with lithium carbonate. A pilot study, Acta Psychiatr Scand 1980;**61**(2):96–102.

12. **Gawin F** and **Kleber H**. Pharmacologic treatments of cocaine abuse, Psychiatr Clin North Am 1986;**9**(3):573–83.

13. **Baldessarini RJ, Tondo L, Floris G**, and **Hennen J**. Effects of rapid cycling on response to lithium maintenance treatment in 360 bipolar I and II disorder patients, J Affect Disord 2000;**61**(1–2):13–22.

14. **Goto S, Terao T, Hoaki N**, and **Wang Y**. Cyclothymic and hyperthymic temperaments may predict bipolarity in major depressive disorder: a supportive evidence for bipolar II1/ 2 and IV, J Affect Disord. 2011;**129**(1–3):34–8.

15. **Peselow ED, Dunner DL, Fieve RR**, and **Lautin A**. Lithium prophylaxis of depression in unipolar, bipolar II, and cyclothymic patients, Am J Psychiatry 1982;**139**(6):747–52.

16. **Rybakowski JK, Dembinska D, Kliwicki S, Akiskal KK**, and **Akiskal HH**. TEMPS-A and long-term lithium response: positive correlation with hyperthymic temperament, J Affect Disord. 2013;**145**(2):187–9.

17. **Semadeni GW.** Clinical study of the normothymic effect of dipropylacetamide, Acta Psychiatr Belg 1976;**76**(3):458–66.

18. **Jacobsen FM.** Low-dose valproate: a new treatment for cyclothymia, mild rapid cycling disorders, and premenstrual syndrome, J Clin Psychiatry 1993;**54**(6):229–34.

19. **Chang KD, Dienes K, Blasey C, Adleman N, Ketter T,** and **Steiner H.** Divalproex monotherapy in the treatment of bipolar offspring with mood and behavioral disorders and at least mild affective symptoms, J Clin Psychiatry 2003;**64**(8):936–42.

20. **Findling RL, Frazier TW, Youngstrom EA, McNamara NK, Stansbrey RJ, Gracious BL,** et al. Double-blind, placebo-controlled trial of divalproex monotherapy in the treatment of symptomatic youth at high risk for developing bipolar disorder, J Clin Psychiatry 2007;**68**(5):781–8.

21. **Montes JM, Saiz-Ruiz J, Lahera G,** and **Asiel A.** Lamotrigine for the treatment of bipolar spectrum disorder: a chart review, J Affect Disord 2005;**86**(1):69–73.

22. **Manning JS, Haykal RF, Connor PD, Cunningham PD, Jackson WC,** and **Long S.** Sustained remission with lamotrigine augmentation or monotherapy in female resistant depressives with mixed cyclothymic-dysthymic temperament, J Affect Disord 2005;**84**(2–3):259–66.

23. **Ghaemi SN** and **Goodwin FK.** Gabapentin treatment of the non-refractory bipolar spectrum: an open case series, J Affect Disord 2001;**65**(2):167–71.

24. **Bisol LW** and **Lara DR.** Low-dose quetiapine for patients with dysregulation of hyperthymic and cyclothymic temperaments, J Psychopharmacol 2010;**24**(3):421–4.

25. **Steele TE** and **Taylor CI.** Hypomania and tricyclic antidepressant choice, Am J Psychiatry 1980;**137**(11):1457–8.

26. **Rounsaville BJ, Sholomskas D,** and **Prusoff BA.** Chronic mood disorders in depressed outpatient diagnosis and response to pharmacotherapy, J Affect Disord 1980;**2**(2):73–88.

27. **Akiskal HS** and **Mallya G.** Criteria for the 'soft' bipolar spectrum: treatment implications, Psychopharmacol Bull 1987;**23**(1):68–73.

28. **Ghaemi SN, Ko JK, Baldassano CF, Kontos NJ,** and **Goodwin FK.** Bipolar spectrum disorder: a pilot study, 155th Annual American Psychiatric Association Meeting; Philadelphia, PA, 2002.

29. **Sharma V, Khan M,** and **Smith A.** A closer look at treatment resistant depression: is it due to a bipolar diathesis?, J Affect Disord 2005;**84**(2–3):251–7.

30. **Shen GH, Sylvia LG, Alloy LB, Barrett F, Kohner M, Iacoviello B,** et al. Lifestyle regularity and cyclothymic symptomatology, J Clin Psychol 2008;**64**(4):482–500.

31. **Totterdell P, Kellett S,** and **Mansell W.** Cognitive behavioural therapy for cyclothymia: cognitive regulatory control as a mediator of mood change, Behav Cogn Psychother 2012;**40**(4):412–24.

32. **Fava GA, Rafanelli C, Tomba E, Guidi J,** and **Grandi S.** The sequential combination of cognitive behavioral treatment and well-being therapy in cyclothymic disorder, Psychother Psychosom 2011;**80**(3):136–43.

33. **Colom F, Vieta E, Sanchez-Moreno J, Palomino-Otiniano R, Reinares M, Goikolea JM,** et al. Group psychoeducation for stabilised bipolar disorders: 5-year outcome of a randomised clinical trial, Br J Psychiatry. 2009;**194**(3):260–5.

34. **Hantouche EG, Majdalani C,** and **Trybou V,** editors. Psychoeducation in group-therapy for cyclothymic patients; a novel approach, IRBD; Rome, 3–5 May 2007.

35. **Hantouche EG** and **Trybou T.** *Live Happily with Ups and Downs* (Paris, France: Odile Jacob; 2011).

36. **Perugi G** and **Akiskal HS.** The soft bipolar spectrum redefined: focus on the cyclothymic, anxious-sensitive, impulse-dyscontrol, and binge-eating connection in bipolar II and related conditions, Psychiatr Clin North Am 2002;**25**(4):713–37.

37. **Perugi G, Akiskal HS, Lattanzi L, Cecconi D, Mastrocinque C, Patronelli A,** et al. The high prevalence of 'soft' bipolar (II) features in atypical depression, Compr Psychiatry 1998;**39**(2):63–71.

38. **Hantouche EG, Angst J, Demonfaucon C, Perugi G, Lancrenon S,** and **Akiskal HS.** Cyclothymic OCD: a distinct form?, J Affect Disord 2003;**75**(1):1–10.

39. **Rihmer Z, Gonda X, Torzsa P, Kalabay L, Akiskal HS,** and **Eory A.** Affective temperament, history of suicide attempt and family history of suicide in general practice patients, J Affect Disord 2013;**149**(1–3):350–4.

40. **Perugi G, Toni C,** and **Akiskal HS.** Anxious-bipolar comorbidity. Diagnostic and treatment challenges, Psychiatr Clin North Am 1999;**22**(3):565–83, viii.

41. **Maremmani I, Perugi G, Pacini M,** and **Akiskal HS.** Toward a unitary perspective on the bipolar spectrum and substance abuse: opiate addiction as a paradigm, J Affect Disord 2006;**93**(1–3):1–12.

42. **Katzow JJ, Hsu DJ,** and **Ghaemi SN.** The bipolar spectrum: a clinical perspective, Bipolar Disord 2003;**5**(6):436–42.

43. Hantouche EG. Pharmacotherapy strategies and psychoeducation for complex cyclothymic patients. The World Psychiatric Association Meeting; **Florence,** Italy 2009.

44. **Perugi G, Fornaro M,** and **Akiskal HS.** Are atypical depression, borderline personality disorder and bipolar II disorder overlapping manifestations of a common cyclothymic diathesis?, *World Psychiatry* 2011;**10**(1):45–51.

45. **Perugi G, Toni C, Passino MC, Akiskal KK, Kaprinis S,** and **Akiskal HS.** Bulimia nervosa in atypical depression: the mediating role of cyclothymic temperament, J Affect Disord 2006;**92**(1):91–7.

46. Ko J, Ghaemi SN, Kontos N, Baldassano C, and Goodwin F. Antidepressant wear off and outcomes in bipolar versus unipolar depression. In: Assocation AP, editor. American Psychiatric Assocation Annual Meeting; Philadelphia, PA, 2002.

47. **Robillard R, Naismith SL, Rogers NL, Scott EM, Ip TK, Hermens DF,** et al. Sleep-wake cycle and melatonin rhythms in adolescents and young adults with mood disorders: comparison of unipolar and bipolar phenotypes, Eur Psychiatry 2013;**28**(7):412–16.

48. **Alatiq Y, Crane C, Williams JM,** and **Goodwin GM.** Dysfunctional beliefs in bipolar disorder: hypomanic vs depressive attitudes, J Affect Disord 2010;**122**(3):294–300.

49. **Perugi G, Toni C, Travierso MC,** and **Akiskal HS.** The role of cyclothymia in atypical depression: toward a data-based reconceptualization of the borderline-bipolar II connection, J Affect Disord 2003;**73**(1–2):87–98.

50. Hantouche EG. Cyclothymia, affective basic temperaments, and schema focused diagnosis: exploring soft bipolarity. The 10th International Review of Bipolar Disorders; Budapest, Hungary, 12–14 May 2010.

Chapter 11

Psychological interventions for early stage bipolar disorder

Jan Scott

Introduction

In young people aged less than 25 years, three of the four most burdensome health problems worldwide are depression, schizophrenia, and bipolar disorder (BD).[1] Such findings emphasize why it is important to provide early intervention for these disorders, in the hope that future generations will experience fewer adverse clinical, functional, social, familial, and economic consequences than the current patient cohort.

Early intervention strategies are more established in psychosis and depression, and now extend beyond treatments for first illness episodes (ie symptom profiles that meet established diagnostic threshold levels) towards individuals deemed 'at high risk' of developing such problems in the future. This strategy is compatible with the philosophy of clinical staging, which suggests that the evolution of severe mental disorders parallels that of chronic medical disorders (such as cancer, diabetes, etc), and as such warrants similar treatment approaches. A staging model attempts to identify where an individual is located on a 'disease continuum' from an asymptomatic state in an individual with enhanced vulnerability for a specific disorder (stage 0) through to end stage disease (stage 4). The application of staging in general medicine has led to the development of interventions for individuals at stage 0 and 1 with the aim of preventing progression to later stages of illness. Furthermore, as shown in Table 11.1, the early stages of conditions such as ischaemic heart disease are often treated with behavioural, psychological, or other non-pharmacological interventions, with the gradual introduction of stage-specific medications and more complex treatments.

In BD, stage 0 can only be identified indirectly (as we have no reliable and specific biomarkers with predictive validity). However, this stage can be represented by asymptomatic offspring of a parent with BD. Stage 1 cases can be recognized by the presence of sub-threshold manic symptoms, brief hypomania, or perhaps by early onset recurrent major depression in an individual with cyclothymia and/or a family history of BD. Individuals in stage 1 do not always seek help for their symptoms, but they may come to the attention of clinical services because of distress and/or reduced functioning. Stage 2 usually signifies the presence of syndromal BD (usually a clinical state fulfilling for the first time the diagnostic criteria for hypomania or mania), while stages 3 and 4 represent progressive phases of an established illness.[2-6]

Table 11.1 The treatment of ischaemic heart disease as an example of a 'clinical staging' approach

Stage	Common characteristics	Typical interventions
Stage 0 (latency or 'at risk')	Increased risk: family history (clinical examination, genetic tests)	Minimize risk of progression, eg. Encourage diet & exercise
Stage 1	Obesity, smoking, high cholesterol	Diet & exercise +/– statins
Stage 2	Increased blood pressure	Anti-hypertensives: eg. beta blockers
Stage 3	Angina	Anti-angina drugs: eg. glyceryl trinitrate (gtn)
Stage 4 (late or end stage)	Heart attack (myocardial infarction)	Surgery to insert cardiac stents (to bypass damaged arteries)

The application of staging models to BD is still in its infancy, but their use has led to discussions about the types of treatment modalities that can be targeted at stage 1, ie interventions for individuals who traditionally have been excluded from mental health services.[7] This is an interesting problem, as it is not appropriate to simply prescribe medications that are used for stage 2 onwards.[3,7] This is for two reasons. First, the individuals do not have syndromal episodes of BD and there is no evidence that the medications used for later stage disease will be helpful. Second, and very importantly, only about 20–30% individuals in stage 1 will ultimately develop BD.[5,8] So, it may be more rationale to either re-deploy existing lower-risk interventions from across mental health, or design new ones with a lower risk-to-benefit ratio than is the accepted norm for cases with established illnesses (ie stage 2 onwards).[7] Although new medications can of course fit into this treatment specification, the 'staging' model of BD has increased interest in the application of psychological treatments for 'at-risk' and first-episode cases.[9,10] As other chapters in this book examine pharmacology for BD, this chapter will explore the therapies being used in young people 'at risk' of or experiencing their first episode of BD.

The chapter begins by identifying the target populations for discussion and then reviews existing indirect evidence about response to therapy in 'early stage' compared with 'later stage' BD. The therapy models that have been specifically tested in young people at high risk of and/or with first-episode BD cases are then described and outcomes briefly noted. The chapter concludes with a description of the strengths and weaknesses of current model and outlines a revised model of intervention that targets more overtly some of the specific, developmentally normal cognitive-emotional and sleep regulation issues that might act as triggers of syndromal episodes of mood disorder in younger as compared with older age groups.

Delineating stage 1 and stage 2 studies of psychological therapies

A broad definition of psychological interventions has been applied in this chapter, namely: 'any non-pharmacological intervention delivered in any format (individual, family, etc), that was used for the purpose of relieving symptoms of mood disturbance or improving functional outcomes in first episode BD cases'.[10] Interventions for at-risk groups were additionally defined as 'incorporating strategies to prevent or delay the onset of a first BD episode'.

To try to find studies in the target populations, stage 1 and 2 were operationalized as:

(i) children and adolescents (young people aged <18 years) deemed at risk of BD, usually because they are the offspring of parent with this disorder, and/or they meet other recognized 'BAR' (bipolar at-risk) criteria;[8,10]

(ii) adolescents and young adults who experience a first episode of 'adult-prototype' BD during the peak period for the onset of BD (age range of about 15–25 years).

In this chapter, the phrase 'first-episode BD' refers mainly to an episode of hypomania or mania but, due to differences in how diagnostic criteria are applied internationally, it also includes some studies of schizo-affective disorder-manic type, psychotic mania and, in a small number of cases, it describes the first episode of affective psychosis.

Publications on children diagnosed with juvenile BD are not reviewed here for several reasons. First, the data on prodromal states, risk syndromes, and rates of transition to stage 2 are primarily focused on adult forms of BD and related disorders.[2,6,8,10] Second, some countries have reported a dramatic increase in the diagnosis of paediatric or juvenile BD, but these changes are not consistent across continents.[11] Furthermore, even in countries with increasing rates, the growth in clinical cases is not matched by similar changes in the rates of BD in the same age groups in carefully executed, large-scale, representative, non-clinical epidemiological studies.[11] Third, and perhaps most relevant to this chapter, it is not yet certain as to how these childhood variants of BD will evolve over time and whether or not they are linked to adult BD.[4] Given these issues, it is difficult to extrapolate from studies of paediatric BD to those of young adults at high risk of, or with first-episode BD.[8,10,11] Having noted these reservations about the reliability and predictive validity of the juvenile BD diagnosis, the design and structure of the psychological interventions employed in these children appear to provide a useful template of how to adapt 'adult' therapy models to the developmental needs of younger patients.[12,13] As such, it is important to acknowledge that several of these models have helped inform the development of interventions now being applied to post-pubertal children and adolescents.[10]

Existing evidence that clinical stage may be associated with therapy outcomes

Clinicians and researchers have only recently begun to explore the utility of clinical staging and early intervention models in BD.[2-6] However, there is an extensive evidence base for the benefits of psychological treatments as an adjunct to medication in BD cases. Although the findings are mainly applicable to adult populations who attend general psychiatry or specialist clinics (ie middle-aged adult populations with long-established BD), it is worthwhile to examine whether there are 'signals' within the previously published research that indicate that response to psychological therapies is influenced by clinical stage.

Post hoc analyses of four randomized controlled trials (RCTs) provide some support for improved outcomes in subgroups defined by course of illness or age.[14–17] An RCT of cognitive behaviour therapy (CBT)[14] and one of group psychoeducation (group PED),[15] both reported that therapy may be more beneficial to individuals with fewer prior illness episodes. Each analysis demonstrated a dose-response pattern, with the greatest level of improvement observed in those with 0–6 prior BD episodes, less evidence of benefit in those with 7–12 BD episodes, and minimal benefit in those with 12 or more prior episodes of BD. A study of family psychoeducation reported similar outcomes.[16] Obviously, number of episodes alone does not define the boundaries of each clinical stage of BD, but it can be viewed as a useful 'proxy' measure.[3,6] Thus, these studies provide indirect evidence to support the notion that lower-risk, higher-benefit treatments are more efficient for individuals at an earlier rather than a later clinical stage.[7]

Kessing et al.[17] also re-analysed the outcomes of an RCT of 158 adults allocated to early intervention at a mood disorder clinic (offering optimized pharmacotherapy and group PED) or to clinics offering standard clinical care. Less than 20% individuals were aged 18–25 years (which undermined the statistical power of the secondary analyses), but outcomes were compared for subgroups defined by age (18–25 versus over 25 years). Overall, hospital admission rates were decreased in all those treated in the mood disorder clinic versus standard treatment. Furthermore, the analysis by age group revealed that this reduction was most marked, although of borderline statistical significance, in the younger age group (hazard ratio 0.33; $p = 0.06$).

Interventions designed for at-risk and first-episode cases

A number of manuals or detailed descriptions are published that give sufficient information about the planned interventions to allow a therapist to deliver a therapy reliably. However, it is noticeable that a number of interventions for individuals with first diagnosis of BD do not state if they are specifically targeted at young people, and some interventions for adolescents do not clarify if they are targeted at first-episode cases. As such this review of interventions includes only those models where outcome data indicate that they have been tested with young people with first-episode disorders. As shown in Table 11.2, interventions are classified according to whether they have been used for individuals at risk, for first-episode BD and for adolescent onset.

Table 11.2 gives an overview of the core elements of the therapies and allows comparison of similarities and differences in the content and targets of the interventions. Although the therapies show many overlaps, the models used in different subgroups are also discussed.

Interventions for individuals at risk of bipolar disorder

Three of the interventions described for use in at-risk populations are based on CBT,[18–20] two use family approaches,[21–22] and one model is based on interpersonal social rhythms therapy (IPSRT).[23]

Pfenning and colleagues[18] describe 'Early-CBT', a group intervention (90 minutes/week for 14 weeks) that includes stress management and problem-solving strategies with elements of mindfulness-based CBT (MBCBT). Modules were also adapted from psychoeducation and other sessions previously used with individuals at risk of developing psychotic disorders. As discussed later in the chapter, Scott[19] describes another CBT model termed CBT-R (CBT-Regulation) to emphasize that it specifically targets deficits in cognitive-emotional regulation, sleep-circadian rhythms, and physical activity. Cotton et al.[20] developed an MBCBT intervention for use with the offspring of bipolar parents who were deemed to be at increased risk because of evidence of mood dysregulation or anxiety problems.

A therapy manual for family focused treatment with 'high-risk' offspring of BD parents (FFT-HR) is available online.[21] The FFT-HR model draws heavily on the techniques used in the FFT approach that were developed for adolescents with BD (FFT-A)[22] but FFT-HR can be used with children aged 9–17 years. It consists of 12 sessions over four months with a module on PED (five sessions), communication enhancement training (three sessions), and problem-solving skills training (three sessions). The main aims of FFT-HR are to support high-risk youth and family members to: (i) identify prodromal symptoms of depressive or (hypo)manic episodes; (ii) differentiate significant mood dysregulation from developmentally appropriate emotional reactivity; (iii) recognize triggers of mood swings; and (iv) build prevention plans to avoid mood escalation.

Multi-family psychoeducational psychotherapy (MF-PEP)[12] is a manualized intervention for children with depressive and bipolar spectrum disorders and their parents. It combines psychoeducation with family therapy and CBT techniques (ie behavioural activation and coping skills, cognitive restructuring). Therapy is delivered over eight sessions lasting 90 minutes each with concurrent parent and child groups. Although mainly targeting younger children, studies report transition rates to BD in those receiving MF-PEP compared with usual treatments.

Goldstein and colleagues[22] report the use of IPSRT with offspring of a parent with BD. The intervention was similar to interpersonal social rhythms therapy for adolescents (IPSRT-A)[24] but consisted of 12 sessions delivered over six months. The IPSRT focus on stabilizing daily rhythms and interpersonal relationships was seen as particularly important for adolescents.

Interventions for first-episode cases

As shown in Table 11.2, three of the interventions described originated from therapy models employed in early intervention in psychosis services[25–27] and have been used with cases of affective and non-affective disorders. The other publication (Jones et al.[28]) described a CBT intervention offered to individuals across a broad age range defined as 'first-diagnosis' BD. The intervention drew on standard CBT approaches

Table 11.2 Comparison of key characteristics of psychological therapies used for at-risk and first-episode bipolar disorder (BD)Regulation

Therapy model*	Format for model for first-episode cases				Components used in therapies for adult cases with established BD & in first-episode cases				Extra components/modifications for first-episode cases			
	Number of sessions	Individual	Group	Family	Psychoeducation	Problem Solving	Relapse prevention techniques	Risk factors for relapse	Developmental adaptations	Social functioning/ relationships	Educational/ vocational functioning	Communication training
At risk												
Group CBT[18]	14		+++		+++	++	++	++	+	+		
CBT-R[19]	24	++			++	++	++	+++	+++	++	+	++
MB-CBT-C[20]	12		++		+	++	+		++			
FFT-HR[21]	12			+++	+++	+++	+++	+++	+++	+	+	+++
IPSRT[22]	12	++			++	+++	++	+++	++	++	+	+
MF-PEP[12]	8		+++	+++	+++	+++	++	++	+	+		+
First episode												
Integrated intervention (EPPIC case management)[25]	Varies ~ 2 yrs	+++			++	+	++	+	+++	+	++	
CBT-based, multimodal therapy[26]	> 22	++		+	+++	+	+++	+++	+++	+++	+++	+

(Continued)

Table 11.2 Continued

Therapy model*	Format for model for first-episode cases				Components used in therapies for adult cases with established BD & in first-episode cases				Extra components/modifications for first-episode cases			
	Number of sessions	Individual	Group	Family	Psychoedu-cation	Problem Solving	Relapse prevention techniques	Risk factors for relapse	Develop-mental adaptations	Social functioning/ relationships	Educational/ vocational functioning	Communi-cation training
HORYZONS (online peer-to-peer modules)[27]	Varies; open access		+++		+++	+	+++		+	+++	+	++
CBT[28]	> 22	+++			+	+++	+++	++				
First episode & adolescent onset												
FFT-A [23]	< 22			+++	++	+++	+	+	+++	+	++	+++
IPSRT-A [24]	< 22	++		+	+	+	++	++	++	+++	++	++
DBT*[29]	> 22	++		+*	++	++	+	+	+++	++	++	+

+++ Module described in intervention manual or publications; + Mentioned as a therapy goal, but limited detail provided about the strategy; ++ Techniques specifically included in the therapy; ++ Techniques specifically included in the therapy;
*DBT also includes a module specifically for parents

CBT = cognitive behaviour therapy; CBT-R = CBT-Regulation; MB-CBT-C = Mindfulness-based CBT children; TEAMS = Thinking Effectively About Mood Swings; EPPIC = Early Psychosis Prevention & Intervention Centre; FFT = FFT-Adolescent; FFT-A = FFT-Adolescent; FFT-HR = FFT-High Risk; IPSRT = Inter-Personal Social Rhythms Therapy; IPSRT-A = Inter-Personal Social Rhythms Therapy-Adolescent; MF-PEP = Multi-Family Psychoeducational Psychotherapy with few modifications, except for some flexibility in location for delivery of therapy (eg offering home-based sessions).

The most well-known early intervention programme was developed at EPPIC[25] in Australia. The approach emerged from the recognition that there were a number of specific challenges and opportunities relevant to working with young people with psychosis including issues of engagement, co-morbidity, and family and developmental factors, which impacted on adaptation to the disorder. The intervention uses a multimodal case-management system (including some group work, and optional individual therapy modules) and the intervention represents a trans-diagnostic approach that targets functional as well as symptomatic recovery.

The manual by Macneil et al.[26] actually evolved largely because of the recognition that the EPPIC approach did not always cater for some of the specific needs of individuals with first-episode BD or affective psychosis. The therapy is longer than many others, but is fairly flexible, and can be adapted according to the clinical/psychological needs of the adolescent and/or the severity of the initial clinical presentation. The interventions used are based mainly on CBT, but also specifically explored 'recovery' concepts; it includes eight possible modules: (i) engagement and formulation; (ii) PED and adaptation; (iii) medication adherence; (iv) specific CBT interventions for (hypo)mania and depression; (v) social rhythm regulation; (vi) relationship and family work; (vii) managing alcohol and substance use (through harm reduction) and other co-morbidities; and (viii) relapse prevention. Macneil et al. also explicitly state that they examine how to cope with prejudice and self-stigma.

Alvarez-Jimenez et al.[27] describes an online series of behavioural interventions integrating: (i) peer-to-peer social networking; (ii) individually tailored interactive psychosocial interventions; and (iii) expert interdisciplinary and peer-moderation, into a package focused on improving long-term outcomes. Although the main clientele for this programme, named HORYZONS, have a first episode of a non-affective psychosis, the individually tailored elements and use of CBT interventions mean that this approach can be applied to BD.

Interventions for adolescent-onset bipolar disorders

Three models were designed for use with adolescents in the first episode of BD or early in the course of the illness.[23,24,29] All three were developed at specialist clinics for this clinical population and all were adapted from therapies used for adults with established BD.

The FFT-A approach specifically targets relapse prevention in adolescents with a diagnosis of BD.[23] The three main modules are as noted for FFT-HR, but are of longer duration. A goal of FFT-A is to decrease stress and interpersonal conflicts by reducing the levels of expressed emotion in the family and by enhancing flexible and adaptive interpersonal patterns. Parents (and if possible, siblings and members of the extended family) are invited to therapy sessions, and families have homework each week.

The IPSRT-A[24] approach emphasizes that interpersonal issues are a risk factor for mood instability in adolescents. The initial, middle, and termination phases are similar in structure to interpersonal therapy for depressed adolescents (IPT-A); however, IPSRT-A is slightly longer (16–18 sessions over 20 weeks) because of the added interventions to increase lifestyle regularity and the increased severity of illness in adolescents with BD. The essential components of IPSRT-A are psychoeducation, interpersonal work, and stabilization of daily social rhythm and sleep. Communication training is included, examining intra-familial communication, but also school- or peer-group interactions.

The dialectical behavioural therapy (DBT) intervention for adolescents with BD[29] is based on the manual by Miller and colleagues,[30] which in turn draws on the DBT approach to emotional dysregulation in adults at risk of repeated self-harm. In DBT for BD, two treatment modalities are proposed: 18 sessions of family skill training (adapted for use with individual family units) and 18 sessions of individual therapy focused on the young person's target behaviours. A unique component of DBT, which is not present in the other therapies reviewed, is the module developed for parents of adolescents with BD that is entitled 'walking the middle path'. This addresses the lack of balance between thoughts and behaviours within the family environment and educates the parents in how to support the adolescent to balance 'change-oriented' with 'acceptance-oriented' skills.

Outcomes

All of the therapy models outlined are being tested in clinical trials, but only six RCTs have been published for the selected sub-groups. If no RCT data are available, outcomes from controlled clinical trials (CCTs) or case series (CS) are reviewed.

At risk

The RCT of MF-PEP[31] is the only study that provides data on 'transition' from at-risk status to BD caseness. The sample comprised of 50 individuals (out of a total of 165 participants) who were deemed at risk of BD because of a depressive spectrum disorder with or without transient manic-like symptoms. Those receiving the MF-PEP were significantly less likely to meet criteria for a bipolar spectrum disorder at follow-up compared with those allocated to the control group (12% v 45%).

The RCT of FFT-HR is the first blinded RCT of a psychosocial intervention for youth at risk for BD.[32] The 40 participants (mean age ~12; 40% medication-free) were randomly allocated to FFT-HR (12 sessions of psychoeducation, communication training, and problem-solving skills) or a brief psychoeducation control condition (1–2 family education sessions). The FFT-HR group demonstrated a more rapid recovery from mood symptoms and longer periods of remission compared with the control group; medication status did not influence outcomes.

The CS of IPSRT[22] and CBT[22,33] represent small-scale studies with mixed outcomes. For example, IPSRT had an important effect on sleep profile in young adults, but less evidence of significant benefits for mood disorders (eg three cases met depression criteria at baseline and four at follow-up).[22] In a broadly defined at-risk group, a CBT model showed only weak effects on manic symptoms;[33] however, the CS of ten offspring of BD parents suggested that MBCBT produced significant reductions in anxiety and associated changes in emotional regulation, but non-significant decreases in depressive or manic symptoms.[20]

First episode

Conus et al.[34] published a follow-up study of 108 individuals (mean age ~22 years; 55% male) who presented with psychotic mania (who were then classified as either BD or schizo-affective disorder). At 12-month follow-up (ie 30 months after entering the EPPIC programme), the BD cases reported better overall outcomes with significantly higher levels of functioning and lower levels of negative symptoms than the group identified as having schizo-affective disorder. However, it is notable that there were a high number of study dropouts.

A CCT described multimodal CBT for first-episode mania and comprised 40 individuals who were concurrently included in a larger-scale open-label RCT of medication.[35] 34 individuals had a diagnosis of 'BD with psychotic symptoms'. The 20 control participants, who received low intensity psychological input (<4 of 8 therapy modules), were matched on key demographic variables with the intervention group. A group by time analysis showed that improvements in depressive symptoms, illness severity, and functioning were significantly greater in the intensive intervention group compared with the control group. In contrast, levels of manic symptoms and overall relapse rates were similar in both groups.

The one-month open feasibility study by Alvarez-Jimenez et al.[27] is unique in its focus and mode of delivery of interventions. Only two cases (out of 20) had an affective psychosis, but the participants demonstrated good uptake of the programme, self-reported improvements in social connectedness, and significant pre-post intervention reductions in depressive symptoms.

Adolescent onset

The first RCT of FFT-A[36] included 58 individuals with a mean age ~15 years; the majority had BD I (n = 38). Group outcomes were similar, although cases allocated to FFT-A recovered from depression significantly earlier (difference ~7 weeks; hazard ratio = 1.85) than those in the control group. In the second, multicentre RCT (n = 145) of similar design,[37] FFT-A showed no benefits in time to recovery or recurrence, nor in percentage of time as well. However, FFT-A did show greater reductions in severity of and weeks without (hypo)manic symptoms.

A small-scale open RCT of IPSRT-A of 17 participants (IPSRT-A = 12; treatment as usual (TAU) = 5)[38] demonstrated significant between group differences in effect size (ES) for changes in depressive (IPSRT-A = 1.8 v TAU = 1.3) and manic symptoms (IPSRT-A = 1.2 v TAU = 0.5), alongside improved social and interpersonal functioning. However, a larger-scale RCT by Inder and colleagues[39] (47 out of 100 were aged <26) of IPRST compared to (SSC) reported no significant differences in outcomes.

A CS of DBT recruited ten individuals (mean age ~16) of whom nine attended >= 90% of scheduled sessions.[29] Significant reductions were noted for depressive (ES = 0.7) but not manic symptoms. Reductions in suicidal ideation, non-suicidal self-injurious behaviour, and emotional dysregulation were also noted.

Strengths and weaknesses

The key therapy approaches that have been employed in established BD cases are described for early-stage BD, and FFT, IPSRT, and CBT models have been developed for use with both at-risk and first-episode subgroups. It is notable that none of the interventions are based on peer-group PED (a commonly used model in adults and established cases of BD), although many approaches incorporate individual PED or group sessions focused on, for example, PED about early warning signs of relapse.

As in the therapies used in adult cases of established BD, all the interventions reviewed included PED about BD, problem-solving skills training, and development of relapse-prevention strategies, and all offered the opportunity for sessions to enhance medication adherence in cases where these treatments were prescribed. Although social rhythm dysregulation is a critical theoretical element of IPSRT-A,[24] nearly all the therapies acknowledge the need to stabilize sleep patterns to try to avert the risk of relapse. Overall, the IPSRT and FFT models have many more similarities than differences to the therapies used with older adults with later-stage BD. However, the CBT models described for early stage BD show less reliance on classical 'Beckian' models and increasingly include mindfulness techniques, use other approaches that target emotional dysregulation (eg DBT), or incorporate multimodal approaches.

Taken together, the outcome data indicate modest benefits from the therapies.[10] Gains reported in open CS without any comparison group or in smaller-scale or single-centre RCTs have not always translated into consistent differences in acute or longer-term outcomes in more methodologically sound studies. Also, where improvements have been associated with therapy, there have often been reductions in depressive but not manic symptoms (or vice versa). The interpretation of the data is hampered by sample heterogeneity, meaning that it is not yet possible to identify whether specific interventions are more effective at different stages of BD (eg early onset or later stages of persistent illness), nor to differentiate clearly between outcomes from different therapies offered at the same stage of illness.

It is tempting to assume that the more limited therapeutic gains seen in early (stage 1/2) compared with more established (stage 3) BD can be explained by extraneous factors or are a consequence of lower 'base rates' of psychopathology or severity of symptomatology in the early stage cases (and hence the possibility that 'floor' effects limit the chances of finding statistically significant differences). However, the alternative explanation is that the models lack active ingredients that may be especially needed in high-risk and first-episode cases.[10,19] For example, most therapies describe age-appropriate modifications such as ensuring that the therapy content, PED modules, and handouts are delivered in an accessible way, using easy-to-understand language. Likewise, therapies give due consideration to maturational level or social context (eg specific sessions focused on the young person's functioning at school, managing peer-group pressures, individuation from parents, etc). However, few interventions explicitly tackle co-morbid substance misuse or consider other overlapping syndromes and symptoms (eg arousal/anxiety, etc).[10] Also, interventions for sleep or emotional regulation do not attend to specific developmental patterns in these phenomena.[40,41] Lastly, and very importantly, there is a lack of targeting of physical health.[10]

A new model

The possibility that the interventions for individuals with emerging BD have paid insufficient attention to developmental trajectories and comorbidities have led us to develop a new therapy model, called CBT-R.[19] The intervention focuses on how to manage risk for a mood disorder, alongside potential triggers for mood, activity, or sleep variations that occur in this age group.[40-42] Two robust prognostic markers in younger people that are putatively linked to underlying pathophysiological mechanisms are disturbed sleep–wake cycle and ruminative thinking style (see Box 11.1).[42]

To date, no psychological treatments for young adults have been adapted explicitly to target these mechanisms simultaneously. The rationale for selecting these phenomena is that both circadian and cognitive-emotional processes are known to undergo predictable, developmental changes (in association with frontal lobe maturation) during adolescence and early adulthood.[42,43] Furthermore, there is evidence of interrelationships between rumination, sleep, behaviour, cognition, and mood (see Table 11.2).[19,42]

We hypothesize that dysregulation of these sleep–wake activity and cognitive-emotional developmental processes will exacerbate or perpetuate current mood symptoms and increase the risk of early transition from stage 1 to stage 2 (or the risk of relapse in stage 2 cases), or will be associated with the evolution of other psychopathology. Consequently, we developed a CBT-R intervention that targets these specific circadian and/or cognitive mechanisms with the goal of increasing the likelihood of sustained stabilization and improved outcomes.[19]

The therapy comprises of four modules that extend for up to 24 sessions. There is some flexibility, as the duration of the first module (problem-solving and engagement) depends on the nature of the problems that led the young person to seek help. The duration of the two main modules are approximately eight sessions each (delivered weekly initially and then every two weeks).

Although CBT-R draws on some of the traditional elements of CBT used in adults, the focus of the CBT-R interventions is shifted to the examination of thinking processes rather than thought content (as cognitive processing style may be a trait marker of risk for psychopathology) and to stabilization of the sleep–wake and physical activity–rest cycles (as opposed to daily activity planning). In this way, the interventions are more clearly derived from theoretical models that take into account important age-related developmental changes in circadian or cognitive-emotional regulation (see Figure 11.1). It is argued that this is necessary as any failure to re-align these systems will exacerbate or perpetuate mood symptoms or act as risk factors that predispose to transition to BD.[19,40-45]

The initial module employs a modified version of behavioural activation (now transformed into behavioural regulation to prevent over-activation in those at risk of hypomania or mania), alongside sessions targeting sleep–wake cycle or circadian regulation.[19] Which interventions are initiated are determined by whether the sleep

Box 11.1 Putative target mechanisms: circadian and cognitive-emotional regulation

(a) Target symptom: sleep; target mechanism: circadian regulation

Prolonged sleep onset latency and delayed sleep phase both peak in young adults (about 14% show these patterns) and show inverse associations with mood and cognitive functioning in non-depressed samples. Further, the degree of circadian disturbance is significantly more marked in those with emerging mood disorders, with >30% young adults with depression showing sleep phase delay according to actigraphy recordings and 60% of those with emerging BD.

Given the overlap between developmental and disease processes, we postulate that age-recognized shifts in circadian regulation act to precipitate or perpetuate illness in individuals at risk of BD or recurrent mood disorders and that targeting these abnormalities can improve outcomes.

(b) Target symptom: rumination; target mechanism: cognitive-emotional regulation

Rumination is defined as a response to negative affect that involves 'repetitively and passively focusing on symptoms of distress and on the possible causes and consequences of the symptoms'. Rumination may comprise of two elements: an adaptive, reflective-distancing component (akin to 'mindfulness') and 'brooding', described as 'getting depressed about being depressed'. It is a critical marker of cognitive-emotional dysregulation as the individuals' focus on their distress (rather than on distraction to reduce dysphoria) and their passivity (rather than active problem-solving to resolve stressors) act together to intensify their negative affect.

Ruminative response style is a robust risk factor for the development and maintenance of psychopathology, especially depression, and recent evidence also implicates rumination in anxiety or co-morbid anxiety-depressive states in younger (but not older) adults and in BDs. Interestingly, those with high levels of rumination also show poorer sleep quality, and abnormal cortisol response to stress. Developmentally, the propensity to rumination peaks during middle and late adolescence (partly because of greater self-focus, etc), and is more common in females.3

disturbance is insomnia (which is often linked to arousal or anxiety), hypersomnia, or prolonged sleep-onset latency with late waking time (which may be a marker of circadian rhythm dysregulation, namely delayed sleep phase). Different modules or combined modules are used to regulate these sleep disturbances, although similar daytime interventions are used to manage physical activity across all cases.[43-45]

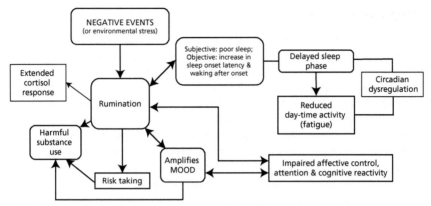

Figure 11.1 Established links between rumination, risk taking, mood, substance use, sleep, and activity

This next module uses rumination-focused CBT (RfCBT).[46,47] Although this model has overlapping elements to mindfulness, we use RfCBT with youth for several reasons. First, it includes functional analysis and more behavioural elements, linking it well with the initial module. Second, it is easier for a wide range of young people to work with RfCBT, as it is more concrete and requires less reliance on some of the more subtle mindfulness skills. Third, the approach is helpful for rumination associated with distress, substance use, anxiety or depressive symptoms, and can also be used to deal with 'positive repetitive self-focused thinking' (positive rumination or 'basking') that has been reported in youth with cyclothymia, brief hypomania, or other bipolar at-risk syndromes.[42]

The RfCBT and the activity-behavioural regulation module can also help tackle risk taking, which is sometimes employed as a maladaptive coping strategy to overcome negative rumination.[48] These modules can be useful in helping to manage potentially harmful substance use and/or risky behaviours associated with sexual activity, etc.[19,42,46]

The final sessions (about four) can be extended over longer periods of time if required and focus on recapping the skills and techniques that have been learnt and developing skills in identifying and managing early warning signs (primarily events, triggers, sleep and behaviour change) that may indicate risk for increases in symptom levels or reductions in functioning.[49,50]

The therapy is longer than many interventions for individuals at risk of BD. However, we suggest that this is helpful because it can take six months to produce a robust and sustained change in cognitive-emotional and sleep-circadian regulation. In addition, some young people prefer to take breaks or have pauses between modules, sometimes to take more time to practise skills from the recent module, sometimes because of ambivalence about the need to continue to attend sessions (which may be linked with 'avoidance' or difficulty in accepting their increased 'risk' status).

Although not tested in an RCT, the preliminary pilot data for this approach in young people at risk of BD (or of recurrent unipolar depression) are encouraging.[19]

Conclusion

Currently, there is insufficient evidence of any major differences in outcomes for early stage BD between individuals offered BD-specific interventions (FFT, CBT, IPSRT) and trans-diagnostic, case-management, or multimodal interventions offered via early intervention in psychosis services (EPPIC case management, HORYZONS). However, a number of challenges remain to be addressed in this field before definitive conclusions can be drawn. These include the need to better understand whether some interventions are most suited to trans-diagnostic samples of young people in the early stages of a range of severe mental disorders and/or to determine whether different psychological interventions are more effective than others for homogenous samples of early stage BD cases.[10] Studies and RCTs of these approaches could help to clarify whether interventions have unique benefits or disorder-specific effects. In addition, given the modest benefits demonstrated with evidence-based therapies that have been adapted for use in at-risk and first-episode and adolescent populations with BD, there is a need to consider additional age- and stage-appropriate modifications. Research on these attempts to modify the developmental trajectory of BD could also provide important insights into mediators and moderators of transitions between the stages of BD.[10]

References

1. **Gore F, Bloem P, Patton G, Ferguson J, Joseph V, Coffey C, Sawyer S,** and **Mathers C.** Global burden of disease in young people aged 10–24 years: a systematic analysis, Lancet, 2011 Jun;**377**(9783):2093–102. Erratum in: Lancet 2011 Aug;378(9790):486.

2. **McGorry PD, Hickie IB, Yung A, Pantelis C,** and **Jackson H.** Clinical staging of psychiatric disorders: a heuristic framework for choosing earlier, safer and more effective interventions, Aust NZJ Psychiatry 2006;**40**(8):616–22.

3. **Berk M, Conus P, Lucas N, Hallam K, Malhi G, Dodd S, Yatham L, Yung A,** and **McGorry P.** Setting the stage: from prodrome to treatment resistance in bipolar disorder, Bipolar Disorder 2007 Nov;**9**(7):671–8.

4. **Duffy A, Alda M, Hajek T, Sherry SB,** and **Grof P.** Early stages in the development of bipolar disorder, J Affect Disord 2010;**121**(1–2):127–35.

5. **Scott J, Leboyer M, Hickie I, Berk M, Kapzinsky F, Frank E, Kupfer D,** and **McGorry P.** Clinical staging in psychiatry: a cross-cutting model of diagnosis with heuristic & practical value, Br J Psychiatry 2013 Apr;**202**(4):243–5.

6. **Scott J, Hickie I,** and **McGorry P.** Invited editorial: Pre-emptive psychiatric treatments: pipe dream or a realistic outcome of clinical staging models?, *Neuropsychiatry* 2012;**2**(4):263–5.

7. **Kapczinski F, Magalhães PV, Balanzá-Martinez V, Dias VV, Frangou S, Gama CS, Gonzalez-Pinto A, Grande I, Ha K, Kauer-Sant'Anna M, Kunz M, Kupka R, Leboyer M, Lopez-Jaramillo C, Post RM, Rybakowski JK, Scott J, Strejilevitch S, Tohen M, Vazquez G, Yatham L, Vieta E,** and **Berk M.** Staging systems in bipolar disorder: an International Society for Bipolar Disorders Task Force Report, Acta Psychiatr Scand 2014 Nov;**130**(5):354–63.

8. **Bechdolf A, Bechdolf A, Ratheesh A, Cotton SM, Nelson B, Chanen AM, Betts J, Bingmann T, Yung AR, Berk M,** and **McGorry PD.** The predictive validity of bipolar

at-risk (prodromal) criteria in help-seeking adolescents and young adults: a prospective study, Bipolar Disord 2014 Aug;16(5):493–504.

9. **Pfennig A, Correll CU, Marx C, Rottmann-Wolf M, Meyer TD, Bauer M,** and **Leopold K.** Psychotherapeutic interventions in individuals at risk of developing bipolar disorder: a systematic review, Early Interv Psychiatry 2014 Feb;8(1):3–11.

10. **Vallarino M, Henry C, Etain B, Gehue L, Macneil C, Scott, E, Barbato A, Conus P, Hlastala S, Fristad M, Miklowitz D,** and **Scott J.** An evidence map of psychosocial interventions for the earliest stages of bipolar disorder, *Lancet Psychiatry* 2015;2(6):548–63.

11. **Douglas J** and **Scott J.** Mania in pre-pubertal children: fact or artefact?, *Bipolar Disorders* 2014;16(1):5–15.

12. **Fristad M, Goldberg-Arnold J,** and **Gavazzi S.** Multifamily psychoeducation groups (MFPG) for families of children with bipolar disorder, *Bipolar Disorder* 2002 Aug;4(4):254–62.

13. **Feeny NC, Danielson CK, Schwartz L, Youngstrom EA,** and **Findling RL.** Cognitive-behavioral therapy for bipolar disorders in adolescents: a pilot study, *Archives of General Psychiatry* 2009 Sep;66(9):1013–21.

14. **Scott J, Paykel E, Morriss R, Bentall R, Kinderman P, Johnson T, Abbott R,** and **Hayhurst H.** Cognitive-behavioural therapy for severe and recurrent bipolar disorders: randomised controlled trial, Br J Psychiatry 2006 Apr;188:313–20.

15. **Colom F, Reinares M, Pacchiarotti I,** et al. Has number of previous episodes any effect on response to group psychoeducation in bipolar patients? A 5-year follow-up post hoc analysis, *Acta Neuropsychiatrica* 2010;22:50–3.

16. **Reinares M, Colom F, Rosa AR,** et al. The impact of staging bipolar disorder on treatment outcome of family psychoeducation, J Affect Disord 2010;123:81–6.

17. **Kessing LV, Hansen HV, Christensen EM, Dam H, Gluud C, Wetterslev J; Early Intervention Affective Disorders (EIA) Trial Group.** Do young adults with bipolar disorder benefit from early intervention?, J Affect Disord 2014 Jan;152–4:403–8.

18. **Pfennig A, Leopold K, Bechdolf A, Correll CU, Holtmann M, Lambert M, Marx C, Meyer TD, Pfeiffer S, Reif A, Rottmann-Wolf M, Schmitt NM, Stamm T, Juckel G,** and **Bauer M.** Early specific cognitive-behavioural psychotherapy in subjects at high risk for bipolar disorders: study protocol for a randomised controlled trial, *Trials* 2014 May;15:161.

19. **Scott J.** Early identification of young people at high risk of recurrent mood disorders: a feasibility study (PB-PG-0609-16166). National Institute for Health Research.

20. **Cotton S, Luberto CM, Sears RW, Strawn JR, Stahl L, Wasson RS, Blom TJ,** and **Delbello MP.** Mindfulness-based cognitive therapy for youth with anxiety disorders at risk for bipolar disorder: a pilot trial, Early Interv Psychiatry 2015 Jan;10–13.

21. **Miklowitz D.** 'FFT-HR: Clinicians Manual for the Family-Focused Treatment of Children and Adolescents at High Risk for Bipolar Disorder' (http://www.sem el.ucla. edu/champ/resources) last accessed 10/08/2015.

22. **Goldstein TR, Fersch-Podrat R, Axelson DA,** et al. Early intervention for adolescents at high risk for the development of bipolar disorder: pilot study of Interpersonal and Social Rhythm Therapy (IPSRT), *Psychotherapy* 2014;51:180–9.

23. **Miklowitz DJ, Biuckians AA,** and **Richards JA.** Early-onset bipolar disorder: a family treatment perspective, Dev Psychopathol 2006;18:1247–66.

24. **Hlastala S** and **Frank E.** Adapting interpersonal and social rhythm therapy to the developmental needs of adolescents with bipolar disorder, *Development and Psychopathology* 2006;**18**(4):1267–88.

25. **Early Psychosis Prevention and Intervention Centre.** *Care Management in Early Psychosis: A Handbook* (Melbourne: EPPIC, 2001).

26. **Macneil CA, Hasty M, Conus P, Berk M,** and **Scott J.** *Bipolar Disorder in Young People: A Psychological Intervention Manual* (Cambridge: Cambridge University Press, 2009).

27. **Alvarez-Jimenez M, Bendall S, Lederman R, Wadley G, Chinnery G, Vargas S, Larkin M, Killackey E, McGorry PD,** and **Gleeson JF.** On the HORYZON: moderated online social therapy for long-term recovery in first episode psychosis, Schizophr Res 2012 Nov (Epub ahead of print).

28. **Jones S** and **Burrell-Hodgson G.** Cognitive-behavioural treatment of first diagnosis bipolar disorder, *Clinical Psychology & Psychotherapy* 2008;**15**:367–77.

29. **Goldstein T, Axelson D, Birmaher B,** and **Brent D.** Dialectical behavior therapy for adolescents with bipolar disorder: a 1-year open trial, *Journal of the American Academy of Child & Adolescent Psychiatry* 2007;**46**:7, 820–30.

30. **Miller A, Rathus S,** and **Linehan M.** *DBT for Suicidal Adolescents* (New York, NY: Guilford Press, 2006).

31. **Nadkarni RB** and **Fristad MA.** Clinical course of children with a depressive spectrum disorder and transient manic symptoms, *Bipolar Disorder* 2010;**12**:494–503.

32. **Miklowitz DJ, Chang KD, Taylor DO,** et al. Early psychosocial intervention for youth at risk for bipolar I or II disorder: a one-year treatment development trial, *Bipolar Disorder* 2011;**13**:67–75.

33. **French P.** Early detection and intervention with mood swings: findings form a single arm psychological therapy trial. International Society of Affective Disorders. Berlin, Germany; 28–30 Apr 2014.

34. **Conus P, Abdel-Baki A, H, Lambert M, McGorry PD,** and **Berk M.** Pre-morbid and outcome correlates of first episode mania with psychosis: Is a distinction between schizoaffective and bipolar I disorder valid in the early phase of psychotic disorders?, *Journal of Affective Disorders* 2010;**126**(1–2):88–95.

35. **Macneil CA, Hasty, Cotton S, Berk M, Hallam K, Kader L, McGorry P,** and **Conus C.** Can a targeted psychological intervention be effective for young people following a first manic episode? Results from an 18-month pilot study, *Early Intervention in Psychiatry* 2012;**6**:4, 380–8.

36. **Miklowitz DJ, Axelson D, Birnnaher B,** et al. Family-focused treatment for adolescents with bipolar disorder: results of a 2-year randomized trial, Arch Gen Psychiatry 2008;**65**:1053–61.

37. **Miklowitz DJ, Schneck CD, George EL,** et al. Pharmacotherapy and family-focused treatment for adolescents with bipolar I and II disorders: a 2-year randomized trial, Am J Psychiatry 2014;**171**:658–67.

38. **Hlastala SA.** Interpersonal and social rhythm therapy for adolescents with bipolar disorder, Annual Convention of the Association for Behavioral and Cognitive Therapies; San Francisco, CA (18–21 Nov 2010).

39. **Inder ML, Crowe MT, Luty SE,** et al. Randomized, controlled trial of Interpersonal and Social Rhythm Therapy for young people with bipolar disorder, *Bipolar Disorder* 2014 Oct.

40. **Aldao A, Nolen-Hoeksema S**, and **Schweizer S**. Emotion-regulation strategies across psychopathology: a meta-analytic review, Clin Psychol Rev 2010 Mar;**30**(2):217–37.

41. **Robillard R, Naismith SL, Rogers NL, Ip TK, Hermens DF, Scott EM**, and **Hickie IB**. Delayed sleep phase in young people with unipolar or bipolar affective disorders, J Affect Disord 2013 Feb;**145**(2):260–3.

42. **Hanlon A, Naismith S, Hickie I**, and **Scott J**. Rumination as a psychological risk factor in staging models. Paper submitted for publication, 2015.

43. **Steinan M, Morken, G, Lagerberg T, Melle I, Andreassen O, Vaaler A**, and **Scott J**. Delayed sleep phase: an important circadian subtype of sleep disturbance in bipolar disorders. Paper submitted for publication, 2015.

44. **Bellivier F, Geoffroy PA, Etain B**, and **Scott J**. Sleep- and circadian rhythm-associated pathways as therapeutic targets in bipolar disorder, Expert Opin Ther Targets 2015 Jun;**19**(6):747–63.

45. **Robillard R, Naismith SL**, and **Hickie IB**. Recent advances in sleep–wake cycle and biological rhythms in bipolar disorder, Curr Psychiatry Rep 2013 Oct;**15**(10):402.

46. **Watkins E, Scott J, Wingrove J**, et al. Rumination-focused cognitive behaviour therapy for residual depression: a case series, Behav Res & Therapy 2007;**45**:2144–54.

47. **Watkins ER, Mullan E, Wingrove J, Rimes K, Steiner H, Bathurst N, Eastman R**, and **Scott J**. Rumination-focused cognitive-behavioural therapy for residual depression: phase II randomised controlled trial, Br J Psychiatry 2011 Oct;**199**(4):317–22.

48. **Pavlickova H, Turnbull OH, Myin-Germeys I**, and **Bentall RP**. The interrelationship between mood, self-esteem and response styles in adolescent offspring of bipolar parents: an experience sampling study, Psychiatry Res 2015 Feb;**225**(3):563–70.

49. **Jackson A, Cavanagh J**, and **Scott J**. A systematic review of early warning signs in affective disorders, J Affect Dis 2003;**74**:209–17.

50. **Scott J**. *Overcoming Mood Swings* (London: Constable Robinson; New York, NY: NYU Press, 2001), 247.

Chapter 12

Psychotherapeutic interventions for bipolar disorder

María Reinares

Introduction

Bipolar disorder is a chronic and recurrent mental illness that may result in a high level of personal, familial, social, and economic burden. The illness is associated with a high co-morbidity and mortality rate, and the risk of recurrences persists even in patients with a good medication adherence. The number of previous episodes is related to a worse quality of life, higher disability, and severe persistent symptoms.[1] Some studies suggest that the higher the number of relapses the greater the deficits in cognition[2] and psychosocial functioning.[3] The advantages of an integrative approach which combines pharmacological treatments with adjunctive psychological interventions would contribute to preventing recurrences and decreasing the burden of bipolar disorder. The reduction of this burden not only implies achieving syndromal recovery but also symptomatic and functional recovery, all essential to improving patients' quality of life and well-being.

Adjunctive psychological interventions would enhance the effect of medication through promoting good adherence, which is often suboptimal in bipolar disorder, and address other aspects that medication alone cannot reach (Box 12.1). Among the latter, training in the detection of early warning signs and coping skills are crucial to control mood fluctuations. Other therapeutic ingredients include education about the illness to correct false beliefs and raise awareness, and reduction of triggering factors such as substance use, irregularity of habits, and stress. Most psychological treatments for bipolar disorder share the previously mentioned components although the emphasis differs depending on the approach. In addition, some treatments also focus on strategies to improve interpersonal relationships and family environment. Cognition and psychosocial functioning are also targets of new approaches.

Despite the importance of empowering patients and their relatives through awareness and proactive behaviours to manage the illness, a recent study[4] reported that only a minority (around 30%) of individuals with bipolar disorder attended psychotherapy services and those who did had greater illness burden (medication side effects, suicide risk and anxiety disorders). These figures contradict the recommendation for introducing the treatment as soon as possible based on the observation

Box 12.1 Ingredients of psychological treatment in bipolar disorder

✓ Education about the illness and its treatment.
✓ Correction of myths, false beliefs, and misattributions.
✓ Replacing self-stigmatization with acceptance and awareness.
✓ Enhancing medication adherence.
✓ Stabilizing sleep/wake cycles and daily routines.
✓ Avoiding substance use.
✓ Promoting healthy habits.
✓ Improving the early detection and treatment of the first signs of relapse.
✓ Training in stress management.
✓ Teaching emotional self-regulation skills.
✓ Improving interpersonal relationships and family environment.
✓ Improving cognitive and psychosocial functioning.
✓ Giving support, psychoeducation, and training to the relatives on strategies to cope with the illness and manage stress.

that bipolar disorder may be a potentially deteriorating illness if not treated early and properly.[5] In addition, some findings have shown that a higher number of previous episodes,[6,7] as well as clinical morbidity and functional impairment[8] may reduce treatment response to psychotherapy. Although more studies in this area are needed, what seems clear is that early diagnosis and treatment would improve the prognosis of the illness. Psychological and psychosocial interventions will undoubtedly play a crucial role across the lifespan of all patients but treatments should be adjusted to the target outcomes which may vary depending on the characteristics of the subjects and the severity of the illness.[9] This chapter explores the role of adjunctive psychotherapy in bipolar disorder.

Adjunctive psychological treatments for bipolar disorders

Box 12.2 lists different adjunctive psychological treatments that have been used in bipolar disorder. Main findings regarding both the most commonly tested interventions as well as other approaches that are currently under study in this population will be discussed.

Cognitive-behavioural therapy (CBT)

The CBT model focuses on the close relationship between thoughts, emotions, and behaviours, and aims at helping the individual to monitor, examine, and change dysfunctional thinking and behaviour associated with undesirable mood states. Mixed findings have been reported regarding the efficacy of adjunctive CBT in bipolar disorder. While positive findings (fewer episodes and days in an episode, less admissions and mood symptoms, and higher social functioning) were obtained in a 12-month

---

Box 12.2 Adjunctive psychological treatments for bipolar disorder

Most commonly tested treatments:
✓ Cognitive-behavioural therapy
✓ Psychoeducation
✓ Interpersonal and social rhythm therapy
✓ Family interventions

Treatments under study:
✓ Cognitive remediation
✓ Functional remediation
✓ Mindfulness-based cognitive therapy
✓ Eye movement desensitization and reprocessing
✓ Dialectical behavioural therapy
✓ Internet-supported psychological interventions

---

study in which 103 bipolar I patients were randomized to 14 sessions of CBT or a control group,[10] at 18-month follow-up the effect of CBT in relapse reduction was not significant.[11] The loss of efficacy throughout the follow-up was also corroborated in the study by Ball et al.,[12] suggesting the need for booster sessions. In contrast to these findings, a study with a follow-up of five years described the benefits in terms of symptoms and social-occupational functioning of an approach that combined CBT and psychoeducation[13] but data on recurrences were not collected. The combination of CBT plus brief psychoeducation was also shown to be superior to brief psychoeducation alone in relation to reducing the number of days of depressed mood.[14] Parikh et al.[15] carried out a randomized controlled trial (RCT) in which 204 bipolar patients received either 20 individual sessions of CBT or six sessions of group psychoeducation, both interventions showed a similar reduction in symptoms and likelihood of relapse. Positive findings have been shown using intensive psychotherapy (30 sessions), in which one type was CBT, in patients with acute bipolar depression.[16] Using a format of cognitive behavioural group therapy, positive results were obtained in symptoms, frequency, and duration of episodes.[17] However, in another study using a similar group format the intervention did not show differences in the occurrence and time to relapse compared with treatment as usual (TAU).[18] Negative findings have also been found in terms of recurrences in an 18-month study by Scott et al.[7] in which CBT (22 sessions) was compared with TAU in a sample of bipolar patients with a highly recurrent course and complex presentations. Interestingly, a post hoc analysis demonstrated that adjunctive CBT was effective only in patients with fewer than 12 previous episodes. Recently, negative findings were described by Meyer and Hautzinger[19] in a two-year study in which 20 sessions of CBT were compared with support therapy. However, the latter also included certain 'active' components (ie information about bipolar disorder and systematic mood monitoring) which might have contributed to these results. CBT was a component of integrated group therapy, an approach designed for bipolar patients with co-morbid substance abuse.[20,21] The intervention had a positive influence on substance abuse but not on affective symptoms. Although all the previous studies were carried out with adult population, a recent review of evidence-based psychosocial treatments concluded that adjunctive CBT was considered to be possibly efficacious in child and adolescent bipolar spectrum disorders.[22]

Psychoeducation

The efficacy of adjunctive group psychoeducation was shown in several trials carried out by Colom et al.[23] with 120 euthymic bipolar patients randomized to 21 sessions of group psychoeducation or non-specific group meetings. The programme consisted of five modules focused on illness awareness, detection of prodroms, adherence enhancement, substance use avoidance, regular habits, and stress management. The benefits of psychoeducation were observed with regard to the percentage, number and time to recurrences, and hospitalizations per patient, both at two-year follow-up[23] and five years.[24] The second study also showed that subjects who received psychoeducation were acutely ill for much shorter periods. The cost efficacy of this intervention has also been proved, particularly in terms of reducing hospitalizations and emergency visits.[25] The findings of Candini et al.[26] supported the hypothesis that 21-session group psychoeducation was an effective way to prevent hospitalization and decrease hospital days in patients with bipolar disorder treated in routine clinical settings. However, a subanalysis of the previously mentioned five-year follow-up study showed that patients with more than seven episodes did not show significant improvement with group psychoeducation in time to recurrence, and those with more than 14 episodes did not benefit from the treatment in terms of time spent ill, highlighting the importance of early intervention.[6] According to these results, in a 12-month study with a similar design but shorter treatment (16 sessions), de Barros et al.[27] found no differences between groups in mood symptoms, psychosocial functioning, and quality of life, except for a subjectively perceived overall clinical improvement by subjects who received psychoeducation. The authors suggested that characteristics of the sample could have explained the findings, as patients with a more advanced stage of disease might have a worse response to psychoeducation.

Positive findings have been found using multicomponent care packages[28,29] in which psychoeducation is a core element. The benefits have specifically been shown regarding manic symptoms[28,29] as well as in relation to social role function and quality of life.[28] The potential to prevent mania, but not depression, and to improve social and occupational functioning was also reported in one of the first RCTs consisting of teaching patients, through 7–12 individual sessions, to identify early symptoms and seek prompt treatment.[30] This study sheds light on the specific impact of one of the main components of psychoeducation: early identification of prodromes.

Recently, a systematic review on psychoeducation[31] indicated that although heterogeneity in the data warrants caution, psychoeducation appeared to be effective in preventing any relapse [n = 7; Odds Ratio: 1.98–2.75; Number Needed to Treat: 5–7] and manic/hypomanic relapses (n = 8; OR: 1.68–2.52; NNT: 6–8) but not depressive relapses. Group, but not individually, delivered interventions were effective against both poles of relapse; the duration of follow-up and hours of therapy explained some of the heterogeneity. Although no consistent effects on mood symptoms, quality of life, or functioning were found, psychoeducation improved medication adherence and short-term knowledge about medication.

Interpersonal and social rhythm therapy (IPSRT)

IPSRT is based on the hypothesis that stressful life events and unstable or disrupted daily routines can lead to circadian rhythm instability and, in vulnerable individuals, to affective episodes. The main study on IPSRT was conducted by Frank et al.[32] with a preventive maintenance phase of two years. This RCT involved 175 acutely bipolar patients and four treatment options, depending on the treatment (IPSRT or intensive clinical management) to which the patient was assigned in the acute and maintenance phase. Although there were no differences between the groups in terms of time to remission nor in the proportion of patients achieving remission, those patients who received IPSRT in the acute treatment phase survived longer without an episode and showed higher regularity of social rhythms. Regularity during acute treatment was associated with reduced likelihood of recurrence during the maintenance phase. Regarding psychosocial functioning,[33] results indicated that subjects particularly women who initially received IPSRT showed faster improvement in occupational functioning; there were no differences between groups at the end of the follow-up. In another trial, intensive psychotherapy (30 sessions), one of whose branches was IPSRT, showed to be more useful than three sessions of psychoeducation on recovery rates, time to recovery, likelihood of being clinically well, and functional outcomes of bipolar outpatients with depression.[16,34] However, recently, Inder et al.[35] randomized a group of 100 bipolar participants, aged 15–36 years with high levels of co-morbidity, to IPSRT (n = 49) or specialist supportive care (n = 51). After treatment, both groups had improved depressive symptoms, social functioning, and manic symptoms.

Family intervention

Several studies support the efficacy of adjunctive family-focused treatment, in comparison with crisis management, in reducing relapses and increasing time to relapse in adults with bipolar disorder.[36,37] This approach consisted of 21 one-hour sessions of psychoeducation, communication-enhancement training, and problem-solving training delivered at home for the patient together with their relatives during the post-episode period. The benefits extended to two-year follow-up and were particularly useful for depressive symptoms and improving medication adherence.[36] The treatment was also shown to reduce hospitalization risk compared with individual treatment.[38] Two RCT studies of adjunctive family-focused treatment for adolescents have been published. One showed positive findings in terms of recovery from depressive symptoms and spending fewer weeks in depressive episodes[39] although no differences in recovery rates and time to recurrences were found. In the second study, time to recovery or recurrence and proportion of weeks ill did not differ between the two treatment groups although secondary analyses revealed that participants in family-focused treatment had less severe manic symptoms during the second year than did those in enhanced care.[40] However, promising findings in terms of symptoms have been described using this treatment in youth at risk of bipolar disorder.[41] In children, other family approaches, such as multifamily psychoeducational psychotherapy[42] and child- and family-focused cognitive-behavioural therapy[43] have shown benefits in reducing symptom severity.

A 12-session group psychoeducation for adults with bipolar disorder and their companions, also resulted in the prevention of relapses, decreased manic symptoms, and improved medication adherence.[44] A multicentre study showed the positive impact of family psychoeducation, delivered to the patients and their relatives, in terms of the improvements of patients' social functioning, patients' depressive symptoms and relatives' burden, compared with the subjects who received TAU.[45]

In acute patients, positive results of adjunctive psychoeducational marital intervention were reported for medication adherence and global functioning but not for symptoms.[46] Similarly, Miller et al.[47] found that neither adjunctive family therapy nor adjunctive multifamily group therapy improved the recovery rate from acute bipolar episodes when compared with pharmacotherapy alone. However, for patients from families with high levels of impairment the addition of any modality of family intervention resulted in a reduction of both the number of depressive episodes and the time spent in depression.[48] Positive findings were found by Miklowitz et al.[16] in a multisite study where 293 acute bipolar depressive outpatients were randomized to three sessions of psychoeducation or up to 30 sessions of three branches of intensive psychotherapy, one of which being family-focused treatment.

Regarding caregiver-focused interventions, a 15-month RCT showed the benefits in the prevention of recurrences of 12 90-minute group sessions of psychoeducation delivered to caregivers of euthymic adults with bipolar disorder. Patients whose caregivers attended group psychoeducation showed a reduced risk of recurrence and a delay in the incidence of recurrence,[49] the intervention being particularly useful for the prevention of hypomanic/manic episodes. Some studies have shown a reduction of the burden perceived by the relatives of bipolar patients after attending caregiver-focused interventions.[50,51,52] Perlick et al.[52] also observed a positive impact on the patients' affective symptoms and the caregivers' health risk behaviour, subjective burden, and depressive symptoms after a family-focused treatment-health promoting intervention compared with a health education intervention delivered via videotapes.

Cognitive remediation

Based on the findings that show the presence of cognitive deficits in a high percentage of patients with bipolar disorder in remission, some authors have started to design interventions aimed at improving both cognitive and functional outcomes in this population. In an open study implementing 14 individual sessions of cognitive remediation for bipolar patients with residual depressive symptoms, Deckersbach and colleagues[53] reported an improvement in residual depressive symptoms, and occupational and psychosocial functioning. Moreover, changes in executive functioning accounted, in part, for the improvements in occupational functioning. Patients with neurocognitive impairment benefited less from the intervention. Recently, Demant et al.[54] carried out a clinical trial with bipolar patients in partial remission and cognitive complaints assigned to 12 weeks' group-based cognitive remediation or standard treatment. Participants were assessed at baseline and weeks 12 and 26. Cognitive remediation (n = 18) had no effect on cognitive or psychosocial functioning compared with standard treatment (n = 22). Only subjective sharpness improved with cognitive remediation at week 12, and quality of life and verbal fluency at week 26 follow-up. The authors suggested that longer-term, more intensive, and individualized cognitive remediation may be necessary to improve cognition in bipolar disorder. More studies are needed in this area.

Functional remediation

Functional remediation consists of an intervention involving neurocognitive techniques and training on attention, memory, and executive functions tasks, and also education on cognition and problem-solving within an ecological framework with the main aim of improving functional outcomes in bipolar disorder. Torrent et al.[55] carried out a multicentre trial with 239 euthymic bipolar patients who had a moderate-severe degree of functional impairment. The sample was randomized into three groups: 21 sessions of group functional remediation, 21 sessions of group psychoeducation, or TAU. Compared with TAU, the functional remediation programme resulted in improving patients' psychosocial functioning. No significant effect of treatment group on the clinical or neurocognitive variables were found at the end of the intervention (six-month), the main effect of time was significant. Similar results, together with an improvement of subdepressive symptoms, were found in a post hoc analysis of 53 euthymic bipolar II patients.[56] Although in the previous studies the interaction between treatment and neurocognitive variables was not significant, a subanalysis that analysed only the subjects from the whole sample who showed cognitive impairment at baseline (two Standard Deviations in at least one cognitive domain) found a positive impact of the intervention on verbal memory.[57] Similarly, a one-year follow-up of the sample used in the original study also detected significant differences in terms of verbal memory and psychosocial functioning.[58] These results suggest that verbal memory seems to be more amenable to treatment than other neurocognitive domains and that the benefits of the intervention on functional outcomes are maintained at least after one-year follow-up.

Mindfulness-based cognitive therapy (MBCT)

In the last decade there has been a proliferation of mindfulness-based interventions, enhancing the ability to focus one's attention on purpose in the present moment and non-judgementally. One of the first controlled studies to assess the efficacy of eight-week sessions of MBCT in a sample of bipolar and unipolar patients was conducted by Williams et al.[59] Their results showed a reduction in anxiety and depressive symptoms in bipolar disorder but only eight patients in each group (MBCT and wait list control) had a diagnosis of bipolar disorder. A reduction in depressive symptoms and anxiety, and an improvement of affective control or emotional regulation have been reported after MBCT in a sample of bipolar patients.[60] Similarly, a decrease in anxiety scores for bipolar patients allocated to MBCT compared with TAU was found in a trial with 95 patients followed over 12 months.[61] However, no differences were observed between groups in the depressive or manic symptoms, time to recurrence, and number of recurrences. It is worth mentioning that when the impact of mindfulness practice was examined, a significant correlation was found between a greater number of days spent meditating during the eight-week MBCT programme and lower depression scores at the end of the follow-up.[62]

Eye movement desensitization and reprocessing (EMDR)

Considering the high frequency of traumatic events in patients with bipolar disorder and its negative impact on the course of the disease, Novo et al.[63] conducted a study in which 14–18 sessions of EMDR were compared with TAU in a sample of 20 bipolar I and II patients with subsyndromal mood symptoms and a history of traumatic events. EMDR uses a standardized eight-phase protocol which involves making side-to-side eye movements while simultaneously focusing on symptoms and experiences related to the traumatic event, incorporating elements of cognitive, interpersonal, and body-centred therapies. At 12 weeks of the follow-up, patients in the treatment group showed a statistically significant improvement in depressive and hypomanic symptoms, symptoms of trauma, and trauma impact compared with the TAU group. Differences, however, disappeared at the end of the follow-up (24 weeks), except for trauma impact that was partly maintained. Further research with bigger samples is required in this area.

Dialectical behaviour therapy

This approach works towards helping subjects increase their emotional and cognitive regulation by learning about the triggers that lead to reactive states and helping to assess which coping skills to apply to avoid undesired reactions. Preliminary results have been obtained by using dialectical behaviour therapy in a few studies carried out with bipolar patients. In a one-year pilot study, Goldstein et al.[64] observed that compared with adolescents receiving an eclectic psychotherapy approach consisting of psychoeducational, supportive, and cognitive behavioural techniques (control group n = 6), adolescents receiving 36 sessions of dialectical behaviour therapy (n = 14) demonstrated significantly less severe depressive symptoms over follow-up, and were nearly three times more likely to show improvement in suicidal ideation. Although there were no between-group differences in manic symptoms or emotional dysregulation with treatment, adolescents receiving dialectical behaviour therapy evidenced improvement from pre- to post-treatment in both manic symptoms and emotional dysregulation. Previously, in a randomized pilot controlled study,[65] 12 weekly sessions of dialectical behavioural therapy skills in a psychoeducational group were also useful for adults with bipolar disorder in terms of reducing depressive symptoms, improving affective control, and mindfulness self-efficacy. Furthermore, group attendees showed a reduction in emergency room visits and mental health-related admissions in the six following months.

Internet-supported psychological interventions

There has gradually been an increasing interest in adopting current technologies into the field of physical and mental health. Several Internet-supported psychological interventions have been designed and are being tested in bipolar disorder.[66] If these interventions delivered through web interfaces and mobile devices prove to be effective they would contribute to reducing the important gap between availability and demand as they have the potential to be delivered anytime and anywhere. Mobile technologies offer the advantage of extending monitoring of daily life outside clinical settings, complementing self-reported measures with continuous objective monitoring in an ecological momentary assessment. However, so far the studies have striking methodological differences in regards to design, quality, and ultimate aims and outcomes. In addition, the reliability of online diagnostic and follow-up assessments scales is not always high. This diversity between studies and the fact that many of them are in a preliminary stage make it difficult at present to draw firm conclusions about the effectiveness of psychological interventions using Internet-supported technologies for bipolar disorder. Nevertheless, most studies support the high rates of retention and adherence, suggesting they may represent a feasible and acceptable method of delivering this kind of interventions.[66] Another issue is to find a balance between the degree of self-management from the patients' side and the level of involvement of the clinicians in the loop in order to obtain necessary feedback, more adequate treatment, and provision of timely interventions thus ensuring patients' safety. Similar to face-to-face psychological treatments, future studies should clarify which components of the programmes are crucial in relation to obtaining expected outcomes, as well as establishing the minimum duration and frequency of online sessions which would guarantee efficacy.

Conclusion and future directions

Most findings indicate the benefits of specific adjunctive psychological treatments in improving the outcomes of bipolar disorder. Despite there being many methodological differences between studies and some discrepant results, findings so far indicate that CBT may be useful to prevent bipolar episodes, especially depression in recovered and less recurrent bipolar patients, although booster sessions might be needed to maintain the benefits and not all trials have shown positive findings. Group psychoeducation seems to have long-lasting prophylactic effects on all sorts of episodes in euthymic patients, while training on prodrome detection as well as systematic care programmes could help to prevent manic episodes. With samples of acutely ill individuals, IPSRT may have an impact on increasing the time without an affective episode, or the recovery rate of depression in the case of intensive treatment. Family intervention seems to have benefits for caregivers and patient outcomes but its potential to prevent manic versus depressive episodes may change according to the treatment format and characteristics of the sample. Functional remediation has shown to improve psychosocial functioning in bipolar patients with high impairment at baseline. The potential impact of functional remediation and cognitive remediation on cognition still requires more research. MBCT appears to be useful in decreasing anxiety symptoms, with some positive findings regarding depressed symptoms and emotional regulation although there is not currently evidence of its efficacy in the prevention of recurrences in bipolar disorder. Studies on the efficacy of EMDR and dialectical behavioural therapy are underway in bipolar disorder. Similarly, the efficacy of psychological interventions using Internet-based technologies is a promising research area but there is still limited evidence available to draw conclusions.

In general, specific adjunctive psychological treatments have shown a positive impact on the prevention of recurrences, the improvement of psychosocial functioning, and aspects of burden and well-being of the patients and their relatives.[9,67] They can also help to decrease the costs related to the illness.[7,15] Some treatments differ from others in their potential to prevent episodes of different polarity.[68] Regarding the maintenance of the effects, in the case of the most commonly tested approaches, the benefits have been proven over one to two years, with only a few studies analysing their efficacy with longer follow-ups of up to five years.[13,24] However, the efficacy of psychological interventions seems to differ depending on the characteristics of the subjects and the course of the illness. Some findings suggest that a higher number of previous episodes[7,6] as well as clinical morbidity and functional impairment[8] may reduce treatment response, underlying the importance of introducing adjunctive therapeutic interventions as soon as possible. It is worth mentioning that most of these studies are based on post hoc analysis and there is a need for prospective longitudinal studies to better assess the association between illness progression and response to treatment. The development of new treatments such as functional remediation[55,58] brings hope to the subset of patients with a higher chronicity. Together with the identification of moderators to the therapeutic response, the mechanism of action of psychological interventions remains unknown although some components (treatment adherence, lifestyle regularity, early detection of prodromes, and stress management), common to most psychotherapies for patients with bipolar disorder, are believed to play an important role. Another aspect to consider refers to the time of implementation of psychological treatments. In most studies, the patients included were in remission or with mild symptoms while in a few studies the intervention was directed at acute patients, which resulted in more discrepant findings. Outcomes vary between studies as well as the length of the intervention and the follow-up. In addition, there is a high heterogeneity in the characteristics of comparison groups which have often not been well matched in terms of intensity of care or contact with the therapist, more attention should be paid to this aspect when interpreting the findings. Studies with less restrictive criteria (ie including patients with co-morbidities) and developed not only in highly specialized centres but in community settings would contribute to reducing the gap between efficacy and effectiveness. What seems clear is that there is a need for designing tailored specific interventions depending on different levels of impairment and the chronicity of the subjects. It is also important to reconcile prevention and remediation strategies and to better determine which individuals with bipolar disorder—and under what conditions—are most likely to benefit from each intervention in order to improve illness prognosis, functional recovery, and quality of life.

References

1. Magalhaes, PV, Dodd, S, Nierenberg, AA, and Berk, M. Cumulative morbidity and prognostic staging of illness in the Systematic Treatment Enhancement Program for Bipolar Disorder (STEP-BD), Aust NZJ Psychiatry 2012;**46**:1058–67.

2. Lopez-Jaramillo, C, Lopera-Vasquez J, Gallo, A, Ospina-Duque, J, Bell, V, Torrent, C, Martinez-Aran, A, and Vieta, E. Effects of recurrence on the cognitive performance of patients with bipolar I disorder: implications for relapse prevention and treatment adherence, Bipolar Disord 2010;**12**:557–67.

3. Rosa, AR, Gonzalez-Ortega, I, Gonzalez-Pinto, A, Echeburua, E, Comes, M, Martinez-Aran, A, Ugarte, A, Fernandez, M, and Vieta, E. One-year psychosocial functioning in patients in the early vs late stage of bipolar disorder, Acta Psychiatr Scand 2012;**125**:335–41.

4. Sylvia, LG, Thase, ME, Reilly-Harrington, NA, Salcedo, S, Brody, B, Kinrys, G, Kemp, D, Shelton, RC, McElroy, SL, Kocsis, JH, Bobo, WV, Kamali, M, McInnis, M, Friedman, E, Tohen, M, Bowden, CL, Ketter, TA, Singh, V, Calabrese, J, Nierenberg, AA, Rabideau, DJ, Elson, CM, and Deckersbach, T. Psychotherapy use in bipolar disorder: Association with functioning and illness severity, Aust NZJ Psychiatry 2015;**49**:453–61.

5. Post, RM, Fleming, J, and Kapczinski, F. Neurobiological correlates of illness progression in the recurrent affective disorders, J Psychiatr Res 2012;**46**:561–73.

6. Colom, F, Reinares, M, Pacchiarotti, I, Popovic, D, Mazzarini, L, Martinez, AA, Torrent, C, Rosa, AR, Palomino-Otiniano, R, Franco, C, Bonnin, CM, and Vieta, E. Has number of previous episodes any effect on response to group psychoeducation in bipolar patients?, *Acta Neuropsychiatrica* 2010;**22**:50–3.

7. Scott, J, Paykel, E, Morriss, R, Bentall, R, Kinderman, P, Johnson, T, Abbott, R, and Hayhurst, H. Cognitive-behavioural therapy for severe and recurrent bipolar disorders: randomised controlled trial, Br J Psychiatry 2006;**188**:313–20.

8. Reinares, M, Colom, F, Rosa, AR, Bonnin, CM, Franco, C, Sole, B, Kapczinski, F, and Vieta, E. The impact of staging bipolar disorder on treatment outcome of family psychoeducation, J Affect Disord 2010;**123**:81–6.

9. Reinares, M, Sanchez-Moreno, J, and Fountoulakis, KN. Psychosocial interventions in bipolar disorder: what, for whom, and when, J Affect Disord 2014;**156**:46–55.

10. Lam, DH, Watkins, ER, Hayward, P, Bright, J, Wright, K, Kerr, N, Parr-Davis, G, and Sham, P. A randomized controlled study of cognitive therapy for relapse prevention for bipolar affective disorder: outcome of the first year, Arch Gen Psychiatry 2003;**60**:145–52.

11. Lam, DH, McCrone, P, Wright, K, and Kerr, N. Cost-effectiveness of relapse-prevention cognitive therapy for bipolar disorder: 30-month study, Br J Psychiatry 2005;**186**:500–6.

12. Ball, JR, Mitchell, PB, Corry, JC, Skillecorn, A, Smith, M, and Malhi, GS. A randomized controlled trial of cognitive therapy for bipolar disorder: focus on long-term change, J Clin Psychiatry 2006;**67**:277–86.

13. Gonzalez, IA, Echeburua, E, Liminana, JM, and Gonzalez-Pinto, A. Psychoeducation and cognitive-behavioral therapy for patients with refractory bipolar disorder: a 5-year controlled clinical trial, Eur Psychiatry 2012.

14. Zaretsky, A, Lancee, W, Miller, C, Harris, A and Parikh, SV. Is cognitive-behavioural therapy more effective than psychoeducation in bipolar disorder?, Can J Psychiatry 2008;**53**:441–8.

15. Parikh, SV, Zaretsky, A, Beaulieu, S, Yatham, LN, Young, LT, Patelis-Siotis, I, Macqueen, GM, Levitt, A, Arenovich, T, Cervantes, P, Velyvis, V, Kennedy, SH, and Streiner, DL. A randomized controlled trial of psychoeducation or cognitive-behavioral therapy in bipolar disorder: a Canadian Network for Mood and Anxiety treatments (CANMAT) study [CME], J Clin Psychiatry 2012;**73**:803–10.

16. Miklowitz, DJ, Otto, MW, Frank, E, Reilly-Harrington, NA, Wisniewski, SR, Kogan, JN, Nierenberg, AA, Calabrese, JR, Marangell, LB., Gyulai, L, Araga, M, Gonzalez, JM, Shirley, ER, Thase, ME, and Sachs, GS. Psychosocial treatments for bipolar depression: a 1-year randomized trial from the Systematic Treatment Enhancement Program, Arch Gen Psychiatry 2007b;**64**:419–26.

17. Costa, RT, Cheniaux, E, Rosaes, PA, Carvalho, MR, Freire, RC, Versiani, M, Range, BP, and Nardi, AE. The effectiveness of cognitive behavioral group therapy in treating bipolar disorder: a randomized controlled study, Rev Bras Psiquiatr 2011;**33**:144–9.

18. Gomes, BC, Abreu, LN, Brietzke, E, Caetano, SC, Kleinman, A, Nery, FG, and Lafer, B. A randomized controlled trial of cognitive behavioral group therapy for bipolar disorder, Psychother Psychosom 2011l;**80**:144–50.

19. Meyer, TD and Hautzinger, M. Cognitive behaviour therapy and supportive therapy for bipolar disorders: relapse rates for treatment period and 2-year follow-up, Psychol Med 2012;**42**:1429–39.

20. Weiss, RD, Griffin, ML, Kolodziej, ME, Greenfield, SF, Najavits, LM, Daley, DC, Doreau, HR, and Hennen, JA. A randomized trial of integrated group therapy versus group drug counseling for patients with bipolar disorder and substance dependence, Am J Psychiatry 2007;**164**:100–7.

21. Weiss, RD, Griffin, ML, Jaffee, WB., Bender, RE, Graff, FS, Gallop, RJ, and Fitzmaurice, GM. A 'community-friendly' version of integrated group therapy for patients with bipolar disorder and substance dependence: a randomized controlled trial, Drug Alcohol Depend 2009;**104**:212–19.

22. Fristad, MA and MacPherson, HA. Evidence-based psychosocial treatments for child and adolescent bipolar spectrum disorders, J Clin Child Adolesc Psychol 2014;**43**:339–55.

23. Colom, F, Vieta, E, Martinez-Aran, A, Reinares, M, Goikolea, JM, Benabarre, A, Torrent, C, Comes, M, Corbella, B, Parramon, G and Corominas, J. A randomized trial on the efficacy of group psychoeducation in the prophylaxis of recurrences in bipolar patients whose disease is in remission, Arch Gen Psychiatry 2003;**60**:402–7.

24. Colom, F, Vieta, E, Sanchez-Moreno, J, Palomino-Otiniano, R, Reinares, M, Goikolea, JM, Benabarre, A and Martinez-Aran, A. Group psychoeducation for stabilised bipolar disorders: 5-year outcome of a randomised clinical trial, Br J Psychiatry 2009;**194**:260–5.

25. Scott, J, Colom, F, Popova, E, Benabarre, A, Cruz, N, Valenti, M, Goikolea, JM, Sanchez-Moreno, J, Asenjo, MA and Vieta, E. Long-term mental health resource utilization and cost of care following group psychoeducation or unstructured group support for bipolar disorders: a cost-benefit analysis, J Clin Psychiatry 2009;**70**:378–86.

26. Candini, V, Buizza, C, Ferrari, C, Caldera, MT, Ermentini, R, Ghilardi, A, Nobili, G, Pioli, R, Sabaudo, M., Sacchetti, E, Saviotti, FM, Seggioli, G, Zanini, A, and de Girolamo, G. Is structured group psychoeducation for bipolar patients effective

in ordinary mental health services? A controlled trial in Italy, J Affect Disord 2013;**151**:149–155.

27. **de Barros, PK, de O Costa, L, Silval, KI, Dias, VV, Roso, MC, Bandeira, M, Colom, F and Moreno, RA.** Efficacy of psychoeducation on symptomatic and functional recovery in bipolar disorder, Acta Psychiatr Scand 2013;**127**:153–8.

28. **Bauer, MS, McBride, L, Williford, WO, Glick, H, Kinosian, B, Altshuler, L, Beresford, T, Kilbourne, AM and Sajatovic, M.** Collaborative care for bipolar disorder: Part II. Impact on clinical outcome, function, and costs, Psychiatr Serv 2006;**57**:937–45.

29. **Simon, GE, Ludman, EJ, Bauer, MS, Unutzer, J and Operskalski, B.** Long-term effectiveness and cost of a systematic care program for bipolar disorder, Arch Gen Psychiatry 2006;**63**:500–8.

30. **Perry, A, Tarrier, N, Morriss, R, McCarthy, E and Limb, K.** Randomised controlled trial of efficacy of teaching patients with bipolar disorder to identify early symptoms of relapse and obtain treatment, BMJ 1999;**318**:149–53.

31. **Bond, K and Anderson, IM.** Psychoeducation for relapse prevention in bipolar disorder: a systematic review of efficacy in randomized controlled trials, Bipolar Disord 2015.

32. **Frank, E, Kupfer, DJ, Thase, ME, Mallinger, AG, Swartz, HA, Fagiolini, AM, Grochocinski, V, Houck, P, Scott, J, Thompson, W and Monk, T.** Two-year outcomes for interpersonal and social rhythm therapy in individuals with bipolar I disorder, Arch Gen Psychiatry 2005;**62**:996–1004.

33. **Frank, E, Soreca, I, Swartz, HA, Fagiolini, AM, Mallinger, AG, Thase, ME, Grochocinski, VJ, Houck, PR and Kupfer, DJ.** The role of interpersonal and social rhythm therapy in improving occupational functioning in patients with bipolar I disorder, Am J Psychiatry 2008;**165**:1559–65.

34. **Miklowitz, DJ, Otto, MW, Frank, E, Reilly-Harrington, NA, Kogan, JN, Sachs, GS, Thase, ME, Calabrese, JR, Marangell, LB, Ostacher, MJ, Patel, J, Thomas, MR, Araga, M, Gonzalez, JM and Wisniewski, SR.** Intensive psychosocial intervention enhances functioning in patients with bipolar depression: results from a 9-month randomized controlled trial, Am J Psychiatry 2007a;**164**:1340–7.

35. **Inder, ML, Crowe, MT, Luty, SE, Carter, JD, Moor, S, Frampton, CM, and Joyce, PR.** Randomized, controlled trial of Interpersonal and Social Rhythm Therapy for young people with bipolar disorder, Bipolar Disord 2014.

36. **Miklowitz, DJ, George, EL, Richards, JA, Simoneau, TL, and Suddath, RL.** A randomized study of family-focused psychoeducation and pharmacotherapy in the outpatient management of bipolar disorder, Arch Gen Psychiatry 2003;**60**:904–12.

37. **Miklowitz, DJ, Simoneau, TL, George, EL, Richards, JA, Kalbag, A, Sachs-Ericsson, N, and Suddath, R.** Family-focused treatment of bipolar disorder: 1-year effects of a psychoeducational program in conjunction with pharmacotherapy; Biol Psychiatry 2000;**48**:582–92.

38. **Rea, MM, Tompson, MC, Miklowitz, DJ, Goldstein, MJ, Hwang,S, and Mintz, J.** Family-focused treatment versus individual treatment for bipolar disorder: results of a randomized clinical trial, J Consult Clin Psychol 2003;**71**:482–92.

39. **Miklowitz, DJ, Axelson, DA, Birmaher, B, George, EL, Taylor, DO, Schneck, CD, Beresford, CA, Dickinson, LM, Craighead, WE, and Brent, DA.** Family-focused treatment for adolescents with bipolar disorder: results of a 2-year randomized trial, Arch Gen Psychiatry 2008;**65**:1053–61.

40. Miklowitz, DJ, Schneck, CD, George, EL, Taylor, DO, Sugar, CA, Birmaher, B, Kowatch, RA, Delbello, MP, and Axelson, DA. Pharmacotherapy and family-focused treatment for adolescents with bipolar I and II disorders: a 2-year randomized trial, Am J Psychiatry 2014;**171**:658–67.

41. Miklowitz, DJ, Schneck, CD, Singh, MK, Taylor, DO, George, EL, Cosgrove, VE, Howe, ME, Dickinson, LM, Garber, J, and Chang, KD. Early intervention for symptomatic youth at risk for bipolar disorder: a randomized trial of family-focused therapy, J Am Acad Child Adolesc Psychiatry 2013;**52**:121–31.

42. Fristad, MA, Verducci, JS, Walters, K, and Young, ME. Impact of multifamily psychoeducational psychotherapy in treating children aged 8 to 12 years with mood disorders, Arch Gen Psychiatry 2009;**66**:1013–21.

43. West, AE, Weinstein, SM, Peters, AT, Katz, AC, Henry, DB, Cruz, RA, and Pavuluri, MN. Child- and family-focused cognitive-behavioral therapy for pediatric bipolar disorder: a randomized clinical trial, J Am Acad Child Adolesc Psychiatry 2014;**53**:1168–78.

44. D'Souza, R, Piskulic, D, and Sundram, S. A brief dyadic group based psychoeducation program improves relapse rates in recently remitted bipolar disorder: a pilot randomised controlled trial, J Affect Disord 2010;**120**:272–6.

45. Fiorillo, A, Del Vecchio, V, Luciano, M, Sampogna, G, De Rosa, C, Malangone, C, Volpe, U, Bardicchia, F, Ciampini, G, Crocamo, C, Iapichino, S, Lampis, D, Moroni, A, Orlandi, E, Piselli, M, Pompili, E, Veltro, F, Carra, G, and Maj, M. Efficacy of psychoeducational family intervention for bipolar I disorder: A controlled, multicentric, real-world study, J Affect Disord 2014;**172C**:291–9.

46. Clarkin, JF, Carpenter, D, Hull, J, Wilner, P, and Glick, I. Effects of psychoeducational intervention for married patients with bipolar disorder and their spouses, Psychiatr Serv 1998;**49**:531–3.

47. Miller, IW, Solomon, DA, Ryan, CE, and Keitner, GI. Does adjunctive family therapy enhance recovery from bipolar I mood episodes?, J Affect Disord 2004;**82**:431–6.

48. Miller, IW, Keitner, GI, Ryan, CE, Uebelacker, LA, Johnson, SL, and Solomon, DA. Family treatment for bipolar disorder: family impairment by treatment interactions, J Clin Psychiatry 2008;**69**:732–40.

49. Reinares, M, Colom, F, Sanchez-Moreno, J, Torrent, C, Martinez-Aran, A, Comes, M, Goikolea, JM, Benabarre, A, Salamero, M, and Vieta, E. Impact of caregiver group psychoeducation on the course and outcome of bipolar patients in remission: a randomized controlled trial, Bipolar Disord 2008;**10**:511–19.

50. Reinares, M, Vieta, E, Colom, F, Martinez-Aran, A, Torrent, C, Comes, M, Goikolea, JM, Benabarre, A, and Sanchez-Moreno, J. Impact of a psychoeducational family intervention on caregivers of stabilized bipolar patients, Psychother Psychosom 2004;**73**:312–19.

51. Madigan, K, Egan, P, Brennan, D, Hill, S, Maguire, B, Horgan, F, Flood, C, Kinsella, A, and O'Callaghan, E. A randomised controlled trial of carer-focussed multi-family group psychoeducation in bipolar disorder, Eur Psychiatry 2012;**27**:281–4.

52. Perlick, DA, Miklowitz, DJ, Lopez, N, Chou, J, Kalvin, C, Adzhiashvili, V, and Aronson, A. Family-focused treatment for caregivers of patients with bipolar disorder, Bipolar Disord 2010;**12**:627–37.

53. Deckersbach, T, Nierenberg, AA, Kessler, R, Lund, HG, Ametrano, RM, Sachs, G, Rauch, SL, and Dougherty, D. RESEARCH: Cognitive rehabilitation for bipolar

disorder: An open trial for employed patients with residual depressive symptoms, CNS Neurosci Ther 2010;**16**:298–307.

54. **Demant, KM, Vinberg, M, Kessing, LV, and Miskowiak, KW.** Effects of short-term cognitive remediation on cognitive dysfunction in partially or fully remitted individuals with bipolar disorder: results of a randomised controlled trial, PLoS One 2015;**10**:e0127955.

55. **Torrent, C, Bonnin, CM, Martinez-Aran, A, Valle, J, Amann, BL, Gonzalez-Pinto, A, Crespo, JM, Ibanez, A, Garcia-Portilla, MP, Tabares-Seisdedos, R, Arango, C, Colom, F, Sole, B, Pacchiarotti, I, Rosa, AR, Ayuso-Mateos, JL, Anaya, C, Fernandez, P, Landin-Romero, R, Alonso-Lana, S, Ortiz-Gil, J, Segura, B, Barbeito, S, Vega, P, Fernandez, M., Ugarte, A, Subira, M, Cerrillo, E, Custal, N, Menchon, JM, Saiz-Ruiz, J, Rodao, JM, Isella, S, Alegria, A, Al-Halabi, S, Bobes, J, Galvan, G, Saiz, PA, Balanza-Martinez, V, Selva, G, Fuentes-Dura, I, Correa, P, Mayoral, M, Chiclana, G, Merchan-Naranjo, J, Rapado-Castro, M, Salamero, M, and Vieta, E.** Efficacy of functional remediation in bipolar disorder: a multicenter randomized controlled study, Am J Psychiatry 2013;**170**:852–9.

56. **Sole, B, Bonnin, CM, Mayoral, M, Amann, BL, Torres, I, Gonzalez-Pinto, A, Jimenez, E, Crespo, JM, Colom, F, Tabares-Seisdedos, R, Reinares, M, Ayuso-Mateos, JL, Soria, S, Garcia-Portilla, MP, Ibanez, A, Vieta, E, Martinez-Aran, A, and Torrent, C.** Functional remediation for patients with bipolar II disorder: improvement of functioning and subsyndromal symptoms, Eur Neuropsychopharmacol 2015;**25**:257–64.

57. **Bonnin, CM, Reinares, M, Martinez-Aran, A, Balanza-Martinez, V, Sole, B, Torrent, C, Tabares-Seisdedos, R, Garcia-Portilla, MP, Ibanez, A, Amann, BL, Arango, C, Ayuso-Mateos, JL, Crespo, JM, Gonzalez-Pinto, A, Colom, F, and Vieta, E.** Effects of functional remediation on neurocognitively impaired bipolar patients: enhancement of verbal memory, Psychol Med 2015;1–11.

58. **Bonnin, CM, Torrent, C, Arango, C, Amann, B, Sole, B, Gonzalez-Pinto, A, Crespo, JM, Tabares-Seisdedos, R, Reinares, M, Ayuso, JL, Garcia-Portilla, MP, Ibanez, A, Salamero, M, Vieta, E, Martinez-Aran, A, and CIBERSAM Functional Remediation Group.** One-year follow-up of functional remediation in bipolar disorder: neurocognitive and functional outcome, Br J Psychiatry 2016; **208**:87–93.

59. **Williams, JM, Alatiq, Y, Crane, C, Barnhofer, T, Fennell, MJ, Duggan, DS, Hepburn, S, and Goodwin, GM.** Mindfulness-based Cognitive Therapy (MBCT) in bipolar disorder: preliminary evaluation of immediate effects on between-episode functioning, J Affect Disord 2008;**107**:275–9.

60. **Ives-Deliperi, VL, Howells, F, Stein, DJ, Meintjes, EM, and Horn, N.** The effects of mindfulness-based cognitive therapy in patients with bipolar disorder: a controlled functional MRI investigation, J Affect Disord 2013.

61. **Perich, T, Manicavasagar, V, Mitchell, PB, Ball, JR, and Hadzi-Pavlovic, D.** A randomized controlled trial of mindfulness-based cognitive therapy for bipolar disorder, Acta Psychiatr Scand 2013b;**127**:333–43.

62. **Perich, T, Manicavasagar, V, Mitchell, PB, and Ball, JR.** The association between meditation practice and treatment outcome in Mindfulness-based Cognitive Therapy for bipolar disorder, Behav Res Ther 2013a;**51**:338–43.

63. **Novo, P, Landin-Romero, R, Radua, J, Vicens, V, Fernandez, I, Garcia, F, Pomarol-Clotet, E, McKenna, PJ, Shapiro, F, and Amann, BL.** Eye movement desensitization and reprocessing therapy in subsyndromal bipolar patients with a history of traumatic events: a randomized, controlled pilot-study, Psychiatry Res 2014;**219**:122–8.

64. Goldstein, TR, Fersch-Podrat, RK, Rivera, M, Axelson, DA, Merranko, J, Yu, H, Brent, DA, and Birmaher, B. Dialectical behavior therapy for adolescents with bipolar disorder: results from a pilot randomized trial, J Child Adolesc Psychopharmacol 2015;25:140–9.

65. Van, DS, Jeffrey, J, and Katz, MR. A randomized, controlled, pilot study of dialectical behavior therapy skills in a psychoeducational group for individuals with bipolar disorder, J Affect Disord 2013:145;386–93.

66. Hidalgo-Mazzei, D, Mateu, A, Reinares, M, Matic, A, Vieta, E, and Colom, F. Internet-based psychological interventions for bipolar disorder: review of the present and insights into the future, J Affect Disord 2015;188:1–13.

67. Reinares, M, Bonnín, CM, Hidalgo-Mazzei, D, Sánchez-Moreno, J, Colom, F, and Vieta, E. The role of family interventions in bipolar disorder: a systematic review, Clin Psychol Rev 2016;43:47–57.

68. Popovic, D, Reinares, M, Scott, J, Nivoli, AM, Murru, A, Pacchiarotti, I, Vieta, E, and Colom, F. Polarity index of psychological interventions in maintenance treatment of bipolar disorder, Psychother Psychosom 2013;82:292–8.

Chapter 13

The role of psychoeducation in the management of bipolar disorder

Francesc Colom

Introduction

Controlling the symptoms of bipolar disorder, establishing a balanced prophylaxis of recurrences, avoiding subthreshold presentations, and reaching functional remission are the very ambitious targets of a utopic bipolar treatment.

Pharmacological treatment is the basis of the treatment of bipolar disorder. However, many of the goals aforementioned can not be reached without adding up evidence-based psychological interventions as well as biophysical treatments.

During the last 15 years, several studies testing the efficacy of psychological interventions have seen the light. However, the evidence for most of them is quite chequered. On the one hand, the promising interpersonal social rhythm therapy has offered only few studies where the main outcome measure hardly changed after treatment. Similarly, the evidence for and against the use of cognitive-behavioural therapy (CBT) has been revealed in a number of studies and a good and convincing cognitive model for bipolar disorder is yet to be defined.

Thus, all the models showing efficacy and cost-efficacy in the prophylaxis of recurrences, include—to one extent or another—psychoeducational ingredients.

A study based on a simple intervention of training patients on early warning sign detection was associated with a significant increase in time to first manic relapse, as well as a 30% decrease in the number of manic episodes, and improvement of social functioning and employment over 18 months.[1] However, the same approach failed to show any significant changes in a larger study with a longer follow-up,[2] indicating that early warning sign recognition is only a part of the scope of topics psychoeducation needs to address.[3] Similarly, despite the fact that psychoeducation helps to improve adherence to lithium in patients with bipolar disorder,[4] adherent patients also benefit from the intervention.[5]

What is psychoeducation?

Psychoeducation is a simple approach aimed at improving the treatment outcome of patients with bipolar disorder and enhancing the prevention of future episodes.

According to most guidelines, it should be offered as an add-on to standard pharma-cotherapy[3] and delivers behavioural training aimed at adjusting patient lifestyle and strategies of coping with bipolar disorder, including enhancement of illness aware-ness, treatment adherence, early detection of relapses, and avoidance of potentially harmful factors such as substance misuse and sleep deprivation.[6] Psychoeducation is an intervention that seeks to empower patients with tools that allow them to be more active in their therapy process. However, it does not represent a therapy option that is based on patient self-help, owing to it being highly structured and requiring a directive influence by a therapist. The Barcelona Bipolar Unit was the first clinic to provide structured, manualized, and evidence-based psychoeducation therapy in a set of modular sessions, which have been used to develop further psychoeducation programmes adapted to satisfy the needs of other bipolar clinics,[5] allowing its imple-mentation worldwide.

Evidence for the efficacy of psychoeducation as a prophylactic add-on

Group-based psychoeducation shows efficacy far beyond that usually seen by the mere supportive role of the group. Psychoeducation is effective as an add-on to main-tenance pharmacotherapy in the prevention of recurrences in bipolar disorder—in particular, episodes of mania/hypomania, mixed episodes, and depression.[5] Psychosocial interventions are by no means substitutes for pharmacotherapy, but they may complement mood stabilizers in protecting patient symptom deterioration, as well as enhance adherence with maintenance treatments.[7,4]

Evidence thus far has shown that psychoeducation in combination with pharma-cotherapy is more effective than pharmacotherapy alone in a number of parameters. Long-term psychoeducation (six months) demonstrated a positive effect on patient adherence to lithium[4] and a significantly lower number of hospitalization and days spent in hospital up to two years, compared with patients receiving a combination of pharmacological treatment and non-structured group meetings.[5] Additionally, the number of total episodes, but also the number of manic, depressive, and mixed episodes individually, was significantly lower in patients receiving psychoeducation both at two-[5] and five-year follow-up.[6] A major reason why psychoeducation appears to be so effective and widely used in bipolar patients is that the intervention reflects a medical model of the illness, thus disregarding stigmatization and perceptional issues; therefore, psychoeducation may appeal to a wider patient population due to its straightforward delivery and common-sense approach.[6]

A replication of the original study by Colom and colleagues supported the pro-gramme's efficacy, as psychoeducated patients had a lower rate and duration of hos-pital admissions.[8]

Despite reports of its prophylactic efficacy, psychoeducation is not effective in treat-ing acute episodes, and may have limitations for use in patients with a higher number of previous manic episodes due, probably, to neuropsychological impairment.[9]

A post hoc analysis of the outcome data from the group psychoeducation trial[9] also pointed at a possible lack of benefit from therapy for those subjects with more than twelve previous episodes, although due to the small sample size of the subgroup used for analysis (n = 24), those results may be as well attributed to a type-II error. As such, there appears to be evidence that the timing of introduction of a psychoeducation package may be important—introducing it early in the course of bipolar disorder may have significant benefits for that individual, but the impact of therapy may be limited in those with an established history of recurrences.[10] This may be related to cognitive impairment, as the number of previous episodes has been reported to be a key factor when it comes to impairment and, interestingly enough, the cut-point explaining most of the neuropsychological impairment would be around ten episodes.[11] However, other studies using a combined approach of psychoeducation plus CBT showed preventive efficacy at long-term (five years) in a sample composed by refractory patients.[12]

One main criticism that may be posed against this 21-session programme is its excessive length that may make its implementation difficult. Several proposals to reduce length have been suggested. However, such shorter programmes do not appear to have an equivalent efficacy. For instance, a six-session programme tested in Turkey was able to improve adherence but not to have impact on relapse prevention.[13]

The efficacy of psychoeducation has, no doubt, some biological underpinnings. It has been reported, for instance, that group psychoeducation normalizes cortisol awakening response.[14] Neuroimaging studies also point out to an increased activity of inferior frontal gyri and a tendency towards decreased activity of right hippocampus and parahippocampal gyrus in psychoeducated patients.[15]

Delivering psychoeducation in everyday practice

Who should deliver psychoeducation?

There is an increasing need to provide educational therapy not only on a specialist level, but also in a primary-care setting. Bipolar clinics offer an environment in which the patient interacts with a variety of health professionals, ranging from mental health nurses to psychologists, psychiatrists, occupational therapists, and pharmacists. Such resources are not available in a primary-care setting, where most patients with bipolar disorder are diagnosed and treated. Therefore, it is important that general practitioners (GPs) are aware of the impact that psychoeducation can have on the recovery process and the improvement in patient quality of life (QoL). It is not necessary for the GP to provide psychoeducation; however, they should be willing to recommend this type of therapy to their patients.

A major advantage of psychoeducation is its relevance and applicability beyond the field of mental health, owing to its simple approach and the fact that most skills required to provide the intervention are transferable to a myriad of other illnesses. The simplicity of psychoeducation allows implementation without long, complex, and thorough training of the therapist. Although the therapist needs to be a clinician (eg psychiatrist, psychologist, nurse), he/she should have specific clinical experience in the field of bipolar disrders rather than being an expert on a certain type of psychotherapy. Due to the nature of the delivery of psychoeducation programmes—group setting—it is important for the therapist to have experience in group work and have several personal characteristics including sense of humour, flexibility, and interpersonal skills.[3]

The proper setting for psychoeducation

Although psychoeducation follows a simple rather than a skilled approach, it is often not easy to implement in an overworked and overwhelmed clinical setting. Psychoeducation based on a diverse team of specialists (including psychiatrists, psychologists, and nurses) lacks complexity for both clinicians and patients, does not require a highly developed theoretical background, and promotes interpersonal skills. This strategy transforms the traditional model of a healing professional and a passive patient, into one of a trusting relationship between patient and clinician, empowering the patient to participate in the treatment process and the clinician to consider patients' choices and perspectives.

Psychoeducation is meaningful in settings where a multidisciplinary team effort is available. A team structure enhances the availability of a member in the patient's team in moments of crisis and ensures that each intervention—eg assessing the early warning signs, changing a medical prescription, controlling sleep habits, or performing an urgent determination of mood-stabilizer serum levels—is performed by a different specialist within the team. By increasing patients' ability to manage their disorder, the goal is to instil a proactive attitude into the patient and help them to develop awareness of when to seek help. The frequency of patients' appointments with their treating psychiatrist should follow an open-door policy, which allows for fewer arranged appointments, but complete flexibility for unscheduled visits or on-call availability upon suspicion of a new episode. In addition, psychoeducation should not be a static treatment, but improved upon on a regular basis, and adjusted in content and application depending on the patient progression, all assessed through a regular review regimen.[3]

What are the core issues to be addressed by psychoeducation?

The intention of psychoeducation sessions is to promote changes in patient behaviours and attitudes in the following areas: the individual's awareness and understanding of bipolar disorder; their adherence to the treatment regimen; the stability of their social and sleep rhythms; reducing any misuse of drugs and/or alcohol; and the individual's ability to recognize and manage the prodrome of bipolar relapse or the internal and external stressors that may increase their vulnerability to future relapse. Often-cited psychosocial influences are stressful life events, family conflict (including high levels of expressed emotion), chronobiological instability (such as social and circadian rhythm disruption), and treatment non-adherence.[16]

Non-adherence to the drug treatment regimen is a common feature among bipolar patients and is the major reason for symptom recurrence. Non-adherence may result from the patient 'feeling under drug control', illness denial, or patients missing their initial manic manifestations. Patients with underlying personality disorders may not be aware of their prodromal symptoms or have difficulties following treatment advice, thus a diagnosis of personality disorder correlates with an increased possibility of non-adherence.[17]

Therefore, it is important to educate patients about the consequences of non-adherence, the effect this has on their own QoL, as well as the effect on their family and friends.

Psychoeducation, more than being a technique, is an attitude when treating the patient, with the underlying aim of improving the relationship between patient and therapist to a level that allows both parties to readjust responsibilities and expertise in the treatment process. This intervention does not cure bipolar disorder, but aids in the elimination of incomprehension and denial, alleviates stigma, deals effectively with guilt, and prevents learned helplessness,[6] factors that seriously impede a patient's physical and mental wellness.

Limitations of psychoeducation and other psychotherapies

As previously discussed, patients with a very high number of episodes may not respond to psychoeducation. This is not surprising, bearing in mind that this sub-group of patients has shown a poor response even to mood stabilizers. Other factors such as co-morbidity may also worsen the response to psychotherapy.

However, patient-related factors are not the only ones to moderate the efficacy of psychoeducation. Moreover, therapist-related factors may be even more determinant.

The therapies that are most effective in treating bipolar disorder are highly structured and based on a coherent stress-vulnerability model that allows the patient to develop a personalized view of their problems and a clear rationale for the interventions made.[4] The therapy promotes independent use of the skills learned, change and progress in therapy are attributed to the patients' self-management skills rather than his/her therapists' skills, and the therapy may enhance the individuals' sense of self-efficacy.[18]

An apparently suitable candidate for therapy may fail to respond if that intervention is not carried out competently. Pooled data from 15 psychotherapy studies suggests there is a significant relationship between the therapist's level of training or experience, the degree of adherence to the treatment manual, the type of therapy used (eg structured brief therapies being superior to psychodynamic therapies) and patient outcomes.[19] Gortner and colleagues (1998)[20] demonstrated a significant correlation between ratings of competency and patient outcome. In a study of 185 depressed patients, individuals treated by senior therapists (>4 years cognitive therapy (CT) experience) showed significantly greater improvement than those treated by novice therapists. Although no study of therapist expertise and competency in appying the psychoeducation model to bipolar disorder has yet been published, most studies do provide data on ratings of these aspects of therapy delivery. It is also clear that the expertise of the therapist is a particularly important determinant of outcome when treating more severe or complex cases.[21] DeRubeis and Feeley[22] demonstrated a significant correlation (r = 0.53) between adherence to symptom focused CT techniques and patient outcomes. However, technical fidelity and competency are not the only important intra-therapy factors, as therapist empathy and the therapeutic alliance both significantly influence outcome of mood disorders.[23] Again, the nature of the therapeutic relationship with an individual with bipolar disorder is critical as many of these individuals resist and challenge a more didactic approach to treatment.[24]

Maintaining a relationship, instigating a logical sequence of interventions, and delivering as much as possible of the planned programme of therapy requires considerable expertise and even under control conditions the median number of sessions attended by participants in clinical trials is about 66% (14 out of 22 sessions) of the allocated course.[25,10] As noted in their meta-analysis of therapy for severe unipolar mood disorders, non-adherence rates with therapy are very similar to non-adherence rates with medication, so a significant limitation will always be that individuals do not totally engage with an apparently effective treatment.[26]

Other aspects limiting a broader implementation of psychoeducation have to do with the huge gap between availability and demand, as psychoeducation is often only available in excellence centres or extremely specialized bipolar units. The number of well-trained therapists is limited and individuals living in broad rural and underserved areas may face extreme difficulties when trying to attend weekly sessions for a very long period. Moreover, in some countries psychoeducation might not be affordable for many affected individuals.

Future directions

There is an emerging interest to explore new approaches to deliver efficacious psychological interventions tailored to individual patient characteristics, overcoming geographic and economic barriers and in a continuous manner.

The Internet has gradually showed a fast and worldwide global expansion in developed countries reaching almost all social, age, ethnic, and educational-level groups through user-friendly interfaces and at low cost. Additionally, access to this resource has moved from desktop computers to nearly everywhere via low-cost smartphones that most people increasingly use for multiple purposes and carry them habitually. This rapid adoption of both the Internet and smartphones has had an impact also on mental health patients, who increasingly seek information and help for their disorders on an everyday basis, increasing the number of resources available.[27] These individuals, who usually suffer from social stigma, found in the Internet a solution for communicating with their peers and obtaining information about their condition in a convenient and moreover in an anonymous way.[28] Furthermore, modern technologies can unobtrusively sense and analyse human behaviour, deliver feedback, and provide behavioural therapy, thus they have been increasingly emphasized for a potential to shift some of the mental healthcare tasks to daily life outside clinical settings and possibly to mitigate today's existing pressure on healthcare systems.[29]

Smartphone-based apps able to capture both subjective and passive data may be able to monitor symptoms and signs and provide tailored psychoeducation.[30]

Conclusion

◆ Pyschological interventions may diminish recurrence rates in a significant subset of patients with bipolar disorder.

◆ Psychological interventions should not be used as a monotherapy, but as add-on strategies to drug treatments.

- Psychological interventions play, mostly, a prophylactic role. Evidence on their efficacy in the management of acute episodes remains scarce.
- The vast majority of efficacious psychological interventions include psychoeducative compounds.
- The basic ingredients of psychoeducation are illness awareness, adherence enhancement, regularity of habits, and identification of warning signs.
- New technologies may play a role in the worldwide dissemination and implementation of psychoeducation to remote and underserved areas.

References

1. **Perry A, Tarrier N, Morris R, McCarthy E, and Limb K.** Randomised controlled trial of efficacy of teaching patients with bipolar disorder to identify early symtoms of relapse and obtain treatment, BMJ 1999;**318**:149–53.
2. **Lobban F, Taylor L, Chandler C, Tyler E, Kinderman P, Kolamunnage-Dona R, Gamble C, Peters S, Pontin E, Sellwood W, and Morriss RK.** Enhanced relapse prevention for bipolar disorder by community mental health teams: cluster feasibility randomised trial, Br J Psychiatry 2010;**196**:59–63.
3. **Colom F.** Keeping therapies simple: psychoeducation in the prevention of relapse in affective disorders, Br J Psychiatry 2011;**198**:338–40.
4. **Colom F and Scott J.** Psychological treatments for bipolar disorders, *Psychiatric Clinics of North America* 2005;**28**:371–84.
5. **Colom F, Vieta E, Martinez-Aran A, Reinares M, Goikolea JM, Benabarre A, Torrent C, Comes M, Corbella B, Parramon G, and Corominas J.** A randomized trial on the efficacy of group psychoeducation in the prophylaxis of recurrences in bipolar patients whose disease is in remission, Arch Gen Psychiatry. 2003;**60**:402–7.
6. **Colom F and Vieta E.** *Kaplan & Sadock's Comprehensive Textbook of Psychiatry* (New York, NY: Williams & Wilkins, 2009).
7. **Miklowitz DJ, George EL, Richards JA, Simoneau TL, and Suddath RL.** A randomized study of family-focused psychoeducation and pharmacotherapy in the outpatient management of bipolar disorder, Arch Gen Psychiatry 2003;**60**:904–12.
8. **Candini V, Buizza C, Ferrari C, Caldera MT, Ermentini R, Ghilardi A, Nobili G, Pioli R, Sabaudo M, Sacchetti E, Saviotti FM, Seggioli G, Zanini A, and de Girolamo G.** Is structured group psychoeducation for bipolar patients effective in ordinary mental health services? A controlled trial in Italy, J Affect Disord 2013;**151**:149–55.
9. **Colom F, Reinares M, Pacchiarotti I, Popovic D, Mazzarini L, Martínez-Arán A, Torrent C, Rosa A, Palomino-Otiniano R, Franco C, Bonnin CM, an dVieta E.** Has number of previous episodes any effect on response to group psychoeducation in bipolar patients? A 5-year follow-up post hoc analysis, Acta Neuropsychiatr 2010;**22**:50–3.
10. **Scott J, Paykel E, Morriss R, Bentall R, Kinderman P, Johnson T, Abbott R, and Hayhurst H.** Cognitive-behavioural therapy for severe and recurrent bipolar disorders: randomised controlled trial, Br J Psychiatry 2006b;**188**:313–20.
11. **Martínez-Arán A, Vieta E, Reinares M, Colom F, Torrent C, Sanchez-Moreno J, Benabarre A, Goikolea JM, Comes M, and Salamero M.** Cognitive function across manic or hypomanic, depressed, and euthymic states in bipolar disorder, Am J Psychiatry 2004;**161**:262–70.

12. González Isasi A, Echeburúa E, Limiñana JM, and González-Pinto A. Psychoeducation and cognitive-behavioral therapy for patients with refractory bipolar disorder: a 5-year controlled clinical trial, Eur Psychiatry 2014;29:134–41.

13. Eker F and Harkın S. Effectiveness of six-week psychoeducation program on adherence of patients with bipolar affective disorder, J Affect Disord 2012;138:409–16.

14. Delle Chiaie R, Trabucchi G, Girardi N, Marini I, Pannese R, Vergnani L, Caredda M, Zerella MP, Minichino A, Corrado A, Patacchioli FR, Simeoni S, and Biondi M. Group psychoeducation normalizes cortisol awakening response in stabilized bipolar patients under pharmacological maintenance treatment, Psychother Psychosom 2013;82:264–6.

15. Favre P, Baciu M, Pichat C, De Pourtalès MA, Fredembach B, Garçon S, Bougerol T, and Polosan M. Modulation of fronto-limbic activity by the psychoeducation in euthymic bipolar patients. A functional MRI study, Psychiatry Res 2013;214:285–95.

16. Pope M, Dudley R, and Scott J. Determinants of social functioning in bipolar disorder, Bipolar Disord 2007 Feb–Mar;9(1–2):38–44.

17. Colom F, Vieta E, Martínez-Arán A, Reinares M, Benabarre A, and Gastó C. Clinical factors associated to treatment non-compliance in euthymic bipolar patients, J Clin Psychiatry 2000;61:549–55.

18. Scott J. Cognitive therapy of affective disorders: a review, Journal of Affective Disorders 1996;37:1–11.

19. Crits-Christoph P, Baranackie K, Kurcias JS, et al. Meta-analysis of therapist effects in psychotherapy outcome studies, Psychotherapy Research 1991;1:81–91.

20. Gortner ET, Gollan JK, Dobson KS, and Jacobson NS. Cognitive-behavioral treatment for depression: relapse prevention. J Consult Clin Psychol. 1998 Apr;66(2):377–84.

21. Davidson K, Scott J, Schmidt U, Tata P, Thornton S, and Tyrer P. Therapist competence and clinical outcome in the POPMACT trial, Psychological Medicine 2004;34:855–63.

22. DeRubeis RJ and Feeley M. Determinants of change in cognitive therapy for depression, Cognitive Therapy and Research 1990;14:469–82.

23. Burns DD and Nolen-Hoeksema S. Therapeutic empathy and recovery from depression in cognitive-behavioural therapy: a structural equation model, Journal of Consulting and Clinical Psychology 1992;60:441–9.

24. Scott J. Psychotherapy for bipolar disorder: an unmet need?, British Journal of Psychiatry 1995;167:581–8.

25. Lam DH, Watkins ER, Hayward P, Bright JA, Wright K, Kerr N, Parr-Davis G, and Sham P. A randomized controlled study of cognitive therapy for relapse prevention for bipolar affective disorder. Outcome of the first year, Arch Gen Psychiatry 2003;60:145–52.

26 DeRubeis RJ, Gelfand LA, Tang TZ, and Simons AD. Medications versus cognitive behaviour therapy for severely depressed outpatients: mega-analysis of four randomised comparisons, American Journal of Psychiatry 1999;156:1007–13.

27. Carras MC, Mojtabai R, Furr-Holden CD, Eaton W, and Cullen BAM. Use of mobile phones, computers and internet among clients of an inner-city community psychiatric clinic, J Psychiatr Pract 2014;20:94–103. doi:10.1097/01.pra.0000445244.08307.84

28. Townsend L, Gearing RE, and Polyanskaya O. Influence of health beliefs and stigma on choosing internet support groups over formal mental health services, Psychiatr Serv 2012;63:370–6. doi:10.1176/appi.ps.201100196

29. Hidalgo-Mazzei D, Mateu A, Reinares M, Matic A, Vieta E, and Colom F. Internet-based psychological interventions for bipolar disorder: review of the present and insights into the future, J Affect Disord 2015a;188:1–13.

30. Hidalgo-Mazzei D, Mateu A, Reinares M, Undurraga J, Bonnín Cdel M, Sánchez-Moreno J, Vieta E, and Colom F. Self-monitoring and psychoeducation in bipolar patients with a smart-phone application (SIMPLe) project: design, development and studies protocols, BMC Psychiatry 2015b;15:52.

Colom F, Vieta E, Sánchez-Moreno J, Palomino-Otiniano R, Reinares M, Goikolea JM, Benabarre A, and Martínez-Arán A. Group psychoeducation for stabilised bipolar disorders: 5-year outcome of a randomised clinical trial, *Br J Psychiatry* 2009;*194*:260–5.

Chapter 14

Functional remediation therapy for bipolar disorder

Carla Torrent, Caterina del Mar Bonnin, and Anabel Martinez-Arán

Psychosocial functioning and bipolar disorder

The concept of functioning is complex and involves different aspects including the capacity of work and study, the capacity to live independently, the capacity to enjoy leisure time, and the capacity to share life with a partner.[1] Bipolar disorder is associated with impairment in a number of areas including cognition and functional impairment, often despite the remission of mood symptoms. Indeed, the World Health Organization ranks bipolar disorder as the sixth leading cause of disability in the world.[2]

Difficulties in psychosocial functioning are especially presented as difficulties in adequate occupational performance and social integration and are presented not only in subtype bipolar I but also in subtype II of the disease.[3] In a study carried out by the National Institute of Mental Health (NIMH) in the United States (US) in the 1970s, less than half of the patients admitted for bipolar disorder returned to work after discharge. At two years, one-third of the patients demonstrated difficulties in work performance, and at five years even the patients who had been compensated in the previous two years presented alterations in social functioning. Along the same line, one study analysing the number of work days lost per year due to physical and mental diseases reported bipolar disorder to be one of the most incapacitating conditions together with neurological disorders and the post-traumatic stress disorder.[4] In another European study including almost 3,500 patients[5] psychiatrists were asked about the occupational situation of the patients one year prior to a manic episode. The results indicated that from 28 to 68% of the patients presented some degree of occupational problems and, among these, 21% were totally unable to work.

Numerous investigations have demonstrated functional impairment in bipolar patients in comparison with both healthy individuals and unipolar patients.[6] Despite the great variability among patients, most (from 30 to 60% of bipolar patients) may present some type of functional impairment.[7] This functional impairment may be prolonged, and may even be present during the periods of euthymia.[8] It is known that more than half of the patients do not recover previous functioning after an affective episode; in general only 40% of patients recover the grade of premorbid functioning during the periods of clinical remission.[9] The difficulties in obtaining functional remission seem to be associated with disease progression; psychosocial adjustment is more preserved in patients with a first episode than in those with more chronic disease, with treatment being more effective in patients in the earlier stages of the disease.[10]

A number of longitudinal studies have shown how functional recovery is much more complicated than clinical remission. One European follow-up study showed that 64% of patients achieved remission two years after an acute episode, but only 34% also achieved functional recovery; that is, they recovered the level of functioning prior to the onset of the disease.[11] In another follow-up study, it was found that 98% of the patients obtained symptomatic recovery at two years. However, only 38% achieved satisfactory functional recovery.[12] In an eight-month follow-up study, Strakowski and colleagues[13] observed that almost all of the patients presented persistent impairment in at least one of the areas of functioning studied and fewer than half achieved adequate functioning in three of the four areas assessed.

The factors involved in functioning remain unclear. According to several studies the most robust clinical predictor of long-term functional impairment is subsyndromal depressive symptoms.[14] These results are especially important, because many patients present depressive symptoms during most of their lives.[15] The rates of functional impairment are quite similar to the number of patients with neurocognitive dysfunction.[16] Indeed, neurocognitive impairment constitutes a central element of bipolar disorder, confirming the association between cognitive performance and psychosocial functioning. Several recent studies have found an interrelation between neurocognitive impairment and functioning in bipolar patients similar to that described in schizophrenia patients.[14]

One of the impaired areas of functioning found in these patients is the occupational area, in which a diminishment has been observed in productivity, with a greater number of days lost over one year and elevated unemployment rates.[17] In a recent study analyses of work functioning indicated that bipolar patients had a greater lifetime histories of unemployment, but also greater incidence of being fired of their jobs.[18] A recent systematic review found that cognitive deficits, depression, and level of education were predictors of employment among bipolar patients.[19] A meta-analysis recently published by Tse and colleagues[20] concludes that patients with positive employment outcomes are more likely to perform well on measures of cognitive performance (eg verbal memory, higher executive function) and have a better course of the illness. With respect to interpersonal relationships, one study carried out by our team reported serious difficulties in maintaining satisfactory sexual relationships, an increase in family and social conflicts, and reduced participation in social activities.[21] With regard to family interaction, the quality of the relations among family members may affect the grade of psychosocial functioning and increase the number of relapses.[22] In a naturalistic trial focusing on the global burden of bipolar disorder the number of depressive episodes, presence of psychotic symptoms during the manic index episode and the body mass index (BMI) at baseline were the best predictors of functional outcome six months after a manic episode.[23]

One of the critical aspects of functioning has to do with its assessment. Investigators traditionally measure one or two elements of functioning without taking all the others into account. The measurements of functioning used in this disorder vary greatly from one study to another; indeed, few measurements have been used by more than one investigator.[24] Functioning may be measured by several scales, the most commonly used being the multidimensional scale for the evaluation of global activity (GAF). Other scales used are the Social Adjustment Scale, the Life Functioning Questionnaire, the Short Form SF-36, and the WHO-DAS. Most of these scales require quite a long time for administration and were not designed specifically to evaluate functional alterations in bipolar disorder or are self-reported questionnaires and their validity is questioned. To this end, the FAST (Functioning Assessment Short Test) was developed for the clinical evaluation of functional impairment presented by patients suffering from mental disorders including bipolar disorder. It is a simple instrument, easy and quick to administer, and evaluates the main difficulties in psychosocial functioning experienced by patients.[25] This is a highly reliable tool to evaluate the objective difficulties presented by patients in psychosocial functioning, an area which has also demonstrated sensitivity to changes in both the short and the long term.[26]

Cognitive functioning in bipolar disorder

Although cognitive and functional impairment appear to be key features of severe mental illnesses, they may not be universal. For example, approximately 20–25% of patients with schizophrenia have been found to have neuropsychological function within normal limits or in patients with bipolar disorder has been found an estimated prevalence between 30 and 62% of bipolar patients performing within normal limits on neuropsychological assessments.[27,28] Recent research suggest the presence of multiple cognitive subgroups in bipolar patients: an intact group with performance comparable with healthy controls on all domains, a selective impairment group with moderate deficits, and a global impairment group with severe deficits across all cognitive domains comparable with deficits in schizophrenia.[29] By subgrouping bipolar patients based on neurocognitive profiles the heterogeneity of the phenotype can be reduced allowing for a more targeted treatment.

According to different studies,[30,31] specific domains of cognitive impairment in bipolar patients include: executive control, verbal learning and memory, working memory, and sustained attention. Cognitive impairments are present already in the early course of bipolar disorder.[32] Moreover, a positive association between neurocognitive dysfunction and functional impairment has been shown in cross-sectional[33] and longitudinal studies.[14] Recent research suggests that cognitive functioning may be differentially related to functional outcomes depending on the severity of the cognitive impairment; this means that cognition may be more strongly related to functional outcomes among individuals with more severe cognitive impairment.[34]

Robinson and Ferrier[35] provided a narrative review of studies that considered the relationship between illness variables and cognitive deficits. They found an association between the number of previous episodes, especially manic ones, with neurocognitive functioning suggesting that successive episodes might be related to a progressive neurocognitive decline. On the contrary, Martino and colleagues[36] did not find that the experience of successive episodes is related to a progressive neuro-cognitive decline, rather it is just that cognitive impairment could be the cause more than the consequence of poorer clinical course; likewise Depp and coworkers[37] suggested the relative independence of mood symptom severity and cognitive abilities.

There are different factors that, directly or indirectly, may influence cognitive functioning in bipolar disorder: the previous history of psychotic symptoms could be associated with poorer cognitive functioning in bipolar patients.[38] However, other recent reports suggest that the presence of prior history of psychotic symptoms was not related to more cognitive dysfunctions.[39] This factor warrants further investigation since research on this issue in bipolar disorder is still very scant.

Regarding the bipolar subtype, bipolar I and II subtypes show cognitive dysfunction; nonetheless, bipolar I subjects are generally more impaired than those with bipolar II disorder.[40,41]

Subdepressive symptomatology has also a negative impact on overall functioning and specifically on occupational functioning and cognitive functioning.[14]

Lifetime duration of bipolar disorder has been associated with cognitive dysfunction. The length of illness negatively correlated with scores on tests of executive function, psychomotor speed, and verbal memory.[42] Verbal memory was the measure that was more consistently associated with the duration of illness. None of the studies have reported any significant associations between duration of euthymia and performance on cognitive tests.[43]

According to several studies cognitive deficits, particularly in the domains of attention, memory, and executive functioning, are related to the number of prior mood episodes, the effects of manic symptomatology on cognition seem stronger than the effects of depressive symptoms.[44] Most studies have reported that those patients with a higher number of hospitalizations showed poorer performance on cognitive measures;[45] it is probable that the number of admissions may constitute an indirect measure of the severity of episodes, as well as of the illness course.

Regarding medication most of the current evidence suggests that the impairment effect appears more related to the illness itself rather than from the effects of pharmacotherapy.

Cognitive remediation in bipolar disorder

At present, the rapid development of investigations in affective disorders has demonstrated qualitatively similar cognitive alterations, albeit of less magnitude, to those of schizophrenia, in other affective disorders such as bipolar disorder. Currently, there is no Food and Drug Administration-approved pharmacological agent for the management of cognitive deficits in bipolar disorder. A number of agents have been tested in the treatment of cognitive deficits in bipolar disorder, with mixed results. It has therefore been suggested that non-pharmacological interventions, such as cognitive remediation and non-invasive brain stimulation techniques, could also have a potential effect on individuals with some type of affective disorder but their role has not yet been properly explored among bipolar patients. Most of the studies have been carried out in mixed samples including affective patients, with schizophrenia and schizoaffectives, making it difficult to draw conclusions. To date, six studies have been undertaken in purely affective patients, and only two of these studies were aimed at bipolar patients. The results of one of the studies, which is an open trial with 18 bipolar individuals and no control group, indicate that an improvement in psychosocial and occupational functioning may be achieved by an intervention focused on both cognitive and residual depressive symptoms. This focus also considers the subdepressive symptomatology since it has been observed that this symptomatology has a close relationship with difficulties in global psychosocial functioning. Nonetheless, in this specific case, it should be taken into account that the beneficial effects of neurocognitive remediation may be confounded with mood improvement.[46] The second study is a randomized controlled trial aiming to investigate the effects of 12 weeks' group-based cognitive remediation on cognitive dysfunction in 46 individuals with bipolar disorder who experienced cognitive difficulties despite being in partial or full remission. The results showed that the short-term group-based cognitive remediation did not seem to improve overall cognitive or psychosocial function in individuals with bipolar disorder. There are some limitations of this study highlighted by the authors: the relatively small sample size; the assessment of cognitive dysfunction was only subjectively reported and the sort duration of the intervention. Probably a longer-term, more intensive, and individualized cognitive remediation may be necessary to improve cognition in bipolar patients. Lately, a new trial has been registered to examine the utility of combining cognitive remediation and d-cycloserine, an NMDA receptor partial agonist, in the treatment of cognitive deficits among individuals with bipolar disorder.[47]

Functional remediation in bipolar disorder

This programme was developed in the Hospital Clínic de Barcelona, with the main objective of treating not only neurocognition but also functional impairment in bipolar disorder. The term functional remediation to refer to an innovative intervention focused especially on the recovery of the psychosocial functioning of the patients through training in the use of neurocognitive skills applied to daily routine. The functional remediation programme is the first approach carried out in the field of bipolar disorder with the aim of improving the psychosocial functioning of these patients. The programme is based on a neurocognitive psychosocial focus including modelling techniques, role playing, self-instructions, verbal instructions, and positive reinforcement, together with metacognition. It includes education on cognitive deficits and their impact on daily life, and provides strategies to manage the cognitive deficiencies in the different cognitive domains, mainly attention, memory, and executive functions.[48] The family is also involved in the process to facilitate the practice of these strategies and for reinforcement. It is important to combine different theories, methodologies, and approaches in order to improve not only the knowledge but also the functioning of these patients, given the complexity and the severity of bipolar disorder.

The efficacy of this programme has been demonstrated in a recent controlled clinical trial comparing three treatments: psychoeducation, functional remediation, and pharmacological treatment only (standard treatment).[49] Ten Spanish centres participated in this multicentre study, recruiting a total of 268 patients. The patients were randomized into three study arms stratified by sex, age, and educational level. Pharmachological treatment was prescribed to the three groups according to local clinical guidelines. The main measure of efficacy consisted of changes observed in psychosocial functioning post-intervention and at one year, assessed with the FAST, with respect to the baseline evaluation.

Thus, once the intervention was completed, the patients were again assessed at a clinical, functional, and neuropsychological level. The results showed an improvement in the functioning of patients participating in the functional remediation group compared with those who did no receive any intervention other than pharmachological treatment. In addition, patients undergoing the functional remediation programme achieved significant improvement in occupational and interpersonal or social functioning compared with those with only the usual pharmacological treatment. Functional improvement was greater with functional remediation than with psychoeducation.[49] The efficacy of the functional remediation intervention programme was maintained at one year of follow-up.[50] The functional remediation programme, therefore, is a promising tool for achieving improvement in functional performance in euthymic bipolar patients. This programme is not a simple training course to improve neurocognition, but rather it aims to provide tools for the patients to manage the difficuties and problems of real life which affect daily functioning. It is important to reduce the impact of bipolar disorder on daily functioning within an ecological framework to thereby increase the well-being of the patients an reduce the costs and social burden of this disease.

The functional remediation programme may improve aspects related to work functioning, increasing economic autonomy and reducing financial dependence. Indeed, approximately 5% of the patients obtained work or improved their occupational performance after the intervention. The interpersonal relationships improve partly by means of the group effect, which facilitates relating to other people, but it should be taken into account that aspects related to memory, strategies for codifying information, and social skills (recognition of emotions, assertiveness) are emphasized.

The patients often have to interact to carry out the exercises or tasks, potentiating the feeling of self-confidence.

With respect to neurocognitive changes, the differences between the three groups were not statistically significant, although the patients in the functional remediation group showed better performance on the learning and verbal memory tests, gaining advantage from the strategies of semantic encoding. Nonetheless, the following cannot be ruled out: the effect of practice as well as other factors must be taken into account, such as that this trial's inclusion criteria required a certain level of functional disability but not necessarily neurospsychological impairment. In an exploratory subanalysis of the main trial[49] with the objective to ascertain whether neurocognitive enhancement was a potential ingredient of functional remediation a total of 188 patients neurocognitively impaired were selected. Functional remediation was effective at improving verbal memory and psychosocial functioning in this sample after six months follow-up.[23]

The object of functional remediation is general functional improvement, not just cognitive improvement. This may explain why improvements in functioning were larger and more significant than neuropsychological changes. The results suggest that even though some cognitive deficits may persist, patients exhibit greater ability and are able to employ more strategies to cope with these deficits in daily life after having received specific training.

The functional remediation programme has proven to be effective in improving the functioning of patients with bipolar I and II disorder,[51] especially in the areas of occupational and social functioning. A combination of pharmacological treatment and functional remediation in patients with relevant difficulties in their daily life could improve the functional prognosis of persons with bipolar disorder. Although the intervention could be implemented at an individual level, the group format may be more effective, not only from an economic point of view, representing an important saving of time, but also because it facilitates interpersonal interaction.

We know that patients with bipolar disorder present deficits in some domains of social cognition (theory of mind and emotional processing) even in phases of euthymia.[52] The deficits in social cognition may lead to poor social functioning, and it is therefore imperative that mental health professionals reach a greater consensus and improvement of methods used in the assessment of the domains of social cognition in bipolar disorder. It is also important that functional/neurocognitive remediation programmes should include interventions directed to improve social cognition.

Patients obtain benefits that improve their functioning from the functional remediation programme, but these effects would most probably be more prolonged and could be generalized to different settings of daily life and to other areas of functioning if the training could be continued, supervised, and monitored by a therapist on completion of the intervention. In this regard, booster sessions every three months or at least twice a year would be very helpful in order to maintain practice and positive results, to review the content, to determine whether the learning has been consolidated, and to establish whether the patients have integrated the new guidelines into their everyday routines.

Structure of the programme

The 21 sessions that constitute the intervention are divided into five blocks or modules (see Box 14.1).

Module 1. This is placed first to allow both patients and relatives to become aware of the cognitive difficulties that may be presented, but also because this module introduces some key concepts that will be more extensively developed in later sessions. For the patients, this psychoeducational work is important as a means of promoting knowledge related to the cognitive limitations they may present, paving the way for de-stigmatization and allowing the limitations to be acted upon.

In addition, it provides a useful way of helping them to understand their problems, while also giving them greater autonomy and preparing the ground for providing

Box 14.1 The structure of the functional remediation programme: 21 sessions, in five modules

Module 1: Training on Neurocognitive Processes

1. Introduction to functional remediation. The role of the family. Enhancing practice and reinforcement.
2. What are the most common cognitive dysfunctions in bipolar disorder?
3. Factors influencing cognitive impairment: myths and realities.

Module 2: Attention

4. What is attention? Strategies for improving it.
5. Strategies to improve attention and their application in daily life.

Module 3: Memory

6. What is memory? Strategies for improving it.
7. Memory: the use of a diary and other external aids.
8. Internal strategies to improve memory.
9. Other mnemonic strategies and their application in daily life.
10. Reading and remembering.
11. Puzzles: retrieving information from the past.

Module 4: Executive Functions

12. Executive functions: self-instructions and self-monitoring.
13. Executive functions: programming and organizing activities.
14. Executive functions: programming activities, establishing priorities, and time management.
15. Executive functions: problem-solving techniques.
16. Executive functions: solving problems.

Module 5: Improving Communication, Autonomy, and Stress Management

17. Managing stressful situations.
18. Training in communication skills.
19. Improving communication.
20. Improving autonomy and functioning.
21. Final session: review of useful strategies.

a set of cognitive techniques and strategies in later sessions. For the relatives, it is important to understand that many of the difficulties presented by the patient originate from the cognitive problems rather than from an attitude, and that participation in an intervention of this type may allow modification of some of these aspects and directly influence the overall functioning of the person with bipolar disorder. It is therefore important to achieve an intermediate point at which acceptance of the disorder is incorporated, restructuring the expectations of the psychosocial functioning of the individual and, in turn, encouraging the performance of tasks to potentiate that person's autonomy without, of course, overburdening the patient.

Module 2. With this module the proper training in cognitive functions starts. Sessions 4 and 5 focus on attention as the basis for other cognitive functions. We explain roughly what attention is, the types of attention (selective, sustained, and divided), and which aspects of daily life are interfered with by deficits in this area. Strategies are provided, to be worked through during the sessions and as part of the homework between the sessions. The main point is to place the emphasis on the importance of attention as a foundation for other areas of cognitive function, and the strategies acquired will be used in subsequent sessions. One such strategy consists of concentrating on one activity, such as a word search, or looking for differences between two images, or a mental calculation task, while having other elements of distraction in parallel, such as noise or background music. Part of the strategy involves taking breaks during attention-straining tasks, and limiting oneself to carrying out one task at a time rather than attempting to multitask a number of activities or initiate new activities before other activities are completed.

Module 3. Includes sessions 6–11 and contains the block devoted to memory. The steps in the process of acquiring and retrieving memory are impacted by the illness, and this module includes various exercises focusing on remembering visual and auditory verbal input, with several strategies to enhance encoding, storage, and recovery of the information. During these sessions, various exercises on remembering visual and auditory verbal input are performed. The group of techniques promotes a more profound processing, elaborating the information so that it acquires a structure with more significance. The main internal techniques to be specifically explained are association, categorization, and narration or story. Other strategies provided are: restitution technique, rhythm and rhyme, repetition technique, method of loci as well as the option of using external aids (diary, clock alarms, information and communication technologies (ICTs), for instance). We will also work on some strategies that allow the reconstruction of information from the past, such as better organizing the memories with well-classified, ordered, and labelled photos, recordings, or videos of important events. The exercises in this module also include a reading task, where patients have to start reading a book and choosing a piece of news in the newspaper to track for several weeks. Before starting the tasks, we refresh memory techniques, such as reading aloud, taking brief notes, and using visual imagery in order to remember instructions and key points.

Module 4. We begin a new block of five sessions in which we work on aspects related to the executive functions. As explained in the first introductory sessions, the executive functions include a group of functions that are usually related mainly to the frontal lobes, and that allow us to organize, plan, and direct our behaviour towards a specific goal and give us the ability to carry it out efficiently.

Thus, these functions allow us to constantly adapt to the changes required by the environment around us. It should be taken into account that many of the cognitive complaints experienced by patients with bipolar disorder are related more to the executive functions than, for example, to true deficits in memory or attention. The main problem is that patients are not aware of these difficulties, or that they do not recognize them as part of their cognitive deficits. During these sessions the nature of these functions is studied in depth and activities are carried out within an ecological setting to learn how to plan, programme, time manage, adapt to unforeseen events, and establish priorities, alongside training in effective problem-solving.

Module 5. The final module integrates aspects of stress management with guidelines for diaphragmatic breathing and muscle-relaxation techniques, followed by two sessions related to training in communication skills, providing some guidelines to improve conversations and enhance assertiveness and reflective listening. The penultimate session aims to reinforce social networking, supplying information concerning activities that may be done in the community.

Finally, in the last session a recap of what has been done is made, and the patients evaluate the intervention.

Conclusions

The fact that the use of cognitive remediation in affective disorders is still at its beginning, provides the opportunity to learn from previously developed experience in the field of schizophrenia. Nevertheless, it should be taken into account that the cognitive deficits in schizophrenic patients are usually of greater severity than those presented by bipolar patients and, thus, the programmes aimed at schizophrenics may not be completely ideal for bipolar patients, being simpler and carrying scarce motivation for participation and poor adherence.

Functional recovery is one of the questions which remains to be solved in the treatment of bipolar disorder. In clinical practice there is a need to reduce the impact of the disability of bipolar patients in order to diminish the suffering and the cost of this disease. Functional remediation seems to be effective in improving the functional outcome of bipolar patients.

Further studies will have to confirm the duration of the effects of the intervention and also to adress the identification of the moderators and mediators in the prediction of functional outcome because this may help to disentangle the complex network of variables that contribute to functional outcome in bipolar disorder.

References

1. **Zarate CA, Jr., Tohen M, Land M**, and **Cavanagh S**. Functional impairment and cognition in bipolar disorder, Psychiatr Q 2000;71:309–29.

2. **Catala-Lopez F, Genova-Maleras R, Vieta E**, and **Tabares-Seisdedos R**. The increasing burden of mental and neurological disorders, Eur Neuropsychopharmacol 2013;**10**.

3. Ruggero CJ, Chelminski I, Young D, and Zimmerman M. Psychosocial impairment associated with bipolar II disorder, J Affect Disord 2007;**104**:53–60.

4. Gitlin MJ, Swendsen J, Heller TL, and Hammen C. Relapse and impairment in bipolar disorder, Am J Psychiatry 1995;**152**:1635–40.

5. Goetz I, Tohen M, Reed C, Lorenzo M, and Vieta E. Functional impairment in patients with mania: baseline results of the EMBLEM study, Bipolar Disord 2007;**9**:45–52.

6. Parker G, Rosen A, Trauer T, and Hadzi-Pavlovic D. Disability associated with mood states and comparator conditions: application of the Life Skills Profile measure of disability, Bipolar Disord 2007;**9**:11–15.

7. Huxley N and Baldessarini RJ. Disability and its treatment in bipolar disorder patients, Bipolar Disord 2007;**9**:183–96.

8. Rosa AR, Franco C, Martinez-Aran A, Sanchez-Moreno J, Reinares M, Salamero M, Arango C, Ayuso-Mateos JL, Kapczinski F, and Vieta E. Functional impairment in patients with remitted bipolar disorder, Psychother Psychosom 2008;**77**:390–2.

9. Tohen M, Bowden CL, Calabrese JR, Lin D, Forrester TD, Sachs GS, Koukopoulos A, Yatham L, and Grunze H. Influence of sub-syndromal symptoms after remission from manic or mixed episodes, Br J Psychiatry 2006;**189**:515–19.

10. Tohen M, Vieta E, Gonzalez-Pinto A, Reed C, and Lin D. Baseline characteristics and outcomes in patients with first episode or multiple episodes of acute mania, J Clin Psychiatry 2010;**71**:255–61.

11. Haro JM, Reed C, Gonzalez-Pinto A, Novick D, Bertsch J and Vieta E. 2-Year course of bipolar disorder type I patients in outpatient care: factors associated with remission and functional recovery, Eur Neuropsychopharmacol 2011;**21**:287–93.

12. Tohen M, Strakowski SM, Zarate C, Jr., Hennen J, Stoll AL, Suppes T, Faedda GL, Cohen BM, Gebre-Medhin P, and Baldessarini RJ. The McLean-Harvard first-episode project: 6-month symptomatic and functional outcome in affective and nonaffective psychosis, Biol Psychiatry 2000;**48**:467–76.

13. Strakowski SM, Williams JR, Fleck DE, and DelBello MP. Eight-month functional outcome from mania following a first psychiatric hospitalization, J Psychiatr Res 2000;**34**:193–200.

14. Bonnin CM, Martinez-Aran A, Torrent C, Pacchiarotti I, Rosa AR, Franco C, Murru A, Sanchez-Moreno J, and Vieta E. Clinical and neurocognitive predictors of functional outcome in bipolar euthymic patients: a long-term, follow-up study, J Affect Disord 2010;**121**:156–60.

15. Judd LL, Akiskal HS, Schettler PJ, Endicott J, Leon AC, Solomon DA, Coryell W, Maser JD, and Keller MB. Psychosocial disability in the course of bipolar I and II disorders: a prospective, comparative, longitudinal study, Arch Gen Psychiatry 2005;**62**:1322–30.

16. Martino DJ, Marengo E, Igoa A, Scapola M, Ais ED, Perinot L, and Strejilevich SA. Neurocognitive and symptomatic predictors of functional outcome in bipolar disorders: a prospective 1 year follow-up study, J Affect Disord 2009;**116**:37–42.

17. Simon GE, Ludman EJ, Unutzer J, Operskalski BH, and Bauer MS. Severity of mood symptoms and work productivity in people treated for bipolar disorder, Bipolar Disord 2008;**10**:718–25.

18. Boland EM, Stange JP, Molz AA, LaBelle DR, Ong ML, Hamilton JL, Connolly SL, Black CL, Cedeno AB, and Alloy LB. Associations between sleep disturbance, cognitive functioning and work disability in bipolar disorder, Psychiatry Res 2015;**10**.

19. Gilbert E and Marwaha S. Predictors of employment in bipolar disorder: a systematic review, J Affect Disord 2013;**145**:156–64.

20. Tse S, Chan S, Ng KL. and Yatham,LN Meta-analysis of predictors of favorable employment outcomes among individuals with bipolar disorder, Bipolar Disord 2014;**16**:217–29.

21. Rosa AR, Reinares M, Franco C, Comes M, Torrent C, Sanchez-Moreno J, Martinez-Aran A, Salamero M, Kapczinski F, and Vieta E. Clinical predictors of functional outcome of bipolar patients in remission, Bipolar Disord 2009;**11**:401–9.

22. Yan LJ, Hammen C, Cohen AN, Daley SE, and Henry RM. Expressed emotion versus relationship quality variables in the prediction of recurrence in bipolar patients, J Affect Disord 2004;**83**:199–206.

23. Bonnin CM, Reinares M, Hidalgo-Mazzei D, Undurraga J, Mur M, Saez C, Nieto E, Vazquez GH, Balanza-Martinez V, Tabares-Seisdedos R, and Vieta E. Predictors of functional outcome after a manic episode, J Affect Disord 2015a;**182**:121–5. doi: 10.1016/j.jad.2015.04.043 (Epub: 2 May 2015, 121–5).

24. Dean BB, Gerner D, and Gerner RH. A systematic review evaluating health-related quality of life, work impairment, and healthcare costs and utilization in bipolar disorder, Curr Med Res Opin 2004;**20**:139–54.

25. Rosa AR, Sanchez-Moreno J, Martinez-Aran A, Salamero M, Torrent C, Reinares M, Comes M, Colom F, Van RW, Ayuso-Mateos JL, Kapczinski F, and Vieta E. Validity and reliability of the Functioning Assessment Short Test (FAST) in bipolar disorder, Clin Pract Epidemiol Ment Health 2007;**3**:5.

26. Rosa AR, Reinares M, Amann B, Popovic D, Franco C, Comes M, Torrent C, Bonnin CM, Sole B, Valenti M, Salamero M, Kapczinski F, and Vieta E. Six-month functional outcome of a bipolar disorder cohort in the context of a specialized-care program, Bipolar Disord 2011;**13**:679–86.

27. Reichenberg A, Harvey PD, Bowie CR, Mojtabai R, Rabinowitz J, Heaton RK, and Bromet E. Neuropsychological function and dysfunction in schizophrenia and psychotic affective disorders, Schizophr Bull 2009;**35**:1022–9.

28. Iverson GL, Brooks BL, Langenecker SA, and Young AH. Identifying a cognitive impairment subgroup in adults with mood disorders, J Affect Disord 2011;**132**:360–7.

29. Burdick KE, Russo M, Frangou S, Mahon K, Braga RJ, Shanahan M, and Malhotra AK. Empirical evidence for discrete neurocognitive subgroups in bipolar disorder: clinical implications, Psychol Med 2014;**44**:3083–96.

30. Bora E, Yucel M, and Pantelis C. Cognitive endophenotypes of bipolar disorder: a meta-analysis of neuropsychological deficits in euthymic patients and their first-degree relatives, J Affect Disord 2009;**113**:1–20.

31. Bourne C, Aydemir O, Balanza-Martinez V, Bora E, Brissos S, Cavanagh JT, Clark L, Cubukcuoglu Z, Dias VV, Dittmann S, Ferrier IN, Fleck DE, Frangou S, Gallagher P, Jones L, Kieseppa T, Martinez-Aran A, Melle I, Moore PB, Mur M, Pfennig A, Raust A, Senturk V, Simonsen C, Smith DJ, Bio DS, Soeiro-de-Souza MG, Stoddart SD, Sundet K, Szoke A, Thompson JM, Torrent C, Zalla T, Craddock N, Andreassen OA, Leboyer M, Vieta E, Bauer M, Worhunsky PD, Tzagarakis C, Rogers RD, Geddes JR, and Goodwin GM. Neuropsychological testing of cognitive impairment in euthymic bipolar disorder: an individual patient data meta-analysis, Acta Psychiatr Scand 2013;**128**:149–62.

32. Torres IJ, DeFreitas CM, DeFreitas VG, Bond DJ, Kunz M, Honer WG, Lam RW, and Yatham LN. Relationship between cognitive functioning and 6-month clinical and functional outcome in patients with first manic episode bipolar I disorder, Psychol Med 2011;**41**:971–82.

33. Martinez-Aran A, Vieta E, Colom F, Torrent C, Sanchez-Moreno J, Reinares M, Benabarre A, Goikolea JM, Brugue E, Daban C, and Salamero M. Cognitive impairment in euthymic bipolar patients: implications for clinical and functional outcome, Bipolar Disord 2004;**6**:224–32.

34. Moore RC, Harmell AL, Harvey PD, Bowie CR, Depp CA, Pulver AE, McGrath JA, Patterson TL, Cardenas V, Wolyniec P, Thornquist MH, Luke JR, Palmer BW, Jeste DV, and Mausbach BT. Improving the understanding of the link between cognition and functional capacity in schizophrenia and bipolar disorder, Schizophr Res 2015;**10**.

35. Robinson LJ and Ferrier IN. Evolution of cognitive impairment in bipolar disorder: a systematic review of cross-sectional evidence, Bipolar Disord 2006;**8**:103–16.

36. Martino DJ, Strejilevich SA, Marengo E, Igoa A, Fassi G, Teitelbaum J, and Caravotta P. Relationship between neurocognitive functioning and episode recurrences in bipolar disorder, J Affect Disord 2013;**147**:345–51.

37. Depp CA, Mausbach BT, Harmell AL, Savla GN, Bowie CR, Harvey PD, and Patterson TL. Meta-analysis of the association between cognitive abilities and everyday functioning in bipolar disorder, Bipolar Disord 2012;**14**:217–26.

38. Martinez-Aran A, Torrent C, Tabares-Seisdedos R, Salamero M, Daban C, Balanza-Martinez V, Sanchez-Moreno J, Manuel GJ, Benabarre A, Colom F, and Vieta E. Neurocognitive impairment in bipolar patients with and without history of psychosis, J Clin Psychiatry 2008;**69**:233–9.

39. Selva G, Salazar J, Balanza-Martinez V, Martinez-Aran A, Rubio C, Daban C, Sanchez-Moreno J, Vieta E, and Tabares-Seisdedos R. Bipolar I patients with and without a history of psychotic symptoms: do they differ in their cognitive functioning?, J Psychiatr Res 2007;**41**:265–72.

40. Sole B, Bonnin CM, Torrent C, Balanza-Martinez V, Tabares-Seisdedos R, Popovic D, Martinez-Aran A, and Vieta E. Neurocognitive impairment and psychosocial functioning in bipolar II disorder, Acta Psychiatr Scand 2012;**125**:309–17.

41. Kessler U, Schoeyen HK, Andreassen OA, Eide GE, Hammar A, Malt UF, Oedegaard KJ, Morken G, Sundet K, and Vaaler AE. Neurocognitive profiles in treatment-resistant bipolar I and bipolar II disorder depression, BMC Psychiatry 2013;**13**:105. doi: 10.1186/1471-244X-13-105, 105–13.

42. Deckersbach T, McMurrich S, Ogutha J, Savage CR, Sachs G, and Rauch SL. Characteristics of non-verbal memory impairment in bipolar disorder: the role of encoding strategies, Psychol Med 2004;**34**:823–32.

43. Thompson JM, Gallagher P, Hughes JH, Watson S, Gray JM, Ferrier IN, and Young AH. Neurocognitive impairment in euthymic patients with bipolar affective disorder, Br J Psychiatry 2005;**186**:32–40.

44. Lopez-Jaramillo C, Lopera-Vasquez J, Gallo A, Ospina-Duque J, Bell V, Torrent C, Martinez-Aran A, and Vieta E. Effects of recurrence on the cognitive performance of patients with bipolar I disorder: implications for relapse prevention and treatment adherence, Bipolar Disord 2010;**12**:557–67.

45. Thompson JM, Hamilton CJ, Gray JM, Quinn JG, Mackin P, Young AH, and Ferrier IN. Executive and visuospatial sketchpad resources in euthymic bipolar disorder: implications for visuospatial working memory architecture, *Memory* 2006;**14**:437–51.

46. Deckersbach T, Nierenberg AA, Kessler R, Lund HG, Ametrano RM, Sachs G, Rauch SL, and Dougherty D. RESEARCH: Cognitive rehabilitation for bipolar disorder: An open trial for employed patients with residual depressive symptoms, CNS Neurosci Ther 2010;**16**:298–307.

47. Breitborde NJ, Dawson SC, Woolverton C, Dawley D, Bell EK, Norman K, Polsinelli A, Bernstein B, Mirsky P, Pletkova C, Grucci F, III, Montoya C, Nanadiego B, Sarabi E, DePalma M, and Moreno F. A randomized controlled trial of cognitive remediation and d-cycloserine for individuals with bipolar disorder, BMC Psychol 2014;**2**:41.

48. Martinez-Aran A, Torrent C, Sole B, Bonnin CM, Rosa AR, Sanchez-Moreno J, and Vieta E. Functional remediation for bipolar disorder, Clin Pract Epidemiol Ment Health 2011;**7**:112–16. doi: 10.2174/1745017901107010112. Epub: 6 June 2011, 112–16.

49. Torrent C, del Mar BC, Martinez-Aran A, Valle J, Amann BL, Gonzalez-Pinto A, Crespo JM, Ibanez A, Garcia-Portilla MP, Tabares-Seisdedos R, Arango C, Colom F, Sole B, Pacchiarotti I, Rosa AR, Ayuso-Mateos JL, Anaya C, Fernandez P, Landin-Romero R, Alonso-Lana S, Ortiz-Gil J, Segura B, Barbeito S, Vega P, Fernandez M, Ugarte A, Subira M, Cerrillo E, Custal N, Menchon JM, Saiz-Ruiz J, Rodao JM, Isella S, Alegria A, Al-Halabi S, Bobes J, Galvan G, Saiz PA, Balanza-Martinez V, Selva G, Fuentes-Dura I, Correa P, Mayoral M, Chiclana G, Merchan-Naranjo J, Rapado-Castro M, Salamero M, and Vieta E. Efficacy of functional remediation in bipolar disorder: a multicenter randomized controlled study, Am J Psychiatry 2013. doi: 10.1176/appi.ajp.2012.12070971, 10.

50. Bonnin CM, Torrent C, Arango C, Amann BL, Sole B, Gonzalez-Pinto A, Crespo JM, Tabares-Seisdedos R, Reinares M, Ayuso-Mateos JL, Garcia-Portilla MP, Ibanez A, Salamero M, Vieta E, Martinez-Aran A, and CIBERSAM Functional Remediation. Functional remediation in bipolar disorder: 1-year follow-up of neurocognitive and functional outcome, Br J Psychiatry 2015b.

51. Sole B, Bonnin CM, Mayoral M, Amann BL, Torres I, Gonzalez-Pinto A, Jimenez E, Crespo JM, Colom F, Tabares-Seisdedos R, Reinares M, Ayuso-Mateos JL, Soria S, Garcia-Portilla MP, Ibanez A, Vieta E, Martinez-Aran A, and Torrent C. Functional remediation for patients with bipolar II disorder: improvement of functioning and subsyndromal symptoms, Eur Neuropsychopharmacol 2015;**25**:257–64..

52. Bora E. Neurodevelopmental origin of cognitive impairment in schizophrenia, Psychol Med 2015;**45**:1–9.

Chapter 15

Predominant polarity, polarity index, and treatment selection in bipolar disorder

Sabrina C. da Costa, Joao L. de Quevedo, and André F. Carvalho

Introduction

Bipolar disorder (BD) is a severe and chronic illness, with an estimated lifetime prevalence of 2.1%, while subthreshold forms of the disorder affect another 2.4% of the general population.[1] According to the World Health Organization (WHO), BD ranks among the ten leading causes of disability-adjusted life years (DALY) in young adults.[2] It is estimated that, even with treatment, about 37% of patients will relapse into an affective episode within one year, while 60% will relapse within two years.[3]

The presentation, course, and co-morbidities seem to be highly heterogeneous among individuals with BD. In addition, certain characteristics of the first major affective episode may delineate subgroups that differ in clinical manifestations and outcomes throughout the course of the illness.[4] BD is highly disabling, and previous studies from the National Institute of Mental Health (NIMH) observed that individuals with BD spend more than half their lifetime with affective symptoms.[5-7] These studies had rated affective symptomatology in a sample that included BD types I and II on a weekly basis; the authors found that depressive episodes and symptoms predominate over the course of BD.[6,7] In addition, a large body of evidence indicates that predominant polarity (PP) (depressive or manic) can be identified in more than half of BD patients; the depressive PP (DPP) occurs more frequently, even though criteria for PP and nomenclatures have varied across different studies.[8-11]

A recent systematic review indicates that several illness characteristics have been found to vary in accordance to PP.[12] The DPP has been associated with a depressive onset of BD, higher number of suicidal attempts, and delayed diagnosis of BD, while the manic PP (MPP) has been associated with earlier age of illness onset, higher prevalence of psychotic features, and higher number of psychiatric hospitalizations.[9-14] The PP has been recently proposed as clinically useful disease specifier, due to its relevance on clinical outcomes and treatment selection during the course of BD.[9-14] Thus, the determination of PP may contribute to the planning of treatment strategies, pharmacological and non-pharmacological, which could be tailored to reflect the specific PP of a given patient.[9-14]

The polarity index (PI) reflects the ratio of the number needed to treat (NNT) for the prevention of depressive episodes and the NNT for the prevention of manic episodes.[15] This emerging concept has allowed the relative ranking of maintenance treatments for BD based on their relative antimanic versus antidepressant efficacy.

This chapter provides a critical overview of evidence of a putative role of PP and the PI in the selection of maintenance pharmacological as well as psychological treatments for BD.

Predominant polarity, polarity index, and treatment selection in bipolar disorder

Since Kraepelin,* significant inter-individual variations during the course of 'manic-depressive insanity' have been acknowledged. In the early 1960s, a sample of 117 manic-depressive patients was prospectively observed, and predominant manic symptoms occurred in 17.9% of patients, while predominant depressive symptoms were present in 25.6%. In this same sample, 56.4% of all individuals had equally pro-nounced mania and depression.† In a different study, a sample of 95 'manic-depressive' inpatients was followed up from 1959 to 1975,[16] and based on the findings from this study, the concept of PP was initially proposed. This study observed that some patients would present a 'nuclear' type of illness (ie, patients who would show both mania and depression requiring hospital admission), while others would have either predomi-nant depression or predominant mania.[16] More recently, the concept of PP has gained renewed interest, and was proposed as a relevant course specifier for BD.[8,9,17-19] Colom and colleagues proposed a threshold of at least two-thirds of lifetime depressive epi-sodes for the definition of a DPP, while at least two-thirds of past episodes satisfy-ing the criteria for mania/hypomania would define an MPP.[18] Even though this last definition proposed by Colom et al. has been frequently adopted among researchers, a uniform operationalizing criteria for PP remains to be established.[12,17,20,21]

The International Society for Bipolar Disorders (ISBD) task force has proposed a nomenclature for course and outcomes for BD. This panel of experts has suggested the use of the concept of PP as a course specifier for BD.[22] In addition, the task force has recommended the adoption of the definition formerly proposed by Colom and colleagues for PP.[22] According to this ISBD task force, the PP of mood epi-sodes may be of critical importance for the long-term management of the disorder.[22] However, there is no currently taxonomic translation for this clinical definition in the *Diagnostic and Statistical Manual of Mental Disorders* (DSM) or *International Classification of Diseases* (ICD) diagnostic guidelines; additionally, mixed states

---

* Kraepelin E. *Manic-Depressive Insanity and Paranoia* (Edinburgh: Livingstone, 1921).

† Leonhard K. Die prapsychotische Temperamente bei den monopolaren und bipolaren pha-sischen Psychosen, Psychiat et Neurol (Basel) 1963;146:105–15.

remain to be encompassed in the current definition of BD.[22] To date, there is not enough evidence to support the inclusion of a predominantly mixed category.[22]

Available data indicate that slightly more than half of BD patients exhibit a specific PP, while a significant proportion of BD patients have an undetermined PP.[9,14,17] Between 45 and 70% of all patients with BD present criteria for PP, while 50–60% of this group has a DPP and 40% present an MPP.[9,14,18] Considering patients with BD as a whole, DPP would account for 25–35% of the cases.[9,18,20] The association between first-episode presentation (depressive versus manic) and subsequent polarity has also been observed, and PP may be a strong predictor of outcome based on this correlation[9,18,20,23] (see Table 15.1).

In a recent naturalistic study of 604 BD patients, 43% (257) of participants with BD I or II presented criteria for PP, being respectively 44.4% MPP (n = 114) and 55.6% DPP (n = 143).[24] The MPP was associated with a higher prevalence of BD I, male gender, younger age of illness onset and first hospitalization, more hospital admissions, a higher prevalence of co-morbid substance misuse, and with a history of psychotic features.[24] A DPP was related to BD II, a depressive onset of illness, stressors at first episode, melancholia, and suicide attempts.[24] In this study, PI was determined, and the net PI, antipsychotics' PI, and mood stabilizer's PI higher in patients with an MPP, indicating a more robust antimanic prophylactic action of the therapeutic regimen. Based on these findings, PP seems to be a predictor of treatment and outcomes, and PI may be taken into account to guide the choice of maintenance therapies for BD.[24] Similar findings have been reported in a different study involving two independent adult samples from France (n = 480) and the United States (US) (n = 714) during the period 1992–2006.[4] Polarity at onset was significantly associated with subsequently PP (P<0.001) in this study. The DPP was associated with a higher density of depressive episodes, suicidal behaviour, and alcohol misuse.[4] A cohort study that investigated 604 BD I and II patients for ten years has observed that women more commonly present DPP, higher prevalence of depressive episodes with psychotic features, and higher prevalence of co-morbid personality disorders.[10] A family history of suicide and lifetime history of suicidality were also more common in this population. In men, MPP occurred more frequently, and presented a more significant history of violent suicide attempts, and substance misuse—more specifically, alcohol and cocaine.[10]

A naturalistic sample of BD I (n = 120) was followed for up to ten years, and of the relationship between a history substance misuse and PP was investigated.[11] In this study, at baseline, DPP was more frequently associated with suicide attempts, family history of affective disorders, and fewer hospitalizations.[11] During the ten-year follow-up, this same group was associated with more mood episodes, higher number of psychiatric hospitalization, and more suicide attempts.[11] At baseline, substance misuse did not significantly differ between bipolar individuals with a either MPP or DPP, while after a ten-year follow-up the rates of substance misuse have decreased significantly only in the MPP type, suggesting that long-term outcomes could be different based on PP, with a DPP presenting worse clinical outcomes and prognosis.[11]

Table 15.1 Findings of PP regarding clinical characteristics and outcomes across different studies

Reference	Sample	Design	Main Findings
Vieta et al., 2009	833 type I BD participants; 788 had baseline and follow-up ratings; DSM-IV criteria	Multicentre RCT Olanzapine, OFC, and placebo	34.1% (n = 269) had a DPP and 12.4% (n = 98) had an MPP. Psychotic features were more common in the DPP. Rapid cycling was more common in the MPP (only in men). In men, an MPP was associated with a greater likelihood for acute treatment response.
Nivoli et al., 2013	604 BD participants (types I, II and NOS); DSM-IV; 332 (55%) females; 407 (67.4%) with type I BD and 201 (32.6%) with type II or type NOS BD; 314 (52.0%) with mood episode and psychotic features and 117 (19.4%) with rapid cycling; Spain	Observational	3 different treatment interventions: 'antimanic stabilization combination', 'antidepressant stabilization combination', and 'anti bipolar II package'. Antimanic stabilization combination was associated with an MPP, while the 'antidepressant stabilization combination' was associated with the DPP.
Popovic et al., 2013	604 type I or II BD participants; included 257 participants with a PP; DSM-IV-TR; Spain	Observational	44.4% (n = 114) had an MPP and 55.6% (n = 143) had a DPP. Polarity index of the therapeutic regimen was significantly higher for the MPP group. The MPP group had higher use of olanzapine, risperidone, and typical antipsychotics. The DPP group had higher use of lamotrigine, antidepressants TCAs, SSRIs, SNRIs, and benzodiazepines. Significantly younger age of onset, younger age at first hospitalization, and higher hospitalization rate were more common among MPP patients.

Notes: PP—predominant polarity; RCT—randomized clinical trial; OFC—olanzapine–fluoxetine combination; DPP—depressive predominant polarity; MPP—manic predominant polarity; TCAs—tricyclic antidepressants; SSRIs—selective serotonin reuptake inhibitors; SNRIs—selective norepinephrine reuptake inhibitors

The diagnostic implications of the predominant polarity have recently been studied in a sample involving 149 euthymic bipolar outpatients.[9] According to this data, patients presenting DPP used to experience longer delays on BD diagnosis, tended to show depressive episodes at first presentation of the illness, earlier age at onset, longer duration of illness, and higher number of suicide attempts when compared with MPP individuals.[9] Furthermore, in a sample of bipolar and unipolar individuals, it was observed that MPP and DPP were similar in scoring higher than unipolar subjects on the hyperthymic/cyclothymic scales of the Temperament Evaluation of the Memphis, Pisa, Paris, and San Diego Autoquestionnaire (TEMPS-A), whereas unipolar depression individuals scored higher on the anxious and depressive scales.[25] These findings, in accordance to previous data in the literature, also support importance of the concept of PP as a disease specifier, and demonstrate the different temperament characteristics of BD subjects.[25]

In a recent cross-sectional study of 278 BD individuals, bipolar patients with MPP have received more antipsychotics and lithium, and this same group presented more psychosis, rapid cycling, stressor precipitants at onset, family history of affective disorders, and a first episode of manic polarity relative to the DPP group.[26] In this study, DPP type was more commonly associated with chronic depression, anxiety co-morbidity, and a higher use of antidepressants, anticonvulsants, and benzodiazepines.[26] In addition, based on this data, temperament may also play a key role in the subtyping of BD patients according to PP, which is in agreement with the current literature; prospective studies are necessary to replicate this findings.[26]

According to the most recent guidelines for the management of patients with BD (Canadian Network for Mood and Anxiety Treatments (CANMAT) 2013), treatment of acute mania remains largely unchanged, being lithium, valproate, and several atypical antipsychotics still the first-line options. Asenapine, paliperidone extended release (ER), and divalproex ER monotherapy, as well as adjunctive asenapine, have been added as part of first-line for acute mania. For bipolar depression, lithium, lamotrigine, and quetiapine monotherapy remains the first-line management, as well as olanzapine in combination with a selective serotonin reuptake inhibitor (SSRI), lithium or divalproex plus SSRI/bupropion. Finally, lithium, lamotrigine, valproate, olanzapine, quetiapine, aripiprazole, risperidone long-acting injection (LAI), and adjunctive ziprasidone continue to be first-line options for maintenance management of BD.[27]

The PI represents the ratio of the NNT for the prevention of depression and the NNT for the prevention of mania. For instance, NNT is an effect-size measure, which can quantify the clinical relevance of a trial outcome. Some drugs, alone or in combination, are more efficacious for the prevention of depressive episodes, while others may be more efficacious for the prophylaxis of manic episodes. Based on this concept, an agent with a PI equal to 1 would have a balanced efficacy for both manic and depressive symptoms, while a PI < 1 would represent greater efficacy in the prevention of depressive episodes, whereas a PI > 1, would signal to more significant antimanic prophylactic effects. In this context, a predominantly antimanic PI (ie, PI > 1) was observed for aripiprazole monotherapy (PI = 12.1),[28] followed by risperidone LAI,[29,30] aripiprazole adjunctive to lithium or divalproex,[31,32] olanzapine monotherapy,[33] ziprasidone adjunctive to lithium or divalproex,[34] adjunctive risperidone LAI,[35] and lithium.[36–39] A PI showing stronger efficacy for the prevention of depressive episodes (ie, PI < 1) was observed for lamotrigine (pooled PI = 0.4),[37,38] followed by olanzapine combined with divalproex,[40] divalproex,[36] and oxcarbazepine combined with lithium.[41] Adjunctive quetiapine[42,43] and quetiapine monotherapy[39] had PIs closest to 1, suggesting a more balanced efficacy for the prevention of both manic and depressive episodes (see Table 15.2).

In a recent systematic review, it was observed that the PP and PI were also relevant for evidence-based maintenance psychological interventions for BD.[44] According

Table 15.2 Polarity index of different interventions

Reference	Intervention	NNT depression	NNT mania	Polarity index
Keck et al., 2007	Aripiprazole monotherapy	73.0	7.0	10.4
Abbar et al., 2011; Woo et al., 2011	Aripiprazole adjunctive to lithium/divalproex-pooled	38.0	9.0	4.2
Bowden et al., 2003; Calabrese et al., 2003	Lamotrigine-pooled	20.2	50.4	0.4
Bowden et al., 2003; Calabrese et al., 2003; Weisler et al., 2011; Bowden et al., 2000	Lithium-pooled	6.1	4.4	1.4
Tohen et al., 2006; Vieta et al., 2012	Olanzapine monotherapy-pooled	17.5	4.4	4.0
Tohen et al., 2004	Olanzapine combined with lithium/divalproex	6.2	11.2	0.5
Vieta et al., 2008	Oxcarbazepine combined with lithium	5.1	8.2	0.6
Weisler et al., 2011	Quetiapine monotherapy	3.3	2.4	1.4
Vieta et al., 2008; Suppes et al., 2009	Quetiapine combined with lithium/divalproex-pooled	5.9	7.1	0.8
Quiroz et al., 2010; Vieta et al., 2012	Risperidone LAI monotherapy-pooled	36.3	4.0	9.1
MacFadden et al., 2009	Adjunctive risperidone LAI	15.8	7.9	2.0
Bowden et al., 2000	Divalproex	10.5	21.3	0.5
Bowden et al., 2010	Ziprasidone Adjunctive to lithium/divalproex	55.1	14.1	3.9
Berwaerts et al., 2012	Paliperidone ER	*17.0*	8.0	N/A

Adapted from *International Journal of Neuropsychopharmacology*, 18, Carvalho A.F et al, 'Treatment implications of predominant polarity and the polarity index: a comprehensive review'. Copyright (2014) with permission from Oxford University Press.

to this study, most psychosocial interventions had a PI < 1, implying better efficacy for the prevention of depressive episodes, including cognitive behavioural therapy (PI ranging from 0.33 to 0.89), family-focused therapy (PI = 0.42), and psychoeducation (PI ranging from 0.73 to 0.78). Enhanced relapse prevention was equally effective for the prevention of depressive and manic episodes (PI = 1.0), whereas brief-technique driven interventions (PI = 3.36) and caregiver group psychoeducation (PI = 1.78) were more efficacious for the prevention of manic episodes.[44]

A post hoc analysis of a previous randomized controlled trial (RCT) comparing olanzapine–fluoxetine combination with either olanzapine alone or placebo for the treatment of bipolar I depression investigated the relationship of PP on treatment response.[45] Of the 833 participants initially enrolled in this trial, 788 subjects had both baseline and follow-up ratings to allow the determination of PP; of these patients, 367 out of 788 (46.6%) could be categorized as having had either DPP (269 out of 788; 34.1%) or MPP (98 out of 788; 12.4%).[45] Additionally, According to the primary outcome, change in the Clinical Global Impression of severity of depressive symptoms (CGI-D),[46] the effect of PP as a predictor was markedly dissimilar between men and women. In women, there were no significant differences in CGI-D scores in accordance with PP, whereas in men MPP type has a significantly better outcome when compared with the predominantly depressive group. Furthermore, MPP in men had better outcomes compared with women with both PP types.[14]

In a recent naturalistic study conducted on a sample of 604 DSM-IV-TR BD patients in Barcelona, different therapeutic regimens were considered: (i) an antimanic stabilization combination, which was characterized by the use of classic thymoleptic medications (ie, lithium, valproate, and carbamazepine), three atypical antipsychotics (clozapine, risperidone and olanzapine), and electroconvulsive therapy; (ii) an antidepressive stabilization combination, including lamotrigine and other atypical antipsychotic agents (notably quetiapine); and (iii) an 'anti-bipolar II package', including antidepressants. Bipolar patients with an MPP were treated mainly with the 'antimanic stabilization combination', whereas BD patients with a DPP were more frequently treated with the 'antidepressive stabilization combination'.[47] The anti-bipolar II package included mainly type-II BD patients with a DPP.[47]

A different sample of 604 DSM-IV-TR BD patients was recently assessed, with findings of 257 of patients presenting a clear PP type (n = 143/55.6% with DPP and n = 114/44.4% with MPP).[24] The total PIs—calculated as mean value of PI of all prescribed mood stabilizers and antipsychotics in each patient—were significantly higher in the predominantly manic group. In addition, the PI of antipsychotics and mood stabilizers taken separately were also higher in the MPP type. The use of antidepressants, lamotrigine and benzodiazepines was more prevalent in the DPP group of patients.[24]

To date, most psychosocial interventions applied in BD management have shown PI < 1, meaning better results for the prevention of depressive relapse, namely cognitive behavioural therapy (PI varying between 0.33 and 0.89), family-focused therapy (PI = 0.42), and psychoeducation (PI ranging from 0.73 to 0.78). Enhanced relapse prevention was equally effective for prevention of manic and depressive episodes (PI = 1.0), while brief-technique driven interventions (PI = 3.36) and caregiver group psychoeducation (PI = 1.78) were more efficacious for relapse preventions of mania.[44] Although several psychosocial interventions have been used as adjunctive practices for maintenance in the course of BD, the current evidence also indicates that adjunctive psychotherapy in the context of individualized long-term treatment of BD appears efficacious for preventing relapse in BD as well.[44]

Finally, it has been previously hypothesized that a lower D2 receptor binding affinity and occupancy would be more relevant than a greater 5-HT(2) receptor action regarding the efficacy of atypical antipsychotics for treatment of bipolar depression.[48] Based on these speculations, a recent study exploring the relationship of D2 receptor affinities[49] and the PI of atypical antipsychotics in monotherapy was conducted, and observed that the higher the D2 receptor binding affinity, the lower the PI of different atypical antipsychotics in monotherapy. In addition, aripiprazole did not seem to follow the same pattern of the other antipsychotics, showing a rather complex mechanism of action,[50] possibly acting either as an antagonist or as an agonist at distinct subpopulations of D2 receptors, a process referred to as functional selectivity.[50] These unique mechanisms may explain the divergent findings related to D2 binding affinity and the PI of this compound.

Limitations of available evidence

Recently, Popovic et al.[51] proposed the PI as a metric parameter for categorizing drug profiles in the relapse prevention of BD. Some limitations to this descriptor have been observed. For instance, PI values are not available for all drugs used in relapse prevention in the course of BD, and in case of polypharmacy, a value for each patient's treatment was calculated as a mean value of all prescribed drugs combined. Furthermore, PI does not reflect pharmacodynamics interactions in the case of polypharmacy. In addition, PIs of drugs used in maintenance treatment of BD were calculated based on current available RCT studies; since well-designed methodological studies are scarce, PI varies among different studies, limiting its applicability and reliability. Finally, mixed episodes have been increasingly emphasized in the current classification of acute episodes in BD, and the fact that PP and PI do not contemplate mixed episodes could also represent a limitation of this metric tool.[52-54]

To date, most studies in PP were performed by the Barcelona Bipolar Disorder Group, and a recent study was conducted in a German sample of 336 BD patients as an attempt to validate the PI.[55] In this study, no significant differences in total PI between DPP and MPP were observed.[55] Even though the PI could not be validated as a numeric expression of efficacy of maintenance treatment under naturalistic conditions, PP has been suggested by this German group as an important specifier for BD, especially regarding maintenance treatment and relapse prevention.[55] Furthermore, it has been taken under consideration that differences in results may be due to differences in prescription patterns between the two groups, as well as sociodemographic and clinical characteristics of the two samples. Limitations of the PI metric were also pointed as playing an important role in these negative findings.[55]

Conclusion

A growing body of evidence suggests that the concepts of PP and PI in BD may have useful applicability for therapeutic and prognostic purposes. As a disease specifier, PP may also aid in the selection of more homogeneous groups of patients for future RCTs for BD. In addition, the PP concept may aid in treatment selection for BD. There is a need to independently replicate existing findings in well-designed prospective studies.

References

1. Merikangas KR, Akiskal HS, Angst J, Greenberg PE, Hirschfeld RMA, Petukhova M, et al. Lifetime and 12-month prevalence of bipolar spectrum disorder in the National Comorbidity Survey replication, Arch Gen Psychiatry 2007 May;64(5):543–52.

2. Mathers CD, Iburg KM, and Begg S. Adjusting for dependent comorbidity in the calculation of healthy life expectancy, Popul Health Metr 2006 Jan;4:4.

3. Gitlin MJ, Swendsen J, Heller TL, and Hammen C. Relapse and impairment in bipolar disorder, Am J Psychiatry 1995 Nov;152(11):1635–40.

4. Etain B, Lajnef M, Bellivier F, Mathieu F, Raust A, Cochet B, et al. Clinical expression of bipolar disorder type I as a function of age and polarity at onset: convergent findings in samples from France and the United States, J Clin Psychiatry 2012;73(4).

5. Judd LL and Akiskal HS. The prevalence and disability of bipolar spectrum disorders in the US population: re-analysis of the ECA database taking into account subthreshold cases, J Affect Disord 2003;73(1–2):123–31.

6. Judd LL, Akiskal HS, Schettler PJ, Endicott J, Leon AC, Solomon DA, et al. Psychosocial disability in the course of bipolar I and II disorders: a prospective, comparative, longitudinal study, Arch Gen Psychiatry 2005;62(12):1322–30.

7. Judd LL, Schettler PJ, Akiskal HS, Maser J, Coryell W, Solomon D, et al. Long-term symptomatic status of bipolar I vs bipolar II disorders, *The International Journal of Neuropsychopharmacology/Official Scientific Journal of the Collegium Internationale Neuropsychopharmacologicum* (CINP) 2003.

8. Baldessarini RJ, Salvatore P, Khalsa HMK, Imaz-Etxeberria H, Gonzalez-Pinto A, and Tohen M. Episode cycles with increasing recurrences in first-episode bipolar-I disorder patients, J Affect Disord 2012;149–54.

9. Rosa AR, Andreazza AC, Kunz M, Gomes F, Santin A, Sanchez-Moreno J, et al. Predominant polarity in bipolar disorder: diagnostic implications, J Affect Disord 2008;107(1–3):45–51.

10. Nivoli AMA, Pacchiarotti I, Rosa AR, Popovic D, Murru A, Valenti M, et al. Gender differences in a cohort study of 604 bipolar patients: the role of predominant polarity, J Affect Disord 2011;133(3):443–9.

11. González-Pinto A, Alberich S, Barbeito S, Alonso M, Vieta E, Martínez-Arán A, et al. Different profile of substance abuse in relation to predominant polarity in bipolar disorder. The Vitoria long-term follow-up study, J Affect Disord 2010;124(3):250–5.

12. Carvalho AF, McIntyre RS, Dimelis D, Gonda X, Berk M, Nunes-Neto PR, et al. Predominant polarity as a course specifier for bipolar disorder: a systematic review, J Affect Disord 2014;56–64.

13. Baldessarini RJ, Undurraga J, Vázquez GH, Tondo L, Salvatore P, Ha K, et al. Predominant recurrence polarity among 928 adult international bipolar I disorder patients, Acta Psychiatr Scand 2012;**125**(4):293–302.

14. Vieta E, Berk M, Wang W, Colom F, Tohen M, and Baldessarini RJ. Predominant previous polarity as an outcome predictor in a controlled treatment trial for depression in bipolar I disorder patients, J Affect Disord 2009;**119**(1–3):22–7.

15. Popovic D, Reinares M, Goikolea JM, Bonnin CM, Gonzalez-Pinto A, and Vieta E. Polarity index of pharmacological agents used for maintenance treatment of bipolar disorder, Eur Neuropsychopharmacol [Internet] 2012;**22**(5):339–46.

16. Angst J. The course of affective disorders, *Psychopathology* 1986;**19**(Suppl 2):47–52.

17. Osher Y, Yaroslavsky Y, el-Rom R, and Belmaker RH. Predominant polarity of bipolar patients in Israel, World J Biol Psychiatry 2000;**1**(4):187–9.

18. Colom F, Vieta E, Daban C, Pacchiarotti I, and Sánchez-Moreno J. Clinical and therapeutic implications of predominant polarity in bipolar disorder, J Affect Disord 2006;**93**(1–3):13–17.

19. Colom F and Vieta E. The road to DSM-V. Bipolar disorder episode and course specifiers, *Psychopathology* 2009;**42**(4):209–18.

20. Daban C, Colom F, Sanchez-Moreno J, García-Amador M, and Vieta E. Clinical correlates of first-episode polarity in bipolar disorder, Compr Psychiatry 2006;**47**(6):433–7.

21. Baldessarini RJ, Salvatore P, Khalsa HMK, Gebre-Medhin P, Imaz H, González-Pinto A, et al. Morbidity in 303 first-episode bipolar I disorder patients, Bipolar Disord 2010;**12**(3):264–70.

22. Tohen M, Frank E, Bowden CL, Colom F, Ghaemi SN, Yatham LN, et al. The International Society for Bipolar Disorders (ISBD) Task Force report on the nomenclature of course and outcome in bipolar disorders, Bipolar Disord 2009;453–73.

23. Perlis RH, Delbello MP, Miyahara S, Wisniewski SR, Sachs GS, and Nierenberg AA. Revisiting depressive-prone bipolar disorder: Polarity of initial mood episode and disease course among bipolar I systematic treatment enhancement program for bipolar disorder participants, Biol Psychiatry 2005;549–53.

24. Popovic D, Torrent C, Goikolea JM, Cruz N, Sánchez-Moreno J, González-Pinto A, et al. Clinical implications of predominant polarity and the polarity index in bipolar disorder: a naturalistic study, Acta Psychiatr Scand 2014;**129**(5):366–74.

25. Mazzarini L, Pacchiarotti I, Colom F, Sani G, Kotzalidis GD, Rosa AR, et al. Predominant polarity and temperament in bipolar and unipolar affective disorders, J Affect Disord 2009;**119**(1–3):28–33.

26. Azorin JM and Adida M, and Belzeaux R. Predominant polarity in bipolar disorders: further evidence for the role of affective temperaments, J Affect Disord 2015;(182):57–63.

27. Yatham LN, Kennedy SH, Parikh SV, Schaffer A, Beaulieu S, Alda M, O'Donovan C, Macqueen G, McIntyre RS, Sharma V, Ravindran A, Young LT, Milev R, Bond DJ, Frey BN, Goldstein BI, Lafer B, Birmaher B, Ha K, and Nolen WA, Berk M. Canadian Network for Mood and Anxiety Treatments (CANMAT) and International Society for Bipolar Disorders (ISBD) collaborative update of CANMAT guidelines for the management of patients with bipolar disorder: update 2013, Bipolar Disord 2013;(15):1–44.

28. Keck PE, Calabrese JR, McIntyre RS, McQuade RD, Carson WH, Eudicone JM, et al. Aripiprazole monotherapy for maintenance therapy in bipolar I disorder: a 100-week, double-blind study versus placebo, J Clin Psychiatry 2007;**68**(10):1480–91.

29. Quiroz JA, Yatham LN, Palumbo JM, Karcher K, Kushner S, and Kusumakar V. Risperidone long-acting injectable monotherapy in the maintenance treatment of bipolar I disorder, Biol Psychiatry 2010;**68**(2):156–62.

30. Vieta E, Montgomery S, Sulaiman AH, Cordoba R, Huberlant B, Martinez L, et al. A randomized, double-blind, placebo-controlled trial to assess prevention of mood episodes with risperidone long-acting injectable in patients with bipolar I disorder, Eur Neuropsychopharmacol 2012;**22**(11):825–35.

31. Abbar M, Khan A, Rollin L, Sanchez R, Carson W, Morris B, et al. P01-186—Efficacy of adjunctive aripiprazole to lithium or valproate in the long-term treatment of mania in subjects with bipolar I disorder (CN138–189), *European Psychiatry* 2011;**186**.

32. Woo YS, Bahk WM, Chung MY, Kim DH, Yoon BH, Lee JH, et al. Aripiprazole plus divalproex for recently manic or mixed patients with bipolar I disorder: a 6-month, randomized, placebo-controlled, doubleblind maintenance trial, Hum Psychopharmacol 2011;**26**(8):543–53.

33. Tohen M, Calabrese JR, Sachs GS, Banov MD, Detke HC, Risser RC, et al. Randomized, placebo-controlled trial of olanzapine as maintenance therapy in patients with bipolar I disorder responding to acute treatment with olanzapine, Am J Psychiatry 2006;**163**(2):247–56.

34. Bowden CL, Vieta E, Ice KS, Schwartz JH, Wang PP, and Versavel M. Ziprasidone plus a mood stabilizer in subjects with bipolar I disorder: a 6-month, randomized, placebo-controlled, double-blind trial, J Clin Psychiatry 2010;**71**(2):130–7.

35. Macfadden W, Alphs L, Haskins JT, Turner N, Turkoz I, Bossie C, et al. A randomized, double-blind, placebo-controlled study of maintenance treatment with adjunctive risperidone long-acting therapy in patients with bipolar I disorder who relapse frequently, Bipolar Disord 2009;**11**(8):827–39.

36. Bowden CL, Calabrese JR, McElroy SL, Gyulai L, Wassef A, Petty F, et al. A randomized, placebo-controlled 12-month trial of divalproex and lithium in treatment of outpatients with bipolar I disorder. Divalproex Maintenance Study Group, Arch Gen Psychiatry 2000.

37. Bowden CL, Calabrese JR, Sachs G, Yatham LN, Asghar SA, Hompland M, et al. A placebo-controlled 18-month trial of lamotrigine and lithium maintenance treatment in recently manic or hypomanic patients with bipolar I disorder. [Erratum appears in Arch Gen Psychiatry 2004 Jul;61(7):680], Arch Gen Psychiatry 2003;**60**(4):392–400.

38. Calabrese JR, Bowden CL, Sachs G, Yatham LN, Behnke K, Mehtonen OP, et al. A placebo-controlled 18-month trial of lamotrigine and lithium maintenance treatment in recently depressed patients with bipolar I disorder, J Clin Psychiatry 2003;**64**(9):1013–24.

39. Weisler RH, Nolen WA, Neijber A, Hellqvist Å, and Paulsson B. Continuation of quetiapine versus switching to placebo or lithium for maintenance treatment of bipolar I disorder (Trial 144: A randomized controlled study), J Clin Psychiatry 2011;**72**(11):1452–64.

40. Tohen M, Vieta E, Goodwin GM, Sun B, Amsterdam JD, Banov M, et al. Olanzapine versus divalproex versus placebo in the treatment of mild to moderate mania: a randomized, 12-week, double-blind study, J Clin Psychiatry 2008;**69**(11):1776–89.

41. **Vieta E, Cruz N, García-Campayo J, de Arce R, Manuel Crespo J, Vallès V**, et al. A double-blind, randomized, placebo-controlled prophylaxis trial of oxcarbazepine as adjunctive treatment to lithium in the long-term treatment of bipolar I and II disorder, Int J Neuropsychopharmacol 2008;**11**(4):445–52.

42. **Vieta E, Suppes T, Eggens I, Persson I, Paulsson B**, and **Brecher M**. Efficacy and safety of quetiapine in combination with lithium or divalproex for maintenance of patients with bipolar I disorder (international trial 126), J Affect Disord 2008;**109**(3):251–63.

43. **Suppes T, Vieta E, Liu S, Brecher M**, and **Paulsson B**. Maintenance treatment for patients with bipolar I disorder: results from a North American study of quetiapine in combination with lithium or divalproex (trial 127), Am J Psychiatry 2009;**166**(4):476–88.

44. **Popovic D, Reinares M, Scott J, Nivoli A, Murru A, Pacchiarotti I**, et al. Polarity index of psychological interventions in maintenance treatment of bipolar disorder, *Psychotherapy and Psychosomatics* 2013;292–8.

45. **Tohen M, Vieta E, Calabrese J, Ketter TA, Sachs G, Bowden C**, et al. Efficacy of olanzapine and olanzapine-fluoxetine combination in the treatment of bipolar I depression, Arch Gen Psychiatry 2003.

46. **Spearing MK, Post RM, Leverich GS, Brandt D**, and **Nolen W**. Modification of the Clinical Global Impressions (CGI) scale for use in bipolar illness (BP): the CGI-BP, Psychiatry Res 1997;**73**(3):159–71.

47. **Alessandra NA, Colom F, Pacchiarotti I, Murru A, Scott J, Valentí M**, et al. Treatment strategies according to clinical features in a naturalistic cohort study of bipolar patients: A principal component analysis of lifetime pharmacological and biophysic treatment options, Eur Neuropsychopharmacol 2013;**23**(4):263–75.

48. **Brugue E** and **Vieta E**. Atypical antipsychotics in bipolar depression: neurobiological basis and clinical implications, Prog Neuropsychopharmacol Biol Psychiatry [Internet] 2007;**31**(1):275–82.

49. **Richtand NM, Welge JA, Logue AD, Keck Jr PE, Strakowski SM**, and **McNamara RK.**. Dopamine and serotonin receptor binding and antipsychotic efficacy, Sect Title Pharmacol 2007;**32**(8):1715–26.

50. **Mailman RB** and **Murthy V**. Third generation antipsychotic drugs: partial agonism or receptor functional selectivity?, Curr Pharm Des 2010;**16**(5):488–501.

51. **Popovic D, Reinares M, Goikolea JM, Bonnin CM, Gonzalez-Pinto A**, and **Vieta E**. Polarity index of pharmacological agents used for maintenance treatment of bipolar disorder, Eur Neuropsychopharmacol J Eur Coll Neuropsychopharmacol [Internet] 2011;**22**:9–11.

52. **Berk M, Dodd S**, and **Malhi GS**. 'Bipolar missed states': the diagnosis and clinical salience of bipolar mixed states, *Australian and New Zealand Journal of Psychiatry* 2005;215–21.

53. **Vieta E** and **Valentí M**. Mixed states in DSM-5: implications for clinical care, education, and research, J Affect Disord 2013;28–36.

54. **Castle DJ**. Bipolar mixed states: still mixed up?, Curr Opin Psychiatry [Internet] 2014;**27**(1):38–42.

55. **Volkert J, Zierhut KC, Schiele MA, Wenzel M, Kopf J**, and **Kittel-Schneider SRA**. Predominant polarity in bipolar disorder and validation of the polarity index in a German sample, BMC Psychiatry 2014;(14):332–8.

Chapter 16

The assessment and management of suicide risk in bipolar disorder

Zoltán Rihmer, Xénia Gonda, and Péter Döme

Introduction

The lifetime prevalence of bipolar spectrum disorders in the general population is ranges from 1.3 to 5.0%.[1,2,3,4,5] Individuals with bipolar disorder (BD) have a life expectancy approximately 9–14 years lower than the general population, while the standardized mortality ratio (SMR) for all-cause mortality for BD is around 2.[6,7,8] Surprisingly, leading causes of lost life years in BDs are rather natural (eg cardiovascular disorders, diabetes mellitus, COPD, influenza, or pneumonia) than unnatural (eg suicide and unintentional injuries).[2,3,4,6,7,8]

At the same time, it is worthy to note that the risk of suicidal behaviour attributable to BD is remarkably high. According to results from different studies, up to 4–19% of patients with BDs ultimately commit suicide, while 20–60% of them attempt suicide at least once in their lifetime.[5,9] Compared with the general population, the risk of dying by suicide (ie SMR for suicide) is about 10–30 times higher in patients with BD.[4,5,7,10] A recent *pooled analysis of studies* reported a suicide rate of 164/100,000/year for patients with BD (when weighted by number of exposure years; number of person years = 1,145,245) which was approximately tenfold higher than in the general population.[9] With few exceptions, available evidence suggests that the risk of death due to suicide attributable to BD is somewhat higher than the corresponding risk attributable to unipolar (major) depressive disorder.[4,9,10,11] Furthermore, since the index diagnosis may change during the long-term course of unipolar depression (MDD) to BD,[4] and in earlier studies bipolar II disorder was not considered a discrete diagnostic entity (thus, it is likely that several bipolar II patients in these studies were included in the MDD group) it seems plausible that the calculations from some previous studies on the difference between suicide risk in BD and MDD could be biased.[12] Suicide risk in BD seems not to differ significantly from the corresponding risk in schizophrenia.[9] A previous suicide attempt is the most powerful single predictor of future completed suicide, particularly in patients with major mood disorders, and current suicidal ideation is the major harbinger of suicidal behaviour.[2,3,13] According to results from several studies, suicide attempts and ideation are also more frequent in BD than in MDD.[3,11,14,15] 'Subthreshold bipolarity' is a debated, diversely defined, and relatively novel concept in psychiatry. The *Diagnostic and Statistical Manual of Mental Disorders* (5th edition) (DSM-5) allows to diagnose certain subthreshold forms of BD under the categories '*Short-duration hypomanic episodes (2–3 days) and major depressive episodes*' and '*Hypomanic episodes with insufficient symptoms and major depressive episodes*'.[16,17] The finding that patients with MDD and subthreshold hypomania (ie those who are suffering from a form of 'subthreshold bipolarity') have higher risk for suicide attempts and ideation than patients with MDD but without subthreshold hypomanic manifestations (ie 'pure' MDD) may also suggest that bipolarity—even at a subthreshold degree—may confer an additional risk of suicidality.[14]

It is important to emphasize that in BD (similarly to some other mental disorders, eg MDD, schizophrenia) the ratio of attempted and completed suicides is about 2–10-times lower than the general population; it is a possible explanation that individuals with BD usually employ suicide methods associated with higher lethality compared with the general population.[9,11,18]

The implementation of effective short- and long-term treatment strategies for BD markedly reduces the risk of suicidal behaviour.[3,4,19,20] Therefore, the early recognition of bipolarity among patients with mood disorders is a key step, which could prevent suicide in this population. In this chapter, we summarize clinically relevant risk and protective factors of suicide in BD. In addition, we briefly discuss the most effective strategies for the management of elevated suicide risk in BD.

Assessment of suicide risk in patients with bipolar disorder

Validated suicide risk assessment tools specifically for BD are currently unavailable for use in primary or specialized care. Notwithstanding the routine screening of risk factor for suicide has uncertain predictive power in BD, a thorough clinical assessment remains an essential step to estimate suicide risk in a given patient with BD.[13,21] The regular assessment of suicide risk is recommended during the long-term care of patients with BD, but it is especially important when a change in the overall clinical picture ensues. The clinical assessment of suicide risk should encompass a thorough examination of the mental state, especially regarding characteristics of the current mood episode. The investigation should also reveal the existence, duration, and intensity of suicidal ideation or plans, the methods intended to be used, access to means (eg guns) as well as the compliance to prescribed medications. In addition, it is essential to gain information about a history of suicidal behaviour (ie the number and degree of violence of previous suicide attempts). Whenever possible, the clinician should obtain the utmost relevant information from family members or friends and eventually from other collateral sources.[18,21] In this chapter, we discuss risk and protective factors for suicidal behaviour, which may aid in estimation of the overall risk of suicidal behaviour in BD.

Suicide risk factors related to the current major mood episode

Suicidal behaviour (completed suicide, suicide attempt) and suicidal ideation in bipolar patients occur mostly during severe pure or mixed major depressive episodes and less frequently in mania with mixed features, but very rare during euphoric mania, hypomania, and euthymia.[2,5,13,15,22,23] Thus, suicidal behaviour in patients with BD seems to be a state- and severity-dependent phenomenon. Compared with pure mania, depressive and mixed episodes carry 18–62 and 27–74 fold higher rates of suicide, respectively.[5,24] Findings from Angst et al.[4] are in line with this evidence (ie they found that SMR for suicide for 'preponderantly manic patients' was 4.7 while the corresponding figures were 10.6 for bipolar II and 13.6 for bipolar I patients). Furthermore, some authors speculate that—in addition to the fact that patients with BD more frequently use violent (ie, highly lethal) suicide methods—elevated suicide risk for BD (when compared with MDD) could also be related to the fact that patients with BD spend more time in depressive and mixed episodes than patients with MDD.[15] However, considering that the majority of patients with BD never commit (and up to 50% of them never attempt) suicide,[2,3] risk factors, other than BD itself, including but not limited to special clinical characteristics as well as personality, familial, and psychosocial risk and protective factors should also play a major contributory role[2,3,25] in suicidal behaviour.

The majority of risk factors for suicide in BD seem to be related to acute phases of the illness (mostly major depressive and mixed affective episodes), but several historical and personality-related factors may also serve as warning signs of high suicide risk. The clinical condition which is the most alarming for suicidal behaviour in BD is a history of recent suicide attempt and the severe (mostly melancholic) major depressive episode, frequently accompanied by hopelessness, guilt, few reasons for living, and marked suicidal ideation[2,3,13,15] as well as agitation and insomnia.[13,25,26] According to the results of Sánchez-Gistau et al.,[27] atypical features of the last depressive episode is significantly associated with a history of suicide attempts among patients with BD.

Recent evidence strongly suggests that a mixed depressive episode labelled as major depressive episode with mixed features in DSM-5 (major depression plus three or more co-occurring intra-depressive hypomanic symptoms; which condition is highly resemble the so-called 'agitated depression'), that is present up to 60% of bipolar I and II depressives,[22,25] substantially increases the risk of both attempted and committed suicide.[5,24] In addition, evidence indicates that mixed affective episodes may carry a higher suicide risk than 'pure' depressive ones,[5,13,14,15,22,23,25,26,28] while some studies have raised the possibility that a history of more mixed and/ or depressive affective episodes could also be associated with higher suicidality in patients with BD.[29,30] These results provide an explanation for the seldomly observed 'antidepressant-induced' suicidal behaviour ie antidepressant monotherapy (antidepressant therapy without concomitant administration of mood stabilizers or atypical antipsychotics), particularly in patients with bipolar spectrum disorders (including 'unipolar' depressives with mixed features) may worsen pre-existing depressive mixed states or generate *de novo* mixed conditions, aggravating the clinical picture and ultimately leading to self-destructive behaviour.[25,26] Therefore, after the commencement of antidepressant treatment the early recognition of symptoms such as agitation, anger, insomnia, and mixed states which may be the harbingers of the previously discussed 'treatment-emergent suicidality' may be essential for suicide prevention among patients with BD.[25,26,31] The role of mood instability in the pathogenesis of suicidal behaviour was also supported by a study, which found that a history of rapid mood switching and panic attacks was associated with an increased likelihood of self-reported suicidal thought or action in patients with BD.[13] However, suicidal behaviour in bipolar patients is not exclusively restricted to depressive and DSM-IV mixed episodes. In contrast to classical (euphoric) mania, where suicidal tendencies are extremely rare, suicidal thoughts and attempts are relatively common in patients with manic episode with mixed features[2,11] supporting the common clinical sense that suicidal behaviour even in BD is linked to depressive symptomatology.[4,11,13]

Although BD, in general, carries a high risk of suicide,[3,11] several studies have shown that bipolar II patients may have even a higher risk of suicide than individuals with BD I.[3,29,32] However, other studies have found that suicide risk does not seem to vary significantly as a function of a bipolar I versus bipolar II diagnosis,[2,4,5,11] while some studies have found the opposite pattern (ie, a higher suicide risk in BD I compared with BD II).[14] Thus, it remains unclear whether there is a difference between the risks of suicide in BD I and BD II.[24]

Bipolar spectrum disorders show a high frequency of psychiatric and medical co-morbidities[1] and it is well documented that co-morbid anxiety/anxiety disorders,[2,3,5,13,32] substance-use disorders,[2,3,5,32] personality—mainly borderline personality—disorders,[3,5,27] attention deficit hyperactivity disorder (ADHD),[33] eating disorders,[24] and serious medical illnesses,[2] particularly in the case of multiple co-morbidities, also increase the risk of all forms of suicidal behaviour. Therefore, a lack of medical and family support and an improper clinical monitoring of the first few days of therapy, when antidepressants usually do not work, or rarely may worsen the depression,[23,26,28] also could contribute to suicide risk.

In adults, the appearance of psychotic states at any time during the course of BD is not a clear risk factor for suicide attempt or death (however, some results suggest such an association in bipolar children).[4,24]

Suicide risk factors related to the prior course of the illness

In regard to suicide risk factors related to the prior course of BD, previous suicide attempt(s), particularly in the case of violent or more lethal methods, is the most powerful single predictor of future attempts and fatal suicide.[2,3,13,15] Bipolar patients in general[34] and bipolar II patients in particular[11] use more violent and more lethal suicide methods than patients with MDD and bipolar I patients, respectively; these associations seem more prominent in males. Therefore, higher rates of suicidal behaviour (mainly completed suicide) in patients with BD than in MDD may be due to a specific effect of BD on males, leading to more dangerous suicidal behaviours.[34]

Other historical variables, including but not limited to an earlier age of illness onset and an early stage of the BD[4,5,11,35] as well as a rapid cycling course, predominant depressive polarity, and multiple (ie great number of prior) admissions to in-patient care[2,4] have also been related to higher risks of both attempted and completed suicide. In accordance to the finding that early stages of the disease are associated with a further increase in suicide risk, a recent study demonstrated that the contribution of suicide to life years lost was highest in young age bands.[8]

A long time lag from initial affective symptoms until a proper diagnosis and/or treatment of BD were also found as risk factors for suicidal behaviour in both prospective and retrospective studies.[29,36]

Some results also indicated that the depressive polarity of the first affective episode (which is typical for bipolar II disorder) is also positively associated with suicidality in BD.[5] Furthermore, depressive polarity of the most recent episode also carries an additional risk of suicidal behaviour in patients with BD.[5]

It is well known that suicide risk is extremely high soon after hospital discharge in psychiatric patients in general, and in affective (including bipolar) disorders patients in particular.[23,37] According to results from Isometsä et al.,[23] the degree of post-discharge risk is highest for depressive episodes followed by mixed and then by manic episodes; at the same time post-discharge risk seem to decline with time more slowly for mixed than for depressive episodes. Other investigations have also revealed that among psychiatric (including bipolar) patients suicide risk is highly elevated during the period immediately after admission.[37]

Suicide risk factors related to personality features and gender

Personality features

Personality characteristics also play a significant role in the development and particularly in the manifestation of suicidal behaviour. The voluminous literature on this subject consistently shows that aggressive/impulsive personality traits[34,38] especially in combination with high level of current hopelessness and pessimism[15,38] markedly increases the risk of suicidal behaviour in patients with BD and other psychiatric disorders. It has also been reported that in bipolar I and II depressed patients the level of impulsivity and the rate of prior suicide attempts increased with increasing number of intra-depressive hypomanic symptoms supporting a relationship between the 'bipolar nature' of depression and impulsive behaviour.[12,39] Irritable mood (a core symptom of mania and hypomania) and anger attacks (inappropriate, sudden spells of anger associated with autonomic arousal and behavioural outbursts) are closely linked and anger attacks seem to be present more frequently in bipolar depression than in unipolar depression.[39] Furthermore, the occurrence of anger attacks during a current unipolar major depressive episode may indicate an underlying bipolarity, since intra-episode 'anger attacks' in a depressive episode are associated with important validating variables indicative of bipolarity (ie early onset of illness, atypical or mixed features of depressive episode, a family history for BD).[39]

Recent studies suggest that affective temperaments may play a role in suicidal behaviour. In contrast to hyperthymic temperament, which seems to be a protective factor against suicidal behaviour,[40,41,42,43] the cyclothymic, irritable, depressive, and anxious affective temperaments were significantly overrepresented in suicide attempters or in mood disorder inpatients with high suicidality.[41,42,43] A cyclothymic affective temperament is particularly indicative of suicidal behaviour on the top of a major mood episode. For example, in patients with a major depressive episode, a cyclothymic personality was significantly related to lifetime and current suicidal behaviour (ideation and attempts) both in adult and paediatric samples.[42,44,45] Compared with bipolar II patients without a cyclothymic temperament (n=120), bipolar II patients with this predominant temperament (n=74) reported more frequent lifetime suicide attempts and current hospitalizations due to suicide risk were also more common among them.[44] Other studies also have shown that bipolar I, bipolar II, and unipolar MDD patients with a cyclothymic temperament have significantly higher rates of prior suicide attempts and lifetime/current suicidal ideation than non-cyclotyhmic patients.[46,47] In addition, a cyclothymic temperament significantly predicted bipolarity and suicide attempts in adult[48,47] and juvenile depressives.[45] A large-scale French study has also found that a cyclothymic temperament was one of the eight risk factors (such as young age at onset, depressive or mixed polarity of the first episode, stressful life events, etc) to be significantly associated with lifetime suicide attempts in patients with bipolar I disorder.[49] A central role of cyclothymic oscillations of mood, thinking, and behaviour in the evolution of suicidal processes has been further supported by studies reporting that a history of rapid mood switching was associated with an increased likelihood of prior suicidal ideation or attempts,[50] and variability in suicidal ideation was a significantly better predictor of prior suicide attempts than duration and intensity of ideation.[51] However, it is worthy of note that the mentioned personality/temperamental characteristics, particularly in their more exuberant forms may become suicide risk factors in BD mainly in the presence of a major mood (mixed depressive or manic) episode. Lastly, most examined literature on a role of affective temperaments as risk factors for suicide in BD derive from cross-sectional studies. Thus, well-designed prospective studies are needed to establish solid causal inferences.

The interaction between personality features and illness characteristics in the emergence of suicidal behaviour is best formulated by Mann et al.[38] in their 'stress-diathesis model'. This model postulates that suicidal behaviour in psychiatric patients is determined not only by the stressor (acute major psychiatric illness), but also by a diathesis, which is in part embedded in one's personality attributes (eg impulsive, aggressive, pessimistic personality traits, and specific affective temperaments).

Gender

The vast majority of suicide victims in the general population are males (eg a male to female rate ratio ranging from 3.6 to 4 has been observed in Europe and the United States), whereas the opposite pattern holds true for suicide attempters.[13,26,52] These differences are smaller in magnitude for patients with BD where the male to female suicide rate ratio is only 1.7 to 1[2,4,5,7,9] suggesting that in individual cases gender is not a significant predictor for committed and attempted suicide in this otherwise high-risk population. Despite this finding, the aforementioned meta-analysis by Schaffer et al.[5] has identified female gender as a risk factor for suicide attempts and male gender as a risk factor for suicide deaths among individuals with BD. In addition, lesbian, gay, bisexual persons, as well as transgender individuals, are at significantly elevated risk of suicidal behaviour, particularly when BD and other significant risk factors for suicide are also present.[53]

Risk factors for suicide related to personal and family history

Several risk factors for suicide related to personal history include the following: (i) early negative life-events (eg, parental loss, isolation, emotional, physical and sexual abuse);[2,3,13,38] (ii) permanent adverse life situations, including unemployment, social isolation, unmarried or divorced status, and a single-parent status;[2,3,13,24] and (iii) acute psychosocial stressors (eg, loss events and financial disasters).[3,13,54] These factors are the most important and clinically useful indicators of possible suicidality, mainly if other risk factors also coexist. However, acute psychosocial stressors seems to be influenced by the victim's own behaviour, particularly in the case of bipolar I disorder.[54] For example, hypomanic or manic episodes frequently lead to aggressive–impulsive behaviour, financial extravagance, or promiscuity. These exuberant set of behaviours may generate several interpersonal conflicts (eg marital breakdown) and new negative life events, which may be related to a higher risk of suicidality in this population.

A family history of suicidal behaviour and/or major mood disorders among first- and second-degree relatives is also a strong risk factor for both attempted and completed suicide in psychiatric patients in general, and in patients with BD in particular.[2,3,5,13,27,38] However, the familial component of suicidal behaviour seems to be partly independent of psychiatric disorders per se. For example, relatives of suicide victims are more than ten times more likely than relatives of comparison subjects to attempt or complete suicide even after controlling for psychopathology.[55] Results of a recent longitudinal study also confirmed that suicidal behaviour among parents with mood disorders conveyed elevated odds for suicidal behaviour among their offspring even after controlling for some other risk factors for suicidality in the offspring.[56]

Box 16.1 summarizes risk factors for suicidality, which could be clinically explored in the context of BD. Suicidal behaviour among patients with BD seems very rare in the absence of major mood episodes. Therefore, suicide risk factors related to depressive episodes and/or mixed states are the most powerful predictors, particularly if other risk factors (and high-lethality suicide methods) are also present. Suicide risk factors are additive: the higher the number of risk factors the higher is the likelihood of suicidal behaviour.

Protective factors for suicide in bipolar disorder

In contrast to the aforementioned risk factors for suicide, only few factors are known to have a protective role against suicidal behaviour. A good family and social support, pregnancy and postpartum period, having a great number of children, holding strong religious beliefs, and restricting access to lethal suicide methods (eg, to reduce domestic and car exhaust gas toxicity and to introduce stricter laws on gun control) whenever possible, seem to have some protective

Box 16.1 Clinically detectable suicide risk factors in bipolar disorders

1. Risk factors related to acute mood episodes

a/Severe major depressive episode

- Current suicide attempt, plan, ideation
- Hopelessness, guilt, few reasons for living
- Agitation, depressive mixed state (DSM-5 major depressive episode with mixed features), insomnia
- Atypical (and perhaps psychotic) features
- Co-morbid Axis I (especially anxiety, eating and substance use disorders and ADHD), Axis II (especially borderline personality disorder) and serious Axis III disorders
- Lack of medical treatment and family/social support
- First few days of the treatment (particularly if appropriate care and co-medication is lacking)
- First few weeks (months) after hospital discharge (especially if hospital admission was due to a depressive or a mixed episode)
- The period immediately after the hospital admission
- (Antidepressant treatment without the use of a concomitant agent with mood-stabilizer property)?

b/Manic or hypomanic episode with mixed features (DSM-5)

2. Risk factors related to prior course of the illness

- Previous suicide attempt/ideation (particularly the violent/highly lethal methods)
- Early onset/early stage of the illness
- Rapid cycling course
- Depressive polarity of the first and/or the most recent episode; predominantly depressive polarity during the prior course
- High number of previous admissions to inpatient care
- Delay in proper diagnosis and/or treatment; lack of treatment

3. Risk factors related to personality features

- Aggressive/impulsive personality traits
- Cyclothymic, irritable, depressive temperament
- Same-sex orientation, bisexuality

4. Risk factors related to personal history

- ◆ Early negative life events (separation, emotional, physical and sexual abuse)
- ◆ Permanent adverse life situations (unemployment, isolation)
- ◆ Acute psychosocial stressors (loss events, financial catastrophe)

5. Risk factors related to family history

- ◆ Family history of mood disorders (first- and second-degree relatives)
- ◆ Family history of suicide and/or suicide attempt (first- and second-degree relatives)

effect.[3] However, the most extensively studied suicide protective factor in major mood disorders has been the acute and long-term pharmacological treatment.[3,4,19,20,13,26]

As suicide is a relatively rare event in the community, it is highly frequent among patients with BD. Most individuals with BD come into contact with different levels of healthcare system some weeks or months before their death.[3,13,19] Thus, healthcare workers may have a primary role in suicide prevention in BD. Unfortunately, less than one-third of bipolar suicide victims and suicide attempters were receiving appropriate pharmacotherapy at the time of the suicide event.[32] Approximately two-thirds of suicide victims die after their first attempt.[13] Thus, the risk of suicide in patients with BD is considerably high even if the patient had never attempted suicide before. A careful examination of all suicide risk and protective factors (see Box 16.1) may aid in the early detection of suicide risk—ideally even before the first suicidal act—and intervene ahead of a patient's first suicide act.

Suicide prevention in bipolar disorder

Several open clinical studies, randomized controlled trials, and meta-analytic reviews consistently have found that long-term treatment with *lithium* markedly reduces the risk of attempted and completed suicide in patients with major mood disorders, including BD I and BD II.[3,4,20,26,31,57,58,59,60] It has also been demonstrated that the discontinuation of lithium treatment in patients with BD leads to an elevated risk of suicidal behaviour in the first year after the discontinuation.[61] This strong antisuicidal effect of lithium seems to be more than the simple result of its episode-prophylactic effect, as it has been reported that during long-term lithium prophylaxis of recurrent bipolar or unipolar affective disorder patients with at least one prior suicide attempt, a significant reduction in the number of suicide attempts was found not only in the excellent responders, but also in moderate responders, and even poor responders.[31] The clinical message of this finding is that in the case of lithium non-response, when the patient has one or more suicide risk factors, instead of switching lithium to another mood stabilizer, the clinician should retain lithium (even on a lower dose) and combine it with other mood stabilizers. The marked antisuicidal effect of lithium in major mood disorders has been further supported in recent years from an epidemiological perspective. Several surveys from different countries have found consistent inverse associations between lithium levels in drinking water and suicide rates.[62] Notwithstanding the acknowledged effect of long-term lithium treatment on suicide prevention, it remains unexplored how fast this antisuicidal effect may appear. Recently, the protocol for a randomized placebo-controlled study was announced aiming to investigate this question during the treatment of depressive episodes with suicidal thoughts/behaviour among patients with MDD or BD.[60] Interestingly, lithium treatment is also associated with reduced all-cause mortality in mood disorders in general and in BD in particular.[59]

The role of *anticonvulsant-type mood stabilizers* in suicide prevention is somewhat contradictory. In 2008, the Food and Drug Administration (FDA) reported an increased risk of suicidality in a non-homogenous group of patients (subjects with 20 different diseases/indications were included in the analysis) under antiepileptic treatment (11 different antiepileptic agents were included). At the same time, the three most commonly used anticonvulsant-type mood stabilizers (divalproex, carbamazepine, and lamotrigine) do not seem to increase suicide risk in BD. Possibly, *divalproex* has rather some suicide preventing effects in the long-term treatment of BD, but this is less supported than antisuicidal effects of lithium.[31,63] A very recent study of 826 patients with BD with an average 3.5 years of follow-up from Finland provided some support for this contention. This study found that treatment with valproic acid was associated with a trend to decreased risk of completed suicide (HR=0.5; p=0.06). On the contrary, however, valproate treatment was associated with elevated risks of suicide attempts in a significant manner.[59] A recently published large-scale study among predominantly male veterans found that the antisuicidal effects of valproic acid were similar to those of lithium in the first year of the treatment.[64] Results of another study also supported that valproic acid is similar to lithium regarding its suicide preventing effects during a 2.5-year follow-up of suicide attempters with BD.[65] Whether anticonvulsants other than valproic acid/divalproex decrease the risk of suicidal behaviour in BD remains unclear.[31,66] However, results of a study by Søndergård et al. tend to support the possibility that all 'classic' mood stabilizers have antisuicidal effects. In this study, authors have investigated the association between continued treatment with mood stabilizers and suicide among all patients discharged from psychiatry hospitals in Denmark as an in- or outpatient between 1995 and 2000 with an *International Classification of Diseases* (10th revision) (ICD-10) diagnosis of BD (n=5,926). The results showed that patients with ≥ 5 prescriptions of mood stabilizers (lithium, divalproex, lamotrigine, oxcarbazepine) had a significantly decreased rate of suicide compared with those patients with a single prescription. In addition, their results provided further evidence that lithium may have superiority in preventing suicide over anticonvulsant mood stabilizers.[57]

A growing body of evidence indicates that *antidepressant (mono)therapy* may worsen the clinical picture as well as the long-term course and outcome of BD. *Antidepressant* (mono)therapy in threshold and subthreshold bipolar depressives—who typically have an early age of illness onset—may lead to antidepressant resistance. In addition, antidepressant monotherapy in these populations may have deleterious consequences in the course of a depressive episode, particularly in adolescents and young adults, not only by inducing (hypo)manic switches, but also leading to a depressive mixed state/agitation, often referred to as 'activation syndrome', which may be a substrate for suicidal behaviour.[19,20,26,28,59] Yerevanian and Choi also concluded in their review that evidence suggests that antidepressant treatment is associated with increased rather than decreased risk of suicidal behaviour in BD.[31] On the contrary, only a few reports (eg ref 67) suggest that antidepressant therapy may be rather protective patients with BD from suicidality. At the same time, the recent task force report of the International Society for Bipolar Disorders (ISBD) also concluded that the evidence of an association of either decreased or increased risk of suicidal behaviour with antidepressant medication in bipolar patients remains inconclusive.[68] However, clinicians may consider to administrate (preferably not dual-action) antidepressants to patients with BD under selected circumstances. Accordingly, antidepressant treatment is recommended for patients with BD: (i) only as an adjuvant therapy (ie concomitant with the administration of agents with mood stabilizing effects); (ii) only for the treatment of a pure depressive episode (ie a depressive episode without agitation and/or other symptoms of mania); (iii) who had previous positive response to antidepressant treatment; and (iv) only for a short period of time. On the other hand, even this adjuvant antidepressant therapy should be avoided: (i) in bipolar patients with a history of rapid cycling; (ii) when previous episodes were predominantly mixed; and (iii) in patients with a previous history of treatment-emerging affective switches. In addition, patients with BD should be closely monitored for emerging signs of (hypo)mania and agitation, in which cases, antidepressant treatment should be suspended.[31,68] At least two studies have demonstrated that the combination of an antidepressant with a mood stabilizer carries a lower risk of suicidal behaviour than antidepressant monotherapy.[31]

In recent years, second-generation (atypical) *antipsychotics* (SGAs) have become ever-increasingly used for the treatment of different mood episodes, and also as maintenance treatments in BD. At the same time, the effects of SGAs on suicidality associated with BD remains more or less unexplored (ie no randomized controlled studies have investigated this issue). It seems that monotherapy with first-generation antipsychotics (FGAs) is associated with a higher risk of suicidality than treatment with second-generation agents (however, this difference dissipated when antipsychotics were used with an adjuvant mood stabilizer). The same study did not find any differences between risperidone, olanzapine, and quetiapine in rates of suicide attempts.[9,20,31,59] SGA or FGA monotherapy seems to be associated with higher risk of suicidality than mood-stabilizer monotherapy or—according to one study—than no therapy.[9,31,69] The combination of antipsychotics with mood stabilizers markedly reduces (but does not eliminate) the elevated risk of suicide seen in patients on antipsychotic monotherapy.[20,69] In spite of limited data, clozapine (with FDA recommendation to reduce repeated suicidality in schizophrenia and schizoaffective disorder) may have protective effects against suicide in BD as well.[9, 31,70]

In conclusion, the ideal long-term pharmacological treatment of BD regarding suicide prevention is mood-stabilizer (preferably lithium) monotherapy. The add-on use of antidepressants or antipsychotics to treat breakthrough depression or mania during the long-term treatment with mood stabilizers should carefully weight for potential risks.[20]

However, it is worthy to note that the antisuicidal effects of long-term treatment with mood stabilizers among patients with BD, although clinically significant,[3,4,20,26,68] is still incomplete. Therefore, the development of novel treatment strategies is a necessary step. As discussed previously, suicidal behaviour is mainly associated with those mood episodes in BD that containing a depressive component. Accordingly, rapid-acting antidepressant agents may promptly mitigate suicidality (eg in emergency settings). In the last decade, several studies were conducted with ketamine, an NMDA receptor antagonist. Promising evidence suggests that a single infusion of ketamine in a subanaesthetic dose may induce a very rapid onset (within approximately 40 minutes) of antidepressive and antisuicidal effects, which typically lasts approximately 3–7 days. Antidepressive and antisuicidal effects were observable in both patients with unipolar or bipolar depression (the danger of manic switch in patients with bipolar depression due to the use of single ketamine infusion with adjuvant mood stabilizer seems to be low). Preliminary evidence suggests that the effect of ketamine on suicidal ideation may be independent of its effect on anxiety and depression.[71,72] It should be emphasized that the effects of ketamine were only investigated regarding suicidal ideation so far, but not regarding suicide attempts and completed suicide.[72] Another mainly unaddressed issue is the prolongation of ketamine's effect over a clinically meaningful period with repeated administration or with the concomitant use of other agents (eg d-cycloserine). The long-term efficacy and safety (regarding, for instance, side effects and addictive potential) of single or repeated ketamine infusions remain largely unknown. Thus, the wide application of ketamine in everyday clinical practice requires additional evidence.[73] In addition, some findings suggest that the use of ketamine for the treatment of psychiatric disorders other than mood disorders (eg in obsessive–compulsive disorder) may be associated with an increase of suicidal ideation, anxiety, and dysphoria. Thus, depressed patients should be investigated for co-morbid psychiatric disorders before the initiation of ketamine treatment.[71] Bearing in mind the potential psychotomimetic side effects of ketamine, other NMDA antagonists have been tested as rapid antisuicidal/antidepressive agents (in an attempt to circumvent ketamine's psychotomimetic effects). Some of these molecules have shown promising rapid antidepressant effects (AZD6765), while others seem devoid of meaningful antidepressant activity (eg memantine).[71,72,74] Similarly to ketamine, nitrous oxide (N_2O; a widely used anaesthetic gas with NMDA receptor antagonist properties but also acting on GABAergic and opioid systems) has shown preliminary but promising rapid-acting antidepressant (which also decreases suicidality) as well.[75] Some agents with primary effects other than NMDA receptor modulation are also under active investigation for rapid antidepressant effects. For instance, scopolamine, a non-selective muscarinic acetylcholine receptor antagonist, with indirect effects on several other neurotransmitter systems (including the NMDA system), seems to be an effective and rapid-acting antidepressant in both recurring MDD and BD. Preliminary results also indicate that scopolamine treatment has antisuicide effects.[71]

Although the efficacy of electroconvulsive therapy (ECT) is well known for the treatment of major mood episodes in BD (ie, depression, mixed episodes, mania), bipolar depression is by far the most common and important indication of ECT in BD. The efficacy of ECT seems similar for unipolar and bipolar depression. From the viewpoint of suicide prevention, since its rapid speed of response ECT is a valuable treatment modality in bipolar patients who are in a severe depressed or in a mixed state.[76,77]

Recently, several effective unspecific ('psychological support', psychoeducation) and specific (cognitive-behavioural therapy, interpersonal and social rhythm therapy, etc) *psychosocial interventions* were developed (or adapted) for the treatment of BD.[3,21,78] These interventions were largely designed for the prevention of relapse/recurrences in BD. However, these psychosocial interventions may be effective for suicide prevention as well. However, up to now there is a dearth of studies which investigated the effect of psychosocial interventions on suicidality in patients with BD.[9,21,79] We identified only two studies with this specific aim; both studies have provided encouraging results.[78,80]

Conclusion

BD is intrinsically associated with an increased risk for suicidality. Therefore, during the long-term treatment of this disorder, clinicians should regularly monitor their bipolar patients for the emergence of suicidal ideation and/or behaviour. This is a crucial step for a rapid and prompt intervention.

The management of suicidality in the context of BD remains a clinical challenge. The long-term treatment with mood stabilizers (preferably lithium) should be prioritized. In addition, the use of antidepressant monotherapy should be avoided by all means (while the use of antidepressants combined with mood stabilizers under certain circumstances may be the subject of careful consideration). Along with pharmaco- and psychotherapeutical approaches for patients with highly elevated suicide risk, the implementation of some practical actions (eg eliminate access to obvious means for suicide; admission to hospital if community-based ongoing monitoring is not available; addressing current use of alcohol and drugs; etc) should also be considered as part of a more comprehensive treatment plan.[21]

References

1. **Rihmer Z** and **Angst J**. Mood disorders—Epidemiology. In: **BJ Sadock, VA Sadock,** and **P Ruiz** (eds): *Kaplan and Sadock's Comprehensive Textbook of Psychiatry, 9th edn* (Philadelphia, PA: Lippincott Williams and Wilkins, 2009), 1645–53.
2. **Hawton K, Sutton** L, **Haw** C, **Sinclair J,** and **Harris** L. Suicide and attempted suicide in bipolar disorder: a systematic review of risk factors, J Clin Psychiatry 2005;**66**:693–704.

3. **Rihmer Z.** Prediction and prevention of suicide in bipolar disorder, Clin Neuropsychiatry 2005;2:48–54.

4. **Angst J, Angst F, Gerber-Werder R,** and **Gamma A.** Suicide in 406 mood-disorder patients with and without long-term medication: a 40 to 44 years' follow-up, Arch Suic Res 2005;9:279–300.

5. **Schaffer A, Isometsä ET, Tondo L, Moreno DH, Turecki G, Reis C, Cassidy F, Sinyor M, Azorin JM, Kessing LV, Ha K, Goldstein T, Weizman A, Beautrais A, Chou YH, Diazgranados N, Levitt AJ, Zarate CA Jr, Rihmer Z,** and **Yatham LN.** International Society for Bipolar Disorders Task Force on Suicide: meta-analyses and meta-regression of correlates of suicide attempts and suicide deaths in bipolar disorder, Bipolar Disord 2015;17:1–16.

6. **Crump C, Sundquist K, Winkleby MA,** and **Sundquist J.** Comorbidities and mortality in bipolar disorder: a Swedish national cohort study, JAMA Psychiatry 2013;70:931–9.

7. **Hayes JF, Miles J, Walters K, King M,** and **Osborn DP.** A systematic review and meta-analysis of premature mortality in bipolar affective disorder, Acta Psychiatr Scand 2015;131:417–25.

8. **Kessing LV, Vradi E, McIntyre RS,** and **Andersen PK.** Causes of decreased life expectancy over the life span in bipolar disorder, J Affect Disord 2015;180:142–7.

9. **Schaffer A, Isometsä ET, Tondo L, Moreno DH, Sinyor M, Kessing LV, Turecki G, Weizman A, Azorin JM, Ha K, Reis C, Cassidy F, Goldstein T, Rihmer Z, Beautrais A, Chou YH, Diazgranados N, Levitt AJ, Zarate CA Jr,** and **Yatham L.** Epidemiology, neurobiology and pharmacological interventions related to suicide deaths and suicide attempts in bipolar disorder: Part I of a report of the International Society for Bipolar Disorders Task Force on Suicide in Bipolar Disorder, Aust NZJ Psychiatry 2015a.

10. **Chesney E, Goodwin GM,** and **Fazel S.** Risks of all-cause and suicide mortality in mental disorders: a meta-review, World Psychiatry 2014;13:153–60.

11. **Tondo L, Lepri B,** and **Baldessarini R.** Suicidal risk among 2,826 Sardinian major affective disorder patients, Acta Psychiatr Scand 2007;116:419–28.

12. **Rihmer Z.** Suicide and bipolar disorder. In: **Zarate CA** and **Manji HK** (eds), *Bipolar Depression: Molecular Neurobiology, Clinical Diagnosis and Pharmacotherapy* (Basel/Boston/Berlin: Birkhäuser Verlag AG, 2009).

13. **Rihmer Z.** Suicide risk in mood disorders, Curr Opin Psychiatry 2007;20:17–22.

14. **Angst J, Cui L, Swendsen J, Rothen S, Cravchik A, Kessler RC,** and **Merikangas KR.** Major depressive disorder with subthreshold bipolarity in the National Comorbidity Survey Replication, Am J Psychiatry 2010;167:1194–201.

15. **Holma KM, Haukka J, Suominen K, Valtonen HM, Mantere O, Melartin TK, Sokero TP, Oquendo MA,** and **Isometsä ET.** Differences in incidence of suicide attempts between bipolar I and II disorders and major depressive disorder, Bipolar Disord 2014;16:652–61.

16. **Mitchell PB.** Bipolar disorder: the shift to overdiagnosis, Can J Psychiatry 2012;57:659–65.

17. **American Psychiatric Association.** *Diagnostic and Statistical Manual of Mental Disorders, 5th Edn* (DSM-5) (Washington, DC: American Psychiatric Association, 2013).

18. **Pompili M, Rihmer Z, Innamorati M, Lester D, Girardi P,** and **Tatarelli R.** Assessment and treatment of suicide risk in bipolar disorders, Expert Rev Neurother 2009;9:109–36.

19. **Rihmer Z.** Pharmacological prevention of suicide in bipolar patients—a realizable target (editorial), J Affect Disord 2007;103:1–3.

20. **Rihmer Z** and **Gonda X**. Pharmacological prevention of suicide in patients with major mood disorders, Neurosci Biobehav Rev 2013;37:2398–403.

21. **Saunders KE** and **Hawton K**. Clinical assessment and crisis intervention for the suicidal bipolar disorder patient, Bipolar Disord 2013;15:575–83.

22. **Judd LL, Schettler PJ, Akiskal H, Coryell W, Fawcett J, Fiedorowicz JG, Solomon DA,** and **Keller MB**. Prevalence and clinical significance of subsyndromal manic symptoms, including irritability and psychomotor agitation, during bipolar major depressive episodes, J Affect Disord 2012;138:440–8.

23. **Isometsä E, Sund R,** and **Pirkola S**. Post-discharge suicides of inpatients with bipolar disorder in Finland, Bipolar Disord 2014;16:867–74.

24. **Schaffer A, Isometsä ET, Azorin JM, Cassidy F, Goldstein T, Rihmer Z, Sinyor M, Tondo L, Moreno DH, Turecki G, Reis C, Kessing LV, Ha K, Weizman A, Beautrais A, Chou YH, Diazgranados N, Levitt AJ, Zarate CA Jr,** and **Yatham L**. A review of factors associated with greater likelihood of suicide attempts and suicide deaths in bipolar disorder: Part II of a report of the International Society for Bipolar Disorders Task Force on Suicide in Bipolar Disorder, Aust NZJ Psychiatry 2015b.

25. **Akiskal HS, Benazzi F, Perugi G,** and **Rihmer Z**. Agitated 'unipolar' depression re-conceptualized as a depressive mixed state: implications for the antidepressant-suicide controversy, J Affect Disord 2005;85:245–58.

26. **Rihmer Z** and **Akiskal HS**. Do antidepressants t(h)reat(en) depressives? Toward a clinically judicious formulation of the antidepressant-suicidality FDA advisory in light of declining national suicide statistics from many countries, J Affect Disord 2006;94:3–13.

27. **Sánchez-Gistau V, Colom F, Mané A, Romero S, Sugranyes G,** and **Vieta E**. Atypical depression is associated with suicide attempt in bipolar disorder, Acta Psychiatr Scand 2009;120:30–6.

28. **Takeshima M** and **Oka T**. Association between the so-called 'activation syndrome' and bipolar II disorder, a related disorder, and bipolar suggestive features in outpatients with depression, J Affect Disord 2013;151:196–202.

29. **Undurraga J, Baldessarini RJ, Valenti M, Pacchiarotti I,** and **Vieta E**. Suicidal risk factors in bipolar I and II disorder patients, J Clin Psychiatry 2012;73:778–82.

30. **Tidemalm D, Haglund A, Karanti A, Landén M,** and **Runeson B**. Attempted suicide in bipolar disorder: risk factors in a cohort of 6,086 patients, PLoS One 2014;9:e94097.

31. **Yerevanian BI** and **Choi YM**. Impact of psychotropic drugs on suicide and suicidal behaviors, Bipolar Disord 2013;15:594–621.

32. **Balázs J, Lecrubier Y, Csiszér N, Koszták J,** and **Bitter I**. Prevalence and comorbidity of affective disorders in persons making suicide attempts in Hungary: importance of the first episode and of bipolar II diagnosis, J Affect Disord 2003;76:113–19.

33. **Lan WH, Bai YM, Hsu JW, Huang KL, Su TP, Li CT, Yang AC, Lin WC, Chang WH, Chen TJ, Tsai SJ,** and **Chen MH**. Comorbidity of ADHD and suicide attempts among adolescents and young adults with bipolar disorder: a nationwide longitudinal study, J Affect Disord 2015;176:171–5.

34. **Zalsman G, Braun M, Arendt M, Grunebaum MF, Sher L, Burke AK, Brent D, Chaudhury SR, Mann JJ,** and **Oquendo MA**. A comparison of the medical lethality of suicide attempts in bipolar and major depressive disorder, Bipolar Disord 2006;8:558–65.

35. **Pompili M, Gonda X, Serafini G, Innamorati M, Sher L, Amore M, Rihmer Z,** and **Girardi P**. Epidemiology of suicide in bipolar disorders: a systematic review of the literature, Bipolar Disord 2013;15:457–90.

36. Altamura AC, Dell'Osso B, Berlin HA, Buoli M, Bassetti R, and Mundo E. Duration of untreated illness and suicide in bipolar disorder: a naturalistic study, Eur Arch Psychiatry Clin Neurosci 2010;**260**:385–91.

37. Hawton K and van Heeringen K. Suicide, Lancet 2009;**373**:1372–81.

38. Mann JJ, Waternaux C, Haas GL, and Malone KM. Toward a clinical model of suicidal behavior in psychiatric patients, Am J Psychiatry 1999;**156**:181–9.

39. Benazzi F. Major depressive disorder with anger: A bipolar spectrum disorder?, Psychother Psychosom 2003;**72**:300–6.

40. Vázquez GH, Gonda X, Zaratiegui R, Lorenzo LS, Akiskal K, and Akiskal HS. Hyperthymic temperament may protect against suicidal ideation, J Affect Disord 2010;**127**:38–42.

41. Pompili M, Rihmer Z, Akiskal HS, Innamorati M, Iliceto P, Akiskal KK, Lester D, Narciso V, Ferracuti S, Tatarelli R, De Pisa E, and Girardi P. Temperament and personality dimensions in suicidal and nonsuicidal psychiatric inpatients, Psychopathology 2008;**41**:313–21.

42. Pompili M, Innamorati M, Rihmer Z, Gonda X, Serafini G, Akiskal H, Amore M, Niolu C, Sher L, Tatarelli R, Perugi G, and Girardi P. Cyclothymic-depressive-anxious temperament pattern is related to suicide risk in 346 patients with major mood disorders, J Affect Disord 2012;**136**:405–11.

43. Rihmer A, Rozsa S, Rihmer Z, Gonda X, Akiskal KK, and Akiskal HS. Affective temperaments, as measured by TEMPS-A, among nonviolent suicide attempters, J Affect Disord 2009;**116**:18–22.

44. Akiskal HS, Hantouche EG, and Allilare JF. Bipolar II with and without cyclothymic temperament: 'Dark' and 'sunny' expressions of soft bipolarity, J Affect Disord 2003;**73**: 49–57.

45. Kochman FJ, Hantouche EG, Ferrari P, Lancrenon S, Bayart D, and Aksikal HS. Cyclothymic temperament as a prospective predictor of bipolarity and suicidality in children and adolescents with major depressive disorder, J Affect Disord 2005;**85**:181–9.

46. Young LT, Cooke RG, Robb JC, and Joffe RT. 'Double bipolar disorder': a separate entity?, Depression 1994/1995;**2**:223–5.

47. Mechri A, Kerkeni N, Touati I, Bacha M, and Gassab L. Association between cyclothymic temperament and clinical predictors of bipolarity in recurrent depressive patients, J Affect Disord 2011;**132**:285–8.

48. Goto S, Terao T, Hoaki N, and Wang Y. Cyclothymic and hyperthymic temperaments may predict bipolarity in major depressive disorder: a supportive evidence for bipolar III1/2 and IV, J Affect Disord 2011;**129**:34–8.

49. Azorin JM, Kaladjian A, Adida M, Hantouche E, Hameg A, Lancrenon S, and Akiskal HS. Risk factors associated with lifetime suicide attempts in bipolar I patients: findings from a French National Cohort, Compr Psychiatry 2009;**50**:115–20.

50. MacKinnon DF, Potash JB, McMahon FJ, Simpson SG, Depaulo JR Jr, and Zandi PP; National Institutes of Mental Health Bipolar Disorder Genetics Initiative. Rapid mood switching and suicidality in familial bipolar disorder, Bipolar Disord 2005;**7**:441–8.

51. Witte TK, Fitzpatrick KK, Joiner TE Jr, and Schmidt NB. Variability in suicidal ideation: a better predictor of suicide attempts than intensity or duration of ideation?, J Affect Disord 2005;**88**:131–6.

52. Värnik P. Suicide in the world, Int J Environ Res Public Health 2012;**9**:760–71.

53. Fritzpatrick KK, Euton SJ, Jones JN, and Schmidt NB. Gender role, sexual orientation and suicide risk, J Affect Disord 2005;87: 35–42.

54. Isometsa E, Heikkinen M, Henriksson M, Aro H, and Lönnqvist J. Recent life events and completed suicide in bipolar affective disorder: a comparison with major depressive disorder in Finland, J Affect Disord 1995;33:99–106.

55. Kim CD, Seguin M, Therrien N, Riopel G, Chawkay N, Lesege AD, and Turecki G. Familial aggregation of suicidal behavior: a family study of male suicide completers from the general population, Am J Psychiatry 2005;162:1017–19.

56. Brent DA, Melhem NM, Oquendo M, Burke A, Birmaher B, Stanley B, Biernesser C, Keilp J, Kolko D, Ellis S, Porta G, Zelazny J, Iyengar S, and Mann JJ. Familial pathways to early-onset suicide attempt: a 5.6-year prospective study, JAMA Psychiatry 2015;72:160–8.

57. Søndergård L, Lopez AG, Andersen PK, and Kessing LV. Mood-stabilizing pharmacological treatment in bipolar disorders and risk of suicide, Bipolar Disord 2008;10:87–94.

58. Cipriani A, Hawton K, Stockton S, and Geddes JR. Lithium in the prevention of suicide in mood disorders: updated systematic review and meta-analysis, BMJ 2013;346:f3646.

59. Toffol E, Hätönen T, Tanskanen A, Lönnqvist J, Wahlbeck K, Joffe G, Tiihonen J, Haukka J, and Partonen T. Lithium is associated with decrease in all-cause and suicide mortality in high-risk bipolar patients: a nationwide registry-based prospective cohort study, J Affect Disord 2015;183:159–65.

60. Lewitzka U, Jabs B, Fülle M, Holthoff V, Juckel G, Uhl I, Kittel-Schneider S, Reif A, Reif-Leonhard C, Gruber O, Djawid B, Goodday S, Haussmann R, Pfennig A, Ritter P, Conell J, Severus E, and Bauer M. Does lithium reduce acute suicidal ideation and behavior? A protocol for a randomized, placebo-controlled multicenter trial of lithium plus Treatment As Usual (TAU) in patients with suicidal major depressive episode, BMC Psychiatry 2015;15:117.

61. Chesin M and Stanley B. Risk assessment and psychosocial interventions for suicidal patients, Bipolar Disord 2013;15:584–93.

62. Vita A, De Peri L, and Sacchetti E. Lithium in drinking water and suicide prevention: a review of the evidence, Int Clin Psychopharmacol 2015;30:1–5.

63. Leon AC, Solomon DA, Li C, Fiedorowicz JG, Coryell WH, Endicott J, and Keller MB. Antiepileptic drugs for bipolar disorder and the risk of suicidal behavior: a 30-year observational study, Am J Psychiatry 2012;169:285–91.

64. Smith EG, Austin KL, Kim HM, Miller DR, Eisen SV, Christiansen CL, Kilbourne AM, Sauer BC, McCarthy JF, and Valenstein M. Suicide risk in Veterans Health Administration patients with mental health diagnoses initiating lithium or valproate: a historical prospective cohort study, BMC Psychiatry 2014;14:357.

65. Oquendo MA, Galfalvy HC, Currier D, Grunebaum MF, Sher L, Sullivan GM, Burke AK, Harkavy-Friedman J, Sublette ME, Parsey RV, and Mann JJ. Treatment of suicide attempters with bipolar disorder: a randomized clinical trial comparing lithium and valproate in the prevention of suicidal behavior, Am J Psychiatry 2011;168:1050–6.

66. Lopez-Castroman J, Courtet P, Baca-Garcia E, and Oquendo MA Identification of suicide risk in bipolar disorder, Bipolar Disord 2015;17:22–3.

67. Leon AC, Fiedorowicz JG, Solomon DA, Li C, Coryell WH, Endicott J, Fawcett J, and Keller MB. Risk of suicidal behavior with antidepressants in bipolar and unipolar disorders, J Clin Psychiatry 2014;75:720–7.

68. Pacchiarotti I, Bond DJ, Baldessarini RJ, Nolen WA, Grunze H, Licht RW, Post RM, Berk M, Goodwin GM, Sachs GS, Tondo L, Findling RL, Youngstrom EA, Tohen M, Undurraga J, González-Pinto A, Goldberg JF, Yildiz A, Altshuler LL, Calabrese JR, Mitchell PB, Thase ME, Koukopoulos A, Colom F, Frye MA, Malhi GS, Fountoulakis KN, Vázquez G, Perlis RH, Ketter TA, Cassidy F, Akiskal H, Azorin JM, Valentí M, Mazzei DH, Lafer B, Kato T, Mazzarini L, Martínez-Aran A, Parker G, Souery D, Ozerdem A, McElroy SL, Girardi P, Bauer M, Yatham LN, Zarate CA, Nierenberg AA, Birmaher B, Kanba S, El-Mallakh RS, Serretti A, Rihmer Z, Young AH, Kotzalidis GD, MacQueen GM, Bowden CL, Ghaemi SN, Lopez-Jaramillo C, Rybakowski J, Ha K, Perugi G, Kasper S, Amsterdam JD, Hirschfeld RM, Kapczinski F, and Vieta E. The International Society for Bipolar Disorders (ISBD) task force report on antidepressant use in bipolar disorders, Am J Psychiatry 2013;170:1249–62.

69. Yerevanian BI, Koek RJ, and Mintz J. Bipolar pharmacotherapy and suicidal behavior. Part 3: Impact of antipsychotics, J Affect Disord 2007;103:23–8.

70. Li XB, Tang YL, Wang CY, and de Leon J. Clozapine for treatment-resistant bipolar disorder: a systematic review, Bipolar Disord 2015;17:235–47.

71. Ballard ED, Richards EM, Ionescu DF, Niciu MJ, Vande Voort J, and Zarate CA Jr. Experimental pharmacologic approaches for the reduction of suicidal ideation and behavior. In: Cannon KE and Hudzik TJ (eds), *Suicide: Phenomenology and Neurobiology.* (New York/Dordrecht/London: Springer, Cham Heidelberg; 2014).

72. Griffiths JJ, Zarate CA Jr, and Rasimas JJ. Existing and novel biological therapeutics in suicide prevention, Am J Prev Med 2014;47:S195–203.

73. Kantrowitz JT, Halberstam B, and Gangwisch J. Single-dose ketamine followed by daily d-cycloserine in treatment-resistant bipolar depression, J Clin Psychiatry 2015;76:737–8.

74. Monteggia LM and Zarate C Jr. Antidepressant actions of ketamine: from molecular mechanisms to clinical practice, Curr Opin Neurobiol 2015;30:139–43.

75. Nagele P, Duma A, Kopec M, Gebara MA, Parsoei A, Walker M, Janski A, Panagopoulos VN, Cristancho P, Miller JP, Zorumski CF, and Conway CR. Nitrous oxide for treatment-resistant major depression: a proof-of-concept trial, Biol Psychiatry 2015;78:10–18.

76. Liebman LS, Ahle GM, Briggs MC, and Kellner CH. Electroconvulsive therapy and bipolar Disorder. In :Yildiz A, Ruiz P, and Nemeroff CB. *The Bipolar Book. History, Neurobiology, and Treatment* (New York, NY: Oxford University Press, 2015).

77. Fink M, Kellner CH, and McCall WV. The role of ECT in suicide prevention, J ECT 2014;30:5–9.

78. Rucci P, Frank E, Kostelnik B, Fagiolini A, Malinger AG, Swartz HA, Thase ME, Siegel L, Wilson D, and Kupfer DJ. Suicide attempts in patients with bipolar I disorder during acute and maintenance phases of intensive treatment with pharmacotherapy and adjunctive psychotherapy, Am J Psychiatry 2002;159:1160–4.

79. Fountoulakis KN, Gonda X, Siamouli M, and Rihmer Z. Psychotherapeutic intervention and suicide risk reduction in bipolar disorder: a review of the evidence, J Affect Disord 2009;113:21–9.

80. Goldstein TR, Fersch-Podrat RK, Rivera M, Axelson DA, Merranko J, Yu H, Brent DA, and Birmaher B. Dialectical behavior therapy for adolescents with bipolar disorder: results from a pilot randomized trial, J Child Adolesc Psychopharmacol 2015;25:140–9.

Chapter 17

Treatment implications for bipolar disorder co-occurring with anxiety syndromes and substance abuse

Gustavo H. Vázquez, Alberto Forte, Sebastián Camino, Leonardo Tondo, and Ross J. Baldessarini

Introduction

Bipolar disorder (BD; types I and II), cyclothymic disorder, and proposed 'bipolar spectrum' disorders with recurrent depression and mild hypomanic symptoms are prevalent, lifelong, episodic illnesses that can have high levels of morbidity, disability, and increased mortality, despite use of available treatments.[1,2,3] BD-I and BD-II carry similar, high risks for suicide.[4] The broad range of BD or bipolar-like syndromes occur at an international lifetime prevalence of 3–10% of the general population.[3,5,6] BD is a leading cause of disability[7] and commonly co-occurs with features of other psychiatric, substance abuse, eating, or personality disorders.[3,8,9] Although not addressed here, diabetes, cardiovascular, and other general medical disorders also occur at higher rates in BD than in the general population, resulting in excess mortality that is similar to suicide and other violent deaths in total deaths/year.[10–12]

Lifetime risk of meeting diagnostic criteria for at least one additional psychiatric syndrome or substanceuse disorder (SUD) with BD averages approximately 65% (but has been up to 80%), with a risk of perhaps 42% for ≥2 other conditions, and of 24% for ≥3 psychiatric or substance-related diagnoses, with some international variations in prevalence (Bauer et al. 2005).[8] The most prevalent psychiatric conditions co-occurring with BD are anxiety syndromes, and SUD, which may be increasing in prevalence.[13,14] Such putative 'co-morbidity' has major clinical and public health significance, with greater overall long-term morbidity and disability, inferior treatmentadherence, increased mortality, and higher costs of care and economic losses due to disability, adding substantially to the high proportion of worldwide illnessburden associated with mood disorders.[7,8]

Co-occurrence of multiple morbid states can be conceptualized as multiple disorders appearing in the same person, as is implied by use of the term 'co-morbidity'

(Feinstein 1970).[15] However, the term can be confusing, particularly when applied to psychiatric illnesses, due to overlap of relatively non-specific symptoms among many syndromes, especially when anxiety or substance abuse and mood disorders are involved.[16-19] A multiple-illness model is strongly encouraged by standard international diagnostic schemes (notably the *Diagnostic and Statistical Manual of Mental Disorders* (DSM) and the *International Classification of Diseases* (ICD)) which define large numbers of putative psychiatric disorders, based largely on descriptive symptomatic criteria of limited specificity that remain biologically unverifiable. Here, by arbitrary convention, we consider BD to be the primary disorder of interest, and anxiety syndromes or SUD as secondary. Clinically, it can be a critical challenge to recognize mood disorders when the presenting problem is anxiety or SUD. Moreover, in otherwise stable, treated BD patients, the secondary problems can be dominant clinically.

An alternative view is that with BD, as a complex disorder, some commonly associated illnesses may fall within the range of manifestations of BD itself, particularly anxiety syndromes.There are potential advantages and disadvantages of either perspective. Multiple-disorder models can tend towards fragmentation of clinical assessment and care, with multiple clinicians focusing narrowly on only some of overall, complex clinical presentations. Alternative, single-illness models including complex presentations may encourage excessive clinical focus on what is presumed to be the primary problem. In psychiatric settings, emphasis is likely to be on the mood disorder, but less on anxiety, personality disorders, substance abuse, or general medical problems. Also not uncommon is overlooking BD itself, especially when it is not fully or typically expressed, and among persons presenting with prominent depression, anxiety, substance abuse, or medical illnesses commanding immediate clinical attention.[1,20] On the contrary, in clinical settings that focus on alcohol- or drug-abuse, substance abuse is likely to be the primary focus. In both settings, there is a risk that some components of the overall clinical presentation will receive less attention or be left to others to address, with a high risk of insufficiently coordinated and balanced therapeutic efforts. There is even a possibility that adequate treatment of BD may be considered sufficient to manage associated morbidities and, conversely, that adequate treatment of substanceabuse itself may resolve many cases of mood disorder. Both of these assumptions can easily be exaggerated, although successful treatment of one problem may improve others.[18] The complexity of BD calls for unusually broad and sophisticated assessments and multimodal treatment programmes, ideally involving more than one clinician with specialized knowledge and experience, particularly when SUD is present. For the present, such integrated, multidisciplinary programmes for evaluation and both short- and long-term care of BD patients are challenging but useful for developing optimal intervention programmes.

Even when recognized, it is typically unclear how to treat complex clinical presentations including anxiety syndromes or substance abuse associated with specific phases of BD. It is especially uncertain when to rely primarily on mood-stabilizing treatments in hopes of ameliorating a range of psychopathological phenomena in BD patients, and when to consider treatments directed at symptoms considered to represent discrete and even separate illnesses.[14] In addition, treatments themselves sometimes produce symptoms that further complicate the conditions being treated. Examples include the mania-inducing or mood-destabilizing actions of antidepressants, and depression-like reactions or restless agitation (akathisia) in response to some antipsychotics (Baldessarini 2013, Baldessarini et al. 2013; Tondo et al. 2010; Vázquez et al. 2013).[21-24] Also, states of acute or chronic intoxication or withdrawal associated with substance abuse can greatly complicate clinical assessment of patients with mood disorders.[18]

Aside from unresolved conceptual questions regarding psychiatric co-morbidity, its diagnostic assessment, and the optimal clinical assessment and treatment of BD with co-morbidity, studies of the prevalence, prognosis, outcome, and effects of treatments in patients meeting standard diagnostic criteria for BD as well as anxiety syndromes or substance abuse remain infrequent.[17,18,25,26] These circumstances encouraged this overview of what is known about the nature, epidemiology, and treatment of patients diagnosed with BD who also manifest anxiety symptoms or syndromes, or substance abuse. We began with extensive computerized searching through August 2015, using the Pubmed/MEDLINE and EMBASE research literature databases, using specific anxiety diagnostic terms and names of commonly abused substances. We screened more than 2,000 report citations, and closely reviewed a total of more than 300 full reports as well as citations found in recent reviews on anxiety or substance use in association with BD.

Anxiety syndromes

Prevalence of anxiety syndromes in BD patients

Anxiety disorders are far more prevalent among BD patients than in the general population, and occur at rates similar to patients diagnosed with unipolar, recurrent major depressive disorders.[27-35] Findings pertaining to prevalence of anxiety syndromes in BD patients derive from both epidemiological[6,27,28,36-42] and clinical studies.[5,8,9,30,31,33,43-58] Approximately half of BD patients studied have met standard diagnostic criteria for at least one anxiety syndrome during their lifetime course.[8,29,41,47,55-59]

We found an average lifetime risk of 47.1% (95% CI: 46.4–53.9) across 32 studies for the presence of at least one anxiety syndrome in BD patients (Table 17.1). Reported prevalence of particular anxiety syndromes in BD patients ranged from 13.2% to 24.0%, and ranked: generalized anxiety ≥ social and specific phobias ≥ panic ≥ posttraumatic stress ≥ obsessive–compulsive syndrome (Table 17.2 and Figure 17.1). These risks are 1.90–8.25 times greater than reported lifetime prevalence for anxiety disorders in the general population (Table 17.2 and Figure 17.1).[5,3,60,61]

Rates of anxiety syndromes were somewhat higher among women than men diagnosed with BD in several studies[41,55,62,63] but not in other findings.[22] Data pooled from these reports indicate that prevalence in women (553/1227; 45.0% [CI: 42.3–47.9]) has averaged 1.43 times higher than in men (262/830; 31.5% [CI: 28.4–34.8]; Table 17.1), paralleling the sexdifference in the general population. In 14 reports on rates of anxiety syndromes in patients with BD subtypes, reported prevalence in BD-I

Table 17.1 Prevalence of all anxiety disorder diagnoses among bipolar disorder subjects

Groups	Studies (n)	Subjects (N)	Mean Prevalence [95% CI]
All bipolar[a]	32	14,316	47.1 [40.3–53.9]
Diagnostic type[b]			
Bipolar I	13	3,019	47.3 [45.5–49.1]
Bipolar II	12	1,438	45.5 [42.9–48.2]
Ratio	—	2.09	1.03
Sex[c]			
Women	5	1,227	45.0 [42.3–47.9]
Men	5	830	31.5 [28.4–34.8]
Ratio	—	1.47	1.43
Current polarity[d]			
Depression	1	106	44.3 [34.7–54.3]
[Hypo]mania	1	44	22.7 [11.5–37.8]
Ratio	—	2.40	1.95

Prevalence is averaged across rates in individual studies.

[a] Cited in text under prevalence of anxiety síndromes, [b] Kessler et al. 1997; Angst et al. 1998; McElroy et al. 2001; Doughty et al. 2004; Simon et al. 2004; Mantere et al. 2006; Merikangas et al. 2007; Albert et al. 2008; Zimmermann et al. 2009; Sala et al. 2012; Das et al. 2013; Baldessarini et al. 2013; Baek et al. 2014; Sala et al. 2014; $\chi2$ = 1.30, p = 0.25, [c]Altshuler et al. 2010; Baldassano et al. 2005; Sala et al. 2012; Baek et al. 2014; Tondo et al. 2013 (unpublished data); $\chi2$ = 37.7, p<0.0001, [d] Mantere et al 2006; $\chi2$ = 6.16, p = 0.01.

(47.3%) and BD-II cases (45.5%) did not differ significantly overall (risk ratio = 1.03; Table 17.2). However, when particular syndromes were considered, phobias were 1.70 times (22.3%/13.1%) more prevalent among BD-I than BD-II patients, whereas panic was found 1.51 times (23.1%/16.6%) more often with BD-II (Table 17.2).

Anxiety symptoms or syndromes, though strongly associated with BD, have been found inconsistently to be antecedents of BD, sometimes years before syndromal presentations of BD.[64,55,65] Such an association is supported by findings that rates of treatment-associated mania or hypomania in placebo-controlled trials of antidepressant treatment for juvenile anxiety disorders were at least as high as in trials for depression.[66] This finding suggests that anxiety as well as depression[22] can sometimes precede as well as follow clinical expression of BD.[9,11,65,67] When followed longitudinally, some BD patients experience anxiety syndromes at a remarkably high proportion of total morbidity.[68–70]

In BD-I patients, anxiety symptoms or syndromes have been associated with an excess of depressive or mixed manic-depressive episodes, long-term, more than with manic or hypomanic illness, and the occurrence of such states was associated with not only a worse long-term prognosis,[2,71] but also with more severe mania (Gonzáles-Pinto et al. 2012).[72] Among BD subjects, anxiety syndromes were associated with current depression, and anxiety symptoms (not syndromes) were associated with greater long-term depressive morbidity.[73] Later excesses of anxiety and depression followed

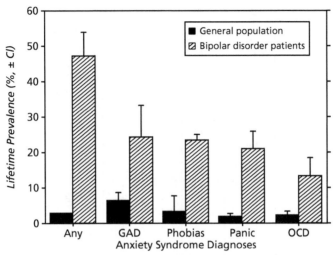

Figure 17.1 Lifetime prevalence (%) of anxiety disorders among bipolar disorder (BD) patients (data from Tables 17.1 and 17.2) versus the general population [Tsuang & Tohen 2002], based on 15–32 epidemiological studies in BD, with 95% confidence intervals (CI). The ratios of risk in bipolar disorder to the general population ranked: any anxiety disorder (16.2) ≥ panic disorder (10.9) ≥ phobias (6.93) ≥ obsessive–compulsive disorder (OCD; 6.35) > generalized anxiety disorder (GAD; 3.79).

first-lifetime illness episodes of anxiety among patients eventually diagnosed with BD.[67] These findings underscore a deficiency in understanding the natural course of anxiety features in BD patients despite their clinical prominence.

Overall, the preceding findings, including the great excess prevalence of anxiety syndromes in BD patients over the general population (Table 17.2), support a strong association of anxiety with depressive, affectively mixed, and perhaps hypomanic phases of BD. These associations are consistent with considering anxiety symptoms to be within the range of symptomatic expression of BD, but do not clarify whether two distinct *disorders* are present or not. Findings that might support the presence of separate, 'co-morbid' anxiety syndromes and BD include observations that nearly half of patients diagnosed with BD never meet diagnostic criteria for an anxiety disorder, and that very few patients with a primary anxiety disorder, even if treated long-term with antidepressants, ever show clinical features of BD.[51,57,74,75]

Association of anxiety with morbidity in BD

Anxiety symptoms and syndromes in BD patients have consistently been associated with younger onset, more mixed-state episodes, and greater overall morbidity, with more hospitalizations and worse overall prognosis, slower or inferior treatment responses, more substance abuse, more rapid cycling, and greater economic costs (for clinical care and disability) than among BD patients without anxiety syndromes.[29,31,38,39,46,47,53–55,57,58,71,74,76–81] Moreover, several studies have found that

Table 17.2 Anxiety syndromes co-occurring with bipolar disorders: prevalence

Syndrome	Mean Prevalence [95% CI]				I/II Risk Ratio
	General Population	All Bipolar (N = 14,448)	Bipolar I (N = 2986)	Bipolar II (N = 926)	
Generalized anxiety	5.70 [5.11–6.29]	24.0 [14.6–33.3]	16.2 [14.9–19.6]	15.5 [10.3–14.6]	1.05
Phobia	12.3 [11.5–13.1]	23.5 [20.8–23.8]	22.3 [20.8–23.8]	13.1 [10.9–15.4]	1.70[a]
Panic	5.70 [5.11–6.29]	20.9 [16.1–25.7]	16.6 [15.3–17.9]	23.1 [20.4–25.9]	0.72[b]
Post-traumatic stress	6.80 [6.02–7.58]	17.1 [8.15–25.9]	14.2 [12.9–15.5]	12.8 [10.8–15.2]	1.11
Obsessive–compulsive	1.60 [1.01–2.19]	13.2 [7.91–18.5]	10.6 [9.60–11.8]	10.6 [8.70–12.7]	1.00
Any anxiety syndrome	28.8 [28.3–29.3]	49.7 [38.3–61.1]	45.5 [9.73–81.3]	46.5 [0–104]	10.9

Data ranked by overall prevalence in BD.[a] Risk of phobia is greater in BD-I; [b] risk of panic is greater in BD-II (both *p*<0.05). Data are from: Angst et al. 1998; Kessler et al. 2005b; Rihmer et al. 2001; McElroy et al. 2001; Simon et al. 2004; Grant et al. 2005; Latalova et al. 2013; Mantere et al. 2006; McIntyre et al. 2006; Merikangas et al. 2007; Albert et al. 2008; Subramainam et al. 2012; Baldessarini et al. 2013; Das et al. 2013; Hernandez et al. 2013; Baek et al. 2014; Shashidhara et al. 2015.Prevalences are 'lifetime' risk except Mantere et al. 2006 involves point-prevalence.The overall excess among BD subjects vs. the general population was 1.73-fold (49.7%/28.8%); this excess ranged from 1.91-fold (phobias), to 8.25-fold (obsessive–compulsive syndrome), and averaged 4.11 [1.02–7.20] for all five anxiety syndrome types.

anxiety symptoms in BD patients were associated with substantially increased risks of suicidal ideation, attempts, and suicides,[29,31,58,82] often in association with a more severely symptomatic illness course and more depression or mixed states, which are risk factors for suicide in BD).[31,38,39,41,46,55,58,83]

Treatments for anxiety syndromes in BD patients

Therapeutics research for anxiety syndromes occurring in BD patients remains extraordinarily underdeveloped (Table 17.3). Recent reviews have identified very few randomized controlled trials of either pharmacotherapies or psychotherapies directed at any type of anxiety morbidity in BD, and even fewer directed at specific anxiety syndromes, or at anxiety in particular phases (depression, mixed states, mania/hypomania, euthymia) or types (I vs II) of BD.[20,74,84]

Despite widespread clinical use of benzodiazepines to treat anxiety symptoms in various circumstances, recent expert taskforce recommendations have positioned them at the lowest level of evidence (anecdotal) for treatment of anxiety syndromes in adults with BD.[84,85] However, several other reviews support their use (particularly clonazepam) for improving a range of acute affective symptoms arising long-term among patients with major affective disorders, without specific evidence of their value for particular anxiety syndromes in BD.[85-87] Benzodiazepines appear not to be inferior to antidepressants for the short-term treatment of patients with primary anxiety disorders.[88] However, we found no studies that specifically evaluated the efficacy and safety of benzodiazepines themselves, or in comparison to alternatives, to treat anxiety symptoms or syndromes in BD patients.

We found no trials testing lithium for effects in anxiety syndromes associated with BD, nor are anticonvulsants with antimanic or mood-stabilizing effects adequately tested for specific effects against anxiety in BD. However, one trial found valproate to be effective for panic syndrome in BD patients, even after poor responses to antidepressants.[89] Also, topiramate (which lacks antimanic or mood-stabilizing effects[21]) as an adjuvant was more effective than placebo in ameliorating obsessive–compulsive symptoms in manic BD patients.[90] Possibly of interest, anxiety syndromes were more prominent among BD patients who had received less mood-stabilizer treatment, although cause–effect relationships in this association are unclear.[77] Studies of potential short- or long-term value of lamotrigine in treating anxiety symptoms in BD patients are notably lacking, although one trial suggested benefits in panic with BD.[91] Although their efficacy in BD in general is not proved (Baldessarini 2013),[21] gabapentin and pregabalin may improve anxiety symptoms in some BD patients.[92]

Some modern antipsychotics may improve anxiety symptoms in BD patients, particularly in low doses, and are generally well tolerated. Added to lithium or as a monotherapy, olanzapine was more effective than lamotrigine against anxiety symptoms in BD patients.[93] Quetiapine has reported beneficial effects in mania and in depressed BD-I or -II patients.[94,95] In a controlled trial, quetiapine also was more effective than valproate or placebo against generalized anxiety or panic in BD patients.[96] However, a comparison of quetiapine-extendedrelease (ER) as a monotherapy or added to a standard mood-stabilizer for acute bipolar depression with co-occurring anxiety

Table 17.3 Treatments for anxiety symptoms or syndromes occurring with bipolar disorder

Treatment	Evidence	Findings	Studies
Antidepressants			
Antidepressants	Case series; trial with OCD (n = 28)	Efficacy uncertain	Perugi et al 2002b; Simon et al. 2004; Schaffer et al. 2007, 2012
Anxiolytics			
Benzodiazepines	Case reports; empirical-clinical use	Appeared to be helpful	Sachs et al. 2003; Winkler et al. 2003; Schaffer et al. 2012
Antipsychotics			
Aripiprazole	Case reports for OCD in BD (N = 3)	Appeared to be effective	Uguz et al. 2010
Lurasidone alone	1 RCT 6 wks) anxiety symptoms in BD-depression (N = 170)	Superior to placebo	Loebel et al. 2014
Lurasidone + Li or VPA	1 RCT (6 wks) anxiety symptoms in BD-depression (N= 348)	Adding drug superior to placebo	Loebel et al. 2014
Olanzapine	1 RCT (8 wks) anxiety symptoms in BD-depression (N = 168)	Drug superior to placebo	Tohen et al. 2007
Olanzapine + fluoxetine	1 RCT (8 wks) anxiety symptoms in BD-depression (N = 31)	Drug superior to placebo or olanzapine alone	Tohen et al. 2007
Quetiapine	4 RCTs (8 wks, 300 or 600 mg/day) anxiety symptoms or GAD in BD-I/II depression (total N = 3317)	Drug superior to placebo or valproate vs generalized anxiety symptoms, not vs GAD	Hirschfeld et al. 2006; Sheehan et al. 2009; Gao et al. 2014
Risperidone	Monotherapy (2.5 mg/day) RCT	Ineffective vs placebo (panic or OCD)	Sheehan et al. 2009
Ziprasidone	Monotherapy (120–160 mg/day) RCT (N = 49)	Ineffective vs. placebo (panic or GAD)	Suppes et al. 2014

Table 17.3 Continued

Treatment	Evidence	Findings	Studies
Anticonvulsants & Lithium			
Gabapentin	Case series (1.3 g/day) add-on (N = 43)	May have reduced anxiety symptoms	Perugi et al. 2002a
Lamotrigine	Case series vs. lithium with panic (N = 164)	May be more effective than lithium	Passmore et al. 2003
Lithium	1 RCT (12 wks), added to olanzapine or valproate vs. anxiety symptoms in euthymic BD (N = 47)	Li + olanzapine superior to Li + valproate	Maina et al. 2008
Pregabalin	Expert opinions	Recommended as possibly useful	Schaffer et al. 2007
Topiramate	1 RCT, 200 mg/day added to lithium or antipsychotic for OCD + mania (N = 39)	Adjunctive drug superior to placebo	Sahraian et a l. 2014
Valproate	Case series BD-II + panic, BD-II added to antidepressants x 3 yrs (total N = 40)	May be effective vs. panic	Baetz et al. 1990; Perugi et al. 2010
Psychosocial Methods			
Psychosocial treatments	4 trials in BD-I + II: CBT vs IPT, CBT vs family therapy, CBT vs psychoeducation, CBT, IPR, or family therapy (total N = 471)	CBT appeared to be particularly effective	Miklowitz et al. 2007; Provencher et al. 2011; Hawke et al. 2013

Abbreviations: BD, bipolar disorder; *CBT*, cognitive-behavioural therapy; *IPT*, interpersonal psychotherapy; *Li*, lithium carbonate; *N* = number of subjects; *OCD*, obsessive–compulsive disorder; *RTC*, randomizedcontrolled trial.

was not more effective than a placebo.[97] In addition, risperidone has been ineffective against panic or obsessive–compulsive syndromes associated with BD,[98] as was ziprasidone for BD with panic or generalized anxiety.[99] Additional promising findings regarding anxiety symptoms arose from trials of lurasidone as a monotherapy or added to lithium or valproate, primarily designed to test for efficacy in depressed BD-I patients.[100] Finally, a small case series suggested beneficial effects of aripiprazole against obsessive–compulsive features in BD patients.[101] All of these findings with pharmacological treatments are preliminary and require extensive additional testing before sound clinical recommendations can be developed.

Studies of psychosocial treatments for coexisting anxiety syndromes and BD also are rare. Psychotherapies appear to reduce anxiety symptoms in BD patients long term.[102,103] Cognitive-behavioural psychotherapy (CBT) is particularly well studied and is effective for primary depressive and anxiety disorders unrelated to BD[104] as well as in BD.[105] CBT also may be as effective, and possibly superior, to interpersonal psychotherapy, family therapy, or psychoeducational programmes for BD patients with anxiety syndromes.[106] Co-occurring anxiety can interfere with overall treatment responses in BD.[20,107] One study found that acutely depressed BD patients with a history of an anxiety syndrome were 26% less likely to recover within 12 months with various psychotherapies, but that effects of such treatments exceeded those of routine care of BD overall.[108]

Comparisons of treatment in primary and BD-associated anxiety

Therapeutic studies of anxiety in BDs are based mainly on secondary analyses of trials designed with other aims.[74,84] They can be supplemented with investigations that evaluate medicines commonly used in the treatment of primary anxiety disorders for effects on anxiety associated with BD, or conversely, using agents commonly used to treat BD for effects in primary anxiety disorders,[20,109] assuming that treatment effects on anxiety in both circumstances are comparable. Treatments tested include antidepressants, lithium, anticonvulsants, antipsychotics, and rarely benzodiazepines or other sedatives. Such studies are few, often poorly designed, and yield limited information.

Antidepressants, including tricyclics, monoamine oxidase inhibitors, serotonin or serotonin-norepinephrinereuptake inhibitors, and mirtazapine are standard treatments for anxiety disorders, as are benzodiazepines, though they vary in efficacy with particular disorders. However, their application for anxiety syndromes in BD remains unstudied. Antidepressants may be avoided due to somewhat exaggerated concern for potential mood-switching and behaviour-destabilizing actions in BD.[22–24,110]

Lithium appears to lack important therapeutic effects in primary anxiety disorders, but has been studied only rarely in few types of anxiety. Nevertheless, there are some indications of possible benefits of lithium treatment in reducing depressive and episodic obsessive–compulsive symptoms when used adjunctively for obsessive–compulsive disorder.[109,111,112] In addition, subtle anxiolytic effects of lithium have been noted in BD patients.[91]

Among anticonvulsants with antimanic or mood-stabilizing effects, carbamazepine has had inconsistent effects in primary panic disorder.[113,114] Lamotrigine may have some benefit for post-traumatic stress disorder and perhaps in obsessive–compulsive disorder.[115] Gabapentin, though of limited benefit in BD, may benefit primary social phobia but perhaps not panic disorder.[116–118] Pregabalin may be effective in social phobia and probably also in generalized anxiety disorder.[116,119] Valproate is not extensively studied in primary anxiety disorders,[20,109,120] but may have benefits in both generalized anxiety and panic disorder.[84,121]

Relatively non-specific anxiety symptoms associated with major affective episodes in BD patients may improve along with other responses to mood stabilizers.[20,74,84] Nevertheless, it is important to reiterate that systematic assessments of mood-stabilizing medicines specifically for effects on anxiety in BD patients remain to be carried out.

There are a few studies of antipsychotics for primary anxiety disorders, with inconsistent effects.[20,109,122] Risperidone was beneficial in controlled trials for primary obsessive–compulsive disorder and post-traumatic stress disorder.[123,124] Olanzapine has shown inconsistent effects in obsessive-compulsive disorder,[125,126] but some efficacy in post-traumatic stress disorder.[127,128] Aripiprazole appeared to be effective for some forms of anxiety in open trials, including for anxiety syndromes associated with major depression,[129] a finding consistent with the strong association of symptoms of anxiety and depressive disorders.[130] Quetiapine has shown inconsistent effects in obsessive–compulsive disorder,[131-133] but has been promising for generalized anxiety disorder.[134] Of note, most of these applications of antipsychotics have been for otherwise poorly treatment-responsive cases, often as adjuncts to other, more standard, antianxiety treatments.

Finally, there are emerging experimental treatments for anxiety or mood disorders.They include antiglutamate agents: riluzole,[135,136] the NMDA-glutamate receptor antagonists memantine[137] and ketamine),[138,139] and repeated transcranial magnetic stimulation (rTMS).[140-142] However, none of these treatments has been tested for anxiety associated with BD.

Conclusions: anxiety

Anxiety symptoms and syndromes are highly prevalent among patients diagnosed with BDs, affecting approximately half of BD-I and BD-II patients at some time. These rates are far higher than the prevalence of anxiety disorders in the general population, consistent with the view that anxiety syndromes and symptoms are part of the spectrum of psychopathology in BD. Anxiety symptoms and syndromes require thoughtful consideration in the comprehensive, flexible, and repeated assessment and treatment of BD patients over time. In addition, mooddisorders including BD should be considered in diagnostic assessments of patients considered to have an anxiety disorder.

Reported prevalence ranked: generalized anxiety ≥ social or specific phobias ≥ panic ≥ post-traumatic stress ≥ obsessive–compulsive syndromes. Co-occurring anxiety syndromes in BD have averaged 43% more prevalent among women than men, but similarly likely in BD-I and BD-II.

Anxiety features have been associated with generally poorer prognosis in BD, including less responsiveness to standard mood-stabilizing agents, greater disability, more substance abuse, and possibly greater risk of suicidal behaviours. However, details of the course and temporal distribution of anxiety phenomena in BD patients, and of their association with particular components of BD require clarification, although selective association of anxiety with depression and perhaps mixed states in BD is suspected.

Associations of anxiety features with adverse clinical outcomes in BD call for therapeutic studies specifically directed at anxiety of particular types associated with BD subtypes (I vs II) and phases (depressive or dysthymic, euthymic, manic or hypomanic, mixed). Emerging, suggestive therapeutic findings pertaining to anxiety in BD include probable benefits of divalproex, lurasidone, olanzapine, quetiaptine, as well as psychotherapies. Prescription of benzodiazepines or antidepressants to treat anxiety symptoms in BD patients appears not to be uncommon clinically, but their use requires critical assessment in individuals over time, with due concern about the potential for intoxication, abuse, and dependence with sedatives, and emotionally or behaviourally destabilizing risks of antidepressants.

Finally, the fundamental conceptual riddle remains as to whether anxiety syndromes co-occurring in BD reflect the range of symptomatic-phenotypic expression of BD, represent separate illnesses (disorders), or are largely an artifact of contemporary categorical diagnostic concepts and methods which encourage continued use of the potentially misleading term 'co-morbidity'.

Substance abuse

Introduction

BD is often associated with SUD in both community and clinical populations.[79,143,144] Among patients with major mood disorders, those with BD have the highest prevalence of co-occurring SUD.[144,145] The basis of this strong association is unclear.[146] Nevertheless, it is highly clinically relevant for association with treatment non-adherence, poor clinical outcome and greater dysfunction, and high risks of premature mortality including by suicide.[17,147,148] Such worsening of morbidity when SUD is present also has important public health implications, given the status of mood disorders as leading contributors to the worldwide burden of all diseases.[149]

Epidemiology

Averages of estimates of lifetime prevalence of various forms of SUD in the general population of the United States (US) and several other developed countries, as well as of their co-occurrence in BD subjects are summarized in Table 17.4. In the general population, prevalence of any form of abuse or dependence on alcohol has averaged 17.6%, with a somewhat lower risk of drug abuse or dependence (12.8%). Risk of any type of SUD in non-clinical populations has averaged 20.2%, ranking: alcohol (17.6%) > cannabis (4.3%) ≥ stimulants (cocaine or amphetamines; 3.2%) ≥ opioids (0.5%). For alcoholism, at least, the risk in the general population is up to three times greater among men.[150,151]

Among BD patients, risk for abuse/dependence on alcohol and several drugs has averaged two to three times greater than in the general population. Compared with unipolar major depression, risks of SUD overall are more than two times greater in both BD-I and BD-II. However, with drugs the excess was 2.7-fold in BD-I but only 1.2-fold in BD-II.[3] For BD-I versus BD-II subjects, the risk ratio for drug abuse averaged 2.3-fold, compared with 1.5-fold for alcohol abuse. SUD involves 33–40% of persons diagnosed with BD.[18,152,153]

Table 17.4 Lifetime prevalence (%) of substance-abuse disorders in patients with bipolar disorder (BD) and the general population

Substance	General Population	Diagnosis		
		Any BD	BD-I	BD-II
Alcohol	17.6 [8.1–27.1]	51.1 [22.3–78.9]	45.2 [33.9–64.5]	35.5 [26.1–44.9]
Cannabis	4.3	27.4 [0–74.8]	41.0 [0–131]	50.0
Stimulants	3.2	13.6 [0–35.1]	24.2	31.8
Opioids	0.5	7.37 [0.7–14.0]	4.6	——
Any drug	12.8 [5.3–20.4]	35.8 [0–125]	44.6 [0–91.0]	24.8 [13.9–35.7]
Any SUD	20.2 [4.6–35.8]	42.3	60.3	40.4

Data from Goodwin & Jamison 2007; Bauer et al. 2005; Cerullo & Strakowski 2007; Do & Mezak 2013; Grant et al. 2004, 2015; Hasin et al. 2007; McElroy et al. 2001; Merikangas et al. 2007; Merikangas & Paksarian 2015; Merikangas & Tohen 2011; Regier et al. 1990). The excess of any SUD in BD over the general population was 2.09 (42.3%/20.2%), and 2.80 for drugs; for the four substance types, this risk ratio averaged 7.06-fold [0–15.5], and ranged from 2.90 (alcohol) to 14.7 (opioids).

Substances most often abused are alcohol and cannabis, followed by cocaine or amphetamines, opioids, and miscellaneous agents. Rates of these associations and related clinical characteristics vary with the substances involved and with BD diagnostic type (Table 17.4).

Substances abused

Alcohol

Abuse of ethanol generally is highly prevalent, affecting 13–18% of the general population of the US.[154,155] The risk is far greater with major mood disorders, involving as many as 45% of BD patients,[40,156] and is similar among BD-I and BD-II.[154] The excess of alcohol abuse among men with BD parallels a twofold excess among men in the general population.[154] Co-occurrence of BD also is high among subjects defined primarily as abusing alcohol.[40,157] Abuse of alcohol with BD-I may anticipate or co-occur more with depressive than manic phases or with anxiety,[158] or with mania–hypomania,[145] and in the general population, there was a correlation between hypomanic symptoms and SUD, even with diagnoses of BD-I and -II excluded.[159] Alcohol abuse in BD also was more likely in association with antisocial personality disorder.[160]

Abuse of alcohol, as with other forms of SUD, is associated with a range of adverse characteristics in BD patients: more severe morbidity, greater dysfunction, more suicidal behaviour, and higher costs of care and greater economic losses due to under-employment.[161] BD patients with alcohol abuse experience illness onset at a younger age, often have psychotic symptoms at the first episode, and more depression later, with poorer functioning.[156] Past and current alcohol-use disorders also were associated with rapid mood cycling and with switching to manic, hypomanic, or mixed states immediately following a major depressive episode.[162] Alcohol abuse or dependence has been associated with at least two-times higher risks of suicide attempts.[156,163-165] Moreover, heavy alcoholabuse (>45.6 g/day) with BD had a higher risk of suicide than with lesser use.[163] Indeed, risk of premature mortality from all causes was increased in BD patients who abused alcohol.[166]

The basis of these co-occurring clinical problems is not clear. Both BD[167,168] and alcoholism[169,170] have strong familial-genetic components, but genetic factors that might be common to both BD and SUD remain to be identified and verified.[171] Efforts to contrast characteristics of cases in which abuse of alcohol has preceded, arisen with, or followed clinical manifestations of BD have yielded little support for specific models of causation. However, patients in whom alcohol abuse preceded overt BD were older at onset and had a better long-term prognosis.[172] It is also plausible that abuse of alcohol (or other substances) may sometimes have a self-medicating role aimed at managing distressing symptoms of BD, particularly in depressive phases, and reckless behaviour in association with manic phases. In general, few studies have assessed changes in alcohol consumption in BD, and they are inconclusive: half find increases with depression and half with mania–hypomania.[3]

Efforts at treating co-occurring BD with alcohol abuse include methods developed separately for each condition. Unfortunately, most of the available research of treatments for SUD or for BD involves samples selected to minimize complexity, tending to exclude cases with both conditions. Lithium and other agents with mood-stabilizing effects have yielded inconsistent findingsin primary alcohola-buse.[173] Encouraging but inconclusive findings involve mood-altering anticonvul-sants.[174] Particularly promising were a few controlled trials of valproate used to treat subjects with co-occurring alcohol abuse and BD, in whom drinking and craving for alcohol were reduced moderately.[161]

Several innovative treatments for alcoholism with co-occurring BD have not yielded conclusive findings. They include such drugs as *acamprosate, clozapine, que-tiapine*, or other *atypical antipsychotics*, or the opioid-antagonists *nalmefene* and *nal-trexone* in a few trials, usually with equivocal changes in alcohol consumption.[18,157,175]

Various forms of supportive, individual, or group psychotherapies or use of 12-step self-help programmes may be beneficial for patients with co-occurring alcohol abuse and BD. Traditionally, these efforts have tended to be organized separately from treat-ment of mood disorders. In addition, there has been a widespread, exaggerated view that many cases of mood disorder may be 'caused' by substance abuse or withdrawal, particularly alcohol. A resulting expectation often has been that resolution of sub-stance abuse might virtually eliminate clinical manifestations of mood disorders and the need for ongoing psychiatric care.[18,145] However, counter to such trends, there has been some movement towards better integration and more comprehensive treatment of patients with mood disorders and abuse of alcohol or other substances.[176]

Cannabis

Regular or daily use of cannabis has been associated with increased incidence of BD but not of unipolar depression, compared with non-users, suggesting a selec-tive association of cannabis use and BD.[177] Cannabis use was six to seventimes more prevalent among BD patients than the general population and was associated with greater disability.[178] Majorities of subjects with BD and cannabis use were male, relatively young, high-school educated, never married, and lived in a rural area.[179] Co-occurring cannabis use was associated with a more severe course of BD ill-ness, as well as additional co-morbidities including abuse of alcohol (66%) or other substances (71%).

With cannabis use, the estimated age at onset of BD was much lower, and was associated with initial manic or psychotic episodes[179] and with earlier hospitaliza-tion.[13] Onset age also was inversely related to the level of cannabis use prior to onset of BD with control for other potentially contributing factors, including sex, bipolar subtype, and family psychiatric or substance-abuse history.[180]

Cannabis use was more likely with initial mania or psychosis in BD, with more manic episodes[13,158] and some later psychotic features, including conceptual disor-ganization, but without delusions, hallucinations, negative symptoms, or impaired daily functioning.[181] BD patients who stopped using cannabis after engaging in treatment showed more symptomatic improvement than those who continued.[181] Sustained cannabis use over a year of follow-up was associated with elevated mood but not with depressive or psychotic symptoms, and with inferior functioning.[182] In addition, use of cannabis by BD subjects versus non-use has been associated with a 2.6-fold higher median number of manic, hypomanic, and depressive episodes/year.[179] Together, these findings support a selective association of cannabis use with mania–hypomania.

Cannabis use is also associated with greater risk of suicide attempts in addition to a relatively severe illness course.[179,183,184] In a meta-analytic review, 559 BD subjects who used cannabis were 44% more likely to attempt suicide than 2,880 who did not.[147] Since depression may not be more likely with cannabis use in BD,[182] an explanation of the association of cannabis use with suicidal behaviour is not well explained. It may reflect overall illness severity and greater dysfunction, fewer supportive social relationships, and inferior adherence to recommended, long-term, mood-stabilizing treatment—all of which are associated with use of cannabis by BD patients.[185]

Despite long suspicion that heavy abuse of cannabis may contribute to development or worsening of mood or psychotic disorders, cause–effect relationships remain unclear.[186] Among the 48% of 144 BD-I patients who used cannabis, in 15%, the BD preceded or was concurrent with use of cannabis, and in 23%, cannabis preceded the mood disorder; in others the sequencing was not clear, so as to leave cause–effect relationships unclear.[187]

Stimulants

World Health Organization (WHO)[188] findings suggest that the lifetime prevalence for use of cocaine is 1–3% of the general population in most developed countries, with higher rates in the US and in countries that produce cocaine, and far higher rates among persons diagnosed with BD. Although mood disorders are commonly associated with abuse of cocaine or other stimulants, particularly methamphetamine, there is a striking paucity of studies focusing on the co-occurrence of stimulant abuse and BD.[189,190] The estimated prevalence of cocaine abuse in BD has ranged from 22%[191] to 30%,[192] with higher rates (30% vs 13%) in BD than with unipolar major depression.[144,193] BD and antisocial personality disorder are notable conditions in which cocaine abuse not only is prevalent, but sometimes more intense than with other psychiatric disorders).[194] The association of stimulantabuse with BD may represent efforts to counter depressive symptoms or to achieve hypomania.

Reports on the treatment of patients with co-occurring BD and abuse of stimulants, especially cocaine are emerging but limited. They support treatment with targeted psychotherapy and use of particular mood-stabilizers, including divalproex, lamotrigine, lithium, or quetiapine,[17,195,196] as well as the mild stimulant-antidepressant bupropion added to mood stabilizers or atypical antipsychotics.[197] Another compound of interest is the dietary supplement *citicoline* (citidine-5'-phosphocholine), a metabolic intermediate in the biosynthesis of phosphatidylcholine from choline.[198] It has mild psychostimulant actions and possible mood-elevating properties. A placebo-controlled trial failed to find that it reduced abuse of methamphetamine or improved cognitive functions in BD patients,[189] although it may have exerted beneficial effects including transient reduction of cocaine use in BD patients.[199]

Opioids

Relatively few studies have focused on the relationship between heroin abuse and BD, despite high rates of opioid abuse in association with mood disorders and with suicidal behaviour.[200] However, evidence concerning the relative risk of opioid abuse and type of mood disorder is inconsistent regarding BD versus major depression.

Among identified heroin addicts, 12–54% have a mood disorder, usually non–bipolar major depression.[144] Among patients with non-bipolar depression, rates of opioid abuse have sometimes exceeded those with BD by more than 50-fold, but with suspicion that depression may have been induced by opioid abuse itself in many cases.[201] However, other studies find the risk of opioid abuse to be greater with BD than in major depression[200,202,203]. Risk of opioid abuse in BD may be especially high in association with prominent aggressive or suicidal behaviours.[200]

It is noteworthy that mania or hypomania can follow withdrawal of opioids.[203] This effect is consistent with evidence of mood-altering effects of some opioids,[204] but with an uncertain relationship to primary BD and representing another potential confounding effect. To further complicate assessment of opioid abuse by BD patients and its clinical significance, relatively high doses (up to 400 mg/day) of methadone were associated with *better* clinical outcomes among heroin-addicted patients with BD-I than among otherwise similar addicts without BD.[205] Uncertainties about relative risks of co-occurrence of opioid abuse with BD versus unipolar major depression and their clinical implications may reflect whether study subjects were from drug abuse samples in whom mood disorders were considered, or from mood-disorder samples in whom opioid abuse was evaluated.

There has been very little specific research on treatments aimed at patients meeting diagnostic criteria for both BD and opioid abuse, and recent expert treatment recommendations have not ventured opinions on the topic.[18,206]

Conclusions: substance abuse

Abuse of single or multiple substances (especially, alcohol, cannabis, stimulants, and opioids) is highly prevalent among mood-disorder patients, and especially those with BD. These co-occurring conditions greatly complicate clinical care of BD patients, contribute importantly to erratic adherence to treatment, lead to more severe illness with adverse outcomes, increase costs of care and of disability, and greatly increase risks of suicide and other forms of violent death, including by apparent accidents. Remarkably, however, in gross disproportion to the importance of the problem, there is a striking paucity of detailed and secure information about the prevalence of specific types of substance abuse among types and phases of BD. There is even less information about optimal treatment based on scientifically rigorous therapeutic trials.[18,152] Notably, fewer than 40% of BD patients with co-occurring SUD were receiving any kind of treatment, and such treatment was 28 times more likely to be located in a psychiatric setting than within a substance-abuse programme.[207] These circumstances severely limit conclusions and recommendations that can be offered.

In large part, lack of research-based information about treatment of BD with co-occurring SUD may arise from the long-dominant tradition of considering psychiatric and substance-use disorders as separate and distinct entities that sometimes may be 'co-morbid'. This view may seem to justify separate research and poorly coordinated clinical programmes, with a notable lack of collaborative integration of research findings and in the design and operation of treatment programmes that address both BD and SUD. That BD patients with co-occurring SUD were treated far more often in a psychiatric than a substance-abuse setting[207] adds to our impression that integration of substance-abuse expertise with comprehensive care of BD patients is uncommon. Indeed, the multiple 'co-morbid' disorder hypothesis may encourage the view that either the substance-abuse or psychiatric side of complex clinical presentations is the responsibility of 'someone else', perpetuating suboptimal or even inadequate clinical care by either psychiatric or substance-abuse experts or programmes, and confusion among non-expert clinicians. Fortunately, there are emerging indications of greater appreciation of the impact of substance abuse on BD and other major psychiatric disorders and of the need for a more collaborative and integrative approach to their study and clinical care.[18,176,206,208]

Concluding remarks

Bipolar disorder is a prevalent, lifelong, major mental illness with high risks of disability and mortality. It is symptomatically complex, changeable over time, and often associated with a range of general medical and psychiatric morbidities, notably including anxiety syndromes and substance abuse. It is unclear whether such co-occurring conditions are best considered 'disorders' that are 'co-morbid' with BD, or simply manifestations of this highly complex disorder. Co-occurring anxiety and substance abuse greatly complicate the course and outcome of BD and present major challenges for clinical management. Selective association of anxiety in BD with depressive and perhaps mixed-dysphoric states is likely, but details of the course, temporal distribution, and mood associations of particular anxiety phenomena in BD patients, and their possible associations with substance abuse all require clarification. Moreover, research supporting sound clinical guidelines for optimal treatment of BD patients who also present additional psychiatric syndromes remains surprisingly limited. Despite the importance of substance abuse in BD, there is a particularly striking paucity of detailed information about prevalence of specific kinds of substance abuse among women versus men or in types and phases of BD. There is even less information about optimal treatment based on sound therapeutic trials—in part as substance abuse is an exclusion criterion for many treatment trials. Such limitations arise in part from the long-dominant tradition of considering psychiatric and substance-use disorders as existing in separate realms, which leads to insufficiently integrated research and clinical programmes. There are indications of growing interest in the impact of substance abuse on BD and in developing more collaborative, integrative approaches to their study and clinical care.

Acknowledgements

Supported in part by a research award from the Aretæus Foundation of Rome and the Lucio Bini Private Donors Research Fund (to LT), by a grant from the Bruce J Anderson Foundation and the McLean Private Donors Research Fund (to RJB).

Disclosures

No author or immediate family member has relationships with corporate or other commercial entities that might represent potential conflicts of interest with the material reported.

References

1. Baldessarini RJ, Vieta E, Calabrese JR, et al. Bipolar depression:overview and commentary, Harv Rev Psychiatry 2010;18:143–57.

2. Forte A, Baldessarini RJ, Tondo L, Vázquez G, Pompili M, and Girardi P. Long-term morbidity in bipolar-I, bipolar-II, and major depressive disorders, J Affect Disord 2015;178:71–8.

3. Goodwin FK and Jamison KR. Comorbidity. Ch 7 in *Manic Depressive Illness*, 2nd edn (New York, NY: Oxford University Press, 2007), 223–45.

4. Tondo L, Pompili M, Forte A, and Baldessarini RJ. Suicide attempts in bipolar disorders: comprehensive review of 101 reports, Acta Psychiatr Scand 2016;133:174–86.

5. Angst J, Cui L, Swendsen JJ, et al. Major depressive disorder with sub-threshold bipolarity in the national comorbidity survey replication, Am J Psychiatry 2010;167:1194–1201.

6. Merikangas KR and Paksarian D. Update on epidemiology, risk factors, and correlates of bipolar spectrum disorder. Ch 2 in Yildiz A, Ruiz P, and Nemeroff CV(eds), *The Bipolar Book* (New York, NY: Oxford University Press, 2015), 21–32.

7. Whiteford HA, Degenhardt L, Rehm J, et al. Global burden of disease attributable to mental and substance-use disorders: findings from the Global Burden of Disease study, Lancet 2013;382:1575–86.

8. Bauer MS, Altshuler L, Evans DR, et al. Prevalence and distinct correlates of anxiety, substance, and combined comorbidity in a multi-site public sector sample with bipolar disorder, J Affect Disord 2005;85:301–15.

9. McElroy SL, Altshuler L, Suppes T, et al. Axis I psychiatric comorbidity and its relationship to historical illness variables in 288 patients with bipolar disorder, Am J Psychiatry 2001;158:420–6.

10. Crump C, Sundquist K, Winkleby MA, et al. Comorbidities and mortality in bipolar disorder: Swedish national cohort study, JAMA Psychiatry 2013;70:931–9.

11. Strakowski SM, Sax KW, McElroy SL, et al. Course of psychiatric and substance-abuse syndromes co-occurring with bipolar disorder after first psychiatric hospitalization, J Clin Psychiatry 1998;59:465–71.

12. Young AH and Grunze H. Physical health of patients with bipolar disorder, Acta Psychatr Scand 2013;Suppl 442:3–10.

13. Minnai GP, Tondo L, Salis P, et al. Secular trends in first hospitalizations for major mood-disorders with comorbid substance-use, Int J Neuropsychopharmacol 2006;9:319–26.

14. Vázquez GH, Tondo L, Undurraga J, and Baldessarini RJ. Nature and management of co-occurring psychiatric ilnesses in bipolar disorder patients: focus on anxiety syndromes. Ch 33 in Yildiz A, Nemeroff C, and Ruiz P (eds), *The Bipolar Book: History, Neurobiology, and Treatment* (New York, NY: Oxford University Press, 2015), 457–70.

15. Feinstein AR. Pre-therapeutic classification of comorbidity in chronic disease, J Chron Dis 1970;23:455–68.

16. Fortin M, Soubhi H, Hudon C, et al. Multimorbidity's many challenges, BMJ 2007;334:1016–17.

17. Salloum I and Ruiz P. Management of comorbid substance or alcohol-abuse [in bipolar disorder]. Ch 35 in Yildiz A, Ruiz P, Nemeroff CB (eds), *The Bipolar Book* (New York, NY: Oxford University Press, 2015), 487–96.

18. **Tolliver BK** and **Anton RF**. Assessment and treatment of mood-disorders in the context of substance-abuse, Dialogues Clin Neurosi 2015;**17**:181–90.

19. **Zimmerman M** and **Mattia JI**. Psychiatric diagnosis in clinical practice: is comorbidity being missed?, Compr Psychiatry 1999;**40**:182–91.

20. **Yatham LN, Kennedy SH, Parikh SV**, et al. Canadian Network for Mood and Anxiety Treatments and International Society for Bipolar Disorders (ISBD) collaborative update of CANMAT guidelines for the management of patients with bipolar disorder, Bipolar Disord 2013;**15**:1–44.

21. **Baldessarini RJ**. *Chemotherapy in Psychiatry*, 3rd edn (New York, NY: Springer Press, 2013).

22. **Baldessarini RJ, Faedda GL, Vázquez GH**, et al. Rate of new onset mania or hypomania in patients diagnosed with unipolar major depression, J Affect Disord 2013;**148**:129–35.

23. **Tondo L, Vázquez GH**, and **Baldessarini RJ**. Mania associated with antidepressant-treatment: comprehensive meta-analytic review, Acta Psychiatr Scand 2010;**121**:404–14.

24. **Vázquez GH, Tondo L, Undurraga J**, et al. Overview of antidepressant treatment in bipolar depression: critical commentary, Intl J Neuropsychopharmacol 2013;**22**:1–13.

25. **Provencher MD, Guimond AJ**, and **Hawke LD**. Comorbid anxiety in bipolar spectrum disorders: a neglected research and treatment issue?, J Affect Disord 2012;**137**:161–4.

26. **Vázquez GH, Baldessarini RJ**, and **Tondo L**. Co-occurrence of anxiety and bipolar disorders: clinical and therapeutic overview,Depression Anxiety 2014a;**31**:196–206.

27. **Chen Y-W** and **Dilsaver SC**. Comorbidity for obsessive-compulsive disorder in bipolar and unipolar disorders, Psychiatry Res 1995a;**59**:57–64.

28. **Chen Y-W** and **Dilsaver SC**. Comorbidity of panic disorder in bipolar illness: evidence from the Epidemiology Catchment Area survey, Am J Psychiatry 1995b;**152**:280–2.

29. **Goldberg D** and **Fawcett J**. Importance of anxiety in both major depression and bipolar disorders, Depress Anxiety 2012;**29**:471–8.

30. **Hernandez J, Cordova M, Ruzek J**, et al. Presentation and prevalence of PTSD in a bipolar disorder population: a STEP-BD examination, J Affect Disord 2013;**150**:450–5.

31. **Koyuncu A, Erlekin E, Binbay A**, et al. Clinical impact of mood-disorder comorbidity on social anxiety disorder, Compr Psychiatry 2014;**55**:363–9.

32. **Merikangas KR** and **Tohen M**. Epidemiology of bipolar disorder in adults and children. Ch 19 in **Tsuang MT, Tohen, MD**, and **Jones PB**(eds), *Textbook of Psychiatric Epidemiology*, 3rd edn (Oxford: Wiley-Blackwell, 2011), 329–42.

33. **Pini S, Cassano GB, Simonini E**, et al. Prevalence of anxiety disorders comorbidity in bipolar depression, unipolar depression and dysthymia, J Affect Disord 1997;**42**:145–53.

34. **Rihmer Z, Szádóczky E, Furedi J**, et al. Anxiety disorders comorbidity in bipolar I, bipolar II and unipolar major depression: results from a population-based study in Hungary, J Affect Disord 2001;**67**:175–9.

35. **Simon NM, Smoller JW, Fava M**, et al. Comparing anxiety disorders and anxiety-related traits in bipolar disorder and unipolar depression, J Psychiatr Res 2003;**37**:187–92.

36. **Angst J**. Emerging epidemiology of hypomania and bipolar II disorder, J Affect Disord 1998;**50**:143–151.

37. **Goodwin RD** and **Hoven CW**. Bipolar-panic comorbidity in the general population: prevalence and associated morbidity, J Affect Disord 2002;**70**:27–33.

38. **Hawke LD, Provencher MD, Parikh SV**, et al. Comorbid anxiety disorders in Canadians with bipolar disorder: clinical characteristics and service use, Can J Psychiatry 2013a;**58**:393–401.

39. **Hawke LD, Velyvis V,** and **Parikh SV.** Bipolar disorder with comorbid anxiety disorders: impact of comorbidity on treatment outcome in cognitive-behavioral therapy and psychoeducation, Int J Bipolar Disord 2013b;**1**:15–21.

40. **Kessler RC, Crum RM, Warner LA,** et al. Lifetime co-occurrence of DSM-III-R alcohol-abuse and dependence with other psychiatric disorders in the National Comorbidity Survey, Arch Gen Psychiatry 1997;**54**:313–21.

41. **Sala R, Goldstein B, Morcillo C,** et al. Course of comorbid anxiety disorders among adults with bipolar disorder in the US population, J Psychiatr Res 2012;**46**:865–72.

42. **Subramaniam M, Abdin E, Vaingankar JA,** et al. Prevalence, correlates, comorbidity and severity of bipolar disorder: results from the Singapore Mental Health study, J Affect Disord 2012;**146**:189–96.

43. **Angst J, Azorin J-M, Bowden CL,** et al. Prevalence and characteristics of undiagnosed bipolar disorder in patients with major depressive episode, Arch Gen Psychiatry 2011;**68**:791–9.

44. **Baek JH, Cha B, Moon E,** et al. The effects of ethnic, social and cultural factors on axis I comorbidity of bipolar disorder: results from the clinical setting in Korea, J Affect Disord 2014;**166**:264–9.

45. **Boylan KR, Bieling PJ, Marriott M,** et al. Impact of comorbid anxiety disorders on outcome in a cohort of patients with bipolar disorder, J Clin Psychiatry 2004;**65**:1106–13.

46. **Butarak SV** and **Koçak OM.** Effects of comorbid anxiety disorders on the course of bipolar disorder-I, Nord J Psychiatry 2015;**3**:1–5.

47. **Castilla-Puentes R, Sala R, Galvez E,** et al. Anxiety disorders and rapid cycling data from a cohort of 8,129 youths with bipolar disorder, J Nerv Ment Dis 2013;**201**:1060–5.

48. **Henry C, van den Bulke D, Bellivier F,** et al. Anxiety disorders in 318 bipolar patients: prevalence and impact on illness severity and response to mood stabilizer, J Clin Psychiatry 2003;**64**:331–5.

49. **Kauer-Sant'Anna M, Kapczinski F,** and **Vieta E.** Epidemiology and management of anxiety in patients with bipolar disorder, CNS Drugs 2009;**23**:953–64.

50. **Kessler RC, Berglund P, Demler O,** et al. Lifetime prevalence and age-of-onset distribution of DSM-IV disorders in the National Comorbidity Survey Replication, JAMA 2005a;**62**:593–602.

51. **Kessler RC, Brandenburg N, Lane M,** et al. Rethinking the duration requirement for generalized anxiety disorder: evidence from the National Comorbidity Survey Replication, Psychol Med 2005b;**35**:1073–82.

52. **Kessler RC, Lane M, Olfson M,** et al. Prevalence, severity, and comorbidity of 12-month DSM-IV disorders in the National Comorbidity Survey Replication, Arch Gen Psychiatry 2005c;**62**:617–27.

53. **Kim Sung-Wan, Berk L, Kulkarni J,** et al. Impact of comorbid anxiety disorders and obsessive–compulsive disorder on 24-month clinical outcomes of bipolar I disorder, J Affect Disord 2014;**166**:243–8.

54. **Paholpak S, Kongsakon R, Pattankumjorn W,** et al. Risk factors for an anxiety disorder comorbidity among Thai patients with bipolar disorder: results from the Thai Bipolar Disorder Registry, Neuropsychiatr Dis Treat 2014;**10**:803–10.

55. **Perich T, Lau P, Hadzi-Pavlovic D,** et al. What clinical features precede the onset of bipolar disorder?, J Psychiatr Res 2015;**62**:71–7.

56. **Perlis RH, Miyahara S, Marangell LB,** et al. Long-term implications of early onset in bipolar disorder: data from the first 1000 participants in the systematic treatment enhancement programfor bipolar disorder (STEP-BD), Biol Psychiatry 2004;**55**:875–81.

57. **Simon NM, Otto MW, Wisniewski SR**, et al. Anxiety disorder comorbidity in bipolar disorder patients: data from the first 500 participants in the systematic treatment enhancement program for bipolar disorder (STEP-BD), Am J Psychiatry 2004;**161**:2222–9.

58. **Shashidhara M, Sushma B, Viswanath B**, et al. Comorbid obsessive–compulsive disorder in patients with bipolar I disorder, J Affect 2015;**174**:367–71.

59. **Gao K, Wang Z, Chen J**, et al. Should an assessment of Axis I comorbidity be included in the initial diagnostic assessment of mood-disorders? Role of QIDS-16-SR total score in predicting number of Axis I comorbidities, J Affect Disord 2013;**148**:256–64.

60. **Merikangas KR and Paksarian D.** Update on epidemiology, risk factors, and correlates of bipolar spectrum disorder. Ch 2 in **Yildiz A, Ruiz P,** and **Nemeroff CV** (eds), *The Bipolar Book* (New York, NY: Oxford University Press, 2015), 21–32.

61. **Tsuang MT and Tohen M.** *Textbook in Psychiatric Epidemiology.* 2nd edn (New York, NY: Wiley-Liss, 2002), 407–20.

62. **Altshuler LL, Kupka RW, Hellemann G**, et al. Gender and depressive symptoms in 711 patients with bipolar disorder evaluated prospectively in the Stanley Foundation bipolar treatment outcome network, Am J Psychiatry 2010;**167**:708–15.

63. **Baldassano CF, Marangell LB, Gyulai L**, et al. Gender differences in bipolar disorder: retrospective data from the first 500 STEP-BD participants, Bipolar Disord 2005;**7**:465–70.

64. **Faedda GL, Serra G, Marangoni C**, et al. Clinical risk factors for bipolar disorders: systematic review of prospective studies, J Affect Disord 2014;**168**:314–21.

65. **Salvatore P, Baldessarini RJ, Khalsa H-MK**, et al. Negative affective features in 516 cases of first psychotic disorder episodes: relationship to suicidal risk, J Depress Anxiety 2013;**27**:2–13.

66. **Offidani E, Fava GA, Tomba E,** and **Baldessarini RJ**. Excessive mood elevation with juvenile antidepressant treatment in depressive versus anxiety disorders: systematic review, Psychother Psychosom 2013a;**82**:132–41.

67. **Baldessarini RJ, Tondo L,** and **Visioli C**. First-episode types in bipolar disorder: predictive associations with later illness, Acta Psychiatr Scand 2014;**129**:383–92.

68. **Freeman MP, Freeman SA,** and **McElroy SL.** Comorbidity of bipolar and anxiety disorders: prevalence, psychobiology, and treatment issues, J Affect Disord 2002;**68**:1–23.

69. **McIntyre RS, Soczynska JK, Beyer JL**, et al. Medical comorbidity in bipolar disorder: re-prioritizing unmet needs, Curr Opin Psychiatry 2007;**20**:406–16.

70. **McIntyre RS, Rosenbluth M, Ramasubbu R**, et al. Managing medical and psychiatric comorbidity in individuals with major depressive disorder and bipolar disorder, Ann Clin Psychiatry 2012;**24**:163–9.

71. **Vieta E. Colom F, CorbellaB**, et al. Clinical correlates of psychiatric comorbidity in bipolar I patients, Bipolar Disord 2001;**3**:253–8.

72. **González-Pinto A, Galán J, Martín-Carrasco M**, et al. Anxiety as a marker of severity in acute mania, Acta Psychiatr Scand 2012;**126**:351–5.

73. **Coryell W, Solomon DA, Fiedorowicz JG**, et al. Anxiety and outcome in bipolar disorder, Am J Psychiatry 2009;**166**:1238–43.

74. **Cazard F and Ferreri F.** [Bipolar disorders and comorbid anxiety: prognostic impact and therapeutic challenges (French)], Encephale 2013;**39**:66–74.

75. **Parker G.** Comorbidities in bipolar disorder: models and management, Med J Austral 2010;**193**(4 Suppl):s18–s20.

76. **Feske U, Frank E, Mallinger AG**, et al. Anxiety as a correlate of response to acute treatment of bipolar I disorder, Am J Psychiatry 2000;**157**:956–62.

77. **Gao K, Kemp DE, Conroy C**, et al. Comorbid anxiety and substance-use disorders associated with a lower use of mood-stabilizers in patients with rapid-cycling bipolar disorder: descriptive analysis of cross-sectional data of 566 patients, Int J Clin Pract 2010;**64**:336–44.

78. **Gaudiano BA** and **Miller IW**. Anxiety disorder comorbidity in bipolar I disorder: relationship to depression severity and treatment outcome, Depress Anxiety 2005;**21**:71–7.

79. **Judd LL** and **Akiskal HS**. Prevalence and disability of bipolar spectrum disorders in the US population: re-analysis of the ECA database taking into account subthreshold cases, J Affect Disord 2003;**73**:123–31.

80. **Keck PE Jr, McElroy SL, Strakowski SM**, et al. Outcome and comorbidity in first- compared with multiple-episode mania, J Nerv Ment Dis 1995;**183**:320–4.

81. **Keck PE Jr, Kessler RC**, and **Ross R**. Clinical and economic effects of unrecognized or inadequately treated bipolar disorder, J Psychiatr Pract 2008;**14**(Suppl 2):31–8.

82. **Simon GE, Hunkeler E, Fireman B**, et al. Risk of suicide attemptand suicide death in patients treated for bipolar disorder I, Bipolar Disord 2007;**9**:526–30.

83. **Angst J, Angst F, Gerber-Werder R**, et al. Suicide in 406 mood-disorder patients with and without long-term medication: 40 to 44 year follow-up, Arch Suicide Res 2005;**9**:279–300.

84. **Schaffer A, McIntosh D, Goldstein BI**, et al. CANMAT task force recommendations for the management of patients with mood-disorders and comorbid anxiety disorders, Ann Clin Psychiatry 2012;**24**:6–22.

85. **Winkler D, Willeit M, Wolf R**, et al. Clonazepam in the long-term treatment of patients with unipolar depression, bipolar or schizoaffective disorder, Eur Neuropsychopharmacol 2003;**13**:129–34.

86. **Morishita S**. Clonazepam as a therapeutic adjunct to improve management of depression: brief review, Hum Psychopharmacol 2009;**24**:191–8.

87. **Sachs GS**. Use of clonazepam for bipolar affective disorder, J Clin Psychiatry 1990;**51**(Suppl):31–4.

88. **Offidani E, Guidi J, Tomba J**, et al. Efficacy and tolerability of benzodiazepines vs. antidepressants in anxiety disorders: systematic review and meta-analysis, Psychother Psychosom 2013b;**82**:355–62.

89. **Perugi G, Frare F, Toni C**, et al. Adjunctive valproate in panic disorder patients with comorbid bipolar disorder or otherwise resistant to standard antidepressants: 3-year 'open' follow-up study, Eur Arch Psychiatry Clin Neurosci 2010;**260**:553–60.

90. **Sahraian A, Bigdeli M, Ghanizadeh A**, et al. Topiramate as an adjuvant treatment for obsessive compulsive symptoms in patients with bipolar disorder: randomized double-blind, placebo-controlled clinical trial, J Affect Disord 2014;**166**:201–5.

91. **Passmore MJ, Garnham J, Duffy A**, et al. Phenotypic spectra of bipolar disorder in responders to lithium versus lamotrigine, Bipolar Disord 2003;**5**:110–14.

92. **Perugi G, Toni C, Frare F**, et al. Effectiveness of adjunctive gabapentin in resistant bipolar disorder: is it due to anxious-alcohol-abuse comorbidity?, J Clin Psychopharmacol 2002a;**22**:584–91.

93. **Tohen M, Calabrese JR, Vieta E**, et al. Effect of comorbid anxiety on treatment response in bipolar depression, J Affect Disord 2007;**104**:137–46.

94. Hirschfeld RMA, Weisler RH, Raines SR, et al. Quetiapine in the treatment of anxiety in patients with bipolar I or II depression: secondary analysis from a randomized, double-blind, placebo-controlled study, J Clin Psychiatry 2006;**67**:355–62.

95. Vázquez GH, Tondo L, Undurraga J, et al. Pharmacological treatment for bipolar depression, Adv Psychiatr Treat 2014b;**20**:193–201.

96. Sheehan DV, Harnet-Sheehan K, Hidalgo RB, et al. Randomized, placebo-controlled trial of quetiapine-XR and divalproex-ER monotherapies in the treatment of the anxious bipolar patient, J Affect Disord 2013;**145**:83–94.

97. Gao K, Wu R, Kemp D, et al. Efficacy and safety of quetiapine-XR as monotherapy or adjunctive therapy to a mood-stabilizer in acute bipolar depression with generalized anxiety disorder and other comorbidities: randomized, placebo-controlled trial, J Clin Psychiatry 2014:75:1062–8.

98. Sheehan DV, McElroy SL, Harnett-Sheehan K, et al. Randomized placebo-controlled trial of risperidone for acute treatment of bipolar anxiety, J Affect Disord 2009;**115**:376–85.

99. Suppes T, Sheehan D, McElroy S, et al.Randomized, double-blind, placebo-controlled study of ziprasidone monotherapy in bipolar disorder with co-occurring lifetime panic or generalized anxiety disorder, J Clin Psychiatry 2014;**75**:1–00.

100. Loebel A, Xu J, Hsu J, Cucchiaro J, and Pikalov A. Development of lurasidone for bipolar depression, Ann NY Acad Sci 2015;**1359**:95–104.

101. Uguz F. Successful treatment of comorbid obsessive-compulsive disorder with aripiprazole in three patients with bipolar disorder, Gen Hosp Psychiatry 2010;**32**:556–8.

102. Fava GA, Bartolucci G, Rafanelli C, et al. Cognitive-behavioral management of patients with bipolar disorder who relapsed while on lithium prophylaxis, J Clin Psychiatry 2001;**62**:556–9.

103. Lam DH, Hayward P, Watkins ER, et al. Relapse prevention inpatients with bipolar disorder: cognitive therapy outcome after two years, Am J Psychiatry 2005;**162**:324–9.

104. Thoma N, Pilecki B, and McKay D. Contemporary cognitive behavior therapy: review of theory, history, and evidence, Psychodyn Psychiatry 2015;**43**:423–61.

105. Stratford HJ, Cooper MJ, Di Simplicio M, et al. Psychological therapy for anxiety in bipolar spectrum disorders: systematic review, Clin Psychol Rev 2015;**35**:19–34.

106. Provencher MD, Hawke LD, and Thienot E. Psychotherapies for comorbid anxiety in bipolar spectrum disorders, J Affect Disord 2011;**133**:371–80.

107. Miklowitz DJ, Otto MW, Frank E, et al. Psychosocial treatments for bipolar depression: one-year randomized trial from the Systematic Treatment Enhancement Program, Arch Gen Psychiatry 2007;**64**, 419–27.

108. Deckersbach T, Peters A, Sylvia L, et al. Do comorbid anxiety disorders moderate the effects of psychotherapy for bipolar disorder?, Am J Psychiatry 2014;**171**:178–86.

109. Singh JB and Zarate C. Pharmacological treatment of psychiatric comorbidity in bipolar disorder: review of controlled trials, Bipolar Disord 2006;**8**:696–709.

110. Pacchiarotti I, Bond DJ, Baldessarini RJ, et al. International Society for Bipolar Disorders (ISBD) task-force report on antidepressant use in bipolar disorders, Am J Psychiatry 2013;**170**:1249–62.

111. McDougle CJ, Price LH, Goodman WK, et al. Controlled trial of lithium augmentation in fluvoxamine-refractory obsessive-compulsive disorder: lack of efficacy, J ClinPsychopharmacol 1991;**11**:175–84.

112. **Pigott TA, Pato MT, L'Heureux F**, et al. Controlled comparison of adjuvant lithium carbonate or thyroid hormone in clomipramine-treated patients with obsessive–compulsive disorder, J Clin Psychopharmacol 1991;**11**:242–8.

113. **Tondo L, Burrai C, Scamonatti L**, et al. Carbamazepine in panic disorder, Am J Psychiatry 1989;**146**:558–9.

114. **Uhde TW, Stein MB, and Post RM**. Lack of efficacy of carbamazepine in the treatment of panic disorder, Am J Psychiatry 1988;**145**:1104–9.

115. **Hertzberg MA, Butterfield MI, Feldman ME**, et al. Preliminary study of lamotrigine for the treatment of posttraumatic stress disorder, Biol Psychiatry 1999;**45**:1226–9.

116. **Mula M, Pini S, and Cassano GB**. Role of anticonvulsant drugs in anxiety disorders: critical review of the evidence, J ClinPsychopharmacol 2007;**27**:263–72.

117. **Pande AC, Davidson JR, Jefferson JW**, et al. Treatment of social phobia with gabapentin: placebo-controlled study, J Clin Psychopharmacol 1999;**19**:341–8.

118. **Pande AC, Pollack MH, Crockett J**, et al. Placebo-controlled study of gabapentin treatment of panic disorder, J Clin Psychopharmacol 2000;**20**:467–71.

119. **Strawn JR and Geracioti TD Jr**. Treatment of generalized anxiety disorder with pregabalin, an atypical anxiolytic, Neuropsychiatr Dis Treat 2007;**3**:237–43.

120. **Bowden CL**. Spectrum of effectiveness of valproate in neuropsychiatry, Expert Rev Neurother 2007;**7**:9–16.

121. **Aliyev NA and Aliyev ZN**. Valproate in the acute treatment of outpatients with generalized anxiety disorder without psychiatric comorbidity: randomized, double-blind placebo-controlled study, Eur Psychiatry 2008;**23**:109–14.

122. **Vulink NCC, Figee M, and Denys D**. Review of atypical antipsychotics in anxiety, Eur Neuropsychopharmacol 2011;**21**:429–449.

123. **Bartzokis G, Lu PH, Turner J**, et al. Adjunctive risperidone in the treatment of chronic combat-related post-traumatic stress disorder, Biol Psychiatry 2005;**57**:474–9.

124. **Reich DB, Winternitz S, Hennen J**, et al. Preliminary study of risperidone in the treatment of post-traumatic stress disorder related to childhood abuse in women, J Clin Psychiatry 2004;**65**:1601–6.

125. **Bystriksky A, Ackerman DL, Rosen RM**, et al. Augmentation of serotonin-reuptake inhibitors in refractory obsessive–compulsive disorder using adjunctive olanzapine: placebo controlled trial, J Clin Psychiatry 2004;**65**:565–8.

126. **Shapira NA, Ward HE, Mandoki M**, et al. Double-blind, placebo-controlled trial of olanzapine addition in fluoxetine-refractory obsessive–compulsive disorder, Biol Psychiatry 2004;**55**:553–5.

127. **Butterfield MI, Becker ME, Connor KM, Sutherland S, Churchill LE, and Davidson JR**. Olanzapine in the treatment of posttraumatic stress disorder: pilot study, Int Clin Psychopharmacol 2001;**16**:197–203.

128. **Stein MB, Kline NA, and Matloff JL**. Adjunctive olanzapine for SSRI-resistant combat-related PTSD: double-blind, placebo-controlled study, Am J Psychiatry 2002;**159**:1777–9.

129. **Katzman MA**. Aripiprazole: clinical review of its use for the treatment of anxiety disorders and anxiety as a comorbidity in mental illness, J Affect Disord 2011;**128**(Suppl 1):S11–S20.

130. **Kessler RC, Berglund P, Demler O**, et al. Epidemiology of major depressive disorder: results from the National Comorbidity Survey Replication, JAMA 2003;**289**:3095–105.

131. **Altmaca M, Kuloglu M, Tezcan E**, et al. Quetiapine augmentation in patients with treatment resistant obsessive–compulsive disorder: single-blind, placebo-controlled study, Int Clin Psychopharmacol 2002;**17**:115–19.

132. **Denys D, de Geus F, van Megen HJ**, et al. Double-blind, randomized, placebo-controlled trial of quetiapine addition in patients with obsessive–compulsive disorder refractory to serotonin reuptake inhibitors, J Clin Psychiatry 2004;**65**:1040–8.

133. **Fineberg NA, Sivakumaran T, Roberts A**, et al. Adding quetiapine to SRI in treatment-resistant obsessive–compulsive disorder: randomized, controlled treatment study, Int Clin Psychopharmacol 2005;**20**:223–6.

134. **Gao K, Sheehan DV**, and **Calabrese JR**. Atypical antipsychotics in primary generalized anxiety disorder or comorbid with mood-disorders, Expert Rev Neurother 2009;**9**:1147–58.

135. **Pittenger C, Coric V, Banasr M**, et al. Riluzole in the treatment of mood and anxiety disorders, CNS Drugs 2008;**22**:761–86.

136. **Zarate CA Jr** and **Manji HK**. Riluzole in psychiatry: systematic review of the literature, Expert Opin Drug MetabToxicol 2008;**4**:1223–34.

137. **Sani G, Serra G, Kotziladis GD**, et al. Role of memantine in the treatment of psychiatric disorders other than the dementias: review of current preclinical and clinical evidence, CNS Drugs 2012;**26**:663–90.

138. **Ionescu D, Luckenbaugh D, Niciu M**, et al. Single infusion of ketamine improves depression scores in patients with anxious bipolar depression, Bipolar Disord 2014;**17**:438–43.

139. **Papolos D, Teicher MH, Faedda GL**, et al. Clinical experience using intranasal ketamine in the treatment of pediatric bipolar disorder/fear of harm phenotype, J Affect Disord 2013;**147**:431–6.

140. **George MS, Padberg F, Schlaepfer TE**, et al. Controversy: repetitive transcranial magnetic stimulation or transcranial direct current stimulation shows efficacy in treatment psychiatric diseases (depression, mania, schizophrenia, obsessive–compulsive disorder, panic, post-traumatic stress disorder), Brain Stimul 2009;**2**:14–21.

141. **Paes F, Machado S, Arias-Carrion O**, et al. Value of repetitive transcranial magnetic stimulation (rTMS) for the treatment of anxiety disorders: integrative review, CNS Neurol Disord Drug Targets 2011;**10**:610–20.

142. **Prasko J, Zalesky R, Bares M**, et al. Effect of repetitive transcranial magnetic stimulation (rTMS) added on to serotonin reuptake inhibitors in patients with panic disorder: randomized, double-blind, sham-controlled study, Neuroendocrinol Lett 2007;**1**:33–8.

143. **Levin FR** and **Hennessy G**. Bipolar disorder and substance-abuse. Biol Psychiatry, 2004;**56**(10):738–48.

144. **Maremmani I, Perugi G, Pacini M**, and **Akiskal HS**. Toward a unitary perspective on the bipolar spectrum and substance-abuse: opiate addiction as a paradigm, J Affect Disord 2006;**93**:1–12.

145. **Grant BF, Stinson FS, Dawson DA**, et al. Prevalence and co-occurrence of substance-use disorders and independent mood and anxiety disorders: results from the National Epidemiologic Survey on Alcohol and Related Conditions (NESARC), Arch Gen Psychiatry 2004;**61**:807–16.

146. **Tohen M, Greenfield SF, Weiss RD**, et al. The effect of comorbid substance-use disorders on the course of bipolar disorder: a review, Harv Rev Psychiatry 1998;**6**:133–41.

147. Carrà G, Bartoli F, Crocamo C, et al. Attempted suicide in people with co-occurring bipolar and substance-use disorders: systematic review and meta-analysis, J Affect Disord 2014:167:125–35.

148. Strakowski SM, DelBello MP, Fleck DE, and Arndt S. Impact of substance-abuse on the course of bipolar disorder, Biol Psychiatry 2000;48:477–85.

149. Murray CJ and Lopez AD. Global mortality, disability, and the contribution of risk factors: Global Burden of Disease Study, Lancet 1997;349:1436–42.

150. Frye MA, Altshuler LL, McElroy SL, et al. Gender differences in prevalence, risk, and clinical correlates of alcoholism comorbidity in bipolar disorder, Am J Psychiatry 2003;160:883–9.

151. Grant BF, Goldstein RB, Saha TD, et al. Epidemiology of DSM-5 alcohol use disorder: results from the National Epidemiologic Survey on Alcohol and Related Conditions III (NESARC), JAMA Psychiatry 2015;72:757–66.

152. Cerullo MA and Strakowski SM. Prevalence and significance of substance-use disorders in bipolar type I and II disorder, Subs Abuse Treat Prevent Policy 2007;2:29–38.

153. Toftdahl NG, Nordentoft M, and Hjorthøl C. Prevalence of substance-use disorders in psychiatric patients: a nationwide Danish population-based study, Soc Psychiatry Psychiatr Epidemiol 2016;51:129–40.

154. Hasin DS, Stinson FS, Ogburn E, and Grant BF. Prevalence, correlates, disability, and comorbidity of DSM-IV alcohol-abuse and dependence in the United States: results from the National Epidemiologic Survey on Alcohol and Related Conditions (NESARC), Arch Gen Psychiatry 2007;64:830–42.

155. Regier DA, Farmer ME, Rae DS, et al. Comorbidity of mental disorders with alcohol and other drug-abuse: results from the Epidemiologic Catchment Area (ECA) study, JAMA 1990;264:2511–18.

156. Cardoso BM, Kauer Sant'Anna M, Dias VV, et. al. The impact of co-morbid alcohol use disorder in bipolar patients, Alcohol 2008;42:451–7.

157. Frye MA and Salloum IM. Bipolar disorder and comorbid alcoholism: prevalence rate and treatment considerations, Bipolar Disord 2006;8:677–85.

158. Baethge C, Hennen J, Khalsa HM, et al. Sequencing of substance-use and affective morbidity in 166 first-episode bipolar I disorder patients, Bipolar Disord 2008;10:738–41.

159. Do EK and Mezuk B. Comorbidity between hypomania and substance-use disorders, J Affect Disord 2013;150:974–80.

160. Peters EN, Schwartz RP, Wang S, et al. Psychiatric, psychosocial, and physical health correlates of co-occurring cannabis use disorders and nicotine dependence, Drug Alcohol Depend 2014;134:228–34.

161. Salloum IM, Cornelius JR, Daley DC, et al. Efficacy of valproate maintenance in patients with bipolar disorder and alcoholism: double-blind placebo-controlled study, Arch Gen Psychiatry 2005;62:37–45.

162. Ostacher MJ, Perlis RH, Nierenberg AA, et al. Impact of substance-use disorders on recovery from episodes of depression in bipolar disorder patients: prospective data from the Systematic Treatment Enhancement Program for Bipolar Disorder (STEP-BD), Am J Psychiatry 2010;167:289–97.

163. Nakaya N, Kikuchi N, Shimazu T, et al. Alcohol consumption and suicide mortality among Japanese men: the Ohsaki Study, Alcohol 2007;41:503–10.

164. **Nery FG, Miranda-Scippa A, Nery-Fernandes F**, et al. Prevalence and clinical correlates of alcohol use disorders among bipolar disorder patients: results from the Brazilian Bipolar Research Network, Compr Psychiatry 2014;**55**:1116–21.

165. **Oquendo MA, Currier D, Liu S-M**, et al. Increased risk for suicidal behavior in comorbid bipolar disorder and alcohol use disorders: results from the National Epidemiologic Survey on Alcohol and Related Conditions (NESARC), J Clin Psychiatry 2010;**71**:902–9.

166. **Yoon Y-H, Chen CM, Y, H-Y**, and **Moss HB**. Effect of comorbid alcohol and drug use disorders on premature death among unipolar and bipolar disorder decedents in the United States, 1999 to 2006, Compr Psychiatry 2011;**52**, 453–64.

167. **Kerner B**. Toward a deeper understanding of the genetics of bipolar disorder, Front Psychiatry 2015;**6**:105–10.

168. **Serretti A** and **Mandelli L**. Genetics of bipolar disorder: genome 'hot regions,' genes, new potential candidates and future directions, Mol Psychiatry 2008;**13**:742–71.

169. **Kendler KS, Schmitt E, Aggen SH**, and **Prescott CA**. Genetic and environmental influences on alcohol, caffeine, cannabis, and nicotine use from early adolescence to middle adulthood, Arch Gen Psychiatry2008;**65**:674–82.

170. **Mayfield RD, Harris RA**, and **Schuckit MA**. Genetic factors influencing alcohol dependence, Br J Pharmacol 2008;**154**:275–87.

171. **Maier W** and **Merikangas K**. Co-occurrence and contransmission of affective disorders and alcoholism in families, Br J Psychiatry 1996;**30**(Suppl):93–100.

172. **Strakowski SM, DelBello MP, Fleck DE**, et al. Effects of co-occurring alcohol-abuse on the course of bipolar disorder following a first hospitalization for mania, Arch Gen Psychiatry 2005;**62**:851–8.

173. **Lejoyeux M** and **Adès J**. Evaluation of lithium treatment in alcoholism, Alcohol 1993;**28**:273–9.

174. **Pani PP, Trogu E, Pacini M**, and **Maremmani I**. Anticonvulsants for alcohol dependence, Cochrane Database Syst Rev 2014;**2**:CD008544.

175. **LeFauve CE, Litten RZ, Randall CL**, et al. Pharmacological treatment of alcohol-abuse/dependence with psychiatric comorbidity, Alcohol Clin Exp Res 2004;**28**:302–12.

176. **Weiss RD, Griffin ML, Jaffee WB**, et al. A 'community-friendly' version of integrated group therapy for patients with bipolar disorder and substance dependence: randomized controlled trial, Drugs Alcohol Depend 2009;**104**:212–19.

177. **Feingold D, Weiser M, Rehm J**, and **Lev-Ran S**. Association between cannabis use and mood-disorders: longitudinal study, J Affect Disord 2014;**172**:211–18.

178. **Agrawal A, Nurnberger JI**, and **Lynskey MT**. Cannabis involvement in individuals with bipolar disorder, Psychiatry Res 2011;**185**:459–61.

179. **Lev-Ran S, Imtiaz S, Rehm J**, and **Le Foll B**. Exploring the association between lifetime prevalence of mental illness and transition from substaznce use to substance use disorders: results from the National Epidemiological Survey of Alcohol and Related Conditions (NESARC), Am J Addict 2013;**22**:93–8.

180. **Lagerberg TV, Kvitland LR, Aminoff SR**, et al. Indications of a dose–response relationship between cannabis use and age at onset in bipolar disorder, Psychiatry Res 2014;**215**:101–4.

181. **Stone JM, Fisher HL, Major B**, et al. Cannabis use and first-episode psychosis: relationship with manic and psychotic symptoms, and with age at presentation, Psychol Med 2014;**44**:499–506.

182. Kvitland LR, Melle I, Aminoff SR, et al. Continued cannabis use at one year follow up is associated with elevated mood and lower global functioning in bipolar I disorder, BMC Psychiatry 2015;**15**:11–20.

183. Kvitland LR, Melle I, Aminoff SR, et al. Cannabis use in first-treatment bipolar I disorder: relations to clinical characteristics, Early Interv Psychiatry 2016;**10**:36–44.

184. Leite RTP, Nogueira S, do Nascimento JPR, et al. Use of cannabis as a predictor of early onset of bipolar disorder and suicide attempts, Neural Plast 2015; [ePub 13 May].

185. Van Rossum I, Boomsma M, Tenback D, et al. Does cannabis use affect treatment outcome in bipolar disorder? A longitudinal analysis, J Nerev Ment Dis 2009;**197**:35–40.

186. Gibbs M, Winsper C, Marwaha S, et al. Cannabis use and mania symptoms: systematic review and meta-analysis, J Affect Disord 2015;**171**:39–47.

187. Strakowski SM, DelBello MP, Fleck DE, et al. Effects of co-occurring cannabis use disorders on the course of bipolar disorder after a first hospitalization for mania, Arch Gen Psychiatry 2007;**64**:57–64.

188. **World Health Organization (WHO).** Cocaine. Available at: http://www.who.int/substance_abuse/facts/cocaine/en/ [accessed 23 Aug 2015].

189. Brown ES and Gabrielson B. Randomized, double-blind, placebo-controlled trial of citicoline for bipolar and unipolar depression and methamphetamine dependence, J Affect Disord 2012;**143**:257–60.

190. Glasner-Edwards S, Mooney LJ, Marinelli-Casey P, et al. Psychopathology in methamphetamine-dependent adults three years after treatment, Drug Alcohol Rev 2010;**29**:12–20.

191. Mirin SM and Weiss RD. Affective illness in substance-abusers, Psychiatr Clin No Am 1986;**9**:503–14.

192. Nunes EV, Quitkin FM, and Klein DF. Psychiatric diagnosis in cocaine abuse, Psychiatry Res 1989;**28**:105–14.

193. Weiss RD, Mirin SM, Griffin ML, and Michael JL. Psychopathology in cocaine abusers: changing trends, J Nerv Ment Dis 1988;**176**:719–25.

194. Ford JD, Gelernter J, DeVoe JS, et al. Association of psychiatric and substance-use disorder comorbidity with cocaine dependence severity and treatment utilization in cocaine-dependent individuals, Drug Alcohol Depend 2009;**99**:193–203.

195. Brown ES, Nejtek VA, Perantie DC, et al. Quetiapine in bipolar disorder and cocaine dependence, Bipolar Disord 2002;**4**:406–11.

196. Brown ES, Perantie DC, Dhanani N, et al. Lamotrigine for bipolar disorder and comorbid cocaine dependence: replication and extension study, J Affect Disord 2006;**93**:219–22.

197. Sepede G, Di Iorio G, Lupi M, et al. Bupropion as an add-on therapy in depressed bipolar disorder type I patients with comorbid cocaine dependence, Clin Neuropharmacol 2014;**37**:17–21.

198. Wignall ND and Brown ES. Citicoline in addictive disorders: review, Am J Drug Alcohol Abuse 2014;**40**:262–8.

199. Brown ES, Todd JP, Hu LT, et al. Randomized, double-blind, placebo-controlled trial of citicoline for cocaine depdence in bipolar I disorder, Am J Psychiatry 2015;**172**:1014–21.

200. Maremmani AGI, Pani PP, Canoniero S, et al. Is the bipolar spectrum the psychopathological substrate of suicidality in heroin addicts?, Psychopathology 2007;**40**:269–77.

201. **Ahmadi J, Majdi B, Mahdavi S,** and **Mohagheghzadeh M.** Mood-disorders in opioid-dependent patients, J Affect Disord 2004;**82**:139–42.

202. **Shabani A, Jolfaei AG, Vazmalaei HA,** et al. Clinical and course indicators of bipolar disorder type I with and without opioid dependence, J Res Med Sci 2010;**15**:20–6.

203. **Shariat SV, Hosseinifard Z, Taban M,** and **Shabani A.** Mania precipitated by opioid withdrawal: a retrospective study, Am J Addict 2013;**22**:338–43.

204. **Carlezon WA Jr, Béguin C,** Knoll At, and **Cohen BM.** Kappa-opioid ligands in the study and treatment of mood-disorders, Pharmacol Ther 2008;**123**:334–43.

205. **Maremmani AGI, Rovai L, Bucciardi S,** et al. Long-term outcomes of heroin dependent, treatment-resistant patients with bipolar 1 comorbidity after admission to enhanced methadone maintenance, J Affect Disord 2013;**151**:582–9.

206. **Beaulieu S. Saury S, Sareen J,** et al. The Canadian Network for Mood and Anxiety Treatments (CANMAT) task force recommendations for the management of patients with mood-disorder and comorbid substance-use disorders, Ann Clin Psychiatry 2012;**24**:38–55.

207. **Kessler RC, Nelson CB, McGonagle KA,** et al. Epidemiology of co-occurring addictive and mental disorders: implications for prevention and service utilization, Am J Orthopsychiatry 1996;**66**:17–31.

208. **Mueser KY** and **Gingerich S.** Treatment of co-occurring psychotic and substance-use disorders, Soc Work Public Health 2013;**28**:424–39.

Chapter 18

The impact of psychiatric co-morbidity in the treatment of bipolar disorder: focus on co-occurring attention deficit hyperactivity disorder and eating disorders

Anna I. Guerdjikova, Paul E. Keck, Jr, and Susan L. McElroy

Introduction

The term 'co-morbidity' was introduced in 1970 by Feinstein to describe the co-occurrence of more than one distinct clinical diagnosis. Bipolar disorder (BD) commonly presents clinically with symptoms of other, co-occurring major psychiatric illnesses, including anxiety, substance use, personality, eating, attention, and impulse control disorders. The presence of more than one psychiatric diagnosis often poses diagnostic and therapeutic challenges. This chapter will review the overlap of BD with attention deficit hyperactivity disorder (ADHD) and with eating disorders (EDs), and will discuss approaches for treating such complicated patients.

Definitions and general prevalences of ADHD and EDs

ADHD is defined by the *Diagnostic and Statistical Manual of Mental Disorder* (5th edition) (DSM-5)[1] as early onset (before 12 years of age) of persistent symptoms of inattention and/or hyperactivity and impulsivity causing impairment of daily functioning in at least two settings. In community studies, the prevalence rate of ADHD is up to 3.4% in children and adolescents and up to 2.5% in adults. Childhood ADHD severity and treatment significantly predicts persistence of ADHD into adulthood.

Anorexia nervosa (AN), bulimia nervosa (BN), and binge eating disorder (BED) are the three major types of EDs defined in the DSM-5. AN is characterized by persistent restriction of food intake leading to significantly low body weight and an intense fear of gaining weight or becoming fat. In BN, individuals engage in recurrent binge eating episodes (eating an unusually large amount of food with a sense of loss of control over eating) followed by inappropriate compensatory weight loss behaviours (such as self-induced vomiting or use of laxatives or diuretics). In addition, self-evaluation in BN is unduly influenced by body shape and weight. BED, a newly recognized DSM-5 ED, is characterized by recurrent episodes of binge eating but without the inappropriate compensatory weight loss behaviours of BN. The estimated lifetime prevalence of AN, BN, and BED (by DSM-IV criteria) are 0.9%, 1.5%, and 3.5% among women, and 0.3% 0.5%, and 2.0% among men, respectively.[2] All three EDs are highly heritable illnesses associated with decreased quality of life, increased disability, and substantial morbidity and mortality.

BD co-morbidity with ADHD and EDs

BD and ADHD

In youths with BD, ADHD has a prevalence rate of up to 48%[3] and conversely, adolescents with ADHD have an increased risk of co-morbid BD.[4] ADHD in paediatric patients with BD negatively affects symptomatology, as well as cognitive, clinical, and global functioning.[5] Among adults with BD, ADHD has a prevalence rate of up to 21%.[6] Among adult patients with ADHD, up to 20% have co-morbid BD.[7] In adults with BD, ADHD is associated with more severe symptoms and clinical course, and poor outcome of both conditions.[8]

BD and EDs

Community studies have found substantial overlap of BN and BED with BD in adults and adolescents. Among adult BD patients, the reported prevalence rates of DSM-5-defined BN, BED, and AN are 15%, 12%, and 0.2% respectively.[9] Controlled family history studies have found elevated rates of BD in the first-degree relatives of individuals with all three types of EDs. Also, a recent study found an increased risk of EDs in the offspring of parents with BD.[10]

BD patients with EDs have shown an earlier age of onset of BD, greater psychiatric co-morbidity, a more severe course of illness, and more weight disturbance than BD patients without an ED.[11-13] Conversely, the presence of BD among ED patients is associated with self-injury, suicide attempts, substance abuse, and treatment resistance of the ED.[14-16]

Presentation of BD with ADHD or an ED

ADHD and BD share numerous features in illness presentation, and thus it can be difficult to distinguish one from the other. For example, both BD and ADHD are associated with emotional dysregulation. The emotional dysregulation of ADHD encompasses a broad range of manifestations, such as affective lability, impulsivity, distractibility, irritability, and frequent mood shifts, and these symptoms also occur in BD. Moreover, BD and ADHD share symptoms such as hyperactivity, increased talkativeness, and sleep disturbances. In paediatric populations in particular, the differential diagnosis between ADHD and BD presents several challenges related to the non-episodic course of BD in youths, to the young age of onset of both disorders, retrospective collateral reports, and possible additional co-morbidities.[5] As a general guidance, the presence of prominent mood, sleep, and aggressive behaviours commonly predict BD, while fidgeting and restlessness, inattentiveness, forgetfulness, and disorganized appearance often points to ADHD. Careful diagnostic assessment over time is usually necessary in order to tease apart the two diagnostic entities and to guide treatment.

Similarly, EDs and BD share a number of symptoms related to eating behaviour and weight dysregulation. Hypomania, mania, and melancholic depression of BD are associated with decreased appetite and weight loss similar to AN, while BD atypical depression is associated with overeating and weight gain, mimicking symptoms of BED. Furthermore, community and clinical studies have shown that BD in adults and youth is associated with elevated rates of overweight and obesity. BD patients with BED or BN have more severe BD symptoms and course of illness, as well as higher mean body mass indices (BMIs) and rates of obesity.

Of note, chronic malnutrition in AN commonly results in moodiness, lack of focus, irritability, and distractibility, thus mimicking symptoms of BD or ADHD. It is thus recommended that a thorough BD versus ADHD differential diagnostic assessment is not performed in underweight patients with AN until sufficient refeeding and weight restoration is achieved.

Treatment

Psychological treatments

There have been no randomized controlled trials (RCTs) of any psychological treatment in patients with BD co-morbid with ADHD or ED. However, certain psychological interventions, briefly described as follows, hold promise when addressing co-morbid mood, attention, and/or eating dysregulation because they are effective in the treatment of BD alone, ADHD alone, or in an ED alone. In general, psychological treatments are not recommended as a monotherapy when treating BD with a co-morbid ADHD or ED and in most cases should be considered as an adjunct to pharmacotherapy.

Psychoeducation

Psychoeducation is a behavioural intervention aimed at increasing the awareness and understanding of illness aetiology, course and treatment. Some of the most helpful psychoeducational techniques focus on enhancement of symptom recognition, early detection of relapse, and treatment adherence. Psychoeducation can be part of individual therapy or applied in a group setting and can target the patient and/or his family.

RCTs have shown that psychoeducation is effective for maintenance of remission in patients with BD and leads to fewer relapses, lower hospitalization rates, and less acuity of illness, probably by enhancing treatment adherence.[17] Similarly, RCTs have shown psychoeducation-reduced symptom severity in paediatric and adult patients with ADHD and also reduced binge eating, BMI, bulimic traits, body dissatisfaction, anxiety, depression, and alexithymia in patients with BED or BN.

Cognitive behaviour therapy (CBT)

Cognitive behaviour therapy (CBT) is one of oldest and most widely used psychological interventions. The comprehensive CBT therapy model teaches patients to pause, re-evaluate, and modify thoughts contributing to maladaptive emotions and behaviours. Regular monitoring and systematic redefining of thoughts is an integral part of the process which also includes ongoing psychoeducation and implementation of environmental modification strategies (ie, organization, scheduling of activities, and problem solving).

RCTs of CBT in BD patients have shown that CBT is effective for acute depressive episodes, and among euthymic patients, for maintenance of remission.[18,19] Similarly, in controlled trials in adolescents and adults with ADHD, CBT resulted in symptom relief,[20-23] especially when combined with pharmacotherapy. Across numerous RCTs, CBT has been established as the 'gold standard' in the treatment of BN and BED and may also be helpful in some patients with AN.

Family-focused therapy (FFT)

Family focused therapy (FFT) provides psychoeducation about the disorder to the whole family. Strategies for problem solving and coping with interfamilial stress are often learned through role-playing. Several RCTs support the effectiveness of FFT for adults with BD.[3] In RCTs in paediatric ADHD, FFT improved medication compliance and ADHD symptoms and reduced family system impairment.[24] FFT is the 'gold standard' in the treatment of EDs in adolescents and young adults, particularly for AN.

Pharmacotherapy

Pharmacotherapy of BD and ADHD

In Table 18.1 and as follows we describe the four RCTs and the five open-label trials exploring treatment of BD co-morbid with ADHD that we were able to locate. All four RCTs were conducted in paediatric samples. To our knowledge, no RCTs in adults with BD and ADHD have yet been performed.

RCTs in BD and ADHD

In the first study, an eight-week open-label trial of divalproex sodium to control manic symptoms was followed by a four-week RCT trial to determine if mixed amphetamine salts were safe and effective for treatment of ADHD symptoms in children and adolescents with BD. Thirty-two (80%) of the 40 patients treated with divalproex sodium alone had at least 50% reduction in Young Mania Rating Scale (YMRS) baseline scores. Only three of these patients achieved a response in ADHD symptoms with divalproex sodium alone. Thirty patients continued in the placebo-controlled crossover trial, and mixed amphetamine salts were found significantly more effective than placebo for ADHD symptoms. No exacerbation of manic symptoms was reported during the double-blind crossover phase of the trial. One patient experienced a manic exacerbation after four weeks of taking

Table 18.1 Randomized and open-label studies of ADHD in patients with co-morbid BD

Study	Number (N) and age of enrolled patients	Drug/dose	Study duration (weeks); study design	Diagnoses	Outcome measure
Controlled Studies					
Scheffer et al., 2005[25]	N = 40 Ages 6–17 years old	Divalproex sodium (mean dose 750 mg/day at the end of OL study) with amphetamine salts (5 mg b.i.d) or placebo	8-week OL divalproex sodium followed by 4-week adjunctive crossover RCT of mixed amphetamine salts or placebo	ADHD and BD I or BD II	Significant improvement in ADHD symptoms as measured with CGI-I scale in divalproex sodium + amphetamine salts as compared with divalproex sodium + placebo
Finding et al., 2007[26]	N = 20 Ages 5–17 year old	1 week of placebo, 1 week of MPH 5 mg b.i.d, 1 week of MPH 10 mg b.i.d, and 1 week of MPH 15 mg b.i.d adjunctive to MS	4-week DB, crossover study	ADHD and bipolar spectrum disorder	Significant improvement in ADHD symptoms as measured with ADHD Rating Scale-IV and Conners' Parent Rating Scale
Tramontina et al., 2009[27]	N = 18 aripiprazole N = 25 placebo Ages 8–17 years old	Aripiprazole (final dose 13.61±5.37 mg) or placebo (final dose 15±3.22 mg)	6-week, RCT, DB	ADHD and BD I or BD II	No significant improvement in ADHD symptoms as measured with SNAP-IV
Zeni et al., 2009[28]	N = 16 Ages 8–17 years old	2 weeks each of MHP (0.3 mg/kg–0.7 mg/kg) or placebo adjunctive to aripiprazole (12.81 mg/day mean dose)	4-week, randomized crossover trial	ADHD and BD I or BD II	No significant effect of MPH over placebo on ADHD symptoms as measured with SNAP-IV was detected

(continued)

Table 18.1 Continued

Study	Number (N) and age of enrolled patients	Drug/dose	Study duration (weeks); study design	Diagnoses	Outcome measure
Open-label studies					
Wilens et al., 2003[29]	N = 36 Ages 19–57 years old	Bupropion SR (370 mg/day average dose) adjunctive to MS or antipsychotic	6-week, OL	ADHD and BD I or BD II	Significant improvement in ADHD symptoms as measured with ADHD Symptom Checklist for DSM-IV and CGI-I
Tramontina et al., 2007[59]	N = 10 Ages 8–17 years of age	Aripiprazole (final dose 11.7±5.57 mg/day)	6-week, OL	ADHD and JBD	Significant improvement in ADHD symptoms as measured with SNAP-IV
Biederman at al., 2008[32]	N = 31 Ages 4–17 years of age	Risperidone monotherapy (0.25 mg.day–2.0mg/day ages 12 and under; 0.5 mg/day–4.0 mg/day ages 13 and older)	8-week, OL	ADHD and BD I, BD II and BD NOS	Significant improvement in ADHD symptoms as measured with ADHD Rating Scale
Chang et al., 2009[33]	N = 12 Ages 6–14 years of age	Atomoxetine (59.2 mg/day mean final dose) adjunctive to MS or antipsychotic	6-week, OL	ADHD and BDI or BDII	Significant improvement in ADHD symptoms as measured with ADHD Rating Scale-IV
McIntyre et al., 2013[30]	N = 40 Ages 18–55 years of age	Lisdexamphetamine (60±10 mg/day average dose) adjunctive to MS, antipsychotic or antidepressant	4-week, OL	ADHD and BD I or BD II	Significant improvement in ADHD symptoms as measured with ADHD Self-Report Scale

MS—mood stabilizer; BD NOS—bipolar disorder, not otherwise specified; DB—double blind; OL—open label; RCT—randomized controlled trial; MPH—methylphenidate; SNAP-IV—Swanson, Nolan, and Pelham Scale-Version IV; CGI-I scale—Clinical Global Impression-Improvement scale; JBD—juvenile bipolar disorder mixed amphetamine salts during an open label extension phase of this study. The manic symptoms resolved within four weeks after mixed amphetamine salts was discontinued.[25]

In the second study, 20 euthymic children and adolescents with BD and ADHD, receiving a stable dose of at least one mood stabilizer, received one week each of placebo, methylphenidate (MPH) 5 mg twice daily, MPH 10 mg twice daily, and MPH 15 mg twice daily using a crossover design. At study's end, and before the blind was broken, a 'best dose week' for each patient was determined. During the best MPH dose treatment ADHD symptoms improved significantly as compared with placebo. Treatment with MPH was generally well tolerated and no mania exacerbations were reported.[26]

In the third study, aripiprazole or placebo was administered in a six-week RCT to acutely manic or mixed children and adolescents with BD and co-morbid ADHD. The group receiving aripiprazole showed significant improvement in BD symptoms. No significant between-group differences, however, were found in ADHD symptoms.[27]

The fourth study was a four-week RCT trial of MPH or placebo combined with aripiprazole performed in 16 children with BD and ADHD. All patients had to have a significant response of their manic symptoms with aripiprazole but still manifest clinically significant symptoms of ADHD to be enrolled. No significant differences between the effects of MPH and placebo were detected in ADHD symptoms. One patient using aripiprazole and MPH discontinued the trial due to the onset of a severe mixed episode.[28]

Open-label studies in BD and ADHD

There have been two open-label studies in adults and three open-label studies in adolescents examining various treatment agents in patients with BD co-morbid with ADHD.

In the first adult study, bupropion was given to 36 euthymic patients with BD receiving mood stabilizers or antipsychotics. ADHD symptoms improved by a mean of 55% during treatment, and hypomanic and depressive symptoms, which were mild at baseline, also improved. Treatment-emergent hypomania was documented in one patient.[29] In the second adult study, 40 patients with stable BD and co-morbid ADHD received adjunctive flexibly dosed lisdexamphetamine (LDX) for four weeks. Significant reduction of both ADHD and residual depressive symptoms were observed. No switches to mania or hypomania were reported.[30]

In the first paediatric study, aripiprazole was administered for six weeks to ten children and adolescents with BD co-morbid with ADHD. Significant improvement in global functioning scores, manic symptoms, and ADHD symptoms were detected. However, in most cases remission in either condition was not achieved.[31] In the second paediatric study, 31 children and adolescents with BD and ADHD received treatment with risperidone monotherapy for eight weeks. Although both hyperactive/impulsive and inattentive ADHD symptoms were significantly improved with risperidone, improvement was modest, and only six patients showed at least 30% reduction in ADHD rating scale scores.[32] The third paediatric study was an eight-week adjunctive trial of atomoxetine in 12 euthymic adolescents with BD and ADHD. Eight of the 12 patients were responders and six were remitters. Two patients discontinued early, one due to hypomanic symptoms at week four and one due to suicidal ideation at week two.[33]

A number of anecdotal case reports in adults with BD and ADHD have reported improvement of ADHD symptomatology on stimulants while mood is carefully managed on a mood stabilizer.[34,35]

Pharmacotherapy of BD with an ED

There have been no RCTs of medication in the treatment of BD patients with a co-morbid ED. However, there are case reports and case series of patients with BD with co-morbid AN responding to lithium;[36] BD with co-morbid BN responding to topiramate;[37] and BD with co-morbid BED responding to topiramate and lamotrigine.[38]

Isolated medications or medication classes

Because of the paucity of RCTs in BD patients with co-occurring ADHD or EDs, we review medications from various classes with preliminary evidence for effectiveness in at least two of these conditions (ie, BD and ADHD or BD and ED), as follows.

Lithium

Lithium is the oldest and best-researched agent in BD, but it has been infrequently tested in ADHD or EDs. In the only RCT of lithium in ADHD we located, lithium (up to 1,200 mg/day) and MPH (up to 40 mg/day) were compared in the treatment of core ADHD symptoms as measured with the Conners' Adult ADHD Rating Scale. Lithium and MPH produced similar improvements in hyperactivity and impulsivity, and on measures of irritability, aggressive outbursts, antisocial behaviour, anxiety, and depression.[39]

Lithium has been tested in single RCTs in the treatment of patients with AN and BN. In patients with AN, lithium was associated with significantly greater weight gain and produced significantly greater improvement on a measure of insight compared with placebo.[40] However, lithium was not efficacious in decreasing purging episodes in BN patients.[41]

Of interest, lithium augmentation of topiramate in 12 patients with BD, BED, and obesity resulted in statistically significant improvement in global severity of mood symptoms as well as reductions in weight and in binge frequency and severity.[42]

Stimulants

Stimulants, including LDX, MPH, dexmethylphenidate, and amphetamine mixed salts, are the most commonly used treatment for ADHD. Their specific mechanism of action is not completely understood but it is thought to be related to presynaptic inhibition of norepinephrine and dopamine reuptake. Stimulants show promise in the treatment of BED and BN as well. Indeed, LDX, is the only medication approved by the Food and Drug Administration (FDA) for the treatment of BED[43] and the second medication approved for the treatment of any ED after fluoxetine received approval for BN in 1996. Regulatory approval of LDX for the treatment of BED was based on a clinical development programme led by Shire Inc that included a placebo-controlled, 11-week, Phase II proof-of-concept trial, testing fixed doses of LDX 30, 50 and 70 mg/day in 217 patients, and two identically designed, placebo-controlled, 12-week, Phase III studies examining LDX 50–70 mg/day across 773 patients.[44] Statistically significant reductions in binge eating days per week, the primary outcome measure, were observed for LDX doses of 50 and 70 mg/day and the tolerability and safety profile of LDX was consistent with previous findings in adults with ADHD. In the only controlled trial, to our knowledge, of stimulants in BN, eight patients with BN received methylamphetamine or placebo intravenously followed by a test meal. Significantly fewer mean (SD) calories were consumed after methylamphetamine and 'the frequency of bulimia' was significantly lower after active drug.[45] Also, in the RCT of LDX in bipolar depression as previously discussed, LDX produced statistically greater improvement in binge eating symptoms than placebo did.[46]

In a recent review by the Canadian Network for Mood and Anxiety Treatments (CANMAT) group, MPH and amphetamine mixed salts were recommended for the treatment of ADHD in adults with BD.[47] This recommendation was based on testing MPH or amphetamine mixed salts adjunctive to mood stabilizer in two studies in adolescents with BD and ADHD, as previously discussed,[25,26] and in one open-label study in adult patients with BD depression without ADHD.[48] Indeed, case reports and open-label data suggest that stimulants might be safe and effective as an adjunctive treatment in adult bipolar depression.[49] In the only RCT we were able to locate, 25 outpatients with BD and syndromal depression received adjunctive LDX or placebo in an eight-week trial. While placebo produced similar rates of improvement in depressive symptoms, LDX was associated with a statistically significant improvement in self-reported depressive symptoms, daytime sleepiness, and binge eating symptoms.[46]

Of interest, one case report described a complicated female patient with BN, bipolar I disorder, cocaine and alcohol dependence, ADHD, and panic disorder who achieved a sustained (>1 year) remission of her BN symptoms and significant improvement of her ADHD disorder symptoms with adjunctive MPH after her bipolar, substance use, and panic disorders were successfully treated with hospitalization, intensive psychotherapy, quetiapine, and lamotrigine.[35]

Non-stimulants

Atomoxetine is a presynaptic selective norepinephrine reuptake inhibitor that is approved for the treatment of ADHD in children and adults in the United States (US). The CANMAT group considers atomoxetine a third-line option in the treatment of BD co-morbid with ADHD.[47] Anecdotal case report data in adults, including one with BD, suggested improvement of hyperactivity and distractibility on 100 mg/day of atomoxetine.[34,50]

To our knowledge atomoxetine has not been explored in AN or BN. It was been tested, however, in a ten-week RCT in 40 patients with BED. Active drug was superior to placebo in decreasing binge eating, global severity of BED, obsessive features of BED, hunger, and body weight.[51]

The literature on stimulants and atomoxetine triggering switches to a manic episode in patients with BD co-occurring with ADHD are mixed and supported by some studies,[52] while others demonstrated no mood symptoms deterioration in stabilized BD patients.[34,48,53] It is recommended that BD patients with ADHD or BED are carefully and continuously monitored for mood instability while treated with stimulants or atomoxetine and that medication is promptly discontinued if hypomanic or manic symptoms occur.

Modafinil and armodafinil

Modafinil and armodafinil are wakefulness provoking agents, structurally unrelated to amphetamine, that are approved in narcolepsy, excessive daytime sleepiness, and shift work sleep disorder. Adjunctive modafinil was compared to placebo in a six-week RCT in 85 patients with BD depression. Modafinil was superior to placebo in for reducing depressive symptoms, and active drug and placebo had similarly low switch rates to hypomania.[54] Modafinil has also demonstrated short-term efficacy in the treatment of adult ADHD in two placebo-controlled studies.[55,56] Additionally, armodafinil was tested in the treatment of BED. In a ten-week controlled trial, 60 patients with BED were treated with armodafinil or placebo. Drug and placebo produced similar rates of improvement in binge eating day frequency, but armodafinil treatment was associated with a statistically significant decrease in binge eating episode frequency, reductions in obsessive–compulsive features of binge eating, and BMI.[57]

Second-generation antipsychotics (SGAs)

SGAs have been tested in a controlled design in BD with co-morbid ADHD in adolescents, as described before, but not in adults. Olanzepine was superior to placebo for weight gain and reduction in obsessive symptoms in a small controlled study in patients with AN.[58] Quetiapine and aripiprazole have been investigated only in open-label trials in AN patients with mixed results, but might hold promise for weight restoration and reduction of obsessive–compulsive symptoms in a carefully selected group of patients with BD co-morbid with AN.[58] By contrast, there are reports of SGAs increasing binge eating behaviour and weight in patients with BED.

Antidepressants

Antidepressant monotherapy is generally contraindicated for treatment of bipolar I depression, but may be used in bipolar II depression. Of note, the CANMAT task force recommends bupropion adjunctive to a mood stabilizer as a first-line of treatment for adult ADHD co-morbid with BD based on the open-label data in adults, as previously discussed,[29] and the possible decreased risk of bupropion triggering mania compared with other antidepressants.

RCTs of antidepressants have been almost uniformly negative for weight restoration and for maintenance of weight restoration in patients with AN. In contrast, antidepressants from various classes have proven efficacious in BN and BED in RCTs. Antidepressants could be used along with mood stabilizers with a low risk of weight gain, appetite stimulation, or binge eating exacerbation in patients with bipolar II disorder and co-morbid BN or BED.

Antiepileptic agents

The thymoleptic properties of two antiepileptic agents, topiramate and zonisamide, in the treatment of patients with BD remain uncertain. Topiramate, however, was not superior to placebo in the treatment of acute bipolar mania in RCTs and its efficacy in treating bipolar depression is unknown. In contrast, in RCTs, topiramate has demonstrated efficacy in the treatment of BN, BED, and obesity and zonisamide was superior to placebo in reducing binge eating and producing weight loss in obese patients with BED.[58] These agents might thus offer promise as adjunctive treatments with mood-stabilizing agents for patients with BD and co-morbid BN and BED.

Substance abuse, misuse, and malingering

When discussing the treatment of BD co-morbid with ADHD with stimulants, the risk of undetected substance use disorder (SUD), misuse, and malingering should be noted. The prevalence of ADHD in patients with SUDs is about three times higher than in the general population and ADHD and BD are both independent risk factors for SUD. Thus, possible drug-seeking behaviour and risk for abuse should be carefully assessed in such patients. Atomoxetine might be a safer choice when treating BD patients with co-morbid ADHD and SUD, considering its lower abuse potential.

The potential misuse of prescribed stimulants in patients with suspected BD requires systematic monitoring. Extended-release stimulants have been reported to have a lower abuse potential than immediate-release stimulants and might be considered when non-stimulant medications fail to treat ADHD symptoms in ADHD with SUD co-morbidity. Malingering can be challenging to detect and it is recommended that prescribers collect diagnostic data from multiple information sources, not limited to patient self-report, to avoid misdiagnosing ADHD, when it is in fact not present. Misuse and malingering are strongly related to SUD and may be particularly frequent in BD patients with ADHD and co-morbid SUD.

Conclusion

Recognition of co-morbid ADHD and ED in patients with BD and vice versa has important implications for treatment. Comprehensive evaluation of patients with BD should include a systematic assessment for ADHD and ED and conversely, patients with ADHD and ED should be assessed for BD. Patients with BD and a co-occurring ADHD and/or ED present with multidimensional problems that most commonly cannot be treated with a single intervention. Such complicated patients often benefit from a team approach to management in order to optimize outcomes. Ideally, a team of professionals, including a psychiatrist, a therapist, and among those with EDs, a dietician, would be available to provide support for the patient and their family.

Overall, the main therapeutic goal in treating patients with BD co-morbid with ADHD or ED is selecting an agent effective in the treatment of both syndromes, or at the minimum, selecting an agent that treats one syndrome without exacerbating the other, either by therapeutic action or side effects.[36] Indeed, the use of certain antipsychotic drugs to control BD symptoms may worsen ADHD and conversely, stimulants or atomoxetine for ADHD treatment may destabilize BD. Similarly, co-morbid BED might be an important reason for weight gain and obesity in BD patients and certain mood-stabilizing and antimanic agents may further exacerbate co-morbid binge eating behaviour and weight gain. Finally, unrecognized BD in ED patients could lead to development of manic symptoms if antidepressants are used to treat BN or BED. Careful diagnosis of presenting and co-morbid conditions is the first step in successful pharmacological management of BD when co-morbid with ADHD or ED.

The treatment of BD co-occurring with ADHD can pose numerous treatment challenges and data on treatment response in adults with this constellation of diagnoses remains very limited. In addition, most pharmacotherapy studies in BD co-morbid with ADHD have been performed in children and adolescents and the results should be carefully interpreted if extrapolated to treatment in adults.

Patients with BD and ADHD should be treated for acute depressive, manic, and mixed states of BD first, before ADHD medication are begun. Indeed, initiating ADHD medications in the absence of mood stabilizers is not recommended. After proper mood stabilization, residual symptoms of ADHD should be addressed accordingly. Certain SGAs might improve both mood and ADHD symptoms, particularly in paediatric populations. Various classes of medications, including stimulants, atomoxetine, bupropion, and wakefulness provoking agents, might hold promise as adjunctive medication in improving ADHD symptoms in euthymic BD patients. Emergence of manic or mixed symptoms should be carefully monitored during treatment of ADHD, and ADHD treatment should be discontinued until BD has stabilized. Clinically, if ADHD is present or *de novo* ADHD symptoms emerge in the course of BD treatment, this should be addressed after proper stabilization of mood. Not appropriately addressing ADHD symptoms during euthymic periods may result in residual symptoms such as difficulties in attention and concentration that could contribute to the impairment in functioning frequently observed during BD remission.

Similarly, treatment of an ED in patients with BD should be done in conjunction with mood stabilization. Selecting a mood stabilizer or antimanic medication with a low risk of causing weight gain in patients with BD and a co-occurring BN or BED is often the critical first step when treating this co-morbidity. When treating BD associated with BN or BED achieving euthymia is often the first step in addressing the eating symptomatology as well. Bipolar depression and BN or BED might improve on antidepressants with a mood-stabilizing agent. Stimulants, adjunctive to mood stabilizers, might be of particular interest to consider when treating BED co-morbid with BD. When treating BD co-morbid with AN, addressing the malnutrition is the primary treatment goal, along with mood stabilization. Mania and AN might improve on lithium and certain atypical antipsychotic medication in addition to carefully monitored refeeding. If lithium is chosen, electrolytes must be carefully monitored.

In summary, BD is frequently co-morbid with ADHD or EDs and the co-occurrence of BD with ADHD or an ED results in worse outcome of both conditions. At present, data on treatment response of BD with co-morbid ADHD or ED, especially in adults, remains very limited. Further treatment research, including RCTs, of these two co-morbidities is greatly needed.

References

1. **APA**. *Diagnostic and Statistical Manual of Mental Disorders* (5th edn), 2013.
2. **Hudson JI, Hiripi E, Pope HG, Jr**, et al. The prevalence and correlates of eating disorders in the National Comorbidity Survey Replication, *Biological Psychiatry* 2007;**61**:348–58.
3. **Frias A, Palma C**, and **Farriols N**. Comorbidity in pediatric bipolar disorder: prevalence, clinical impact, etiology and treatment, *Journal of Affective Disorders* 2015;**174**:378–89.
4. **Biederman J, Faraone S, Milberger S**, et al. A prospective 4-year follow-up study of attention-deficit hyperactivity and related disorders, *Archives of General Psychiatry* 1996;**53**:437–46.
5. **Marangoni C, De Chiara L**, and **Faedda GL**: Bipolar disorder and ADHD: comorbidity and diagnostic distinctions, *Current Psychiatry Reports* 2015;**17**:604.
6. **Kessler RC, Adler L, Barkley R**, et al. The prevalence and correlates of adult ADHD in the United States: results from the National Comorbidity Survey Replication, *The American Journal of Psychiatry* 2006;**163**:716–23.
7. **Wingo AP** and **Ghaemi SN**. A systematic review of rates and diagnostic validity of comorbid adult attention-deficit/hyperactivity disorder and bipolar disorder, *The Journal of Clinical Psychiatry* 2007;**68**:1776–84.
8. **Perugi G** and **Vannucchi G**. The use of stimulants and atomoxetine in adults with comorbid ADHD and bipolar disorder, *Expert Opinion on Pharmacotherapy* 2015;**16**:2193–204.
9. **McElroy SL, Crow S, Blom TJ**, et al. Prevalence and correlates of DSM-5 eating disorders in patients with bipolar disorder, *Journal of Affective Disorders* 2015;**191**:216–21.
10. **Bould H, Koupil I, Dalman C**, et al. Parental mental illness and eating disorders in offspring, *The International Journal of Eating Disorders* 2015;**48**:383–91.
11. **Wildes JE, Marcus MD**, and **Fagiolini A**. Prevalence and correlates of eating disorder co-morbidity in patients with bipolar disorder, *Psychiatry Res* 2008;**161**:51–8.
12. **McElroy SL, Frye MA, Hellemann G**, et al. Prevalence and correlates of eating disorders in 875 patients with bipolar disorder, *Journal of Affective Disorders* 2011;**128**:191–8.
13. **McElroy SL, Crow S, Biernacka JM**, et al. Clinical phenotype of bipolar disorder with comorbid binge eating disorder, *Journal of Affective Disorders* 2013;**150**:981–6.
14. **Stein D, Lilenfeld LR, Wildman PC**, et al. Attempted suicide and self-injury in patients diagnosed with eating disorders, *Compr Psychiatry* 2004;**45**:447–51.
15. **Simpson SG, al-Mufti R, Andersen AE**, et al. Bipolar II affective disorder in eating disorder inpatients, *The Journal of Nervous and Mental Disease* 1992;**180**:719–22.

16. **Campos RN, Dos Santos DJ, Cordas TA**, et al. Occurrence of bipolar spectrum disorder and comorbidities in women with eating disorders, *International Journal of Bipolar Disorders* 2013;**1**:25.

17. **Swartz HA and Swanson J**. Psychotherapy for bipolar disorder in adults: a review of the evidence, *Focus* 2014;**12**:251–66.

18. **Jones SH, Smith G, Mulligan LD**, et al. Recovery-focused cognitive-behavioural therapy for recent-onset bipolar disorder: randomised controlled pilot trial, *The British Journal of Psychiatry: the Journal of Mental Science* 2015;**206**:58–66.

19. **Lam DH, Hayward P, Watkins ER**, et al. Relapse prevention in patients with bipolar disorder: cognitive therapy outcome after 2 years, *The American Journal of Psychiatry* 2005;**162**:324–9.

20. **Vidal R, Castells J, Richarte V**, et al. Group therapy for adolescents with attention-deficit/hyperactivity disorder: a randomized controlled trial, *Journal of the American Academy of Child and Adolescent Psychiatry* 2015;**54**:275–82.

21. **Young S, Khondoker M, Emilsson B**, et al. Cognitive-behavioural therapy in medication-treated adults with attention-deficit/hyperactivity disorder and co-morbid psychopathology: a randomized controlled trial using multi-level analysis, *Psychological Medicine* 2015;**45**:2793–804.

22. **Knouse LE and Safren SA**. Current status of cognitive behavioral therapy for adult attention-deficit hyperactivity disorder, *The Psychiatric Clinics of North America* 2010;**33**:497–509.

23. **Safren SA, Sprich S, Mimiaga MJ**, et al. Cognitive behavioral therapy vs relaxation with educational support for medication-treated adults with ADHD and persistent symptoms: a randomized controlled trial, *JAMA: the Journal of the American Medical Association* 2010;**304**:875–80.

24. **Pfiffner LJ and Haack LM**. Behavior management for school-aged children with ADHD, *Child and Adolescent Psychiatric Clinics of North America* 2014;**23**:731–46.

25. **Scheffer RE, Kowatch RA, Carmody T**, et al. Randomized, placebo-controlled trial of mixed amphetamine salts for symptoms of comorbid ADHD in pediatric bipolar disorder after mood stabilization with divalproex sodium, *The American Journal of Psychiatry* 2005;**162**:58–64.

26. **Findling RL, Short EJ, McNamara NK**, et al. Methylphenidate in the treatment of children and adolescents with bipolar disorder and attention-deficit/hyperactivity disorder, *Journal of the American Academy of Child and Adolescent Psychiatry* 2007;**46**:1445–53.

27. **Tramontina S, Zeni CP, Ketzer CR**, et al. Aripiprazole in children and adolescents with bipolar disorder comorbid with attention-deficit/hyperactivity disorder: a pilot randomized clinical trial, *The Journal of Clinical Psychiatry* 2009; **70**:756–64.

28. **Zeni CP, Tramontina S, Ketzer CR**, et al. Methylphenidate combined with aripiprazole in children and adolescents with bipolar disorder and attention-deficit/hyperactivity disorder: a randomized crossover trial, *Journal of Child and Adolescent Psychopharmacology* 2009;**19**:553–61.

29. **Wilens TE, Prince JB, Spencer T**, et al. An open trial of bupropion for the treatment of adults with attention-deficit/hyperactivity disorder and bipolar disorder, *Biological Psychiatry* 2003;**54**:9–16.

30. **McIntyre RS, Alsuwaidan M, Soczynska JK**, et al. The effect of lisdexamfetamine dimesylate on body weight, metabolic parameters, and attention deficit

hyperactivity disorder symptomatology in adults with bipolar I/II disorder, *Human Psychopharmacology* 2013;**28**:421–7.

31. **Tramontina S, Zeni CP, Pheula GF**, et al. Aripiprazole in juvenile bipolar disorder comorbid with attention-deficit/hyperactivity disorder: an open clinical trial, *CNS Spectrums* 2007;**12**:758–62.

32. **Biederman J, Hammerness P, Doyle R**, et al. Risperidone treatment for ADHD in children and adolescents with bipolar disorder, *Neuropsychiatric Disease and Treatment* 2008;**4**:203–7.

33. **Chang K, Nayar D, Howe M**, et al. Atomoxetine as an adjunct therapy in the treatment of co-morbid attention-deficit/hyperactivity disorder in children and adolescents with bipolar I or II disorder, *Journal of Child and Adolescent Psychopharmacology* 2009;**19**:547–51.

34. **Castaneda R, Levy R, Hazzi C**, et al. Treating adult attention deficit hyperactivity disorder in hospitalized psychiatric patients, *General Hospital Psychiatry* 2008;**30**:572–7.

35. **Guerdjikova AI and McElroy SL**. Adjunctive methylphenidate in the treatment of bulimia nervosa co-occurring with bipolar disorder and substance dependence, *Innovations in Clinical Neuroscience* 2013;**10**:30–3.

36. **McElroy SL, Kotwal R, Keck PE, Jr**, et al. Comorbidity of bipolar and eating disorders: distinct or related disorders with shared dysregulations?, *Journal of Affective Disorders* 2005;**86**:107–27.

37. **Barbee JG**. Topiramate in the treatment of severe bulimia nervosa with comorbid mood disorders: a case series, *The International Journal of Eating Disorders* 2003;**33**:468–72.

38. **Yamamoto T, Kanahara N, Hirai A**, et al. Lamotrigine in binge-eating disorder associated with bipolar II depression and treatment-resistant type 2 diabetes mellitus: a case report, *Clinical Neuropharmacology* 2013;**36**:34–5.

39. **Dorrego MF, Canevaro L, Kuzis G**, et al. A randomized, double-blind, crossover study of methylphenidate and lithium in adults with attention-deficit/hyperactivity disorder: preliminary findings, *The Journal of Neuropsychiatry and Clinical Neurosciences* 2002;**14**:289–95.

40. **Gross HA, Ebert MH, Faden VB**, et al. A double-blind controlled trial of lithium carbonate primary anorexia nervosa, *Journal of Clinical Psychopharmacology* 1981;**1**:376–81.

41. **Hsu LK, Clement L, Santhouse R**, et al. Treatment of bulimia nervosa with lithium carbonate. A controlled study, *The Journal of Nervous and Mental Disease* 1991;**179**:351–5.

42. **Kotwal R, Guerdjikova A, McElroy SL**, et al. Lithium augmentation of topiramate for bipolar disorder with comorbid binge eating disorder and obesity, *Human Psychopharmacology* 2006;**21**:425–31.

43. FDA. FDA approval of Vyvanse (retrieved 2/12/15).

44. **McElroy SL, Hudson J, Ferreira-Cornwell MC**, et al. Lisdexamfetamine dimesylate for adults with moderate to severe binge eating disorder: results of two pivotal phase 3 randomized controlled trials, *Neuropsychopharmacology: Official Publication of the American College of Neuropsychopharmacology* 2015.

45. **Ong YL, Checkley SA, and Russell GF**. Suppression of bulimic symptoms with methylamphetamine, *The British Journal of Psychiatry: the Journal of Mental Science* 1983;**143**:288–93.

46. **McElroy SL, Martens BE, Mori N**, et al. Adjunctive lisdexamfetamine in bipolar depression: a preliminary randomized, placebo-controlled trial, *International Clinical Psychopharmacology* 2015;**30**:6–13.

47. **Bond DJ, Hadjipavlou G, Lam RW**, et al. The Canadian Network for Mood and Anxiety Treatments (CANMAT) task force recommendations for the management of patients with mood disorders and comorbid attention-deficit/hyperactivity disorder, *Annals of Clinical Psychiatry: Official Journal of the American Academy of Clinical Psychiatrists* 2012;**24**:23–37.

48. **El-Mallakh RS**. An open study of methylphenidate in bipolar depression, *Bipolar Disorders* 2000;**2**:56–9.

49. **Dell'Osso B, Ketter TA, Cremaschi L**, et al. Assessing the roles of stimulants/stimulant-like drugs and dopamine-agonists in the treatment of bipolar depression, *Current Psychiatry Reports* 2013;**15**:378.

50. **Kraemer M, Uekermann J, Wiltfang J**, et al. Methylphenidate-induced psychosis in adult attention-deficit/hyperactivity disorder: report of 3 new cases and review of the literature, *Clinical Neuropharmacology* 2010; **33**:204–6.

51. **McElroy SL, Guerdjikova A, Kotwal R**, et al. Atomoxetine in the treatment of binge-eating disorder: a randomized placebo-controlled trial, *The Journal of Clinical Psychiatry* 2007;**68**:390–8.

52. **Post RE** and **Kurlansik SL**. Diagnosis and management of adult attention-deficit/hyperactivity disorder, *American Family Physician* 2012;**85**:890–6.

53. **Lydon E** and **El-Mallakh RS**. Naturalistic long-term use of methylphenidate in bipolar disorder, *Journal of Clinical Psychopharmacology* 2006;**26**:516–18.

54. **Frye MA, Grunze H, Suppes T**, et al. A placebo-controlled evaluation of adjunctive modafinil in the treatment of bipolar depression, *The American Journal of Psychiatry* 2007;**164**:1242–9.

55. **Turner DC, Clark L, Dowson J**, et al. Modafinil improves cognition and response inhibition in adult attention-deficit/hyperactivity disorder, *Biological Psychiatry* 2004;**55**:1031–40.

56. **Taylor FB** and **Russo J**. Efficacy of modafinil compared to dextroamphetamine for the treatment of attention deficit hyperactivity disorder in adults, *Journal of Child and Adolescent Psychopharmacology* 2000;**10**:311–20.

57. **McElroy SL, Guerdjikova AI, Mori N**, et al. Armodafinil in binge eating disorder: a randomized, placebo-controlled trial, *International Clinical Psychopharmacology* 2015;**30**:209–15.

58. **McElroy SL, Guerdjikova AI, Mori N**, et al. Psychopharmacologic treatment of eating disorders: emerging findings, *Current Psychiatry Reports* 2015;**17**:35.

59. **Tramontina S, Zeni CP, Pheula G**, et al. Topiramate in adolescents with juvenile bipolar disorder presenting weight gain due to atypical antipsychotics or mood stabilizers: an open clinical trial, *Journal of Child and Adolescent Psychopharmacology* 2007;**17**:129–34.

Chapter 19

Bidirectional relationships between general medical conditions and bipolar disorder: treatment considerations

Nefize Yalin, Danilo Arnone, and Allan Y. Young

Mortality in bipolar disorder

Bipolar disorder (BD) is one of the leading mental health diseases responsible for significant levels of disability and excess mortality.[1] All-cause mortality rates are twofold higher than the general population with an estimated reduction in life expectancy in BD in the range of 8.5–19.8 years.[2] Although excess mortality in BD has often been associated with 'unnatural' causes such as suicide or accidents,[3] recent evidence suggests that bipolar spectrum disorders are also associated with a 1.64-fold increase in mortality rates secondary to a range of 'natural' causes.[4]

In terms of specific causes of mortality in BD, the commonest conditions include circulatory disorders (eg cardiovascular and cerebrovascular), and a range of multi-system disorders which span from endocrine and metabolic to respiratory and neo-plastic.[3] Studies investigating mortality risk in patients with BD in comparison with the general population suggest a significant increase in relative risk for both men and women. More specifically for women and men respectively a 1.67–2.14 and 1.58–1.73-fold increase has been described for circulatory diseases,[5,6] 2.17–3.2 and 2.87–3.1 for respiratory system diseases,[4,6] and 2.01–2.8 and 2.47–3.2 for endocrine and metabolic conditions.[4,6] Specific medical conditions leading to mortality in BD include ischaemic heart diseases, cerebrovascular diseases, diabetes mellitus, chronic obstructive pulmonary disease, and influenza.[4,5]

Co-morbid general medical conditions in bipolar disorder

The occurrence of physical morbidity (one condition or more) is a frequent event in BD described in the range of 32.4–100% in clinical surveys.[7–10] It is believed that physical co-morbidity significantly contributes not only to the excess mortality measured in BD but also to its premature manifestation.[3]

A range of clinical and epidemiological factors are considered as predictors of higher rates of physical co-morbidity in BD. These include advancing age, female

Table 19.1 Mean prevalence of co-morbid general medical conditions in bipolar disorder

Co-morbid Condition	Mean Prevalence of Medical Co-morbidity	Range across the Studies	References
At least one co-morbid general medical condition	70.62%	32.40–100%	(7–14, 16, 18, 19)
Any circulatory diseases	16.23%	1.2–34.8%	(8, 11, 13, 14, 18, 19)
Ischaemic heart diseases	6.48%	1.2–10.6%	(9, 16, 18, 19, 21, 23)
Stroke	1.7%	1.4–1.9%	(9, 16, 19, 22)
Hypertension	21.49%	10.4–34.80%	(7, 9, 10, 12, 16, 18, 19, 23)
Diabetes mellitus type II	9.4%	Meta-analysis result	(39)
Dyslipidemia	18.64%	12.5–23.40%	(9, 16, 18, 19, 37)
Obesity	35.90%	28.9–44.4%	(11, 31-35)
Overweight	35.8%	32–39%	(31, 32, 34)
Metabolic syndrome	37.3%	Meta-analysis result	(42)
Any thyroid diseases	9.70%	4.6–14.6%	(9, 11, 12, 18)
Hypothyroidism	8.18%	6.1–10%	(9, 16, 19, 22)
Hyperthyroidism	0.3%		(19)
Any neurological diseases	19.05%	10.7–37.3%	(8, 13, 14, 19)
Migraine	34.8%	Meta-analysis result	(49)
Epilepsy	2.86%	1.8–4.2%	(12, 19, 22)
Multiple sclerosis	0.4%		(9)
Any gastrointestinal diseases	21.3%	7.3–36.4%	(8, 11, 13, 14, 19)
Peptic ulcer	8.13%	4.5–10.8%	(7, 10, 19)
Irritable bowel disease	3.65%	1.6–5.7%	(12, 22)
Any respiratory diseases	21.54%	2.9–71.82%	(8, 9, 11, 13, 14, 19)

(continued)

Table 19.1 Continued

Co-morbid Condition	Mean Prevalence of Medical Co-morbidity	Range across the Studies	References
Chronic obstructive pulmonary disease	9%	6.6–12.9%	(9, 12, 16, 19, 22)
Asthma	10.77%	3–20.1%	(9, 10, 16, 18, 19, 22)
Any infectious & parasitic diseases	7.6%		(14)
Human immuno-deficiency virus	1.28%	0.1–2.8%	(9, 14, 16, 19)
Hepatitis C virus	7.1%	1.9–13.5%	(9, 14, 19)
Any cancers	3.78%	2.8–4.5%	(12, 14, 16, 18)

sex, history of attempted suicide and physical abuse, low income, longer and more severe depressive episodes, higher duration of untreated illness, ten or more recurrences during the course of illness, childhood onset, presence of co-morbid anxiety and substance misuse disorders.[7,8,10–15] The presence of physical co-morbidity is also responsible for greater levels of disability and dependency, low levels of employment suitability, higher psychiatric consultation and hospitalization rates, and increased refractoriness for the treatment of depressive mood states.[10,11,15] Physical co-morbidities reported to occur more frequently in BD than expected in the general population include circulatory and related precursor diseases, asthma and chronic obstructive pulmonary disease, migraine, epilepsy/seizures, multiple sclerosis, gastric ulcer, irritable bowel syndrome, thyroid diseases, human immune deficiency virus (HIV) and hepatitis C virus (HCV) infection. (Table 19.1).[7,9,10,12,16,17] These are described in more detail as follows.

Circulatory and related precursor diseases

As for the general population, circulatory disorders are one of the leading causes of mortality and morbidity in BD. The reported prevalence in BD patients ranges between 1.2% and 34.8%.[8,11,13,14,18,19] These higher rates are mainly associated with accelerated atherosclerosis,[20] resulting particularly in ischaemic heart diseases and stroke as cardiovascular and cerebrovascular morbidity.[9,16] The prevalence of ischaemic heart diseases and stroke has been reported as being 1.2–10.6% and 1.4–1.9% respectively.[9,16,18,19,21–23] The National Epidemiologic Survey on Alcohol and Related Conditions (NESARC) study showed that ischaemic heart diseases are approximately five times higher in BD patients compared with controls.[23] Follow-up results of the NESARC study indicated that patients with BD were at a 2–3-fold increased risk of developing any cardiovascular disease and were diagnosed 14–17 years earlier compared with matched controls.[24] The occurrence of ischaemic strokes was also reported to be higher in BD with a 1.74-fold increased risk compared with the general population.[25]

The observation that the risk of developing ischaemic heart disease is higher in younger than older BD patients in comparison with their counterparts in general population[21] has resulted in BD being proposed as one of the moderate-risk conditions for atherosclerosis and early diagnosis of cardiovascular diseases among youth.[20] Clinical and epidemiological factors associated with greater occurrence of co-morbid cardiovascular diseases in BD include longer duration of depressive episodes,[26] female sex,[27] increased manic/hypomanic symptom burden and type I illness.[28] An anticipated earlier onset of ischaemic stroke has also been reported in BD and a greater risk of manifesting has been associated with male gender, presence of a lower socio-economic status and co-occuring medical co-morbidity.[29]

It is well established that hypertension, obesity, diabetes mellitus type II, dyslipidemia, and metabolic syndrome are leading precursor illnesses for circulatory diseases.[30]

Obesity and excess weight are frequently determined in BD in a large number of cases (28.9–44.4% and 32–39% respectively).[11,31-35] These appear to be related with pharmacological treatment of BD and occurring more frequently with advancing age.[33,34] Obesity and excess weight are also associated with a range of negative outcomes in BD, such as decreased global and cognitive functioning and life satisfaction, increased disability,[35,36] early onset of BD symptoms,[34] increased duration and hospitalization rates in depressive episodes,[33] and presence of psychiatric and medical co-morbidity.[32-34]

Higher prevalence rates of hypertension in BD are reported in several nationwide epidemiologic studies with rates varying between 10.4% and 34.80%.[7,9,10,12,16,18,19,23] There is a twofold increased hypertension risk in patients with BD compared with the general population with an earlier onset than expected.[23]

Dyslipidemia has also been shown to be more prevalent in BD patients compared with the general population with prevalence rates varying between 12.5% and 23.4%.[9,16,18,19,37] The incidence rates of dyslipidemia are approximately 1.5 times higher in the bipolar population[37] and tend to be more frequent with advancing age and in men.[37,38]

The association between BD and diabetes mellitus type II is well established. A recent meta-analysis revealed that BD patients have double the risk of diabetes mellitus type II compared with controls with a prevalence of 9.4%.[39] The presence of co-morbid diabetes mellitus in BD has been shown to be more frequent with advancing age, later age of disease onset, lower level of education,[40] a more chronic course with higher rates of rapid cycling, and non-response to lithium treatment.[41]

Metabolic syndrome, defined as a composite measure of vascular risk factors (abdominal obesity, hypertriglyceridemia, low high-density lipoprotein levels, hypertension and insulin resistance), has been reported to be twofold higher in BD patients compared with controls with a prevalence of 37.3%.[42] Similarly to other degenerative vascular risk factors, metabolic syndrome is more frequent with advancing age[43] and antipsychotic treatment[42] and it results in a number of negative clinical outcomes, including higher number of hospitalizations[44] and history of suicide attempts.[45]

Thyroid diseases

Thyroid diseases have consistently been reported as more common in BD compared with the general population with reported prevalence rates between 4.6% and 14.6%.[9,11,12,18] These higher rates are mainly attributable to hypothyroidism with prevalence rates between 6.1% and 10%[9,16,19,22] while prevalence of hyperthyroidism is as low as 0.3%.[22]

The prevalence of thyroid diseases in BD is related with poorer response to standard treatments and more frequent with advancing age and in women.[46] In particular, hypothyroidism is associated with negative clinical outcomes in BD including rapid cycling and cognitive decline.[47,48]

Neurologic diseases

Migraine, epilepsy/seizures, and multiple sclerosis are the most frequently reported co-morbid neurological disorders in BD patients.[17] A recent meta-analysis suggests a pooled prevalence of migraine as high as 34.8% in BD with higher rates of co-morbidity in type II rather than type I disorders.[49] Of importance, migraine appears to cluster with greater frequency with other physical co-morbidities in BD[50] and is associated with lower economic status[51] and a range of negative outcomes including earlier age at onset,[51] more severe and frequent depressive episodes,[50] co-morbid anxiety disorders, and suicidal behaviour.[51]

Prevalence of multiple sclerosis and epilepsy in BD patients is reported to be higher than the general population with rates between 0.4% and 1.8–4.2% respectively.[9,12,19,22] Nationwide cohort studies indicate a four-times higher risk for epilepsy[52] and two-times higher risk for multiple sclerosis[53] in BD. More studies are warranted in this area to understand the temporal relationship and the impact of these diseases on BD course.

Gastrointestinal and respiratory diseases

The prevalence of any gastrointestinal co-morbidity is reported to be between 7.3% and 36.4% in BD.[8,11,13,14,19] Peptic ulcer and irritable bowel syndrome are the leading causes of these higher rates with a prevalence of 4.5–10.8%[7,10,19] and 1.6–5.7%[12,22] respectively.

The prevalence of pulmonary diseases in BD has been reported between 2.9% and 71.82% with a mean rate of approximately 20%.[8,9,11,13,14,19] Asthma and chronic obstructive pulmonary disease contribute the most with prevalence rates of 3–20.1%[9,10,16,18,19,22] and 6.6–12.9%[9,12,16,19,22] respectively.

Despite the significant prevalence of these conditions in BD, there is paucity of studies available. Longitudinal studies are warranted to better understand the temporal association of gastrointestinal and respiratory diseases with BD.

Infectious diseases

Individuals with BD are at risk of infectious diseases largely due to substance use disorders (SUDs) and high-risk sexual behaviours.[17] The overall prevalence of infectious and parasitic diseases is reported as 7.6% in BD.[14] HIV and HCV infection are the most frequent infectious diseases co-morbid to BD. Prevalence rates for HIV and HCV infection are reported between 0.1% and 2.8% and 1.9% and 13.5% respectively.[9,14,16,19] HIV infection in BD is associated with an escalation in clinically significant cognitive decline,[54] enhanced impairment in daily functioning,[54] and decreased adherence to treatment for both HIV and BD.[55] Further studies are necessary to investigate the link between BD and infectious diseases.

Neoplastic diseases

Thus far, studies conducted on the co-morbidity between cancer and BD have reached inconsistent results with different prevalence rates ranging between 2.8% and 4.5%.[12,14,16,18] Although some nationwide cohort studies have reported no increased risk of neoplastic morbidity,[5] other studies have suggested a 1.39 to 2.6-times higher overall cancer risk in BD patients.[56,57] Notably, a significant increase of female-hormone-regulated cancers such as breast, cervical, and uterine cancers and tobacco and alcohol-related cancers is shown in patients with BD.[56]

Underlying causes of elevated co-morbidity between general medical conditions and bipolar disorder

The increased prevalence of medical conditions and related higher mortality reported in BD are most likely a multifactorial phenomenon driven by both multiple causality and possible bilateral directionality (Figure 19.1). Bipolar illness has been reported

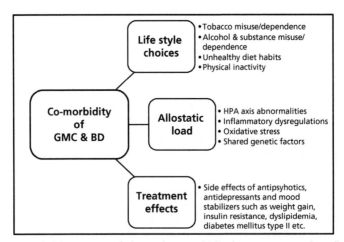

Figure 19.1 Underlying causes of elevated co-morbidity between general medical conditions (GMCs) and bipolar disorder (BD)

to contribute to the worsening of physical health and of pre-existing general medical conditions as well as associated with newly developed physical disorders during the course of the illness itself.[58,59]

Lifestyle choices

Detrimental lifestyle choices impacting on physical health such as increased tobacco consumption, a sedentary lifestyle, substance misuse, and unhealthy diet habits have been described in BD.[58]

Tobacco use is a known cause of highly co-morbid medical conditions in BD, including different types of cancers, circulatory and respiratory diseases, diabetes mellitus, and peptic ulcer.[60] Lifetime smoking rates in BD are approximately 3.5 times increased and patients tend to be more nicotine dependent and have lower cessation rates compared with the general population.[61]

Substance and alcohol use disorders are known risk factors for cancers, diabetes mellitus, hypertension, circulatory, respiratory, liver, and sexually transmitted diseases.[62] The co-morbidity of any substance use is very common in BD with a lifetime prevalence rate of approximately 50%.[63]

Physical inactivity and unhealthy dietary choices contribute to the development of circulatory and related diseases and diabetes mellitus.[64] It has been shown that patients with BD are more likely to report poor exercise habits and suboptimal eating behaviours, such as infrequent walking, less than two regular daily meals, and having difficulty in obtaining or cooking food.[64]

In conclusion, there is an established relationship between BD and day-to-day lifestyle choices that might inadvertently increase health hazards, thus predisposing to general medical conditions with increased frequency compared with the general population.

Allostatic load and bipolar disorder

The over-activity of physiological systems in an effort to adapt to environmental challenges has been described in the literature as 'allostatic load' resulting in 'nitrosative' stress affecting a range of bodily functions, resulting in DNA damage, endothelial dysfunction, decrease in inflammatory response, and telomere shortening.[65,66] Furthermore, allostatic load leading to a more frequent occurrence of oxidative phenomena across body systems is believed to contribute to the onset or to the accelerated evolution of the wide range of medical conditions observed in BD with a higher frequency compared with the general population.[65,66] Hence, this line of research suggests that the overall risk of developing or worsening of common medical conditions, such as cardiovascular disease, might be influenced by factors intrinsic to the adaptive pathophysiology of BD which are likely to be particularly evident in more severe forms of the illness.[66-68]

Neuropsychological stress is often described in clinical presentations of BD in conjunction with a heightened function of the hypothalamic pituitary adrenal (HPA) axis. Stress can affect glucocorticoid signalling and cardio-metabolic physiological responses so that excessive HPA axis activity can increase the allostatic load in BD inducing obesity, insulin resistance, glucose intolerance, dyslipidemia, hypertension, and telomere shortening.[69] Telomere shortening, considered a proxy for aging, has been associated with general medical conditions in BD possibly related to physical degeneration.[17,65] A higher allostatic load might contribute to explain the increased risk of mortality, cognitive impairment, and a general decline in physical functioning, including cardiovascular diseases, as shown in longitudinal population studies.[67] It has been shown that intracellular glucocorticoid and mineralocorticoid receptors share complex interactions with hetero-dimers, co-activators, and co-repressors cascading into genetic and epigenetic modifications affecting transcription factors in approximately 30% of genes affecting a range of biological functions.[69] Furthermore, there is evidence for exaggerated HPA-axis activity in BD synergistic with an overactive inflammatory system. For example, it has been shown that a blunted neuroendocrine response can coexist with T cells glucocorticoid receptor resistance and increased lymphocyte signalling following a stress challenge.[70,71] These studies support the notion that allostatic load, modulated by the contributions of multiple system interactions, might be contributing not only to the pathogenesis of BD but also to co-morbid general medical conditions.[65] For instance, the role of the immune system and a pro-inflammatory response in BD has recently been investigated as an independent contributing factor not only to the aetiology of the disorder but also as a potential independent variable to the development of general medical conditions.[66] Inflammation is implicated in mechanisms involved in endothelial dysfunction, plaque formation, and related complications (eg rupture and thrombosis), atherosclerosis, hypertension, diabetes, and obesity.[68] It has also been shown that aberrant inflammatory processes take place in the central nervous system and in the periphery of individuals with BD.[67,68] Early reports of higher presentations of autoimmune conditions in BD (eg autoimmune thyroiditis)[72] have now expanded into the observation of accentuated responses in a range of components of the immune system.[73] These include markers of systemic inflammation (eg high-sensitivity C-reactive protein (hsCRP)), linked with an increased risk of developing atherogenesis and plaque formation[68] and also peripheral cytokines. Increases in peripheral levels of hsCRP have been demonstrated in bipolar mania.[74] Peripheral pro-inflammatory cytokines such as interleukin (IL) 2 and 4 have been shown to be elevated in BD in the manic phase, while IL 6 has been shown to be preferentially elevated in the depressed state of BD.[75] Furthermore IL 2, 6, and tumour necrosis factor (TNF) receptor availability in BD have been shown to correlate with body mass index, leptin circulating levels, circulating lipids, and medication status.[76] Other peripheral inflammatory markers shown to be increased in BD include TNF α, IL 1, 4, and 8.[65,66]

In summary, allostatic load (ie, expression of adaptive changes occurring in BD) could further contribute to not just the pathogenesis of mood disorders but also the biological underpinnings of the high frequency of general medical conditions, particularly in relation to atherosclerosis and vascular disorders. Another important clinical phenomenon is the observation of the presence of cognitive impairment with illness progression also potentially associated with allostatic load.[77] Recent research findings suggest a correlation between general medical conditions and cumulative measures of illness burden (eg greater chronicity and higher number of episodes[65,77]).

Pharmacological treatment

The excess of general medical conditions and mortality associated with BD antecede modern psychopharmacology. Nevertheless, some pharmacological treatments have the potential to increase the risk of developing or worsening general medical conditions in view of their association with metabolic and endocrine effects, weight gain (defined as a minimum of ≥7% increase compared with baseline weight), obesity, diabetes mellitus type II and cardiovascular diseases.[78-80] Recognized contributory factors include the dose of the psychotropic drugs, concurrent medications and their side effects and potential interactions, diet, lifestyle, and physical activity levels.[81] Examples of compounds used as first-and second-line treatment options in BD treatment and their common potential contribution to general medical conditions are described as follows.

Lithium

Lithium is widely used in the treatment of BD and it is associated with impaired nephrogenic functions, hypothyroidism, hyperparathyroidism, and weight gain in terms of major adverse effects.[82]

Clinical hypothyroidism is nearly six times higher and thyroid-stimulating hormone increases on average by 4.00 iU/mL in lithium-treated patients compared with placebo.[82] Lithium-induced hypothyroidism is more prevalent in women and most of the patients are diagnosed in the first years of lithium treatment.[82] Lithium treatment also causes a 10% increase in calcium and parathyroid hormone in patients with normal baseline levels compared with controls.[82]

Reduced glomerular filtration rate by –6.22 mL/min to –10.3 mL/min and urinary concentrating ability by 15% of normal maximum were shown in lithium-treated patients.[82] Although these impairments may not be clinically significant in most of the patients, progress to nephrogenic diabetes insipidus and chronic interstitial nephropathy are seen in some cases.[80] However, end-stage renal disease is rare but may occur after long-term lithium treatment.[80]

Weight gain in lithium-treated patients is described as a dose-dependent side effect, particularly evident in the first two years of treatment, and is present in more than 70% of treated individuals with 30% reaching obesity.[79] Animal studies have indicated that this effect is mediated by an increase in glucagon release and consequent hypoinsulinemic and hyperglycaemic effects.[83] This phenomenon has been shown to be particularly pronounced in case of insulin resistance, so that effective glycaemic control is particularly important in diabetic bipolar patients treated with lithium.[83] As the weight gain effects of lithium appear dose-dependent, plasma lithium levels below 0.8 mmol/l are less likely to cause metabolic perturbation.[79]

Sodium valproate

Sodium valproate has been associated with weight gain in 3–20% of people treated[79] and body weight increases occur as early as after two to three months of treatment and may continue without plateau for months or years throughout treatment.[80] Maintenance serum levels have been described in the range of 85 +/– 30 μ/ml for divalproex and levels above 125 μ/ml have been associated with more frequently occurring weight gain suggesting the importance of considering the minimum effective dose (especially in prophylaxis) to minimize the occurrence of dose-related side effects.[79,84] Valproate treatment is also associated with higher plasma insulin levels indicating possible development of insulin resistance, higher triglyceride and lower HDL-C levels as dyslipidemic disturbances distinct from weight gain effects.[85]

Second-generation antipsychotics with mood-stabilizing properties

Second-generation antipsychotics, increasingly used in the treatment of BD, have been associated with weight gain, insulin resistance, diabetes mellitus, and also hyperlipidemia, which in turn potentially contributing to sensitizing patients to overall metabolic dysregulation.[78] Clozapine and olanzapine are considered the greatest contributors, followed by quetiapine, risperidone, paliperidone, and asenapine as moderate contributors to weight gain.[78] Aripiprazole, lurasidone, and ziprasidone generally associated with body weight effect of a smaller magnitude.[78] Olanzapine-induced weight gain has been shown to be common and in the range of 2.5 kg in efficacy studies in bipolar mania, of a greater magnitude of sodium valproate, and more pronounced when used as adjuvant treatment rather than monotherapy (20% vs 6%).[79] Weight increase associated with quetiapine administration has been described to be equivalent to 7% of the initial body weight, in the range of 2.6 kg in treatment studies in bipolar mania,[86] and of a similar magnitude to sodium valproate.[79] Efficacy studies indicate that clozapine's metabolic effects tend to be progressive over longer periods of duration of treatment resulting in 10–20% increments of initial pre-treatment weight.[79,87] Risperidone-induced weight gain shown in RCTs appears to be less significant compared with other similar antipsychotics with a mean increase in weight equivalent to 2.9 kg compared with 4.45 kg for clozapine, and 4.15 kg for olanzapine.[79,88] Treatment studies suggest that asenapine weight gain is four-times higher and paliperidone is two-times higher compared with placebo, in the range of 7% increase, significant in the first three months of treatment and progressive for a year.[89] Metabolic effects of ziprasidone and aripiprazole have been shown to be minimal[90, 91] and these two compounds should be considered as an option when a relatively more weight neutral compound is indicated.[92]

Second-generation antipsychotics are also risk factors for lipid abnormalities and diabetes mellitus. Clozapine and olanzapine are associated with the highest risk for lipid abnormalities and diabetes mellitus followed by quetiapine.[78,92] Effects of the other second-generation antipsychotics on lipid and glucose metabolism are reported to be mild or minimal.[78,89]

All antipsychotics have the potential to reduce the seizure threshold and increase the risk of sudden cardiac death in a dose-related fashion most likely related to their propensity to increase the corrected QT interval.[78] This risk should be always taken into account and particularly in cases of family histories of sudden cardiac death.[78]

Lamotrigine

Clinical studies in lamotrigine treated BD patients suggest weight changes similar to placebo-treated groups both in monotherapy and as adjunctive treatment.[79] It follows that the impact of lamotrigine on weight gain and body metabolism is generally considered minimal and this compound can be useful in case of medical co-morbidity when clinically indicated.[79]

Carbamazepine

The association between carbamazepine and weight gain is mostly based on epilepsy studies rather than observations in bipolar patients and indicates possible weight gain in treated patients.[79] Potential mechanisms for weight gain include appetite stimulation, fluid retention, changes in lipid profile and oedema.[79]

Antidepressants

Antidepressants are not the treatment of choice in BD despite being not uncommonly co-prescribed with mood stabilizers in the treatment of bipolar depression. Among the antidepressants often prescribed in BD, selective serotonin re-uptake inhibitors (SSRIs) have been associated with weight loss in the acute treatment phase (aside paroxetine which has been linked with weight gain) and weight gain is described in SSRIs maintenance phase.[79,93] Bupropion has been associated with weight loss and venlafaxine is believed not to cause significant weight variations.[79,93] Mirtazapine and tricyclic antidepressants are known to induce weight gain.[79,93] Furthermore, venlafaxine is frequently associated with dose-dependent hypertension and tricyclic antidepressants and bupropion are known for epileptogenic potential.[94,95]

Treatment implications

Minimizing health risks

Management of lifestyle choices which cause health risks is most advisable. Smoking, unhealthy diets, and a sedentary lifestyle can be modified with targeted interventions which can include simple education of patients and carers, and participation in more complex behavioural programmes for cessation of smoking and/or substance misuse and dietary advise.[78,96]

Assessment and monitoring of physical health

It is important to systematically assess the health of individuals with BD. This is particularly relevant when psychotropic medication is prescribed and imperative when physical health is likely to be affected.[78] This should be conducted in conjunction with assessing generic and specific lifestyle risks and use of substances (eg smoking, alcohol use, etc). This aspect of care is important to emphasize in view of the evidence of healthcare disparities in mental health.[97]

In order to establish concomitant risk factors, personal and family histories can help to detect the presence of diabetes mellitus, high blood pressure, and vascular diseases including ischaemic events.[78] Relevant prescribed medication should be assessed for potential interactions and potentiation of metabolic effects. Baseline measures should include weight measurement, blood pressure, and waist circumference.[78,98] With regard to weight measurement, waist circumference appears to be a better predictor than body mass index for insulin resistance, hyperlipidemia, and hypertension.[78] Full blood count, fasting glucose, fasting lipid profile, electrolytes, liver enzymes, serum bilirubin and creatinine, prothrombin time and partial thromboplastin time, eGFR, urinanalysis, urine toxicology for substance use, thyroid stimulating hormone, and prolactin levels should be performed before initiation of psychotropic treatment for BD.[98] Abnormalities in haemoglobin A1c (HbA1c) has been suggested as a more sensitive approach to detect patients likely to develop diabetes and its measurement can be added to routine analyses.[99] Baseline electrocardiography should complete the assessment especially in cases of patients with risk factors such as QTc prolongation, arrhythmias, and family history of sudden cardiac death.[78,98]

Health monitoring is an essential component of the management of BD and should be part of a regular comprehensive programme of regular medical follow-ups on a yearly basis.[96] With regard to pharmacological management, in the absence of any abnormalities detected at baseline, good practice suggests a minimum frequency of follow-ups at six weeks, three months, and six months after baseline assessment and on yearly basis subsequently. If risk factors are identified at baseline and/or abnormalities are detected, the frequency may vary in relation to specific needs of the individual with a tendency to be more frequent.[78] Electrocardiography is also tailored on individual needs such as the presence of significant abnormalities, history or risks of sudden cardiac death, and specialist advice.[78]

Pharmacological optimization

It is essential that pharmacological prescribing is tailored on specific patients' needs by taking into account any significant general medical condition. Consideration should be given to minimizing poly-pharmacy and pharmacological potentiation of unwanted effects by combining psychotropic drugs with compounds which could increase health-risk parameters. In case of significant general medical problems or in the presence of significant health risks, it is generally advisable to switch to compounds with the least effect on metabolism, weight, and cardiac conductivity.[78]

Pharmacological management of general medical conditions

Similar to the general population, specific treatments to address general medical conditions including statins, antihypertensive treatment, and hypoglycaemic drugs might be indicated, especially in cases when lifestyle changes have not proven sufficiently effective to obtain normalization.[78]

Conclusion

In summary, BD is associated with an excess of medical conditions and increased premature mortality compared with the general population. Awareness of medical co-morbidity and a systematic approach to the physical needs of patients are important components of the treatment provided. Attention to modifiable risk factors and pharmacological optimization can help, improving clinical outcome and quality of life of patients. It is important for future studies to devote attention to the physical health of patients and to consider longitudinal designs and operationalized criteria to systematically evaluate physical health and its temporal relationship with the onset and progression of mood symptoms, and factors implicated in improving outcome of medical morbidity in BD.

References

1. Whiteford HA, Degenhardt L, Rehm J, Baxter AJ, Ferrari AJ, Erskine HE, et al. Global burden of disease attributable to mental and substance use disorders: findings from the Global Burden of Disease Study 2010, *Lancet* 2013;**382**:1575–86.

2. Chesney E, Goodwin GM, and Fazel S. Risks of all-cause and suicide mortality in mental disorders: a meta-review, *World Psychiatry: Official Journal of the World Psychiatric Association* 2014;**13**:153–60.

3. Roshanaei-Moghaddam B and Katon W. Premature mortality from general medical illnesses among persons with bipolar disorder: a review, *Psychiatric Services* 2009;**60**:147–56.

4. Osby U, Brandt L, Correia N, Ekbom A, and Sparen P. Excess mortality in bipolar and unipolar disorder in Sweden, *Archives of General Psychiatry* 2001;**58**:844–50.

5. Crump C, Sundquist K, Winkleby MA, and Sundquist J. Comorbidities and mortality in bipolar disorder: a Swedish national cohort study, *JAMA Psychiatry* 2013;**70**:931–9.

6. Laursen TM, Munk-Olsen T, Nordentoft M, and Mortensen PB. Increased mortality among patients admitted with major psychiatric disorders: a register-based study comparing mortality in unipolar depressive disorder, bipolar affective disorder, schizoaffective disorder, and schizophrenia, *The Journal of Clinical Psychiatry* 2007;**68**:899–907.

7. Perron BE, Howard MO, Nienhuis JK, Bauer MS, Woodward AT, and Kilbourne AM. Prevalence and burden of general medical conditions among adults with bipolar I disorder: results from the National Epidemiologic Survey on Alcohol and Related Conditions, *The Journal of Clinical Psychiatry* 2009;**70**:1407–15.

8. Kemp DE, Gao K, Ganocy SJ, Caldes E, Feldman K, Chan PK, et al. Medical and substance use comorbidity in bipolar disorder, *Journal of Affective Disorders* 2009;**116**:64–9.

9. Kilbourne AM, Cornelius JR, Han X, Pincus HA, Shad M, Salloum I, et al. Burden of general medical conditions among individuals with bipolar disorder, *Bipolar Disorders* 2004;**6**:368–73.

10. McIntyre RS, Konarski JZ, Soczynska JK, Wilkins K, Panjwani G, Bouffard B, et al. Medical comorbidity in bipolar disorder: implications for functional outcomes and health service utilization, *Psychiatric Services* 2006;**57**:1140–4.

11. Thompson WK, Kupfer DJ, Fagiolini A, Scott JA, and Frank E. Prevalence and clinical correlates of medical comorbidities in patients with bipolar I disorder: analysis of acute-phase data from a randomized controlled trial, *The Journal of Clinical Psychiatry* 2006;**67**:783–8.

12. Smith DJ, Martin D, McLean G, Langan J, Guthrie B, and Mercer SW. Multimorbidity in bipolar disorder and undertreatment of cardiovascular disease: a cross sectional study, BMC Med 2013;**11**:263.

13. Maina G, Bechon E, Rigardetto S, and Salvi V. General medical conditions are associated with delay to treatment in patients with bipolar disorder, *Psychosomatics* 2013;**54**:437–42.

14. Beyer J, Kuchibhatla M, Gersing K, and Krishnan KR. Medical comorbidity in a bipolar outpatient clinical population, *Neuropsychopharmacology* 2005;**30**:401–4.

15. Kemp DE, Gao K, Chan PK, Ganocy SJ, Findling RL, and Calabrese JR. Medical comorbidity in bipolar disorder: relationship between illnesses of the endocrine/metabolic system and treatment outcome, *Bipolar Disorders* 2010;**12**:404–13.

16. Carney CP and Jones LE. Medical comorbidity in women and men with bipolar disorders: a population-based controlled study, *Psychosomatic Medicine* 2006;**68**:684–91.

17. McIntyre RS, Soczynska JK, Beyer JL, Woldeyohannes HO, Law CW, Miranda A, et al. Medical comorbidity in bipolar disorder: re-prioritizing unmet needs, *Current Opinion in Psychiatry* 2007;**20**:406–16.

18. Sylvia LG, Shelton RC, Kemp DE, Bernstein EE, Friedman ES, Brody BD, et al. Medical burden in bipolar disorder: findings from the Clinical and Health Outcomes Initiative in Comparative Effectiveness for Bipolar Disorder study (Bipolar CHOICE), *Bipolar Disorders* 2015;**17**:212–23.

19. Fenn HH, Bauer MS, Altshuler L, Evans DR, Williford WO, Kilbourne AM, et al. Medical comorbidity and health-related quality of life in bipolar disorder across the adult age span, *Journal of Affective Disorders* 2005;**86**:47–60.

20. Goldstein BI, Carnethon MR, Matthews KA, McIntyre RS, Miller GE, Raghuveer G, et al. Major depressive disorder and bipolar disorder predispose youth to accelerated atherosclerosis and early cardiovascular disease: a scientific statement from the American Heart Association, *Circulation* 2015;**132**:965–86.

21. Huang KL, Su TP, Chen TJ, Chou YH, and Bai YM. Comorbidity of cardiovascular diseases with mood and anxiety disorder: a population based 4-year study, *Psychiatry and Clinical Neurosciences* 2009;**63**:401–9.

22. Schoepf D and Heun R. Bipolar disorder and comorbidity: increased prevalence and increased relevance of comorbidity for hospital-based mortality during a 12.5-year observation period in general hospital admissions, *Journal of Affective Disorders* 2014;**169**:170–8.

23. Goldstein BI, Fagiolini A, Houck P, and Kupfer DJ. Cardiovascular disease and hypertension among adults with bipolar I disorder in the United States, *Bipolar Disorders* 2009;**11**:657–62.

24. Goldstein BI, Schaffer A, Wang S, and Blanco C. Excessive and premature new-onset cardiovascular disease among adults with bipolar disorder in the US NESARC cohort, *The Journal of Clinical Psychiatry* 2015;**76**:163–9.

25. Prieto ML, Cuellar-Barboza AB, Bobo WV, Roger VL, Bellivier F, Leboyer M, et al. Risk of myocardial infarction and stroke in bipolar disorder: a systematic review and exploratory meta-analysis, *Acta Psychiatrica Scandinavica* 2014;**130**:342–53.

26. Fiedorowicz JG, Jancic D, Potash JB, Butcher B, and Coryell WH. Vascular mortality in participants of a bipolar genomics study, *Psychosomatics* 2014;**55**:485–90.

27. Fiedorowicz JG, He J, and Merikangas KR. The association between mood and anxiety disorders with vascular diseases and risk factors in a nationally representative sample, J Psychosom Res 2011;**70**:145–54.

28. Fiedorowicz JG, Solomon DA, Endicott J, Leon AC, Li C, Rice JP, et al. Manic/ hypomanic symptom burden and cardiovascular mortality in bipolar disorder, *Psychosomatic Medicine* 2009;**71**:598–606.

29. Wu HC, Chou FH, Tsai KY, Su CY, Shen SP, and Chung TC. The incidence and relative risk of stroke among patients with bipolar disorder: a seven-year follow-up study, *PLoS One* 2013;**8**:e73037.

30. National Cholesterol Education Program Expert Panel on Detection E, Treatment of High Blood Cholesterol in A. Third Report of the National Cholesterol Education Program (NCEP) Expert Panel on Detection, Evaluation, and Treatment of High Blood Cholesterol in Adults (Adult Treatment Panel III) final report, *Circulation* 2002;**106**:3143–421.

31. de Almeida KM, de Macedo-Soares MB, Kluger Issler C, Antonio Amaral J, Caetano SC, da Silva Dias R, et al. Obesity and metabolic syndrome in Brazilian patients with bipolar disorder, Acta Neuropsychiatr 2009;**21**:84–8.

32. Calkin C, van de Velde C, Ruzickova M, Slaney C, Garnham J, Hajek T, et al. Can body mass index help predict outcome in patients with bipolar disorder?, *Bipolar Disorders* 2009;**11**:650–6.

33. Goldstein BI, Liu SM, Zivkovic N, Schaffer A, Chien LC, and Blanco C. The burden of obesity among adults with bipolar disorder in the United States, *Bipolar Disorders* 2011;**13**:387–95.

34. Gurpegui M, Martinez-Ortega JM, Gutierrez-Rojas L, Rivero J, Rojas C, and Jurado D. Overweight and obesity in patients with bipolar disorder or schizophrenia compared with a non-psychiatric sample, *Progress In Neuro-Psychopharmacology & Biological Psychiatry* 2012;**37**:169–75.

35. McElroy SL, Kemp DE, Friedman ES, Reilly-Harrington NA, Sylvia LG, Calabrese JR, et al. Obesity, but not metabolic syndrome, negatively affects outcome in bipolar disorder, *Acta Psychiatrica Scandinavica* 2015. doi: 10.1111/acps.12460. [Epub ahead of print]

36. Yim CY, Soczynska JK, Kennedy SH, Woldeyohannes HO, Brietzke E, and McIntyre RS. The effect of overweight/obesity on cognitive function in euthymic individuals with bipolar disorder, Eur Psychiatry 2012;**27**:223–8.

37. Hsu JH, Chien IC, and Lin CH. Increased risk of hyperlipidemia in patients with bipolar disorder: a population-based study, *General Hospital Psychiatry* 2015;**37**:294–8.

38. Vemuri M, Kenna HA, Wang PW, Ketter TA, and Rasgon NL. Gender-specific lipid profiles in patients with bipolar disorder, *Journal of Psychiatric Research* 2011;**45**:1036–41.

39. Vancampfort D, Mitchell AJ, De Hert M, Sienaert P, Probst M, Buys R, et al. Prevalence and predictors of type 2 diabetes mellitus in people with bipolar disorder: a systematic review and meta-analysis, *The Journal of Clinical Psychiatry* 2015.

40. Kim B, Kim S, McIntyre RS, Park HJ, Kim SY, and Joo YH. Correlates of metabolic abnormalities in bipolar I disorder at initiation of acute phase treatment, Psychiatry Investig 2009;**6**:78–84.

41. Calkin CV, Ruzickova M, Uher R, Hajek T, Slaney CM, Garnham JS, et al. Insulin resistance and outcome in bipolar disorder, *The British Journal of Psychiatry: the Journal of Mental Science* 2015;**206**:52–7.

42. Vancampfort D, Vansteelandt K, Correll CU, Mitchell AJ, De Herdt A, Sienaert P, et al. Metabolic syndrome and metabolic abnormalities in bipolar disorder: a meta-analysis of prevalence rates and moderators, *The American Journal of Psychiatry* 2013;**170**:265–74.

43. Salvi V, D'Ambrosio V, Bogetto F, Maina G. Metabolic syndrome in Italian patients with bipolar disorder: a 2-year follow-up study, *Journal of Affective Disorders* 2012;**136**:599–603.

44. McIntyre RS, Woldeyohannes HO, Soczynska JK, Miranda A, Lachowski A, Liauw SS, et al. The rate of metabolic syndrome in euthymic Canadian individuals with bipolar I/II disorder, *Advances in Therapy* 2010;**27**:828–36.

45. Fagiolini A, Frank E, Scott JA, Turkin S, Kupfer DJ. Metabolic syndrome in bipolar disorder: findings from the Bipolar Disorder Center for Pennsylvanians, *Bipolar Disorders* 2005;**7**:424–30.

46. Bauer M, Glenn T, Pilhatsch M, Pfennig A, and Whybrow PC. Gender differences in thyroid system function: relevance to bipolar disorder and its treatment, *Bipolar Disorders* 2014;**16**:58–71.

47. Bauer MS, Whybrow PC, and Winokur A. Rapid cycling bipolar affective disorder. I. Association with grade I hypothyroidism, *Archives of General Psychiatry* 1990;**47**:427–32.

48. Martino DJ and Strejilevich SA. Subclinical hypothyroidism and neurocognitive functioning in bipolar disorder, *Journal of Psychiatric Research* 2015;**61**:166–7.

49. Fornaro M and Stubbs B. A meta-analysis investigating the prevalence and moderators of migraines among people with bipolar disorder, *Journal of Affective Disorders* 2015;**178**:88–97.

50. Brietzke E, Moreira CL, Duarte SV, Nery FG, Kapczinski F, Miranda Scippa A, et al. Impact of comorbid migraine on the clinical course of bipolar disorder, Compr Psychiatry 2012;**53**:809–12.

51. Nguyen TV and Low NC (2013): Comorbidity of migraine and mood episodes in a nationally representative population-based sample, *Headache* **53**:498–506.

52. Wotton CJ and Goldacre MJ. Record-linkage studies of the coexistence of epilepsy and bipolar disorder, *Social Psychiatry and Psychiatric Epidemiology* 2014;**49**:1483–8.

53. Johansson V, Lundholm C, Hillert J, Masterman T, Lichtenstein P, Landen M, et al. Multiple sclerosis and psychiatric disorders: comorbidity and sibling risk in a nationwide Swedish cohort, Mult Scler 2014;**20**:1881–91.

54. Posada C, Moore DJ, Deutsch R, Rooney A, Gouaux B, Letendre S, et al. Sustained attention deficits among HIV-positive individuals with comorbid bipolar disorder, J Neuropsychiatry Clin Neurosci 2012;**24**:61–70.

55. Moore DJ, Posada C, Parikh M, Arce M, Vaida F, Riggs PK, et al. HIV-infected individuals with co-occurring bipolar disorder evidence poor antiretroviral and psychiatric medication adherence, AIDS Behav 2012;**16**:2257–66.

56. Hung YN, Yang SY, Huang MC, Lung FW, Lin SK, Chen KY, et al. Cancer incidence in people with affective disorder: nationwide cohort study in Taiwan, 1997–2010, *The British Journal of Psychiatry: the Journal of Mental Science* 2014;**205**:183–8.

57. McGinty EE, Zhang Y, Guallar E, Ford DE, Steinwachs D, Dixon LB, et al. Cancer incidence in a sample of Maryland residents with serious mental illness, *Psychiatric Services* 2012;**63**:714–17.

58. Kupfer DJ. The increasing medical burden in bipolar disorder, JAMA 2005;**293**:2528–30.

59. Kisely SR and Goldberg DP. The effects of physical illness on psychiatric disorder, *Journal of Psychopharmacology* 1993;**7**:119–25.

60. *The Health Consequences of Smoking—50 Years of Progress: A Report of the Surgeon General* (Atlanta, GA; 2014).

61. Jackson JG, Diaz FJ, Lopez L, and de Leon J. A combined analysis of worldwide studies demonstrates an association between bipolar disorder and tobacco smoking behaviors in adults, *Bipolar Disorders* 2015;**17**:575–97.

62. Schulte MT and Hser Y-I. Substance use and associated health conditions throughout the lifespan, *Public Health Reviews* 2014;**35**.

63. Pettinati HM, O'Brien CP, and Dundon WD. Current status of co-occurring mood and substance use disorders: a new therapeutic target, *The American Journal of Psychiatry* 2013;**170**:23–30.

64. Kilbourne AM, Rofey DL, McCarthy JF, Post EP, Welsh D, and Blow FC. Nutrition and exercise behavior among patients with bipolar disorder, *Bipolar Disorders* 2007;**9**:443–42.

65. Kapczinski F, Vieta E, Andreazza AC, Frey BN, Gomes FA, Tramontina J, et al. Allostatic load in bipolar disorder: implications for pathophysiology and treatment, *Neuroscience and Biobehavioral Reviews* 2008;**32**:675–92.

66. Perugi G, Quaranta G, Belletti S, Casalini F, Mosti N, Toni C, et al. General medical conditions in 347 bipolar disorder patients: clinical correlates of metabolic and autoimmune-allergic diseases, *Journal of Affective Disorders* 2015;**170**:95–103.

67. Goldstein BI, Kemp DE, Soczynska JK, and McIntyre RS. Inflammation and the phenomenology, pathophysiology, comorbidity, and treatment of bipolar disorder: a systematic review of the literature, *The Journal of Clinical Psychiatry* 2009;**70**:1078–90.

68. Leboyer M, Soreca I, Scott J, Frye M, Henry C, Tamouza R, et al. Can bipolar disorder be viewed as a multi-system inflammatory disease?, *Journal of Affective Disorders* 2012;**141**:1–10.

69. Walker BR. Glucocorticoids and cardiovascular disease, *Eur J Endocrinol* 2007;**157**:545–59.

70. Wieck A, Grassi-Oliveira R, do Prado CH, Rizzo LB, de Oliveira AS, Kommers-Molina J, et al. Differential neuroendocrine and immune responses to acute psychosocial stress in women with type 1 bipolar disorder, Brain Behav Immun 2013;**34**:47–55.

71. Knijff EM, Breunis MN, van Geest MC, Kupka RW, Ruwhof C, de Wit HJ, et al. A relative resistance of T cells to dexamethasone in bipolar disorder, *Bipolar Disorders* 2006;**8**:740–50.

72. Kupka RW, Breunis MN, Knijff E, Ruwhof C, Nolen WA, and Drexhage HA. Immune activation, steroid resistancy and bipolar disorder, *Bipolar Disorders* 2002;**4**(Suppl 1):73–4.

73. Strawbridge R, Arnone D, Danese A, Papadopoulos A, Herane Vives A, and Cleare AJ. Inflammation and clinical response to treatment in depression: a meta-analysis, *European Neuropsychopharmacology: the Journal of the European College of Neuropsychopharmacology* 2015;**25**:1532–43.

74. Dickerson F, Stallings C, Origoni A, Boronow J, and Yolken R. Elevated serum levels of C-reactive protein are associated with mania symptoms in outpatients with bipolar disorder, *Progress in Neuro-psychopharmacology & Biological Psychiatry* 2007;**31**:952–5.

75. Brietzke E, Stertz L, Fernandes BS, Kauer-Sant'anna M, Mascarenhas M, Escosteguy Vargas A, et al. Comparison of cytokine levels in depressed, manic and euthymic patients with bipolar disorder, *Journal of Affective Disorders* 2009;**116**:214–17.

76. Tsai SY, Chung KH, Huang SH, Chen PH, Lee HC, and Kuo CJ. Persistent inflammation and its relationship to leptin and insulin in phases of bipolar disorder from acute depression to full remission, *Bipolar Disorders* 2014;**16**:800–8.

77. **Vieta E, Popovic D, Rosa AR, Sole B, Grande I, Frey BN**, et al. The clinical implications of cognitive impairment and allostatic load in bipolar disorder, Eur Psychiatry 2013;**28**:21–9.

78. **De Hert M, Detraux J, van Winkel R, Yu W**, and **Correll CU**. Metabolic and cardiovascular adverse effects associated with antipsychotic drugs, Nat Rev Endocrinol 2012;**8**:114–26.

79. **Torrent C, Amann B, Sanchez-Moreno J, Colom F, Reinares M, Comes M**, et al. Weight gain in bipolar disorder: pharmacological treatment as a contributing factor, *Acta Psychiatrica Scandinavica* 2008;**118**:4–18.

80. **Murru A, Popovic D, Pacchiarotti I, Hidalgo D, Leon-Caballero J**, and **Vieta E**. Management of adverse effects of mood stabilizers, Curr Psychiatry Rep 2015;**17**:603.

81. **Correll CU, Lencz T**, and **Malhotra AK**. Antipsychotic drugs and obesity, Trends Mol Med 2011;**17**:97–107.

82. **McKnight RF, Adida M, Budge K, Stockton S, Goodwin GM**, and **Geddes JR**. Lithium toxicity profile: a systematic review and meta-analysis, *Lancet* 2012;**379**:721–8.

83. **Hermida OG, Fontela T, Ghiglione M**, and **Uttenthal LO**. Effect of lithium on plasma glucose, insulin and glucagon in normal and streptozotocin-diabetic rats: role of glucagon in the hyperglycaemic response, Br J Pharmacol 1994;**111**:861–5.

84. **Bowden CL**. Valproate, *Bipolar Disorders* 2003;**5**:189–202.

85. **Chang HH, Yang YK, Gean PW, Huang HC, Chen PS**, and **Lu RB**. The role of valproate in metabolic disturbances in bipolar disorder patients, *Journal of Affective Disorders* 2010;**124**:319–23.

86. **Bowden CL, Grunze H, Mullen J, Brecher M, Paulsson B, Jones M**, et al. A randomized, double-blind, placebo-controlled efficacy and safety study of quetiapine or lithium as monotherapy for mania in bipolar disorder, *The Journal of Clinical Psychiatry* 2005;**66**:111–21.

87. **Umbricht DS, Pollack S**, and **Kane JM**. Clozapine and weight gain, *The Journal of Clinical Psychiatry* 1994;**55**(Suppl B):157–60.

88. **Guille C, Sachs GS**, and **Ghaemi SN**. A naturalistic comparison of clozapine, risperidone, and olanzapine in the treatment of bipolar disorder, *The Journal of Clinical Psychiatry* 2000;**61**:638–42.

89. **De Hert M, Yu W, Detraux J, Sweers K, van Winkel R**, and **Correll CU**. Body weight and metabolic adverse effects of asenapine, iloperidone, lurasidone and paliperidone in the treatment of schizophrenia and bipolar disorder: a systematic review and exploratory meta-analysis, *CNS Drugs* 2012;**26**:733–59.

90. **Keck PE, Jr, Marcus R, Tourkodimitris S, Ali M, Liebeskind A, Saha A**, et al. A placebo-controlled, double-blind study of the efficacy and safety of aripiprazole in patients with acute bipolar mania, *The American Journal of Psychiatry* 2003;**160**:1651–8.

91. **Keck PE, Jr, Versiani M, Potkin S, West SA, Giller E, Ice K**, et al. Ziprasidone in the treatment of acute bipolar mania: a three-week, placebo-controlled, double-blind, randomized trial, *The American Journal of Psychiatry* 2003;**160**:741–8.

92. **Baptista T, De Mendoza S, Beaulieu S, Bermudez A**, and **Martinez M**. The metabolic syndrome during atypical antipsychotic drug treatment: mechanisms and management, *Metabolic Syndrome and Related Disorders* 2004;**2**:290–307.

93. **Fava M**. Weight gain and antidepressants, *The Journal of Clinical Psychiatry* 2000;**61**(Suppl 11):37–41.

94. **Ruffmann C, Bogliun G**, and **Beghi E**. Epileptogenic drugs: a systematic review, *Expert Review of Neurotherapeutics* 2006;**6**:575–89.

95. **Stahl SM, Grady MM, Moret C**, and **Briley M**. SNRIs: their pharmacology, clinical efficacy, and tolerability in comparison with other classes of antidepressants, CNS Spectr 2005;**10**:732–47.

96. **Young AH** and **Grunze H**. Physical health of patients with bipolar disorder, Acta Psychiatr Scand 2013 Suppl;3–10.

97. **M DEH, Correll CU, Bobes J, Cetkovich-Bakmas M, Cohen D, Asai I**, et al. Physical illness in patients with severe mental disorders. I. Prevalence, impact of medications and disparities in health care, *World Psychiatry: Official Journal of the World Psychiatric Association* 2011;**10**:52–77.

98. **Yatham LN, Kennedy SH, Schaffer A, Parikh SV, Beaulieu S, O'Donovan C**, et al. Canadian Network for Mood and Anxiety Treatments (CANMAT) and International Society for Bipolar Disorders (ISBD) collaborative update of CANMAT guidelines for the management of patients with bipolar disorder: update 2009, *Bipolar Disorders* 2009;**11**:225–55.

99. **Manu P, Correll CU, van Winkel R, Wampers M**, and **De Hert M**. Prediabetes in patients treated with antipsychotic drugs, *The Journal of Clinical Psychiatry* 2012;**73**:460–6.

Chapter 20

The treatment of bipolar disorder in women

Danielle Balzafiore, Thalia Robakis,
Sarah Borish, Vena Budhan,
and Natalie Rasgon

Introduction

Bipolar disorder (BD) is a chronic and often disabling mental illness characterized by the occurrence of recurrent episodes of depression and elevation over the course of an individual's lifetime.[1] Half of patients will suffer from another episode within one year of recovery from a mood episode,[2] and more than 90% of patients who have a single manic episode will have recurrent episodes throughout their life.[1] As a result, the economic burden of BD is substantial.[3,4] In the United States (US) alone, national projections on the impact of BD on the labour force are estimated to be as high as $14.1 billion.[5] Internationally, lifetime prevalence rates of bipolar I disorder, bipolar II disorder, and subthreshold BD are 0.6%, 0.4%, and 1.4%, respectively. Twelve-month prevalence rates of bipolar I disorder, bipolar II disorder, and subthreshold BD are 0.4%, 0.3%, and 0.8%, respectively.[6]

While the lifetime and 12-month prevalence of BD is similar between males and females, studies have identified gender differences in clinical presentation and course, which may contribute to differences in treatment response.[7,8] Reproductive hormones may influence BD course, particularly in women, and emerging lines of evidence support a relationship between the menstrual cycle and reproductive events with mood symptoms.[9,10] Thus, the management of BD in women requires gender-specific information in order to enhance treatment outcomes.[7,11]

Gender differences in the clinical presentation of bipolar disorder

Most, but not all studies, suggest that women may have a later age of BD onset compared with men.[12,13] These findings may be secondary to differences associated with bipolar subtype, notably, that bipolar I disorder occurs at an earlier age than bipolar II disorder.[1] Males' first mood episode is more likely to be manic, and conversely, females' first episode is more likely to be major depressive.[14] Similarly, females may be more likely than males to be diagnosed with bipolar II disorder.[15]

However, these findings are not consistent across the literature, and some studies have shown no significant gender differences in bipolar subtype.[9] Females are also more likely than males to experience mixed episodes[13] and rapid cycling.[15] Both mixed episodes and rapid cycling have been associated with poorer BD prognosis.[16,17]

Research evaluating whether depressive episodes are more prevalent among females has yielded variable results.[8] However, females with BD are consistently more likely than males to report a lifetime experience of depression rather than discrete depressive episodes.[9,18] Results from one longitudinal study that included 80 BD outpatients[9] indicated that women reported depression (28.3% vs 17.0%) and large fluctuations in mood over three months more frequently than men.

Further, females often have patterns of medical co-morbidity that differ from males.[1] There is some evidence suggesting that females compared to males may display higher rates of endocrine/metabolic disorders,[12] abdominal obesity,[19] and appetite and weight changes.[14] Of note, elevated body mass index has been shown to be a significant predictor of diminished response to combined treatment with lithium and valproate.[20]

Rasgon et al.[21] evaluated metabolic function in 103 women with BD compared to 36 age-matched healthy controls and found that women with BD demonstrated worse metabolic biomarkers compared with healthy controls. Specifically, women with BD had higher levels of fasting insulin, fasting plasma glucose, and homeostatic assessment of insulin resistance scores and greater body mass index and waist circumference compared with women without BD. Family history of type 2 diabetes mellitus was associated with significantly worse metabolic biomarkers among women with BD but not among healthy controls. While second-generation antipsychotics, which are commonly used to treat BD, are known to promote metabolic dysfunction, in this study medication type was not associated with metabolic biomarkers, suggesting that metabolic dysfunction in women with BD may not be entirely the result of pharmaceutical treatment. Rather, metabolic dysfunction may be an integral aspect of the pathophysiology in a subset of women with BD.[21]

In addition to medical correlates, gender differences in psychiatric co-morbidities may also impact treatment. Among patients with BD, eating disorders are more prevalent among females[22,23] and may be associated with a more severe bipolar course, including earlier age of onset,[22-24] greater number of depressive and mood episodes,[23,24] higher rates of rapid cycling,[23] more severe depressive symptoms,[22] and suicide attempts.[23,24]

The longitudinal consequences of co-morbid eating disorders in females with BD remain to be definitively established. However, studies evaluating the influence of co-morbid eating disorders in patients with unipolar depression provide some evidence that co-morbid eating disorders may be associated with an increased risk for depression recurrence and relapse, as well as a diminished response to antidepressant treatment.[25,26]

We recently evaluated the effects of lifetime eating disorder co-morbidity on the clinical course and longitudinal outcomes in patients with BD.[27] Among 503 BD outpatients, 76 (15.1%) reported a lifetime history of an eating disorder. Bipolar disorder outpatients with versus without co-morbid eating disorders were more often female (86.8% vs 53.2%), and median time to recovery from depression for patients with an eating disorder was approximately twice as long (454 vs 230 days) as patients without co-morbid eating disorders. Additional research is warranted to ascertain the influence of co-morbid eating disorders on BD illness course and treatment outcomes.

Thus, BD manifests somewhat differently among males and females, with respect to timing of onset, symptom profile, and medical and psychiatric co-morbidities. The astute clinician will take this information into account so as to be able to counsel each patient according to his or her individual risk profile.

Mood cycling and the female reproductive cycle

The average age of the first BD episode ranges from age 18 to the late 20s,[1] placing women at risk for mood episodes across the reproductive years.[28] Several lines of research support an interaction between reproductive events and increased risk for affective symptoms, both in women generally, and particularly in women with BD. Beginning in puberty, girls are at increased risk for depression,[29] and throughout the reproductive cycle, women with mood disorders are more susceptible to premenstrual mood changes compared to healthy peers.[10,30]

Reciprocally, a number of women with BD meet diagnostic criteria for premenstrual dysphoric disorder (PMDD),[31] a severe form of premenstrual syndrome marked by emotional lability, low mood, and/or anxiety. Symptoms begin during the late luteal phase of the menstrual cycle and remit at onset of menses or shortly after.[1] With the release of the *Diagnostic and Statistical Manual of Mental Disorders* (5th edition) (DSM-5), PMDD moved from the appendix to primary syndromes.[1] It remains unclear whether PMDD in women with BD should be considered a separate diagnostic entity from BD with menstrual entrainment of mood cycles; further research in this area is urgently required.[32] Nonetheless, the distinction may have important implications for treatment.

A common and effective means of treating PMDD is the use of selective serotonin reuptake inhibitors (SSRIs) given during the luteal phase only.[33] However, Dias and colleagues highlight the need for caution regarding the use of antidepressants to manage luteal-phase mood symptoms among women with BD.[31] Bipolar depression may be less likely to respond to treatment with canonical antidepressants, and furthermore, antidepressants can precipitate manic switching and cycle acceleration,[34] suggesting that alternative treatments may be warranted for women with menstrually entrained bipolar mood cycling.

There is some evidence that oral contraceptives (OCPs) may assist with PMDD symptom management.[30] However, using mood stabilizers and OCPs concurrently requires caution as mood stabilizers may influence the metabolism of OCPs.[7] OCPs have been shown to reduce the effective serum levels of both valproate and lamotrigine.[35] Conversely, carbamazepine, oxcarbazepine, and topiramate have been shown to induce cytochrome P450 3A4, leading to enhanced metabolism of both the estrogenic and progestogenic components of OCPs and thus reducing their effectiveness.[36,37]

In women whose mood-stabilizing therapy is insufficient to control their menstrually entrained cycling, a switch of mood stabilizer should be considered before the addition of an OCP to the regimen, particularly if the mood stabilizer in question is known to interfere with the metabolism of the OCP. In cases where the OCP reduces serum levels of the mood stabilizer, regular monitoring of mood stabilizer serum levels in combination with clinical judgement should be sufficient to establish an appropriate and effective dose. It should be noted that some evidence suggests that lamotrigine on its own may be of particular utility for reducing the amplitude of mood variability across the menstrual cycle.[38]

Beyond menstrually entrained cycling, menstrual abnormalities are also commonly reported among women with BD and require consideration in the management of affective symptoms. In some cases the menstrual abnormality may predate the bipolar illness. For example, in one study approximately 50% of women with BD reported menstrual abnormalities including menorrhagia, amenorrhoea, and irregular periods, prior to initiating treatment of mood symptoms.[39] Alternatively, menstrual abnormalities may also emerge pursuant to treatment with mood stabilizers. In particular, valproate compounds have been found to exacerbate pre-existing menstrual abnormalities as well as precipitate new onset of menstrual abnormalities in women without previous symptoms.[40] Valproic acid has also been associated with the onset of polycystic ovary syndrome, one of the most common endocrinopathies among women, more so than any other mood stabilizer[39,40] and represents a significant consideration with respect to treatment for women with BD.

Thus, the mood cycling evident in BD has many points of intersection with the menstrual cycle. Bipolar mood cycles may be entrained with the menstrual cycle, and menstrual abnormalities may predate the diagnosis and treatment of BD in a significant subset of women. Additionally, the pharmacological effects of mood stabilizers on the metabolism of OCP and the functioning of the female reproductive cycle are important to take into account when selecting appropriate treatment agents for women with BD.

Treatment of bipolar disorder during pregnancy and postpartum

The management of BD during the perinatal period, including preconception, pregnancy, and postpartum, requires a careful approach to optimize the maintenance of mood stability while minimizing the potential for adverse fetal effects conferred by mood-stabilizing medications.[7,41]

Manifestations of bipolar disorder in the perinatal period

The issue of whether pregnancy is protective against mood episode relapse is controversial; however, when considered collectively, pregnancy does not appear to increase risk for mood symptoms in women with BD.[11] Viguera et al.[42] found that risk for mood episode recurrence was twofold greater among pregnant women who discontinued a mood stabilizer, particularly abruptly, compared with those who continued throughout the pregnancy. Predictors of illness recurrence during pregnancy included a bipolar II disorder diagnosis, an earlier age of BD onset and illness duration, a greater number of prior recurrences, antidepressant use, and use of anti-convulsants compared with lithium.

In contrast, postpartum is a period of clearly elevated risk for mood episodes in women with pre-existing BD.[43] Approximately 40–67% of women with BD report experiencing postpartum mania or depression.[29,44] Additionally, women without a previous BD diagnosis may present for the first time with postpartum depression. This population is prone to being diagnosed and treated as unipolar, leading to the phenomenon of apparent treatment resistance. One investigation of this phenomenon found that over half of women diagnosed with treatment-resistant postpartum depression in fact had bipolar features that had been missed by the treating clinicians.[45] Identifying clinical indicators of possible BD for women with new onset postpartum depression is imperative because failure to properly diagnose postpartum BD may delay the initiation of appropriate treatment, lead to inappropriate treatment, or result in polypharmacy and treatment refractoriness.[46]

Additionally, while postpartum psychosis is rare in the general population, affecting one to two childbearing women per thousand, about 26% of childbearing women with BD experience psychosis during the postpartum period.[47] Severe postpartum manic and psychotic symptoms are highest in the first two weeks postpartum among women with BD.[48] Hallucinations and delusions in postpartum psychosis are often related to the infant, and in rare cases, may contribute to a risk of harm to the infant.[49] The most serious consequence of postpartum psychotic symptoms is the possibility of infanticide and suicide.

Therefore, the possibility of pregnancy needs to be considered in treating all women with BD during the reproductive years, and issues surrounding contraception and family planning are central to treatment management.[41] Preconception planning should involve comprehensive prenatal counselling at least three months before pregnancy. Discussions should focus on the known possible risks of taking medications during pregnancy, as well as risks to both the mother and unborn child should bipolar decompensation occur, and the risk of genetic transmission of BD to the child.[7] Folate supplementation is also recommended three months before conception and continuing into the first trimester of pregnancy to reduce the risk of neural tube defects.[7]

Mood-stabilizing medication during pregnancy

The quality of data on psychotropic medication use during pregnancy is compromised by complex ethical issues that preclude the conduction of randomized trials.[50] Thus, the best available information comes from large observational studies. However, since the underlying mental illness is in itself associated with negative outcomes for the neonate, including reduced birth weight and increases in obstetric complications,[51] those studies that have not controlled for the underlying mental illness are very difficult to interpret.

Optimal decision-making on the use of psychotropic medication during pregnancy in women with BD requires a careful risk–benefit analysis for each patient.[7,11] Monotherapy is preferable whenever possible.[52] The teratogenic effects of valproate and carbamazepine are well documented in the literature.[7] Lithium was initially thought to produce a major increase in the risk of Ebstein's anomaly; however, more recent and better-designed investigations have revised these estimates greatly downward.[53,54] While some elevated risk for cardiac anomaly may remain, the absolute risk remains small. With appropriate monitoring (including fetal echocardiography and level II ultrasound), lithium may be a reasonable choice in pregnancy among women who have failed to achieve mood stabilization with alternative agents.[54]

Studies of antipsychotics in pregnancy are limited by small sample sizes, non-randomized design, ubiquitous polypharmacy, and difficulty controlling for the underlying mental illness. The best available information does not suggest that increases in congenital malformation rates accrue to antipsychotics as a class, although available samples are underpowered to detect increases among rare malformations.[51,55] Increases in rates of preterm birth with first-generation antipsychotics[55] and in rates of gestational diabetes with second-generation antipsychotics[56] are supported. Quetiapine has been documented to have lower rates of placental passage than comparable medications,[57] suggesting that in the absence of efficacy data, it is a reasonable first choice. However, when efficacy data are available for a given agent, this should take top priority in agent selection for the patient.

For mothers concerned about medication exposure to the infant, electroconvulsive therapy (ECT) represents one potential treatment for perinatal mood disruption or psychosis. Several large case series support its overall safety and efficacy in pregnant populations.[58,59] Studies also provide support for the beneficial effects of ECT in the treatment of postpartum psychosis.[60,61]

Transcranial magnetic stimulation (TMS) is a newer neurostimulatory approach that may also be of interest for women who wish to avoid medications. Studies on its use in BD are extremely limited and preliminary,[62] and none have been conducted in pregnant women. However, pilot data support the tolerability and a reasonable degree of efficacy of TMS in pregnant women with unipolar depression.[63,64]

Other non-pharmacological approaches such as interpersonal and social rhythm therapy,[65] cognitive behavioural therapy, and family focused therapy[66] have shown good efficacy and may be helpful for reducing medication burden. Interventions should be aimed at maintaining a regular schedule of daily activities and stability in personal relationships.[67] Other brief interventions to improve and maintain mental health for women with BD during the perinatal period include fostering family collaboration to promote maternal self-care, adequate maternal nutrition, adult socialization, and breaks from childcare.[47] Though the use of dietary supplements with pharmacological treatment is common among patients with BD,[68] findings from one recent review do not provide evidence for efficacy in treating bipolar depression.[69] Additionally, dietary supplementation may present danger to special populations, including pregnant women.[70]

Mood-stabilizing medication during postpartum

The management of BD in women during the postpartum period involves unique treatment challenges because both untreated symptoms and treatments pose risks. In most cases, the potential risks of untreated symptoms outweigh risks of carefully selected medications with close monitoring.[47] Decision-making regarding breast-feeding is central to treatment management during the postpartum period.

Although breastfeeding is associated with many potential benefits to both the mother and child, it requires unique considerations in mothers diagnosed with BD due to its association with sleep disruption, which consequently increases the mother's vulnerability to relapse.[71] Pregnant women with BD should be counselled about the importance of maintaining their sleep well in advance of parturition and be encouraged to plan collaboratively for this need with their partners and other available support persons. New mothers with BD may also be encouraged to consider the relative benefits of full-time breastfeeding versus supplementing breast milk with formula or full-formula feeding to facilitate night-time feeds by alternative support persons.[46]

Another important issue related to breastfeeding is concern of infant toxicity due to exposure to various mood stabilizers in the breast milk. All psychotropic drugs used to treat BD are excreted to some degree in breast milk and therefore present some risk to the infant during the breastfeeding period.[72] The American Academy for Pediatrics recommends determining whether medication is truly necessary, choosing the safest drug, and encourages consultation between the paediatrician and the mother's physician to discuss medications to which an infant is exposed and the potential side effects.[7]

Among mood-stabilizing agents, valproate is not appropriate for use in lactating mothers due to evidence of reduced full-scale IQ scores in their children at age three.[73] Meador and colleagues did not detect any negative effect of carbamazepine or lamotrigine on IQ at three years.[73] However, clinicians should monitor for hepatotoxicity and haematological toxicity in infants of mothers on carbamazepine and for skin rash in infants of mothers on lamotrigine. Similarly, lithium may be problematic in lactation due to a narrow toxic–therapeutic window and potential wide swings in serum levels related to immature clearance capacities in infants. While most breastfeeding babies do not experience adverse effects from maternal lithium use, toxicity is possible, especially if infants become dehydrated.[47] However, some authors have suggested that close monitoring of serum lithium levels in mother and infant can permit breastfeeding.[74]

Outcome data for the use of atypical antipsychotics in lactation are limited; however, typically infant serum levels range from undetectable to <10% of maternal levels. In an olanzapine surveillance study, the most commonly reported adverse events were somnolence (3.9%), irritability (2%), tremor (2%), and insomnia (2%), although the majority reported no adverse events (82.3%).[75] It is worthwhile to consider that following birth the infant is bigger, the liver is more developed, and drug delivery is generally less via lactation than it was via placenta. Thus, if a mother was taking a given medication during pregnancy, the major exposure has already occurred and avoidance of breastfeeding has limited impact on drug exposure, and important benefits may be lost.

In general, treatment decisions about medication use in postpartum should be based on the mother's clinical status and previous course, regardless of breastfeeding status. The mother's health and stability should always take priority over the feeding method of the infant. For mothers considering breastfeeding while taking medications, suitable clinical characteristics include stable maternal mood, a simple medication regimen, adherence to infant-monitoring recommendations, a healthy infant, and a collaborative paediatrician.[74]

Overall, the perinatal period, and the postpartum period in particular, represents a significant challenge for maintenance of stability in BD. Risks associated with effective therapies must be balanced against the risks associated with uncontrolled mood cycling in the mother. The safety of mother and newborn should always be the top priority in the treatment and management of BD in the perinatal period.

Treatment of bipolar disorder during menopause

The menopausal transition can also be a time of change in the observed patterns of mood cycling for patients with BD. Overall, studies have indicated that approximately 20–50% of women with BD report intense mood symptoms during the menopausal transition.[29] The menopausal transition may also precipitate a new onset or worsening of BD symptoms, including increased irritability, depressive symptoms, and hypomania/mania, increased frequency of depressive episodes, greater rates of rapid cycling, and severe emotional distress.[29,76] More recent research also suggests a gradient of worsening mood state in women with BD from the premenopausal to perimenopausal to postmenopausal state.[77]

Research evaluating the treatment of BD during the menopause transition is limited. There are few studies looking at the use of hormone therapy in BD, and findings related to possible benefits in treatment are mixed. There is some evidence that suggests that women using hormone therapy are less likely to report intensifying mood symptoms during perimenopause compared with non-users.[29] However, Marsh et al.[77] found that compared with non-users, the use of hormone therapy in perimenopausal and postmenopausal women did not predict the number of visits presenting in a depressed state.

Vasomotor symptoms are a common complaint for perimenopausal women, and some of the most commonly used treatments include psychoactive medications such as SSRI antidepressants, venlafaxine or desvenlafaxine, and gabapentin.[78] These are often prescribed by gynaecologists or primary-care physicians who may be unaware of the potential for these medications to affect mood equilibrium in patients with BD. While most antidepressants are safe for use in bipolar women, they require concurrent treatment with a mood stabilizer as unopposed antidepressant treatment may precipitate mania. In patients with rapid cycling, antidepressants have the potential to worsen the rapid cycling even when used in concert with a mood stabilizer.[79]

Gabapentin, while of relatively lower efficacy as a mood stabilizer[80] may nonetheless be of use as an adjunct to an effective mood-stabilizing regimen, and certainly presents much less risk of precipitating mania or rapid cycling than the antidepressants, as previously discussed. In general, to avoid mood disruptions resulting from outside prescriptions, careful review of medications from all providers at each visit and open communication among treating providers are essential.

Sleep is often disrupted in perimenopausal women, and this can constitute a trigger for mood episodes;[71] thus, interventions to target regular sleep and avoidance of circadian disruption can be helpful in this population. Overall, more research is needed to understand the unique presentation of BD during the menopausal transition as well as potential treatments.

Conclusion

Sex-specific effects in the clinical presentation and course of BD in women have important treatment implications for the management of symptoms across the menstrual cycle and reproductive lifespan.[7,11] Women differ from men in the age of onset, clinical pattern of symptoms, and rates and types of psychiatric co-morbidities.

For many women with BD, periods of hormonal fluctuation appear to present a unique risk for affective symptoms,[29] thus making treatment challenging. Women with BD compared to without are particularly vulnerable to premenstrual mood symptoms,[31] menstrual abnormalities, and polycystic ovary syndrome.[39] Treatments may involve both psychotropic and gynaecological expertise, and patients benefit from collaborative care among their specialist providers.

Management of BD in the perinatal period entails many complex decisions. The postpartum period in particular is a time of greatly elevated risk for mood episodes. Use of psychotropic medication in pregnancy and lactation requires a careful risk–benefit analysis for each patient.[7,11] While maintenance of mood stability is the primary goal, medications must be carefully selected to minimize risk of adverse fetal and neonatal outcomes. Behavioural and social interventions should be targeted to minimize stress and prioritize optimal sleep and regular habits.

Lastly, women with BD may be at risk for a worsening illness course during the menopausal transition.[76,77] Pharmacological approaches to mood stabilization are not greatly different in this population, but the elevated risk for sleep impairments should be recognized and any disruption promptly treated.

References

1. **American Psychiatric Association.** *Diagnostic and Statistical Manual of Mental Disorders*, 5th edn (Washington, DC: American Psychiatric Association; 2013).

2. **Solomon DA, Keitner GI, Miller IW, Shea MT,** and **Keller MB.** Course of illness and maintenance treatments for patients with bipolar disorder, J Clin Psychiatry 1995;**56**(1):5–13.

3. **Jin H** and **McCrone P.** Cost-of-illness studies for bipolar disorder: systematic review of international studies, *PharmacoEconomics* 2015;**33**(4):341–53.

4. **Miller S, Dell'Osso B,** and **Ketter TA.** The prevalence and burden of bipolar depression, J Affect Disord 2014;**169**(Suppl 1):S3–11.

5. **Kessler RC, Akiskal HS, Ames M, Birnbaum H, Greenberg P, Hirschfeld RM,** et al. Prevalence and effects of mood disorders on work performance in a nationally representative sample of US workers, Am J Psychiatry 2006;**163**(9):1561–8.

6. **Merikangas KR, Jin R, He JP, Kessler RC, Lee S, Sampson NA,** et al. Prevalence and correlates of bipolar spectrum disorder in the world mental health survey initiative, Arch Gen Psychiatry 2011;**68**(3):241–51.

7. **Burt VK and Rasgon N.** Special considerations in treating bipolar disorder in women, Bipolar Disord 2004;**6**(1):2–13.

8. **Diflorio A and Jones I.** Is sex important? Gender differences in bipolar disorder, Int Rev Psychiatry 2010;**22**(5):437–52.

9. **Rasgon N, Bauer M, Grof P, Gyulai L, Elman S, Glenn T,** et al. Sex-specific self-reported mood changes by patients with bipolar disorder, J Psychiatr Res 2005;**39**(1):77–83.

10. **Payne JL, Roy PS, Murphy-Eberenz K, Weismann MM, Swartz KL, McInnis MG,** et al. Reproductive cycle-associated mood symptoms in women with major depression and bipolar disorder, J Affect Disord 2007;**99**(1–3):221–9.

11. **Ketter TA, Rasgon NL,** and **Vemuri M.** Treatment of women with bipolar disorder. In: **Ketter TA** (ed), *Advances in Treatment of Bipolar Disorder* (Washington, DC: American Psychiatric Publishing; 2015), 199–216.

12. **Azorin JM, Belzeaux R, Kaladjian A, Adida M, Hantouche E, Lancrenon S,** et al. Risks associated with gender differences in bipolar I disorder, J Affect Disord 2013;**151**(3):1033–40.

13. **Grant BF, Stinson FS, Hasin DS, Dawson DA, Chou SP, Ruan WJ,** et al. Prevalence, correlates, and comorbidity of bipolar I disorder and axis I and II disorders: results from the National Epidemiologic Survey on Alcohol and Related Conditions, J Clin Psychiatry 2005;**66**(10):1205–15.

14. **Kawa I, Carter JD, Joyce PR, Doughty CJ, Frampton CM, Wells JE,** et al. Gender differences in bipolar disorder: age of onset, course, comorbidity, and symptom presentation, Bipolar Disord 2005;7(2):119–25.

15. **Schneck CD, Miklowitz DJ, Calabrese JR, Allen MH, Thomas MR, Wisniewski SR,** et al. Phenomenology of rapid-cycling bipolar disorder: data from the first 500 participants in the Systematic Treatment Enhancement Program, Am J Psychiatry 2004;**161**(10):1902–8.

16. **Baldessarini RJ, Salvatore P, Khalsa HM,** and **Tohen M.** Dissimilar morbidity following initial mania versus mixed-states in type-I bipolar disorder, J Affect Disord 2010;**126**(1–2):299–302.

17. **Degenhardt EK, Gatz JL, Jacob J,** and **Tohen M.** Predictors of relapse or recurrence in bipolar I disorder, J Affect Disord 2012;**136**(3):733–9.

18. **Miquel L, Usall J, Reed C, Bertsch J, Vieta E, Gonzalez-Pinto A,** et al. Gender differences in outcomes of acute mania: a 12-month follow-up study, Arch Womens Ment Health 2011;**14**(2):107–13.

19. **van Winkel R, De Hert M, Van Eyck D, Hanssens L, Wampers M, Scheen A,** et al. Prevalence of diabetes and the metabolic syndrome in a sample of patients with bipolar disorder, Bipolar Disord 2008;**10**(2):342–8.

20. **Kemp DE, Gao K, Chan PK, Ganocy SJ, Findling RL,** and **Calabrese JR.** Medical comorbidity in bipolar disorder: relationship between illnesses of the endocrine/ metabolic system and treatment outcome, Bipolar Disord 2010;**12**(4):404–13.

21. **Rasgon NL, Kenna HA, Reynolds-May MF, Stemmle PG, Vemuri M, Marsh W,** et al. Metabolic dysfunction in women with bipolar disorder: the potential influence of family history of type 2 diabetes mellitus, Bipolar Disord 2010;**12**(5):504–13.

22. Jen A, Saunders EF, Ornstein RM, Kamali M, and McInnis MG. Impulsivity, anxiety, and alcohol misuse in bipolar disorder comorbid with eating disorders, Int J Bipolar Disord 2013;1:13.

23. McElroy SL, Frye MA, Hellemann G, Altshuler L, Leverich GS, Suppes T, et al. Prevalence and correlates of eating disorders in 875 patients with bipolar disorder, J Affect Disord 2011;128(3):191–8.

24. Brietzke E, Moreira CL, Toniolo RA, and Lafer B. Clinical correlates of eating disorder comorbidity in women with bipolar disorder type I, J Affect Disord 2011;130(1–2):162–5.

25. Jang S, Jung S, Pae C, Kimberly BP, Craig Nelson J, and Patkar AA. Predictors of relapse in patients with major depressive disorder in a 52-week, fixed dose, double blind, randomized trial of selegiline transdermal system (STS), J Affect Disord 2013;151(3):854–9.

26. Mischoulon D, Eddy KT, Keshaviah A, Dinescu D, Ross SL, Kass AE, et al. Depression and eating disorders: treatment and course, J Affect Disord 2011;130(3):470–7.

27. Balzafiore DR, Kim H, Goffin KC, Rasgon NL, Miller S, Wang PW, et al. Prevalence and clinical characteristics of lifetime eating disorders comorbidity in bipolar disorder patients. Poster session presented at: International Society for Bipolar Disorders; 3–6 June 2015; Toronto, Ontario.

28. Yonkers KA, Wisner KL, Stowe Z, Leibenluft E, Cohen L, Miller L, et al. Management of bipolar disorder during pregnancy and the postpartum period, Am J Psychiatry 2004;161(4):608–20.

29. Freeman MP, Smith KW, Freeman SA, McElroy SL, Kmetz GE, Wright R, et al. The impact of reproductive events on the course of bipolar disorder in women, J Clin Psychiatry 2002;63(4):284–7.

30. Rasgon N, Bauer M, Glenn T, Elman S, and Whybrow PC. Menstrual cycle related mood changes in women with bipolar disorder, Bipolar Disord 2003;5(1):48–52.

31. Dias RS, Lafer B, Russo C, Del Debbio A, Nierenberg AA, Sachs GS, et al. Longitudinal follow-up of bipolar disorder in women with premenstrual exacerbation: findings from STEP-BD, Am J Psychiatry 2011;168(4):386–94.

32. Teatero ML, Mazmanian D, and Sharma V. Effects of the menstrual cycle on bipolar disorder, Bipolar Disord 2014;16(1):22–36.

33. Yonkers KA, Halbreich U, Freeman E, Brown C, Endicott J, Frank E, et al. Symptomatic improvement of premenstrual dysphoric disorder with sertraline treatment. A randomized controlled trial. Sertraline Premenstrual Dysphoric Collaborative Study Group, JAMA 1997;278(12):983–8.

34. Ghaemi SN, Rosenquist KJ, Ko JY, Baldassano CF, Kontos NJ, and Baldessarini RJ. Antidepressant treatment in bipolar versus unipolar depression, Am J Psychiatry 2004;161(1):163–5.

35. Herzog AG, Blum AS, Farina EL, Maestri XE, Newman J, Garcia E, et al. Valproate and lamotrigine level variation with menstrual cycle phase and oral contraceptive use, Neurology 2009;72(10):911–14.

36. Andreasen AH, Brosen K, and Damkier P. A comparative pharmacokinetic study in healthy volunteers of the effect of carbamazepine and oxcarbazepine on cyp3a4, Epilepsia 2007;48(3):490–6.

37. Nallani SC, Glauser TA, Hariparsad N, Setchell K, Buckley DJ, Buckley AR, et al. Dose-dependent induction of cytochrome P450 (CYP) 3A4 and activation of pregnane X receptor by topiramate, Epilepsia 2003;44(12):1521–8.

38. **Robakis TK, Holtzman J, Stemmle PG, Reynolds-May MF, Kenna HA, amd Rasgon NL.** Lamotrigine and GABAA receptor modulators interact with menstrual cycle phase and oral contraceptives to regulate mood in women with bipolar disorder, J Affect Disord 2015;**175**:108–15.

39. **Rasgon NL, Altshuler LL, Fairbanks L, Elman S, Bitran J, Labarca R,** et al. Reproductive function and risk for PCOS in women treated for bipolar disorder, Bipolar Disord 2005;**7**(3):246–59.

40. **Joffe H, Cohen LS, Suppes T, McLaughlin WL, Lavori P, Adams JM,** et al. Valproate is associated with new-onset oligoamenorrhea with hyperandrogenism in women with bipolar disorder, Biol Psychiatry 2006;**59**(11):1078–86.

41. **Meltzer-Brody S** and **Jones I.** Optimizing the treatment of mood disorders in the perinatal period, Dialogues Clin Neurosci 2015;**17**(2):207–18.

42. **Viguera AC, Whitfield T, Baldessarini RJ, Newport DJ, Stowe Z, Reminick A,** et al. Risk of recurrence in women with bipolar disorder during pregnancy: prospective study of mood stabilizer discontinuation, Am J Psychiatry 2007;**164**(12):1817–24; quiz 923.

43. **Viguera AC, Nonacs R, Cohen LS, Tondo L, Murray A,** and **Baldessarini RJ.** Risk of recurrence of bipolar disorder in pregnant and nonpregnant women after discontinuing lithium maintenance, Am J Psychiatry 2000;**157**(2):179–84.

44. **Di Florio A, Forty L, Gordon-Smith K, Heron J, Jones L, Craddock N,** et al. Perinatal episodes across the mood disorder spectrum, JAMA Psychiatry 2013;**70**(2):168–75.

45. **Sharma V, Khan M, Corpse C,** and **Sharma P.** Missed bipolarity and psychiatric comorbidity in women with postpartum depression, Bipolar Disord 2008;**10**(6):742–7.

46. **Kelly E** and **Sharma V.** Diagnosis and treatment of postpartum bipolar depression, Expert Rev Neurother 2010;**10**(7):1045–51.

47. **Miller LJ, Ghadiali NY, Larusso EM, Wahlen KJ, Avni-Barron O, Mittal L,** et al. Bipolar disorder in women, Health Care Women Int 2015;**36**(4):475–98.

48. **Doyle K, Heron J, Berrisford G, Whitmore J, Jones L, Wainscott G,** et al. The management of bipolar disorder in the perinatal period and risk factors for postpartum relapse, Eur Psychiatry 2012;**27**(8):563–9.

49. **Spinelli MG.** Postpartum psychosis: detection of risk and management, Am J Psychiatry 2009;**166**(4):405–8.

50. **Babu GN, Desai G,** and **Chandra PS.** Antipsychotics in pregnancy and lactation, Indian J Psychiatry 2015;**57**(Suppl 2):S303–7.

51. **Boden R, Lundgren M, Brandt L, Reutfors J, Andersen M,** and **Kieler H.** Risks of adverse pregnancy and birth outcomes in women treated or not treated with mood stabilisers for bipolar disorder: population based cohort study, BMJ 2012;**345**:e7085.

52. **Sadowski A, Todorow M, Yazdani Brojeni P, Koren G,** and **Nulman I.** Pregnancy outcomes following maternal exposure to second-generation antipsychotics given with other psychotropic drugs: a cohort study, BMJ Open 2013;**3**(7).

53. **Cohen LS, Friedman JM, Jefferson JW, Johnson EM,** and **Weiner ML.** A reevaluation of risk of in utero exposure to lithium, JAMA 1994;**271**(2):146–50.

54. **Diav-Citrin O, Shechtman S, Tahover E, Finkel-Pekarsky V, Arnon J, Kennedy D,** et al. Pregnancy outcome following in utero exposure to lithium: a prospective, comparative, observational study, Am J Psychiatry 2014;**171**(7):785–94.

55. **Lin HC, Chen IJ, Chen YH, Lee HC,** and **Wu FJ.** Maternal schizophrenia and pregnancy outcome: does the use of antipsychotics make a difference?, Schizophr Res 2010;**116**(1):55–60.

56. **Boden R, Lundgren M, Brandt L, Reutfors J**, and **Kieler H**. Antipsychotics during pregnancy: relation to fetal and maternal metabolic effects, Arch Gen Psychiatry 2012;**69**(7):715–21.

57. **Newport DJ, Calamaras MR, DeVane CL, Donovan J, Beach AJ, Winn S**, et al. Atypical antipsychotic administration during late pregnancy: placental passage and obstetrical outcomes, Am J Psychiatry 2007;**164**(8):1214–20.

58. **Anderson EL** and **Reti IM**. ECT in pregnancy: a review of the literature from 1941 to 2007, Psychosom Med 2009;**71**(2):235–42.

59. **Leiknes KA, Cooke MJ, Jarosch-von Schweder L, Harboe I**, and **Hoie B**. Electroconvulsive therapy during pregnancy: a systematic review of case studies, Arch Womens Ment Health 2015;**18**(1):1–39.

60. **Babu GN, Thippeswamy H**, and **Chandra PS**. Use of electroconvulsive therapy (ECT) in postpartum psychosis—a naturalistic prospective study, Arch Womens Ment Health 2013;**16**(3):247–51.

61. **Focht A** and **Kellner CH**. Electroconvulsive therapy (ECT) in the treatment of postpartum psychosis, J ECT 2012;**28**(1):31–3.

62. **Cretaz E, Brunoni AR**, and **Lafer B**. Magnetic seizure therapy for unipolar and bipolar depression: a systematic review, Neural Plast 2015;**2015**:521398.

63. **Hizli Sayar G, Ozten E, Tufan E, Cerit C, Kagan G, Dilbaz N**, et al. Transcranial magnetic stimulation during pregnancy, Arch Womens Ment Health 2014;**17**(4):311–15.

64. **Kim DR, Epperson N, Pare E, Gonzalez JM, Parry S, Thase ME**, et al. An open label pilot study of transcranial magnetic stimulation for pregnant women with major depressive disorder, J Womens Health (Larchmt) 2011;**20**(2):255–61.

65. **Frank E, Swartz HA**, and **Kupfer DJ**. Interpersonal and social rhythm therapy: managing the chaos of bipolar disorder, Biol Psychiatry 2000;**48**(6):593–604.

66. **Marangell LB**. Current issues: women and bipolar disorder, Dialogues Clin Neurosci 2008;**10**(2):229–38.

67. **Sharma V, Burt VK**, and **Ritchie HL**. Bipolar II postpartum depression: detection, diagnosis, and treatment, Am J Psychiatry 2009;**166**(11):1217–21.

68. **Bauer M, Glenn T, Conell J, Rasgon N, Marsh W, Sagduyu K**, et al. Common use of dietary supplements for bipolar disorder: a naturalistic, self-reported study, Int J Bipolar Disord 2015;**3**(1):29.

69. **Rakofsky JJ** and **Dunlop BW**. Review of nutritional supplements for the treatment of bipolar depression, Depress Anxiety 2014;**31**(5):379–90.

70. **Kroll DJ**. ASHP statement on the use of dietary supplements, Am J Health Syst Pharm 2004;**61**(16):1707–11.

71. **Plante DT** and **Winkelman JW**. Sleep disturbance in bipolar disorder: therapeutic implications, Am J Psychiatry 2008;**165**(7):830–43.

72. **Thomas P** and **Severus WE**. Managing bipolar disorder during pregnancy and lactation: is there a safe and effective option? Eur Psychiatry 2003;**18**(Suppl 1):3S–8S.

73. **Meador KJ, Baker GA, Browning N, Clayton-Smith J, Combs-Cantrell DT, Cohen M**, et al. Cognitive function at 3 years of age after fetal exposure to antiepileptic drugs, N Engl J Med 2009;**360**(16):1597–1605.

74. **Viguera AC, Newport DJ, Ritchie J, Stowe Z, Whitfield T, Mogielnicki J**, et al. Lithium in breast milk and nursing infants: clinical implications, Am J Psychiatry 2007;**164**(2):342–5.

75. **Brunner E, Falk DM, Jones M, Dey DK,** and **Shatapathy CC.** Olanzapine in pregnancy and breastfeeding: a review of data from global safety surveillance, BMC Pharmacol Toxicol 2013;**14**:38.

76. **Marsh WK, Templeton A, Ketter TA,** and **Rasgon NL.** Increased frequency of depressive episodes during the menopausal transition in women with bipolar disorder: preliminary report, J Psychiatr Res 2008;**42**(3):247–51.

77. **Marsh WK, Ketter TA, Crawford SL, Johnson JV, Kroll-Desrosiers AR,** and **Rothschild AJ.** Progression of female reproductive stages associated with bipolar illness exacerbation, Bipolar Disord 2012;**14**(5):515–26.

78. **Drewe J, Bucher KA,** and **Zahner C.** A systematic review of non-hormonal treatments of vasomotor symptoms in climacteric and cancer patients, SpringerPlus 2015;**4**:65.

79. **El-Mallakh RS, Vohringer PA, Ostacher MM, Baldassano CF, Holtzman NS, Whitham EA,** et al. Antidepressants worsen rapid-cycling course in bipolar depression: a STEP-BD randomized clinical trial, J Affect Disord 2015;**184**:318–21.

80. **Geddes JR** and **Miklowitz DJ.** Treatment of bipolar disorder, Lancet 2013;**381**(9878):1672–82.

Chapter 21

The treatment of bipolar disorder in children and adolescents

Philip Hazell

Introduction

Bipolar disorder (BD) affects about 1% of adolescents[1] provided one accepts that most experience manic episodes of less than four days duration.[2] The prevalence of BD among prepubertal children is unknown, but case series have been described.[3] BD accounted for 18.1% of paediatric hospitalizations for mental health disorder in the United States (US) in 2009, compared with 44.1% for unipolar depression and 12.1% for psychosis.[4] The grandiosity, euphoria, increased energy, distractibility, pressured thought, pressured speech, and impaired judgement, which are typical of adult mania are also seen in young people with mania, but manifestations seem age-dependent.[5] While manic episodes in adults are often of rapid onset and are characterized by a distinct alteration in mental state and function, the distinction in children is typically less clear. After commencement, manic symptoms in children and adolescents tend to follow a more chronic course, with bursts of mania interspersed with dysphoria or depression. In a four-year prospective longitudinal study of 86 subjects with a manic episode at intake, 87% achieved remission, but 64% of those achieving remission relapsed.[6] Mean episode duration for the index episode of mania was 79.2 +/– 66.7 consecutive weeks.[6] Children with BD are further differentiated from adolescents with the condition by having more continuous irritability, and more likely being male.[3] As co-morbidity with attention deficit hyperactivity disorder (ADHD), conduct disorder (CD), or anxiety problems is common, 'interepisode' functioning in a young person with BD may still be impaired. Children and adolescents presenting for acute treatment of mania may not have new or recent onset problems, but rather a worsening of difficulties that have been present for some time. As such, samples of children and adolescents recruited for acute treatment studies are not directly comparable with samples of adults recruited for clinical trials of acute mania.

The treatment of BD in children and adolescents is similar to the treatment of adults with the condition, but some differences emerge. Children and adolescents are more likely than adults to experience a protracted and poorly differentiated prodrome in which symptoms of other mental disorders may be prominent. As a result the management of the emergent BD is often a matter of modifying rather than initiating treatment. Treatment requires the engagement and cooperation of parents or caregivers. The disorder usually disrupts school attendance and academic performance, therefore the clinician must also liaise with educational providers. In some cases, behaviours exhibited by the young person may overwhelm the capacity of parents and caregivers, even in the absence of indications for hospitalization. In these situations the clinician may need to liaise with welfare services to arrange alternative accommodation. As is the case with unipolar depression, the evidence base for treating BD in children and adolescents is much narrower than it is for adults. However, there are now several randomized control trials (RCTs) for the treatment of acute mania with more in the pipeline.

National Institute for Health and Clinical Excellence[7] and American Academy of Child and Adolescent Psychiatry[8] guidelines for the assessment and treatment of BD in children and adolescents are in need of updating. That said, clinicians can be poorly adherent to the existing guidelines. A study of administrative claims data, for example, found that only 20% of children and adolescents with BD received recommended treatment within 90 days of diagnosis, while 24% received contraindicated treatment such as antidepressant monotherapy.[9] There is international variation in the approach to treatment. For example, first line management for mania is an antipsychotic agent in some countries, and a mood stabilizer in others.[10] There is also variability in the approaches to management between different treatment centres within the same country. Guidelines recommend that acute presentations of mania in young people should be managed in hospital if the patient is at risk of suicide.[8,7] Clark adds that in a first episode presentation hospitalization is useful to undertake the necessary baseline investigations.[11] Other options include partial hospitalization, assertive outreach, and outpatient treatment. Many of the clinical trials reported in this chapter were conducted in outpatient samples which may raise questions about the severity, and even primary nature, of the illness. However, outpatient treatment of acute mania in children and adolescents does appear to be common clinical practice, and may also be a reflection of the acute on chronic nature of manic presentations in the youth.

Early intervention

Early intervention in the context of BD refers to the recognition and management of individuals at high risk of developing the condition, and those with early manifestations of the illness. Some authors also include treatment of a first episode of BD within the early intervention framework.[12,13] In this chapter, first-episode mania will be discussed in the section on the treatment of acute mania. Owing to the gradual onset of bipolar symptoms in most young patients[14] the distinction between prodrome and first episode can, however, be blurred. Many young patients with an evolving BD will be in treatment already for a co-morbid condition such as anxiety, ADHD, CD or substance use disorders.

Potential indicators for early intervention include presence of: a positive family history for BD, prodromal symptom complex, neurobiological markers, endophenotypic markers, or temperamental features.[15] Characterization of the bipolar

prodrome is still in the development phase.[16] Candidate features of the bipolar prodrome are summarized with commentary in Table 21.1.

A retrospective study of 52 youths (16.2 ± 2.8 years) with an established diagnosis
of bipolar I found a gradual onset of symptoms in nearly 90% of the sample. Of those
with a gradual onset, two-thirds had a slow deterioration in symptoms prior to the
first index episode, with the remainder having a rapid deterioration.[14] The prodromal symptom complex comprised a mixture of non-specific general psychopathology such as a drop in school performance, subthreshold depressive symptoms, and
subthreshold mania symptoms such as racing thoughts, increased energy or goal-
directed behaviour, and overtalkativeness.[14] The significance of the high proportion

Table 21.1 Candidate features of the prodrome to bipolar disorder

Candidate prodromal feature	Comment
Subthreshold mania symptoms	Present for two or more consecutive days, but less than four days. The greater the number of symptoms, intensity, and duration the more likely the individual is to develop a full-blown bipolar episode. Needs to be distinguished in young people from elation caused, for example, by the completion of national examinations.
Depressive symptoms	Present for at least a week. Depression is a common disorder among young people hence relatively few experiencing these features alone will develop a full-blown bipolar episode.
Mood lability	Dysregulated mood is a feature of many mental disorders. In milder forms it is also a normal manifestation of adolescence. Is of greater significance if severe and of rapid onset.
Irritability	Irritability is a feature of many mental disorders. In milder forms it is also a normal manifestation of adolescence. Is of greater significance if severe and of rapid onset.
Anxiety/worry	Anxiety is a common disorder among young people hence relatively few experiencing these features alone will develop a full-blown bipolar episode.
Energy changes	In the absence of other features of subthreshold mania or depression.
Anger aggressiveness	In the absence of other features of subthreshold mania or depression.
Sleep disturbance	In the absence of other features of subthreshold mania or depression.
Features of attention deficit hyperactivity disorder	Especially if the symptoms are of atypically late onset; for example, occurring for the first time during adolescence.
Decline in academic/ occupational function and social function	Can be a signal of the onset of other disorders.

Adapted from *Bipolar Disorder*, 16, Malhi GS et al, 'Predicting bipolar disorder on the basis of
phenomenology: implications for prevention and early intervention', pp. 455–570. Copyright (2013) with
permission from John Wiley and Sons

reporting a gradual onset of problems is the opportunity it affords for recognition and intervention to inhibit or delay the first index episode.

Definitive treatment recommendations for the management of the prodrome to BD in children and adolescents would be premature, as more work is required to establish the sensitivity and specificity of the prodromal symptom complex. However, potential interventions recommended for the high-risk and prodromal group include self-help and mental health literacy, family psychoeducation, substance use reduction, cognitive behaviour therapy (CBT), and supportive counselling.[17] A systematic review concluded that family and child-focused interventions trialled in this context are of uncertain benefit.[18] In most circumstances the family and child-focused interventions included in the review were adjunctive to other treatment such as pharmacotherapy. In contrast, Cotton et al.[19] reported a pilot study of mindfulness-based cognitive therapy to youth with anxiety disorders and at risk for BD who were mostly not medicated. Participants experienced a reduction in anxiety and an improvement in emotion regulation but it is uncertain what protection the intervention afforded against the onset of bipolar symptoms. Pharmacotherapy has been advocated in high risk individuals and those experiencing a prodromal symptom complex on the theoretical grounds that some medications may be neuroprotective, thus delaying or suppressing the onset of acute symptoms.[20] To date, however, there has been no empirical research to support the practice. Similarly, there has been interest in complementary medicine, particularly Omega-3 fatty acid preparations, as a protective strategy in the bipolar prodrome but supporting evidence is still lacking.

Acute mania

A review of the acute treatment of mania in children and adolescents[21] concluded that second-generation antipsychotic (SGA) monotherapy is effective while current data do not support the use of mood-stabilizer (MS) monotherapy. Data for combination therapies are limited, and it is uncertain if they afford advantage over SGA monotherapy in the acute phase of treatment. Omega-3 fatty acids and psychosocial treatments are of uncertain benefit. Electroconvulsive therapy (ECT) is reserved for treatment-refractory mania. This section of the chapter updates the 2012 review.

An updated search of PubMed and the Clinical Trials databases identified four published randomized placebo controlled trials of SGA (aripiprazole (2), olanzapine, risperidone) and three unpublished trials (asenapine (NCT01349907, http://www.clinicaltrials.gov), quetiapine, ziprasidone). Since publication of the 2012 review, trials of paliperidone (NCT00592358, http://www.clinicaltrials.gov) and ziprasidone (NCT01117220, http://www.clinicaltrials.gov) have been terminated without results. Sample sizes ranged from 41 (aripiprazole 1) to 395 (asenapine). Participants were typically 10–17 years old, met criteria for BD type I (the aripiprazole trials also enrolled participants with BD type II), and were experiencing a manic or mixed episode. Trials commonly permitted ADHD, ODD, CD, and anxiety co-morbidity but excluded other psychiatric conditions. It was not clear in most cases if patients were naïve to antipsychotic medication. Acute trials ranged in duration from 21 to 42 days, but one of the aripiprazole trials was extended for a total of 30 weeks.[22] Three trials (aripiprazole

2, asenapine, and quetiapine) randomized participants to fixed doses of medication, while other trials titrated doses based on clinical efficacy and tolerability. The smaller aripiprazole trial permitted concurrent treatment with psychostimulants. Response in each of the trials was defined as a 50% reduction in scores on the Young Mania Rating Scale (YMRS). All trials favoured active treatment over placebo and differences in response rates were statistically significant. Response rates to active treatment ranged from 49% to 89%, while response to placebo ranged from 22% to 52%. Numbers needed to treat (NNT) for each trial and medication dose are summarized in Table 21.2.

Three reviews[23,24,25] of the tolerability of SGAs in children and adolescents approached the topic in different ways. Liu et al.[24] combined data from open-label and RCTs to provide a descriptive report of common adverse events for each drug. These data, augmented with data about asenapine, are summarized in Table 21.3. Fraguas et al.[23] reviewed open-label and randomized trials of SGA for both schizophrenia and bipolar spectrum disorders, focusing on weight gain, metabolic and cardiovascular parameters, prolactin levels, and extrapyramidal symptoms. Consistent with the descriptive data reported in Table 21.3, in RCTs for BD Fraguas et al.[23] found statistically significant increases in body mass index (BMI) for olanzapine and higher doses of risperidone, but not for aripiprazole, quetiapine, and lower doses of risperidone. Drug-placebo differences in mean glucose levels were non-significant for olanzapine and risperidone and unavailable for other SGA. Mean cholesterol level increases for aripiprazole, olanzapine, quetiapine, and risperidone were non-significant. Increases

Table 21.2 Numbers needed to treat (NNT) estimates derived from randomized controlled trials of second-generation antipsychotics for mania in children and adolescents

Medication	Daily dose	Duration of treatment	NNT
Aripiprazole 1	5–20 mg	42 days	3
Aripiprazole 2	10 mg	28 days	6
Aripiprazole 2	30 mg	28 days	3
Asenapine	5 mg	21 days	7
Asenapine	10 mg	21 days	4
Asenapine	20 mg	21 days	5
Olanzapine	2.5–20 mg	21 days	4
Quetiapine	400 mg	21 days	4
Quetiapine	600 mg	21 days	5
Risperidone	0.5–2.5 mg	21 days	3
Risperidone	3-6 mg	21 days	3
Ziprasidone	2.5–20 mg	21 days	4

Table 21.3 Adverse events described from open-label and randomized controlled trials of second-generation antipsychotics for mania in children and adolescents

Medication	Adverse events
Aripiprazole	Sedation, gastrointestinal complaints, cold symptoms, headache, extrapyramidal symptoms
Asenapine	Somnolence, sedation, oral hypoaesthesia, fatigue
Olanzapine	Sedation, cold symptoms, increased appetite, weight gain
Quetiapine	Sedation, gastrointestinal complaints, weight gain
Risperidone	Sedation, headaches, increased appetite, weight gain
Ziprasidone	Sedation, headaches, dizziness

Data from *Journal of the American Academy of Child & Adolescent Psychiatry*, 50, 2011, Liu HY et al, 'Pharmacologic treatments for pediatric bipolar disorder: a review and meta-analysis', pp. 749–762.

in mean triglyceride levels were statistically significant for olanzapine but non-significant for aripiprazole, quetiapine, and risperidone. Increases in mean prolactin levels were statistically significant for olanzapine and risperidone, and non-significant for quetiapine. Where available, rates of dystonia, rigidity, tremor, and akathisia were mildly elevated compared with placebo, but no difference reached statistical significance. Correll et al.[25] examined placebo-controlled trials for bipolar mania in both children and adults. The authors were able to calculate weighted numbers needed to harm (NNH) for several adverse outcomes across five RCTs for SGA. For the purposes of comparison in this chapter the NNH for each outcome was rounded up to the next whole number, and are presented along with data for MSs in Table 21.6.

MSs with or without antipsychotics have traditionally been used in the treatment of various phases of BD.[8] Evidence of their efficacy in the acute treatment of mania in children and adolescents comes predominantly from open-label trials and a few RCTs. Efficacy of MSs in children and adolescents with BD has been the subject of recent reviews and the following summary of their efficacy in mania is derived from them and supplemented by more recent trials.[25,26,27,24,28]

Liu et al. found three published randomized placebo-controlled trials of MSs (one each for extended release valproate, oxcarbazepine, and topiramate) for acute mania in children and adolescents[24] (see Table 21.4).

Trials of carbamazepine (NCT0018170) and lithium (NCT00442039) have been listed on the Clinical Trials Register (http://www.clinicaltrials.gov) as completed but

Table 21.4 Numbers needed to treat (NNT) estimates derived from randomized controlled trials of mood stabilizers for mania in children and adolescents

Medication	Mean daily dose	Duration of treatment	NNT
Extended-release valproate	1286 mg	28 days	100
Oxcarbazepine	1515 mg	49 days	6
Topiramate	278 mg	28 days	8

no results are listed. Sample sizes for the published studies ranged from 56 (topiramate) to 150 (extended release valproate). Participants were between 10–17 years old in the extended release valproate trial with the oxcarbazepine and topiramate trials extending down to seven years and six years, respectively. Participants met criteria for type I BD and were experiencing a manic or mixed episode. The trials commonly permitted ADHD, ODD, CD, and anxiety co-morbidity but excluded other psychiatric conditions. Trials ranged in duration from 28 to 49 days. The trials also permitted concurrent treatment with psychostimulant and rescue medications such as lorazepam. Response in two trials (extended release valproate and oxcarbazepine) was defined as a 50% reduction in scores on the YMRS whereas in the topiramate trial response was defined as much improved or very much improved on the Clinical Global Impression (CGI) scale. None of the trials favoured active treatment over placebo as differences in response rates failed to achieve statistical significance. Response rates to active treatment ranged from 24% to 42%, while response to placebo ranged from 22% to 26%. NNT are summarized in Table 21.4. Liu et al.[24] also identified a randomized placebo-controlled discontinuation trial of lithium, where randomization occurred after at least four weeks of treatment for mania. The difference in the rate of relapse between the group maintained on lithium and the group switched to placebo was not statistically significant. The finding is difficult to interpret, because patients were permitted to receive concurrent treatment with an antipsychotic medication (haloperidol or risperidone) if they were aggressive or experiencing psychotic symptoms.

There were no RCTs comparing other MSs (carbamazepine, standard release valproate, and lamotrigine) with placebo in the acute treatment of mania in children and adolescents. There were, however, eight monotherapy open-label trials including three with lithium, three with standard-release valproate, and one each with carbamazepine extended release and lamotrigine.[26,24] Sample sizes ranged from 30 to 100. Participant ages ranged from four to 19 years. Participants met criteria for type I BD in most trials and were experiencing a manic or mixed episode. Trials commonly permitted ADHD, ODD, CD, anxiety co-morbidity but excluded other psychiatric conditions and ranged in duration from two to 26 weeks. The lithium trials used target serum levels of 0.6 to 1.2 mEq/L and the divalproex sodium trials target levels at 80 to 125 µg/ml. Response rates (50% reduction in scores on the YMRS, plus in one study improved or very much improved on the CGI) ranged from 44% to 73%. These trials did not report on remission rates.

The adverse effects of MS use in children and adolescents has been the subject of recent reviews.[25,24] Relative to SGAs, there are fewer trials and less systematic data about adverse events. The combined adverse event data from open-label trials and RCTs are reported for each drug in Table 21.5.

Using NNH as a metric, relative to SGAs MSs were less likely to cause somnolence but more likely to cause insomnia and discontinuation owing to intolerability (summarized in Table 21.6).[25] Using weighted mean difference as a metric, weight gain was considerably less with MSs (effect size 0.10, 95% CI –0.12 to 0.33) than SGAs (effect size 0.53, 95% CI 0.41 to 0.66). Metabolic data have not been routinely collected in RCTs of MSs, therefore comparison with SGAs is not possible. No trials of lithium were included in the analysis conducted by Correll et al.,[25] but owing to its

Table 21.5 Adverse events described from open-label and randomized controlled trials of mood stabilizers for mania in children and adolescents

Medication	Adverse events
Lithium carbonate	Nausea, vomiting, increased appetite, weight gain, headaches, and stomach aches
Sodium valproate/ valproic acid/divalproex sodium	Sedation, gastrointestinal upset, headaches, dizziness, stomach pain, tremor, weight gain, decrease in mean platelet count, and increase in mean ammonia level
Carbamazepine	Nausea and sedation
Oxcarbazapine	Dizziness, nausea, somnolence, diplopia, fatigue, and rash
Lamotrigine	Gastrointestinal symptoms, headaches, and skin rashes
Topiramate	Decreased appetite, nausea, and weight loss

Data from *Journal of the American Academy of Child & Adolescent Psychiatry*, 50, 2011, Liu HY et al, 'Pharmacologic treatments for pediatric bipolar disorder: a review and meta-analysis', pp. 749–762.

properties lithium deserves special mention. Lithium has a low therapeutic index requiring regular monitoring of serum levels to ensure the drug dose is not too high. Toxicity can also occur if the patient becomes dehydrated (a risk for young physically active patients). Adverse effects are generally directly related to serum lithium concentrations. Common adverse effects seen even in the therapeutic range are listed in Table 21.5. More serious effects include renal dysfunction leading to polyuria, cardiovascular effects including arrhythmia, neurological effects, and thyroid suppression.

Three RCTs have compared MSs with each other or with SGAs in the acute treatment of mania in children and adolescents.[27,24,29] One RCT (50 people aged 12–18 years with mania treated for four weeks) found an 84% response rate in patients

Table 21.6 Weighted estimates for numbers needed to harm (NNH) for adverse events in randomized controlled trials of second-generation antipsychotics and mood stabilizers for mania

	SGAs	MSs
Somnolence	5	10
Insomnia	100	16
Akathisia	21	–
Extrapyramidal side effects	8	–
>7% weight gain	10	–
Hyperprolactinaemia	8	–
Discontinuation due to intolerability	21	10

Data from *Bipolar Disorders*, 12, 2010, Correll CU et al, 'Antipsychotic and mood stabilizer efficacy and tolerability in pediatric and adult patients with bipolar I mania: a comparative analysis of acute, randomized, placebo-controlled trials', pp. 116–141.

treated with quetiapine group compared with a 56% response rate in those treated with divalproex. In addition, the quetiapine group showed a more rapid resolution of manic symptoms.[24] One RCT (66 children and adolescents with mania treated for six weeks) found a 78.1% response/62.5% remission rate for those treated with risperidone compared with a 45.5% response/33.3% remission rate for those treated with valproate.[29] One RCT (279 people aged six to 15 years with mania treated for eight weeks) found response rates to risperidone, lithium, or valproate of 68.5%, 35.6%, and 24% respectively.[27] NNT for SGAs versus MSs are summarized in Table 21.7. A differing line of evidence involving retrospective analysis of claims data found patients receiving MS or SGA monotherapy had similar rates of hospital admission, but those initiated on an SGA were less likely to discontinue treatment (hazard ratio 0.63, 95% CI 0.42–0.96).[30]

One systematic review identified one RCT of combination pharmacotherapy.[24] This RCT (30 people aged 12–18 years with mania treated for six weeks) found an 87% response rate in patients treated with a combination of quetiapine plus divalproex compared with a 53% response rate in those treated with placebo plus divalproex with an NNT of 3 for the combination versus monotherapy.[24] The systematic review also found open-label studies for lithium plus divalproex, lithium plus risperidone, olanzapine plus topiramate, and an MS combined with another MS, psychostimulant, antipsychotic, or antidepressant.[24] A quasi-randomized study compared risperidone plus divalproex with risperidone plus lithium. Response rates ranged from 70.6% to 89.5%. Although some of these trials followed unsatisfactory response to monotherapy, comparison with monotherapy is not valid as the clinical improvements may have been a function of time on treatment or the natural history of the condition rather than specific benefits of combined therapy.

RCTs of the novel treatments riluzole (NCT00805493) and intranasal ketamine (NCT01504659) were registered with clinicaltrials.gov but have been terminated.

An RCT of flax oil (rich in Omega-3 fatty acids) in 51 young people with active bipolar symptoms found no advantage of active treatment over placebo in moderating symptoms over 16 weeks.[31] Only a quarter of the actively treated participants achieved a change in eicosapentaenoic acid (serum marker of Omega-3 fatty acid levels) the investigators considered adequate enough to be of benefit, therefore the findings are difficult to interpret.

Table 21.7 Numbers needed to treat (NNT) estimates derived from randomized controlled head-to-head comparison trials of mood stabilizers versus second-generation antipsychotics for mania in children and adolescents

Medication	Mean daily dose	Duration of treatment	NNT
Quetiapine vs divalproex	422 mg vs 101 µg/ml	28 days	4
Risperidone vs divalproex	1.4 mg vs 96 µg/ml	42 days	3
Risperidone vs lithium	2.6 mg vs 1.09 mEq/L	42 days	3
Risperidone vs divalproex	2.6 mg vs 113.6 µg/ml	42 days	2

Hazell and Jairam[21] found no recent studies reporting efficacy and safety of ECT for mania in children or adolescents. One small RCT (n = 18) directed to adolescent outpatients within three months of an acute manic, mixed, or depressive episode found dialectical behaviour therapy in combination with pharmacotherapy was no better than treatment as usual for reducing severity and duration of manic symptoms.[32]

Co-morbidity in children and adolescents with BD is common and most recent treatment trials as previously discussed permit ADHD, ODD, CD, obsessive–compulsive disorder, and anxiety co-morbidities making results more generalizable to clinical populations. However, these clinical studies have excluded participants with developmental disabilities, anorexia nervosa, schizophrenia, ongoing substance use disorder, major medical or neurological condition, and pregnancy.[27,24] One RCT and one open-label trial have found that ADHD co-morbidity did not reduce the antimanic response of SGAs (aripripazole and risperidone) and in fact risperidone demonstrated some efficacy in reducing ADHD symptoms as well.[33,24] A secondary analysis of an olanzapine trial for mania in children and adolescents found that 20 of the 52 subjects with mania had co-morbid OCD and their antimanic response to olanzapine was significantly worse than that of the subjects who did not have co-morbid OCD.[34]

Current data demonstrate that all SGAs so far evaluated are more likely than placebo to induce a clinically significant reduction in core symptoms of mania in children and adolescents. The data are encouraging but some questions still remain. We do not have good information about expected time to response, nor do we know what proportion of those deemed non-responders at study endpoint might be expected to respond with continuing treatment. Following on from this we do not have data to inform the decision of when to switch to an alternative agent, or when to augment treatment with an MS. The trials have involved outpatients or a combination of inpatients and outpatients. It is uncertain whether the results generalize to a more severely ill inpatient population. As noted by Pavuluri,[35] clinical trials have other limitations such as self-selection into studies, use of rescue medications which may mask the efficacy of the study drug, the impact of untreated co-morbidities, and the probability that the blind will be broken owing to the side effect profiles of the treatment. None of the reviews published to date has examined the impact of study quality on estimates of efficacy.

There is limited evidence to separate the evaluated SGAs in terms of efficacy, given the NNT estimates for optimal doses of each compound range from 3 to 4. Time to response analyses might in future separate the drugs, but this is unlikely. Attention naturally then shifts to tolerability, where data on some variables do separate the drugs. Most striking are the differential effects on weight gain, which are greatest for olanzapine and least for ziprasidone. During the relatively short period of acute stabilization of a manic episode, however, this should be of less concern than it is for continuation treatment. Weight gain can be minimized in the inpatient setting by optimizing the ward diet and encouraging the patients remain active.

The NNTs of SGAs versus MSs are similar to SGAs versus placebo, and RCTs to date have not found MSs to separate statistically from placebo in terms of response rates. Thus, the data does not support the use of MS monotherapy in the treatment of mania in children and adolescents. Combination therapy appears to be common in clinical practice.[36] Open-label evidence indicates that SGA + lithium/valproate and perhaps lithium + valproate combinations are effective in the acute treatment of mania in children and adolescents. Clinicians may have other reasons for prescribing combination therapy during the acute phase of treatment; for example, the early initiation of prophylaxis. Data for alternative and psychosocial treatments and ECT are too limited to allow comment on their role in acute treatment.

Bipolar depression

Depression is a common first manifestation of emergent BD, and youth with established BD spend more time in the depressed polarity than in hypomania or mania.[37] Distinguishing bipolar depression from unipolar depression prior to the onset of mania symptoms is a clinical challenge. A systematic review found that bipolar depression in youth was distinguished from unipolar depression by higher levels of depression severity, associated impairment, psychiatric co-morbidity with ODD, CD, and anxiety disorders, and family history of mood and disruptive behaviour disorders in first-degree relatives.[38] These features align with but are not identical to the characteristics of depression in youth that predict switching from depression to mania. Switching is predicted by a positive family history of mood disorders, emotional and behavioural dysregulation, subthreshold mania, and psychosis.[39] Not recognizing that these features signal the possibility of bipolar depression may lead to the initiation of antidepressant monotherapy, which is associated with a higher risk of manic switching than are other pharmacological treatments.[40]

RCTs for the treatment of bipolar depression in youth are few. Unlike studies in adult populations, RCTs of quetiapine and of extended-release quetiapine found no differences in response and remission rates of acute depression associated with bipolar I disorder in adolescents.[41,42] Significantly more adolescents with bipolar depression treated with a combination of olanzapine and fluoxetine achieved response and remission criteria than those treated with placebo over eight weeks.[43] The NNT for remission was 7. The rationale for combining an SGA with a serotonin reuptake inhibitor is to protect the patient against manic switching, owing to the antimanic properties of the antipsychotic. Fluoxetine is the antidepressant of first choice for depressed young people owing to its favourable safety and efficacy record. Olanzapine, on the other hand, would not be the first choice of SGA owing to its propensity to cause weight gain and metabolic effects. But the industry sponsor for the study was seeking Food and Drug Administration (FDA) approval for this specific treatment combination to extend its indication for bipolar depression to the paediatric age range. The active treatment group, as expected, gained more weight (average 4.4 kg) and was more likely to have abnormal lipid studies. Switching to mania was low (one patient). An alternative strategy is to combine an antidepressant with an MS, but there are no clinical trials in children and adolescents to support this practice.

A review of psychosocial treatments for paediatric bipolar spectrum disorders found no treatments specifically directed to bipolar depression.[44] That said, psychosocial treatments for BD often address the depressive as well as manic phases of the illness. RCTs are limited but the review identified one trial of family focused treatment (FFT) versus family education control for young people in the early phases of BD which found a significantly faster time to recovery from depressive symptoms in the experimental group.[44] An RCT of child- and family focused CBT versus psychotherapy as usual in 7–13 year olds with BD favoured the experimental treatment on parent-rated but not clinician-rated depression measures.[45] One small RCT (n = 18) directed to adolescent outpatients within three months of an acute manic, mixed, or depressive episode found dialectical behaviour therapy in combination with pharmacotherapy was superior to treatment as usual for reducing severity and duration of depressive symptoms.[32]

Relapse prevention

Relapse rates of BD in children and adolescents are at least as high as they are in adults.[46] A naturalistic study found 12 of 13 adolescents with BD who were poorly adherent to lithium treatment relapsed within 18 months, compared with 9 of 24 who were adherent to treatment.[47] Keeping a young person with BD well demands the application of the full range of specialist clinical skills, including the maintenance of a therapeutic alliance, individual psychological support, motivational interventions, attention to physical well-being and lifestyle, education and support of family or carers, liaison with education providers and other key people in the young person's life, and the capacity to monitor and fine-tune pharmacotherapy. Adolescents with BD may, similar to those with chronic medical conditions, erroneously believe that if they do not take treatment, they do not have a disorder. Adolescents may also ignore health-promoting advice about sleep, exercise, diet, and moderation of substance use through denial, or because they confuse it with parental overcontrol. I have resorted at times to using phrases with patients such as 'Everything is negotiable. Except your medication'.

Of the guidelines cited earlier in the chapter, one recommends monotherapy with an MS for relapse prevention[8] while the other recommends monotherapy with an SGA.[7] There is limited evidence to support either recommendation. The gold standard for establishing efficacy in relapse prevention is the rate of relapse and relative time to relapse after one or more treatments have been discontinued using randomized double-blind methodology. Two such trials were identified in a review.[46] In one trial, patients stabilized on a combination of lithium and divalproex were randomized to withdraw from one or other drug. There was no difference in rates of relapse (approximately 65%) or time to relapse (average 16 weeks). In another trial, patients stabilized on aripiprazole were randomized to continue on the study drug or switch to placebo. Time to discontinuation owing to a mood event was significantly longer in those maintained on aripiprazole compared with those switched to placebo (25.9 ± 5.5 weeks versus 3 ± 0.6 weeks, p <0.01) but discontinuation rates were high (80% and 100% respectively). An unpublished trial (NCT00723450, http://

www.clinicaltrials.gov) of lamotrigine augmentation of existing pharmacotherapy (unspecified) found longer mean time to a bipolar event in those who continued with the study drug compared with those who switched to placebo, but the difference was statistically non-significant (136 ± 15 days versus 107 ± 14 days, p = 0.07). Open-label studies exist for lithium and quetiapine but the findings are difficult to interpret.[46]

On the basis of existing evidence there is slightly more support for SGA monotherapy than there is for MS monotherapy to prevent the relapse of BD in children and adolescents, but there is a major knowledge gap in this area. There are no systematic data to inform combination treatments, or the optimal duration of any form of pharmacotherapy. The American Academy of Child and Adolescent Psychiatry guideline recommends at least 12 to 24 months of maintenance pharmacotherapy following an index episode[8] while the National Institute for Health and Clinical Excellence guideline recommends up to five years of maintenance treatment in patients who carry risk factors for relapse such as frequent episodes, previous psychotic episodes, substance misuse, ongoing stress, and poor social support.[7] Risks of relapse, particularly if they occur during important periods such as studying for and sitting national exams or moving away from home to attend tertiary education, need to be balanced against the risk of longer-term exposure to medication.

Refractory bipolar disorder

BD is considered refractory when a patient is experiencing a severe and sustained episode of mania or depression that has been unresponsive to standard medication therapies.[8] For mania this means not responding to a trial of at least one SGA in adequate doses combined with an MS in adequate doses for an adequate duration. For bipolar depression this means not responding to a trial of a combination of antidepressant and SGA with or without an MS, all in adequate doses. Such patients would usually be treated in an inpatient setting, preferably a high-severity or intensive care unit with staff skilled in the care children and adolescents who are severely unwell. The National Institute for Health and Clinical Excellence[7] and American Academy of Child and Adolescent Psychiatry[8] both recommend ECT for refractory mania and bipolar depression, although there is an absence of empirical evidence to support the practice. Indicators for ECT include physical compromise owing to dehydration, malnutrition, and exhaustion, severe and persistent psychotic symptoms, and unrelenting suicidality. Clinicians are advised to consult their local health authority guidelines concerning the assessment and consenting process for ECT in minors, as there is regional variation. Scheffer et al. developed a three-step algorithm for the management of treatment-resistant mania or mixed episode.[48] The three steps comprise: (i) removal of potentially destabilizing agents such as antidepressants, gamma aminobutyric acid agonists, and psychostimulants; (ii) optimization of antimanic agents; and (iii) use of a limited number of MSs. In an open-label study (n = 120) of people aged 6–17 years, three-quarters of the participants had achieved remission after six months of treatment informed by the algorithm. In refractory mania or mixed episode, clinicians might follow such an algorithm but move to ECT if the patient becomes critically unwell.

Concluding remarks

The treatment of BD in children and adolescents shares much in common with the treatment of adults with the condition, but there are important differences. As with the management of any child and adolescent mental health disorder, engagement and involvement of the patient's family is critical to successful intervention. Liaison with other key stakeholders such as education providers is also important. There is no definitive treatment for bipolar prodrome symptoms in children and adolescents, although candidate interventions include self-help, psychoeducation, individual therapy, and family interventions. Low-dose pharmacotherapy options have also been considered on theoretical grounds but evidence to support the practice is lacking. Most treatment research has focused on the management of acute mania, where pharmacotherapy is the dominant therapeutic modality. Evidence favours SGA monotherapy over MS monotherapy for time to response and efficacy, but not tolerability. There is no evidence indicating combination therapy is superior to monotherapy in the acute phase of mania. Empirical evidence for the treatment of bipolar depression is limited, with preliminary data favouring a combination of SGA and antidepressant over monotherapy with an SGA. There is consensus that antidepressant monotherapy is contraindicated owing to the risk of triggering a switch to mania. Concurrent family therapy may hasten recovery. SGA monotherapy may be effective in relapse prevention, while limited evidence suggests MS monotherapy may be ineffective. Guidelines endorse ECT for refractory mania and bipolar depression but there is no clinical trial evidence to support the practice. The development of algorithms to guide the management of all phases of BD is a work in progress.

References

1. **Pfeifer JC, Kowatch RA,** and **DelBello MP.** Pharmacotherapy of bipolar disorder in children and adolescents: recent progress, *CNS Drugs* 2010;**24**:575–93.
2. **Stringaris A, Santosh P, Leibenluft E,** et al. Youth meeting symptom and impairment criteria for mania-like episodes lasting less than four days: an epidemiological enquiry, *Journal of Child Psychology & Psychiatry & Allied Disciplines* 2010;**51**:31–8.
3. **Masi G, Perugi G, Millepiedi S,** et al. Developmental differences according to age at onset in juvenile bipolar disorder, *Journal of Child & Adolescent Psychopharmacology* 2006;**16**:679–85.
4. **Bardach NS, Coker TR, Zima BT,** et al. Common and costly hospitalizations for pediatric mental health disorders, *Pediatrics* 2014;**133**:602–9.
5. **Geller B** and **Luby J.** Child and adolescent bipolar disorder: a review of the past 10 years, *Journal of the American Academy of Child & Adolescent Psychiatry* 1997;**36**:1168–76.
6. **Geller B, Tillman R, Craney JL,** et al. Four-year prospective outcome and natural history of mania in children with a prepubertal and early adolescent bipolar disorder phenotype, *Archives of General Psychiatry* 2004;**61**:459–67.
7. **National Collaborating Centre for Mental Health.** *The Management of Bipolar Disorder in Adults, Children and Adolescents in Primary and Secondary Care* (London: Gaskell, 2006).

8. **McClellan J, Kowatch R, Findling RL**, et al. (2007) Practice parameter for the assessment and treatment of children and adolescents with bipolar disorder.[Erratum appears in J Am Acad Child Adolesc Psychiatry. 2007 Jun;46(6):786]. *Journal of the American Academy of Child & Adolescent Psychiatry* **46**: 107–125.

9. **Dusetzina SB, Gaynes BN, Weinberger M**, et al. Receipt of guideline-concordant pharmacotherapy among children with new diagnoses of bipolar disorder, *Psychiatric Services* 2011;**62**:1443–9.

10. **Diler R.** *Pediatric Bipolar Disorder. A Global Perspective* (New York, NY: Nova Science, 2006).

11. **Clark A.** Proposed treatment for adolescent psychosis. 2: bipolar illness, *Advances in Psychiatric Treatment* 2001;**7**:143–9.

12. **Berk M, Hallam K, Malhi GS**, et al. Evidence and implications for early intervention in bipolar disorder, *Journal of Mental Health* 2010;**19**:113–26.

13. **Macneil CA, Hallam K, Conus P**, et al. Are we missing opportunities for early intervention in bipolar disorder?, *Expert Review of Neurotherapeutics* 2012;**12**:5–7.

14. **Correll CU, Hauser M, Penzner JB**, et al. Type and duration of subsyndromal symptoms in youth with bipolar I disorder prior to their first manic episode, *Bipolar Disorders* 2014;**16**:478–92.

15. **Pavuluri MN.** Effects of early intervention on the course of bipolar disorder: theories and realities, *Current Psychiatry Reports* 2010;**12**:490–8.

16. **Malhi GS, Bargh DM, Coulston CM**, et al. Predicting bipolar disorder on the basis of phenomenology: implications for prevention and early intervention, *Bipolar Disorders* 2014;**16**:455–70.

17. **Berk M, Berk L, Dodd S**, et al. Stage managing bipolar disorder, *Bipolar Disorders* 2014;**16**:471–7.

18. **Frias A, Palma C,** and **Farriols N.** Psychosocial interventions in the treatment of youth diagnosed or at high-risk for pediatric bipolar disorder: a review of the literature, *Rev Psiquiatr Salud Ment* 2015; doi:10.1016/j.rpsm.2014.11.002.

19. **Cotton S, Luberto CM, Sears RW**, et al. Mindfulness-based cognitive therapy for youth with anxiety disorders at risk for bipolar disorder: a pilot trial, *Early Intervention in Psychiatry* 2015; doi: 10.1111/eip.12216.

20. **Salvadore G, Drevets WC, Henter ID**, et al. Early intervention in bipolar disorder, part II: therapeutics, *Early Intervention in Psychiatry* 2008;**2**:136–46.

21. **Hazell P** and **Jairam R.** Acute treatment of mania in children and adolescents, *Current Opinion in Psychiatry* 2012;**25**:264–70.

22. **Findling RL, Correll CU, Nyilas M**, et al. Aripiprazole for the treatment of pediatric bipolar I disorder: a 30-week, randomized, placebo-controlled study, *Bipolar Disorders* 2013;**15**:138–49.

23. **Fraguas D, Correll CU, Merchan-Naranjo J**, et al. Efficacy and safety of second-generation antipsychotics in children and adolescents with psychotic and bipolar spectrum disorders: comprehensive review of prospective head-to-head and placebo-controlled comparisons, *European Neuropsychopharmacology* 2011;**21**:621–45.

24. **Liu HY, Potter MP, Woodworth KY**, et al. Pharmacologic treatments for pediatric bipolar disorder: a review and meta-analysis, *Journal of the American Academy of Child & Adolescent Psychiatry* 2011;**50**:749–62.e739.

25. **Correll CU, Sheridan EM,** and **DelBello MP.** Antipsychotic and mood stabilizer efficacy and tolerability in pediatric and adult patients with bipolar I mania: a

comparative analysis of acute, randomized, placebo-controlled trials, *Bipolar Disorders* 2010;**12**:116–41.

26. **Findling RL, Kafantaris V, Pavuluri M**, et al. Dosing strategies for lithium monotherapy in children and adolescents with bipolar I disorder, *Journal of Child & Adolescent Psychopharmacology* 2011;**21**:195–205.

27. **Geller B, Luby J, Joshi P**, et al. A randomized controlled trial of risperidone, lithium, or divalproex sodium for initial treatment of bipolar I disorder, manic or mixed phase, in children and adolescents, *Archives of General Psychiatry* 2012.

28. **Thomas T, Stansifer L**, and **Findling RL**. Psychopharmacology of pediatric bipolar disorders in children and adolescents, *Pediatric Clinics of North America* 2011;**58**:173–87.

29. **Pavuluri MN, Passarotti AM, Lu LH**, et al. Double-blind randomized trial of risperidone versus divalproex in pediatric bipolar disorder: fMRI outcomes, *Psychiatry Research* 2011;**193**:28–37.

30. **Chen H, Mehta S, Aparasu R**, et al. Comparative effectiveness of monotherapy with mood stabilizers versus second generation (atypical) antipsychotics for the treatment of bipolar disorder in children and adolescents, *Pharmacoepidemiology & Drug Safety* 2014;**23**:299–308.

31. **Gracious BL, Chirieac MC, Costescu S**, et al. Randomized, placebo-controlled trial of flax oil in pediatric bipolar disorder, *Bipolar Disorders* 2010;**12**:142–54.

32. **Goldstein TR, Fersch-Podrat RK, Rivera M**, et al. Dialectical behavior therapy for adolescents with bipolar disorder: results from a pilot randomized trial, *Journal of Child and Adolescent Psychopharmacology* 2015;**25**:140–9.

33. **Biederman J, Hammerness P, Doyle R**, et al. Risperidone treatment for ADHD in children and adolescents with bipolar disorder, *Neuropsychiatric Disease and Treatment* 2008;**4**:203–7.

34. **Joshi G, Mick E, Wozniak J**, et al. Impact of obsessive–compulsive disorder on the antimanic response to olanzapine therapy in youth with bipolar disorder, *Bipolar Disorders* 2010;**12**:196–204.

35. **Pavuluri M**. Pharmacologic treatments for pediatric bipolar disorder (letter), *Journal of the American Academy of Child and Adolescent Psychiatry* 2011;**50**:1290.

36. **Constantine RJ, Boaz T**, and **Tandon R**. Antipsychotic polypharmacy in the treatment of children and adolescents in the fee-for-service component of a large state Medicaid program, *Clinical Therapeutics* 2010;**32**:949–59.

37. **DeFilippis MS** and **Wagner KD**. Bipolar depression in children and adolescents, *CNS Spectrums* 2013;**18**:209–13.

38. **Uchida M, Serra G, Zayas L**, et al. Can unipolar and bipolar pediatric major depression be differentiated from each other? A systematic review of cross-sectional studies examining differences in unipolar and bipolar depression, *Journal of Affective Disorders* 2015;**176**:1–7.

39. **Uchida M, Serra G, Zayas L**, et al. Can manic switches be predicted in pediatric major depression? A systematic literature review, *Journal of Affective Disorders* 2014;**172c**:300–6.

40. **Bhowmik D, Aparasu RR, Rajan SS**, et al. Risk of manic switch associated with antidepressant therapy in pediatric bipolar depression, *Journal of Child and Adolescent Psychopharmacology* 2014;**24**:551–61.

41. **DelBello MP, Chang K, Welge JA**, et al. A double-blind, placebo-controlled pilot study of quetiapine for depressed adolescents with bipolar disorder, *Bipolar Disorders* 2009;**11**:483–93.

42. **Findling RL, Pathak S, Earley WR**, et al. Efficacy and safety of extended-release quetiapine fumarate in youth with bipolar depression: an 8-week, double-blind, placebo-controlled trial, *Journal of Child and Adolescent Psychopharmacology* 2014;**24**:325–35.

43. **Detke HC, DelBello MP, Landry J**, et al. Olanzapine/fluoxetine combination in children and adolescents with bipolar I depression: a randomized, double-blind, placebo-controlled trial, *Journal of the American Academy of Child and Adolescent Psychiatry* 2015;**54**:217–24.

44. **Fristad MA** and **MacPherson HA**. Evidence-based psychosocial treatments for child and adolescent bipolar spectrum disorders, *Journal of Clinical Child and Adolescent Psychology* 2014;**43**:339–55.

45. **West AE, Weinstein SM, Peters AT**, et al. Child- and family-focused cognitive-behavioral therapy for pediatric bipolar disorder: a randomized clinical trial, *Journal of the American Academy of Child and Adolescent Psychiatry* 2014;**53**:1168–78;1178.e1161.

46. **Diaz-Caneja CM, Moreno C, Llorente C**, et al. Practitioner review: long-term pharmacological treatment of pediatric bipolar disorder, *Journal of Child Psychology & Psychiatry & Allied Disciplines* 2014;**55**:959–80.

47. **Strober M, Morrell W, Lampert C**, et al. Relapse following discontinuation of lithium maintenance therapy in adolescents with bipolar I illness: a naturalistic study, *The American Journal of Psychiatry* 1990;**147**:457–61.

48. **Scheffer RE, Tripathi A, Kirkpatrick FG**, et al. Guidelines for treatment-resistant mania in children with bipolar disorder, *Journal of Psychiatric Practice* 2011;**17**:186–93.

Chapter 22

The treatment of bipolar disorder in the elderly

Gilberto Sousa Alves, Felipe Kenji Sudo, and Johannes Pantel

Introduction

Bipolar disorder (BD) is an extremely disabling condition characterized by periodic mood changes, euphoria, and disinhibition, usually accompanied by cognitive and functional impairment. The estimated prevalence of BD in adult life may range from 2.8 to 6.5%.[1] In the aged population, the prevalence is not fully known. The Epidemiologic Catchment Area study, which involved more than 20,000 outpatients, estimated 0.2% in the 45–64-year-old group,[2] while another study, with a population-based sample, found a prevalence rate of 0.6% in adults aged 65 or older.[3] The neurobiology of BD in elderly patients remains largely disputed, with changes in brain structure and connectivity, particularly in frontal and temporal lobes, being regarded as major neuroanatomical aspects,[4] while genetic and environmental factors seem to be associated in a lesser extension with clinical features. Vascular changes in small vessels, commonly associated with depressive symptoms, rarely lead to maniac symptoms, although the occurrence of heart attacks, thalamic ischaemia, for example, can be in a few cases associated with the outbreak of mood symptoms. With regards to the classification systems, the *Diagnostic and Statistical Manual of Mental Disorders* (5th edition) (DSM-5) and the *International Classification of Diseases* (10th revision) (ICD-10),[5,6] clinical features of BD in the elderly and other age groups are described essentially identical.

A large number of studies have reported cognitive changes among elderly patients with BD. The mostly compromised domains were processing speed and cognitive function. It seems that this cognitive pattern is a candidate trait feature of BD in general, and some evidence has been collected on a worse of such functional deficits in older patients.[7] Mortality rates, including death related to suicidal behaviour, are higher among elderly BD patients when compared with the general population.[8] Evidence also reported a higher use of outpatient psychogeriatric and daily clinic services among BD patients when compared with subjects with unipolar depression.[9]

In this chapter, a review of the current evidence for treating BD in the elderly is summarized, and new perspectives of treatment addressed.

General recommendations for the therapeutic intervention in old-age BD

Peculiarities of BD among elderly patients

The initial therapeutic approach must take into consideration the multiple aspects that differentiate the clinical picture of old-age BD from findings in younger adults. While less is known on the role of medication in neuronal connectivity, clinical experience testifies the higher number of adverse effects among elderly BD subjects, including tardive dyskinesia, dizziness, and sedation. Bioavailability of psychotropic medication may be altered by gastrointestinal absorption, reduced muscle mass associated with higher percentage of fat in human body, reduced first-pass hepatic metabolism and hepatic biotransformation, as well as a decreased serum albumin. Taking together, age-related pharmacokinetic changes justify the well-known recommendation of 'start low, go slow' in the vast majority of cases. Another difficulty is that the occurrence of depressive symptoms in BD is usually more frequent than either hypomanic or maniac features, which eventually can mask treatment effects.[10] Conversely, up to 25% of patients diagnosed with major depressive disorder (MDD) may show features of BD.[11] Furthermore, geriatric BD tend to have lower qualification and are more likely to present with depressive polarity of first episode.[12]

As in young and adult patients, the recognition of typical maniac symptoms in the elderly patient is a primary need for proper diagnosis: racing thoughts, pressure speech, distractibility, affective instability, increased energy and activity, and reduced length of sleep may lead to reconsideration of the diagnosis of BD in patients previously categorized as MDD.[13]

Ascertaining the differential diagnosis

The management of BD in the elderly may be difficult by multiple issues[14] (see Table 22.1). One must carefully consider the occurrence of a medical co-morbidity in the differential diagnosis. In addition, there is a risk of co-morbidity with some dementia syndromes, particularly frontotemporal dementia (FTD) and Alzheimer's dementia.[15] Misdiagnosis with FTD may often occur, even though it is less discussed by the literature.[15] In addition, a higher occurrence of cerebrovascular risk factors and white-matter hyperintensities has been reported in late-onset BD.[16] The so-called secondary mania may be suspected in subjects with no history of mood disorder and may be associated with systemic infections, such as influenza, St Louis type A encephalitis and Q fever and other medical aetiologies (Table 22.1). Taken together, these issues strongly support the need of a rigorous medical and neurological examination, particularly for the first-time treated patient.

Another difficulty is that the first diagnosis of affective disorder among relatively young older people may be often depression, while maniac features have been reported as a tardive feature, that usually appears up to ten years after the onset.[17] Treatment for BD must consider the efficacy of pharmacological agents during different phases of the disease, including periods of euthymia in which relapse prevention strategies can be applied. Optimal management of BD requires a careful multidimensional

Table 22.1 Initial approach and treatment management of geriatric BD

What to investigate	What to rule out
Suicidal thoughts or attempts	Environment factors, co-morbid personality disorder
Depressive or maniac episodes throughout life	Anxiety and somatic disorders
History of mood disorders in the family	Unipolar depression
Impulsivity, aggressive behaviour	Thyroid dysfunction, frontotemporal dementia medication misuse
Personality trait-markers	Borderline, schizoid personality; alcohol or drug abuse
Current or recent use of corticosteroids and other medications	Lupus, withdraw symptoms of corticoid, supra adrenal suppression, Graves' disease; investigate use of anabolic drugs, amphetamine, amantadine, St John's wort, thyroid supplements
Atypical symptoms: syncope, balance or gait disorder, loss of urinary control, weight loss	Frontal lobe tumours, vascular ischaemia, Parkinson syndrome, metastases, subarachnoid bleeding, meningiomas, encephalitis due to influenza, St Louis type A encephalitis or Q fever

investigation. Preferably, treatment should be preceded by a detailed clinical assessment, in which the mental health professional can formulate a syndromic diagnosis and screen for risk situations, such as suicidal ideation and aggressive behaviour. Where risk is identified, a management plan should be developed (hospitalization or day treatment, for instance) and reviewed throughout the treatment.[18] After that, the assessment of signs and symptoms can be performed and the use of rating scales to quantify severity of the acute episode and to check for treatment response is advised. A medical examination should be conducted to identify co-morbidities and differential diagnoses. Behavioural disturbances may warrant immediate administration of pharmacological agents, even before the comprehensive psychiatric assessment can be undertaken, to ensure the patient's safety.[19]

Establishing compliance to treatment

Although data suggested that the adequate management of BD was associated with improvement in the quality of life, social and physical functioning of patients, poor compliance have been recognized as a major challenge for clinicians assisting those individuals. Suboptimal adherence may range from 20 to 69% in this population and it may be associated with lack of insight into the need for medications, desire to avoid medication side effects, co-morbidity with substance abuse, and cognitive deficits observed in older BD subjects.[20] When compared with younger BD subjects, older patients tend to present a lesser knowledge on mood disorders in general and more negative views on the need to use it.[21,22] Therefore, general treatment recommendations for BD commonly highlight the importance of early establishing a stable therapeutic alliance between the professional and the patient. Monitoring the patient's satisfaction during the treatment, evaluating the psychosocial context, the support network and the coping styles may contribute to adherence to treatment and it may allow the detection of environmental factors contributing to the illness.[19] Psychosocial strategies (commented in more detail in the further topics) are effective and should be considered alongside pharmacological treatment.

Identifying potential risks and complication prior to therapy

Overall, age itself has been regarded as a distinguished risk factor for drug-associated side effects, including the higher risk of falls and hip or femur fractures, acute renal failure, and Parkinson-similar symptoms. Older adults are thus at increased risk for developing several adverse reactions, mostly related to medication toxicity, presence of a co-morbid disease process, and use of multiple medications. Patient safety should be a major concern in those cases. Medication management requires monitoring of safe therapeutic serum levels, as well as rapidly detecting side effects.[23] One recent review have also defined one group with possible distinct neuropathology and clinical features, the older-age BD (OABD), defined as individuals aged over 60 years and that might represent as much as 25% of total BD population.[24] However, the OABD categorization still awaits evidence on controlled psychosocial studies and large-scale prospective pharmacological intervention.[24]

Some particularities in managing old age BD require close monitoring. Older BD subjects are among the higher-risk groups for developing metabolic syndrome, mainly those using olanzapine or clozapine.[25] The risk for medication-induced cognitive disorders should also be considered, especially when polypharmacy and higher doses are applied.[26] Interestingly, growing evidence supports the effects of chronic lithium intake in slowing the progression of neurodegeneration in BP patients with high risk for developing Alzheimer's disease.[27] Risk of fall may be increased in inpatients using lithium, anticonvulsants, antipsychotics, and antidepressants.[28] Conversely, anticonvulsant use may increase over twofold the risk for bone fracture in older subjects.[29]

Treatment of old-age BD

The need to promote a rational use of medication and non-pharmacological intervention has justified the development of guidelines for the treatment of BD in adults. As a result, publications from the American Psychiatric Association, the Canadian Network for Mood and Anxiety Treatments (CANMET), and the World Federation of Societies of Biological Psychiatry (WFSBP) have achieved increasing popularity. Some of the major issues underlined by guidelines are safety, tolerability, and potentially undesirable interactions. The recommendation level (RG) may combine the optimal levels of safety and tolerability. The level 1 would be prescribing a drug with the highest rating in both scores. Usually, when all the drugs of the RG 1 failed, it is recommended shifting to RG of 2, then 3, 4, or 5.[10]

The following recommendations for the management of older BD patients were based on clinical guidelines,[30,11,31,32] results from mixed population studies, and a small series of cases[33] and reports on effectiveness and tolerability of agents in this population. Of 998 clinical trials assessing BD registered in the American Clinical Trial Registry, only nine specifically recruited older patients.[34] Of note, differences in pharmacokinetics, psychiatric and general medical co-morbidities, and the concurrent use of multiple medications are some of the factors that may influence the treatment response and tolerability, and should be considered by clinicians when assisting those patients.

Taken together, the current evidence points to the lack of evidence-based treatment guidelines and randomized controlled studies to provide safe and effective recommendation of lithium, valproate, and other mood stabilizers in old-age BD treatment. In spite of that, a great deal of effort has been done by some reviews[35,36,37,38] to sum up the evidence on the management and treatment of BD in the elderly.

Pharmacological treatment

Emergency management of acute mania

When oral therapy is possible, atypical antipsychotics, including risperidone, olanzapine and quetiapine, and valproate should be considered in the early treatment of acute agitation. Benzodiazepines (clonazepam and lorazepam) should not be used in monotherapy, but can be useful adjuncts to sedate agitated patients. In patients who refuse oral medications, intramuscular olanzapine, ziprasidone and aripiprazole, or a combination of haloperidol and a benzodiazepine may be considered in line with the relevant legal regulations. Intravenous sodium valproate or oral divalproex extended release (ER) have shown to improve acute mania in recent studies. Antidepressants should be tapered and discontinued.[11,32]

Management of acute mania

Untreated manic subjects or those using other medications should be initiated with first-line agents (Figure 22.1). First-line agents for management of acute mania in monotherapy include lithium, valproate (or divalproex and divalproex ER), olanzapine, risperidone, quetiapine (and quetiapine XR), aripiprazole, asenapine, ziprasidone, and paliperidone ER. For dysphoric or mixed mania, valproate or carbamazepine or atypical antipsychotics may have better efficacy than lithium.[39,40,41] Valproic acid may be preferred to lithium in secondary mania, particularly due to stroke and dementia, subjects with renal failure and cardiac disorders, whereas lithium may be more secure in individuals with liver diseases and in patients using warfarin.[40,42] Carbamazepine should be used with caution, due to drug interactions and risk for Steven-Johnson syndrome.[30] Genotyping HLA-B-1502 has been advised to reduce the risk for hypersensitivity reactions when using carbamazepine.[30] Oxcarbazepine produces less drug interactions, but risk of hyponatremia and inconclusive results from studies evaluating its effect on mania has lowered it to a third-line option.[32] As mentioned, olanzapine and clozapine should be avoided in patients with risk for metabolic syndrome.[30]

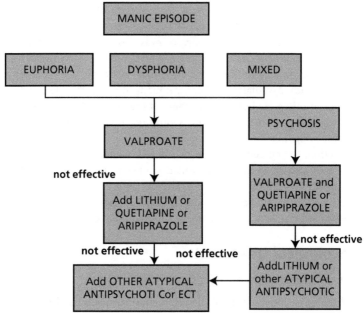

Figure 22.1 Algorithm for Manic episode in older BD patients
Data from World *Journal of Biological Psychiatry*, 11, 2010, Grunze H et al, 'The World Federation of Societies of Biological Psychiatry (WFSBP) Guidelines for the Biological Treatment of Bipolar Disorders: Update 2010 on the treatment of acute bipolar depression', pp. 81–109; data from *Bipolar Disorder*, 15, 2013, Yatham L.N et al, 'Canadian Network for Mood and Anxiety Treatments (CANMAT) and International Society for Bipolar Disorders (ISBD) collaborative update of CANMAT guidelines for the management of patients with bipolar disorder', pp. 1–44.

Risperidone is categorized as first-line in one guideline,[40] but extrapyramidal effects may worsen motor function in elderly individuals, and only limited data exists on its efficacy in mixed states. Ziprasidone can be effective, but potential cardiac toxicity should be a concern when administering to older subjects.[40] Moreover, the tolerability of lithium is lower in the elderly and neurotoxicity occurs at concentrations considered safe in general adult populations. Lithium clearance decreases with age due to less efficient glomerular filtration. In addition, drugs commonly used by older people, such as thiazide diuretics, angiotensin-converting enzyme (ACE) inhibitors, and non-steroidal anti-inflammatory drugs, can increase serum lithium concentrations.[43]

Although less than 10% of patients in acute mania receive monotherapy, researchers have recommended that clinicians should avoid combination therapy in older BD subjects, so that drug interactions and side effects could be minimized.[30,40] Only when patients are uncontrolled on monotherapy with a first-line agent in optimal dosage, the next step should be switching to or adding on an alternative first-line agent. Combination of lithium with valproate may have 1.5-fold better efficacy than monotherapy with either drug.[30] Other first-line adjunctive therapy includes combinations of the following agents with lithium or divalproex: risperidone, quetiapine, olanzapine, aripiprazole, or asenapine. Studies suggested that about 20% more patients could respond with combined therapy than with mood-stabilizer monotherapy.[32]

Patients who are intolerant or irresponsive to monotherapy and combined therapy with first-line agents should then receive a second-line agent. Second-line therapy includes agents in monotherapy (carbamazepine, carbamazepine ER, haloperidol, and electroconvulsive therapy—ECT) or combined therapy (lithium + divalproex). Although ECT can be an effective option for treating acute mania, research studies have not be rigorous; therefore, more data are needed to include it among first-line intervention. Haloperidol has shown to be more effective in acute mania than lithium, divalproex, quetiapine, aripiprazole, ziprasidone, carbamazepine, asenapine, and lamotrigine. However, several authors advised that the use of haloperidol should be restricted to short periods, since it may increase risk of a depressive episode.[30,32]

Third-line options have shown to be beneficious in small trials, but further studies are still needed to recommend their formal application. Those agents are, in monotherapy, chlorpromazine, clozapine, oxcarbazepine, and tamoxifen. Third-line combined strategies include lithium or divalproex + haloperidol, lithium + carbamazepine, and adjunctive tamoxifen.[32]

Agents that presented negative results in trials and therefore are not recommended for the management of acute mania are gabapentin, topiramate, lamotrigine, verapamil, and tiagabine. Combinations that fail to show benefits in manic states are: risperidone + carbamazepine and olanzapine + carbamazepine.[30,32] The latter combined therapy can possible increase in the risk of dyslipidemia and weight gain; therefore, it should not be used in older overweight BD patients.[30]

Antidepressants should be discontinued and factors that can perpetuate manic symptoms, such as prescribed medication, illicit-drug use/abuse, or an endocrine disorder, should be ruled out. Patients should be advised to avoid stimulants, such as caffeine and alcohol, and gradually decrease nicotine use.[32] Hypnotics and sedatives should be discontinued as soon as symptoms improve.[11]

The STEP-AD study reported that older BD patients who achieved remission used 689 (±265) mg/day of lithium, which is close to the minimum dose recommended for young BD adults. Valproate was also used in lower doses in elders with BD than in younger subjects, but the mean daily doses were within the recommended range for young adults.[44]

Management of acute bipolar depression

Drug-free patients should start with a first-line agent (Figure 22.2). According to the CANMAT guideline, first-line agents in monotherapy are lithium, lamotrigine, quetiapine, and quetiapine XR;[32] however, the Taiwan consensus included only quetiapine as first-line agent for acute bipolar depression.[30] The British Association of Psychopharmacology recommended quetiapine and lamotrigine as first-line options.[11] Previous response to a medication appears to be a strong predictor for treatment success.[45] Combined first-line strategies include: lithium or divalproex + SSRI, olanzapine + SSRI, lithium + divalproex, and lithium or divalproex + bupropion.[32] The WFSBP contraindicated lithium in monotherapy for bipolar depression due to inconclusive data; on the other hand, the combination of lithium and lamotrigine was considered the first choice when monotherapy fails.[45] Quetiapine and quetiapine XR were accepted as a first-option agent in all guidelines.

Controversy in this field is abundant. A recent meta-analysis reported that statistical superiority of active agents over placebo was identified in only half of the trials.

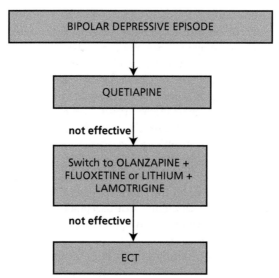

Figure 22.2 Algorithm for depressive episode in older BD patients
Data from *World Journal of Biological Psychiatry*, 11, 2010, Grunze H et al, 'The World Federation of Societies of Biological Psychiatry (WFSBP) Guidelines for the Biological Treatment of Bipolar Disorders: Update 2010 on the treatment of acute bipolar depression', pp. 81–109; data from *Neural Regeneration Research*, 8, 2013, Zhang, Y et al, 'Antidepressants for bipolar disorder: A meta-analysis of randomized, double-blind, controlled trials', pp. 2962–2974.

Evidence was stated as inconsistent, unfavourable or poorly studied for several treatments. For instance, authors reported that there was no well conducted study showing efficacy of lithium in acute bipolar depression.[46] A multisite prospective trial of lamotrigine showed significant improvement in depression (57.4% of remission and 64.8% of response) and improvement in functional status in bipolar depressed elders.[17] Nonetheless, the need to administer it slowly to avoid dermatological side effects might make it difficult to employ in acute bipolar phases. Valproate has been poorly studied up to the present in this phase of the disease. Quetiapine has proven to be superior to placebo in five clinical trials, although effect-sizes were moderate. Combination of olanzapine + fluoxetine achieved the higher effect-size for the management of bipolar depression in a recent meta-analysis, although methodological issues and the high dropout rate (38.5%) may have influenced the results.[46]

Use of antidepressants in acute bipolar depression has been a long-standing object of debate. Antidepressants in monotherapy have been regarded as contraindicated in patients with BD because of the weak evidence of efficacy.[45] A large randomized placebo-controlled trial assessing antidepressant monotherapy in bipolar depression—the EMBOLDEN II (Efficacy of Monotherapy Seroquel in Bipolar Depression) study—did not evidence superiority of 20 mg of paroxetine over placebo as measured by the Montgomery-Åsberg Depression Rating Scale (MADRS), after eight weeks.[47] Overall, the combination of olanzapine–fluoxetine has been indicated for BD, although there is no specification of such use for geriatric BD.[48] Conversely, a recent meta-analysis of randomized, double-blind, controlled trials concluded that antidepressants were not superior to placebo in the treatment of bipolar depression.[49] The research evidence about the risk of switching to mania with antidepressants is inconsistent.[30]

Managing mixed mania state

Recommendations for mixed mania have been regarded for most of the literature as tentative, particularly due to imprecise definition of mixed state.[10] Patients classified as showing mixed states may present more severe depressive episodes and somewhat milder manic states than those presenting mania solely.

Some evidence indicates more benefit of valproate than lithium in mixed manic states, but this evidence remains disputed.

Maintenance therapy

Continuation period is defined as the first six months following the acute episode, whereas maintenance period refers to months 6–12 after remission of acute symptoms.[30] There is currently no international consensus for the indication of the maintenance treatment. While North American guidelines suggested that maintenance phase treatment should be adopted after every episode, European recommendations indicated the need for it only after the second episode and with an interval of < three years between the two episodes. The WFSBP guidelines recommended maintenance therapy only for: (i) patients with a first episode, severe symptoms, and psychiatric family history; (ii) those with a second episode, with a psychiatric family history or severe symptoms; and (iii) those with a third episode.[30]

According to the British Association of Psychopharmacology, the Taiwan consensus, and the CANMAT group, lithium, valproate, olanzapine, and quetiapine (for both depression and mania), as well as lamotrigine (for preventing depression) and risperidone long-acting injection (LAI) are considered the first-line monotherapy options for maintenance treatment of BD. The WFSBP guidelines did not include valproate as a first-line choice and considered lithium as the highest effective option for long-term relapse prevention, especially for the indicators 'any episode' or mania.[31] The CANMAT also included ziprasidone for preventing manic episodes, whereas the British and the WFSBP recommendations included aripiprazole to prevent mania.[11,31] Aripiprazole may also have some effect in preventing rapid cycling.[31] Quetiapine, risperidone LAI (mania), aripiprazole (mania), and ziprasidone (mania) are also recommended as adjunctive therapy with lithium or divalproex. Adjunctive treatment with topiramate, oxcarbazepine, and gabapentin has yielded inconsistent results.[30,32]

The role of antidepressants in the maintenance phase is debatable, considering that more than 50% of the patients may have residual depressive symptoms.[50] However, evidence is still weak to recommend the long-term use of antidepressants in BD.[31]

Managing adverse reactions of therapy

As a general rule, the clinician must be aware of the pharmacological issues involving bioavailability and interaction between different drug classes. Common and rare adverse events must be monitored carefully in the first weeks of treatment.

Concerning the choice of the optimal mood stabilizer, the increased rate of side effects has demotivated many clinicians to continue prescribing lithium therapy for BD in the elderly. It is estimated that for every new prescription of lithium, there were at least three others of valproate.[33] In fact, important aspects have encouraged clinicians to prefer the valproate therapy prescriptions. One example is the effect of lithium on thyroid function. Although evidence on this issue remains disputed, ageing has been regarded as one important contributor to affect body pharmacokinetics by reducing the clearance and distribution of lithium. Previous evidence reported a twofold higher prevalence of hypothyroidism among BD,[51] even though no evidence agreement has been accomplished and negative results could also be noted.[52] In addition, the monitoring of drug interactions is a point of major concern, since a considerable number of medications may diminish lithium urine excretion and increase the risk of neurotoxicity, including ACE, furosemide, thiazide diuretics, and non-steroidal anti-inflammatories (Table 22.2). More often, lithium-related complications comprise renal dysfunction, dermal reactions, reduced magnesium and calcium uptake, elevated plasmatic levels of calcium and magnesium, and weight gain.

A general approach to some common problems reported alongside old-age BD treatment is briefly summarized in Table 22.2.

Non-pharmacological treatment

ECT and repetitive transcranial magnetic stimulation (rTMS)

When applied according to the current standards, ECT is considered a low-risk procedure in older subjects, although transient increase in blood pressure and in myocardial oxygen demand can occur.[53] Depressed older patients are treated with ECT more often than younger individuals, due to the poor tolerance to pharmacotherapy, the need for rapid response in frail subjects, and the higher frequency of treatment resistance and psychotic symptoms. One study assessing effectiveness of acute and maintenance ECT in elderly subjects reported a decrease in the hospitalization rates and in the admission days.[54]

Limited data exists on the use of ECT in old manic patients, but anecdotal clinical experience recommends its use, especially in severe and refractory cases.[55,42] rTMS may be a substitute for ECT. However, amount and quality of evidence on rTMS in this patient group is low and a single-blind study did not show comparable efficacy.[30]

Psychotherapy and psychosocial interventions

While pharmacotherapy is considered the first-line treatment, most of the guidelines recommended that ongoing psychotherapy and psychosocial rehabilitation should be performed. Among interventions suited for older BD patients, cognitive behaviour therapy (CBT) and interpersonal and social rhythm therapy (IPSRT) are the most recommended due to the presence of a stronger psychoeducational component than other methods.[56] Interpersonal therapy and family focused therapy were also included in clinical recommendations.[11]

Table 22.2 Management of physical conditions often present in treatment of geriatric BD

Be cautious with	How to manage
Reduced biotransformation	• Prefer using lorazepam instead of diazepam • Avoid use of Cytochrome P450 inducers (CBZ) • Poor metabolism of CYP1A2 may be a problem among 12% of elderlies
Reduced bioavailability	• Monitor mood-stabilizer levels every 1–2 weeks during the first two months; keep lower serum levels in the elderly: lithium (0.4–1 mEq/L), valproate (65–90 µg/mL) • Rate renal clearance, serum BUN and creatinine every 1–3 months after baseline
Frailty	• Avoid severe sedation • Monitor risk of falls • Family counselling • Consider hospital admission • Reduce at the lowest effective dosage possible antipsychotic or mood stabilizer • Physiotherapy
Metabolic disease	• Prefer short-term use of olanzapine in case of diabetes (switch to other antipsychotic when it is possible)
Pharmacological interactions	• CBZ + Ca^{++} channel blockers = risk of CBZ toxicity; monitor CBZ levels • Lithium + non-steroidal anti-inflammatories| methyldopa |loop diuretic |COX-2 inhibitors = risk of lithium toxicity; avoid combination or monitor carefully blood lithium • Valproate + meropenem/imipenem = decrease valproate level. Avoid this combination • Valproate + sulfonylureas (glimepiride) = decrease valproate levels; risk of hypoglycaemia; decrease valproate levels • Warfarin-antidepressants = risk of bleeding; avoid or decrease warfarin level
Toxicity signals	• Impaired cognition, coarse tremor, lethargy, weakness, hyperreflexia, ataxia, dysarthria, bradycardia, hypotension, oliguria, fever • Monitor closely vital signals, diuresis, neurological level • Reduce drastically or suspend the mood stabilizer • Consider admission when depressed conscious level, worse of symptoms • Administer drug monitoring
Decrease of renal function	• Adjust daily dosage of lithium to lower levels • Monitor glomerular filtration in case of pre-existing renal impairment

A relatively small number of controlled studies support specific biologic or psychosocial interventions for either acute or long-term care of elderly patients with BD. Furthermore, the lack of greater sample sizes, homogeneous age groups, multiple medications in use, and medical co-morbidities might be potential confounders on most of these studies.

Psychotherapy for BD subjects aims at decreasing both overt and mild/subclinical symptoms and improving quality of life. Identifying and coping with prodromal symptoms through CBT has shown to enhance treatment compliance and maintain social rhythm stability.[57] Moreover, teaching individuals about the relationship between stress, the environmental context, and the rupture of sleep/wake cycles on the one hand, and the onset of symptoms on the other hand can prevent the trigger factors associated with vulnerability for mood episodes and positively influence long-term course of the disease.[56]

To sum up, more studies on psychotherapy and other non-pharmacological intervention are required to comprehend the role of these interventions on the course of BD. Whenever possible, family members and caregivers should be encouraged to participate in the treatment and should receive continuous information and counselling from specialists.

Concluding remarks

In despite of the emerging evidence brought by literature, therapeutic efforts targeting depressive and maniac symptoms in old-age BD are still limited by some important gaps in the efficacy, safety, and tolerability of medications. In addition, mixed or unclear clinical presentation of BD in the elderly and the neurobiological mechanisms associated with the disorder remain disputed and shall be clarified by future research. Treatment guidelines reassemble the current evidence and may provide a more rational intervention on acute or long-lasting symptoms. Elderly patients with BD must be cautiously accompanied in relation to drug compliance, titration schema, and clinical and laboratory examination. Whenever possible, family members or caregivers should be involved in the treatment process. Ethical issues involving patrimony and profession may eventually lead to forensic evaluation.

References

1. Bauer M, and Pfennig A. Epidemiology of bipolar disorders, *Epilepsia* 2005;**46**(Suppl 4):8–13.

2. Regier DA, Boyd JH, Burke JD, Rae DS, Myers JK, Kramer M, Robins LN, George LK, Karno M, and Locke BZ. One-month prevalence of mental disorders in the United States. Based on five Epidemiologic Catchment Area sites, Arch Gen Psychiatry 1988;**45**:977–86.

3. Préville M, Boyer R, Grenier S, Dubé M, Voyer P, Punti R, Baril M-C, Streiner DL, Cairney J, and Brassard J. Scientific Committee of the ESA Study. The epidemiology of psychiatric disorders in Quebec's older adult population, Can J Psychiatry Rev Can Psychiatr 2008;**53**:822–32.

4. **Oertel-Knöchel V, Reuter J, Reinke B, Marbach K, Feddern R, Alves G, Prvulovic D, Linden DEJ, and Knöchel C.** Association between age of disease-onset, cognitive performance and cortical thickness in bipolar disorders, J Affect Disord 2015. doi: 10.1016/j.jad.2014.10.060

5. *Diagnostic and Statistical Manual of Mental Disorders* (Amer Psychiatric Pub Incorporated, 2013).

6. *The ICD-10 Classification of Mental and Behavioural Disorders: Clinical Descriptions and Diagnostic Guidelines* (World Health Organization, 1992).

7. **Gunning-Dixon FM, Murphy CF, Alexopoulos GS, Majcher-Tascio M, and Young RC.** Executive dysfunction in elderly bipolar manic patients, Am J Geriatr Psychiatry Off J Am Assoc Geriatr Psychiatry 2008;**16**:506–12. doi: 10.1097/JGP.0b013e318172b3ec

8. **Dhingra U, and Rabins PV.** Mania in the elderly: a 5–7 year follow-up, J Am Geriatr Soc 1991;**39**:581–3.

9. **Bartels SJ, Forester B, Miles KM, and Joyce T.** Mental health service use by elderly patients with bipolar disorder and unipolar major depression, Am J Geriatr Psychiatry Off J Am Assoc Geriatr Psychiatry 2000;**8**:160–6.

10. **Bowden CL.** Pharmacological treatments for bipolar disorder: present recommendations and future prospects. In: *Behavioral Neurobiology of Bipolar Disorder and its Treatment* (Springer Science & Business Media; 2010).

11. **Goodwin GM, Consensus Group of the British Association for Psychopharmacology.** Evidence-based guidelines for treating bipolar disorder: revised second edition— recommendations from the British Association for Psychopharmacology, J Psychopharmacol Oxf Engl 2009;**23**:346–88. doi: 10.1177/0269881109102919

12. **Nivoli AMA, Murru A, Pacchiarotti I, Valenti M, Rosa AR, Hidalgo D, Virdis V, Strejilevich S, Vieta E, and Colom F.** Bipolar disorder in the elderly: a cohort study comparing older and younger patients, Acta Psychiatr Scand 2014;**130**:364–73. doi: 10.1111/acps.12272

13. **Goldberg JF, Perlis RH, Bowden CL, Thase ME, Miklowitz DJ, Marangell LB, Calabrese JR, Nierenberg AA, Sachs, and GS.** Manic symptoms during depressive episodes in 1,380 patients with bipolar disorder: findings from the STEP-BD, Am J Psychiatry 2009;**166**:173–81. doi: 10.1176/appi.ajp.2008.08050746

14. **Abou-Saleh MT, Katona CLE, and Kumar A.** *Principles and Practice of Geriatric Psychiatry* (John Wiley & Sons, 2011).

15. **Neary D, Snowden JS, Gustafson L, Passant U, Stuss D, Black S, Freedman M, Kertesz A, Robert PH, Albert M, Boone K, Miller BL, Cummings J, and Benson DF.** Frontotemporal lobar degeneration: a consensus on clinical diagnostic criteria, *Neurology* 1998;**51**:1546–54.

16. **Aylward EH, Roberts-Twillie JV, Barta PE, Kumar AJ, Harris GJ, Geer M, Peyser CE, Pearlson GD.** 1994. Basal ganglia volumes and white matter hyperintensities in patients with bipolar disorder. Am. J Psychiatry **151**, 687–693.

17. **Sajatovic M, Gildengers A, Jurdi RK Al, Gyulai L, Cassidy KA, Greenberg RL, Bruce ML, Mulsant BH, Have T Ten, and Young RC.** Multisite, open-label, prospective trial of lamotrigine for geriatric bipolar depression: a preliminary report, Bipolar Disord 2011;**13**:294–302. doi: 10.1111/j.1399-5618.2011.00923.x

18. **Sajatovic M, Herrmann N, and Shulman K.** Acute mania and bipolar affective disorder. In: *Principles and Practice of Geriatric Psychiatry* (John Wiley & Sons, 2011).

19. **Malhi GS, Adams D, Lampe L, Paton M, O'Connor N, Newton LA, Walter G, Taylor A, Porter R, Mulder RT, and Berk M.** Northern Sydney Central Coast Mental Health Drug & Alcohol, NSW Health Clinical Redesign Program, CADE Clinic, University of Sydney. Clinical practice recommendations for bipolar disorder, Acta Psychiatr Scand 2009;Suppl 27–46. doi: 10.1111/j.1600-0447.2009.01383.x

20. **Depp CA, Cain AE, Palmer BW, Moore DJ, Eyler LT, Lebowitz BD, Patterson TL, and Jeste DV.** Assessment of medication management ability in middle-aged and older adults with bipolar disorder, J Clin Psychopharmacol 2008;**28**:225–9. doi: 10.1097/JCP.0b013e318166dfed

21. **Kessing LV.** Diagnostic subtypes of bipolar disorder in older versus younger adults, Bipolar Disord 2006;**8**:56–64. doi: 10.1111/j.1399-5618.2006.00278.x

22. **Schaub RT, Berghoefer A, and Müller-Oerlinghausen B.** What do patients in a lithium outpatient clinic know about lithium therapy?, J Psychiatry Neurosci JPN 2001;**26**:319–24.

23. **Sherrod T, Quinlan-Colwell A, Lattimore TB, Shattell MM, and Kennedy-Malone L.** Older adults with bipolar disorder: guidelines for primary care providers J Gerontol Nurs 2010;**36**:20–7; quiz 28–9. doi:10.3928/00989134-20100108-05

24. **Sajatovic M, Strejilevich SA, Gildengers AG, Dols A, Jurdi RK Al, Forester BP, Kessing LV, Beyer J, Manes F, Rej S, Rosa AR, Schouws SN, Tsai S-Y, Young RC, and Shulman KI.** A report on older-age bipolar disorder from the International Society for Bipolar Disorders Task Force, Bipolar Disord 2015. doi: 10.1111/bdi.12331

25. **McIntyre RS, Danilewitz M, Liauw SS, Kemp DE, Nguyen HTT, Kahn LS, Kucyi A, Soczynska JK, Woldeyohannes HO, Lachowski A, Kim B, Nathanson J, Alsuwaidan M, and Taylor VH.** Bipolar disorder and metabolic syndrome: an international perspective, J Affect Disord 2010;**126**:366–87. doi:10.1016/j.jad.2010.04.012

26. **Diniz BS, Nunes PV, Machado-Vieira R, and Forlenza OV.** Current pharmacological approaches and perspectives in the treatment of geriatric mood disorders, Curr Opin Psychiatry 2011;**24**:473–7. doi: 10.1097/YCO.0b013e32834bb9bd

27. **Kessing LV, Forman JL, and Andersen PK.** Does lithium protect against dementia?, Bipolar Disord 2010;**12**:87–94. doi: 10.1111/j.1399-5618.2009.00788.x

28. **Lavsa SM, Fabian TJ, Saul MI, Corman SL, and Coley KC.** Influence of medications and diagnoses on fall risk in psychiatric inpatients, Am J Health-Syst Pharm AJHP Off J Am Soc Health-Syst Pharm 2010;**67**:1274–80. doi: 10.2146/ajhp090611

29. **Mezuk B, Morden NE, Ganoczy D, Post EP, and Kilbourne AM.** Anticonvulsant use, bipolar disorder, and risk of fracture among older adults in the Veterans Health Administration, Am J Geriatr Psychiatry Off J Am Assoc Geriatr Psychiatry 2010;**18**:245–55. doi: 10.1097/JGP.0b013e3181bf9ebd

30. **Bai Y-M, Chang C-J, Tsai S-Y, Chen Y-C, Hsiao M-C, Li C-T, Tu P, Chang S-W, Shen WW, and Su T-P.** Taiwan consensus of pharmacological treatment for bipolar disorder, J Chin Med Assoc JCMA 2013;**76**:547–56. doi: 10.1016/j.jcma.2013.06.013

31. **Grunze H, Vieta E, Goodwin GM, Bowden C, Licht RW, and Möller H-J, Kasper S.** WFSBP Task Force on Treatment Guidelines for Bipolar Disorders. The World Federation of Societies of Biological Psychiatry (WFSBP) guidelines for the biological treatment of bipolar disorders: update 2012 on the long-term treatment of bipolar disorder, World J Biol Psychiatry Off J World Fed Soc Biol Psychiatry 2013;**14**:154–219. doi: 10.3109/15622975.2013.770551

32. Yatham LN, Kennedy SH, Parikh SV, Schaffer A, Beaulieu S, Alda M, O'Donovan C, Macqueen G, McIntyre RS, Sharma V, Ravindran A, Young LT, Milev R, Bond DJ, Frey BN, Goldstein BI, Lafer B, Birmaher B, Ha K, Nolen WA, and Berk M. Canadian Network for Mood and Anxiety Treatments (CANMAT) and International Society for Bipolar Disorders (ISBD) collaborative update of CANMAT guidelines for the management of patients with bipolar disorder: update 2013, Bipolar Disord 2013;15:1–44. doi: 10.1111/bdi.12025

33. Shulman KI. Lithium for older adults with bipolar disorder: Should it still be considered a first-line agent?, *Drugs Aging* 2010;27:607–15. doi: 10.2165/11537700-000000000-00000

34. Health, US National Institutes of, 4 August. Clinical trials on geriatric bipolar disorder. [Online document]. Available at: https://clinicaltrials.gov/ct2/results?term=Geriatric+Bipolar+Disorder+AND+treatment&Search=Search.

35. Aziz R, Lorberg B, and Tampi RR. Treatments for late-life bipolar disorder, Am J Geriatr Pharmacother 2006;4:347–64. doi: 10.1016/j.amjopharm.2006.12.007

36. Sajatovic M, Madhusoodanan S, and Coconcea N. Managing bipolar disorder in the elderly: defining the role of the newer agents, *Drugs Aging* 2005;22:39–54.

37. Shulman KI, and Herrmann N. The nature and management of mania in old age, Psychiatr Clin North Am 1999;22:649–65, ix.

38. Young RC, Gyulai L, Mulsant BH, Flint A, Beyer JL, Shulman KI, and Reynolds CF. Pharmacotherapy of bipolar disorder in old age: review and recommendations, Am J Geriatr Psychiatry Off J Am Assoc Geriatr Psychiatry 2004;12:342–57. doi: 10.1176/appi.ajgp.12.4.342

39. Ceron-Litvoc D, Soares BG, Geddes J, Litvoc J, and de Lima MS. Comparison of carbamazepine and lithium in treatment of bipolar disorder: a systematic review of randomized controlled trials, Hum Psychopharmacol 2009;24:19–28. doi: 10.1002/hup.990

40. Grunze H, Vieta E, Goodwin GM, Bowden C, Licht RW, Moller H-J, and Kasper S. The World Federation of Societies of Biological Psychiatry (WFSBP) guidelines for the biological treatment of bipolar disorders: update 2009 on the treatment of acute mania, World J Biol Psychiatry Off J World Fed Soc Biol Psychiatry 2009;10:85–116. doi: 10.1080/15622970902823202

41. Smith LA, Cornelius V, Warnock A, Tacchi MJ, and Taylor D. Acute bipolar mania: a systematic review and meta-analysis of co-therapy vs monotherapy, Acta Psychiatr Scand 2007;115:12–20. doi: 10.1111/j.1600-0447.2006.00912.x

42. Marín-Mayor JL-Á. LF, and Agüera-Ortiz M. *Abordaje terapéutico del trastorno bipolar en ancianos: tratamientos específicos y características especiales, Psicogeriatría* 2009;1(2):115–25.

43. Sproule BA, Hardy BG, and Shulman KI. Differential pharmacokinetics of lithium in elderly patients, *Drugs Aging* 2000;16:165–77.

44. Jurdi RK Al, Marangell LB, Petersen NJ, Martinez M, Gyulai L, and Sajatovic M. Prescription patterns of psychotropic medications in elderly compared with younger participants who achieved a 'recovered' status in the systematic treatment enhancement program for bipolar disorder. Am J Geriatr Psychiatry Off J Am Assoc. Geriatr Psychiatry 2008;16:922–33. doi: 10.1097/JGP.0b013e318187135f

45. Grunze H, Vieta E, Goodwin GM, Bowden C, Licht RW, Möller H-J, and Kasper S. The World Federation of Societies of Biological Psychiatry (WFSBP) Guidelines for the

Biological Treatment of Bipolar Disorders: Update 2010 on the treatment of acute bipolar depression, World J Biol Psychiatry 2010;11:81–109. doi: 10.3109/15622970903555881

46. **Selle V, Schalkwijk S, Vázquez GH, and Baldessarini RJ.** Treatments for acute bipolar depression: meta-analyses of placebo-controlled, monotherapy trials of anticonvulsants, lithium and antipsychotics, *Pharmacopsychiatry* 2014;47:43–52. doi: 10.1055/s-0033-1363258

47. **McElroy SL, Weisler RH, Chang W, Olausson B, Paulsson B, Brecher M, Agambaram V, Merideth C, Nordenhem A, and Young AH.** EMBOLDEN II (Trial D1447C00134) Investigators. A double-blind, placebo-controlled study of quetiapine and paroxetine as monotherapy in adults with bipolar depression (EMBOLDEN II), J Clin Psychiatry 2010;71:163–74. doi: 10.4088/JCP.08m04942gre

48. **Pacchiarotti I, Bond DJ, Baldessarini RJ, Nolen WA, Grunze H, Licht RW, Post RM, Berk M, Goodwin GM, Sachs GS, Tondo L, Findling RL, Youngstrom EA, Tohen M, Undurraga J, González-Pinto A, Goldberg JF, Yildiz A, Altshuler LL, Calabrese JR, Mitchell PB, Thase ME, Koukopoulos A, Colom F, Frye MA, Malhi GS, Fountoulakis KN, Vázquez G, Perlis RH, Ketter TA, Cassidy F, Akiskal H, Azorin J-M, Valentí M, Mazzei DH, Lafer B, Kato T, Mazzarini L, Martínez-Aran A, Parker G, Souery D, Özerdem A, McElroy SL, Girardi P, Bauer M, Yatham LN, Zarate CA, Nierenberg AA, Birmaher B, Kanba S, El-Mallakh RS, Serretti A, Rihmer Z, Young AH, Kotzalidis GD, MacQueen GM, Bowden CL, Ghaemi SN, Lopez-Jaramillo C, Rybakowski J, Ha K, Perugi G, Kasper S, Amsterdam JD, Hirschfeld RM, Kapczinski F, and Vieta E.** The International Society for Bipolar Disorders (ISBD) Task Force Report on Antidepressant Use in Bipolar Disorders, Am J Psychiatry 2013;170:1249–62. doi: 10.1176/appi.ajp.2013.13020185

49. **Zhang Y, Yang H, Yang S, Liang W, Dai P, Wang C, and Zhang Y.** Antidepressants for bipolar disorder: a meta-analysis of randomized, double-blind, controlled trials, Neural Regen Res 2013;8:2962–74. doi: 10.3969/j.issn.1673-5374.2013.31.009

50. **Arvilommi P, Suominen K, Mantere O, Leppämäki S, Valtonen HM, and Isometsä E.** Maintenance treatment received by patients with bipolar I and II disorders—a naturalistic prospective study, J Affect Disord 2010;121:116–26. doi: 10.1016/j.jad.2009.05.005

51. **Juurlink DN, Mamdani MM, Kopp A, Rochon PA, Shulman KI, and Redelmeier DA.** Drug-induced lithium toxicity in the elderly: a population-based study, J Am Geriatr Soc 2004;52:794–8. doi: 10.1111/j.1532-5415.2004.52221.x

52. **Kupka RW, Nolen WA, Post RM, McElroy SL, Altshuler LL, Denicoff KD, Frye MA, Keck Jr, PE, Leverich GS, Rush AJ, Suppes T, Pollio C, and Drexhage HA.** High rate of autoimmune thyroiditis in bipolar disorder: lack of association with lithium exposure, Biol Psychiatry 2002;51:305–11. doi: 10.1016/S0006-3223(01)01217-3

53. **Kelly KG, and Zisselman M.** Update on electroconvulsive therapy (ECT) in older adult, J Am Geriatr Soc 2000;48:560–6. doi: 10.1111/j.1532-5415.2000.tb05005.x

54. **Shelef A, Mazeh D, Berger U, Baruch Y, and Barak Y.** Acute electroconvulsive therapy followed by maintenance electroconvulsive therapy decreases hospital re-admission rates of older patients with severe mental illness, J ECT 2015;31:125–8. doi: 10.1097/YCT.0000000000000197

55. **Lisanby SH.** Electroconvulsive therapy for depression, N Engl J Med 2007;357:1939–45. doi: 10.1056/NEJMct075234

56. Frank E, Swartz HA, and **Kupfer DJ**. Interpersonal and social rhythm therapy: managing the chaos of bipolar disorder, Biol Psychiatry 2000;**48**:593–604.

57. **Lam DH, Watkins ER, Hayward P, Bright J, Wright K, Kerr N, Parr-Davis G,** and **Sham P**. A randomized controlled study of cognitive therapy for relapse prevention for bipolar affective disorder: outcome of the first year, Arch Gen Psychiatry 2003;**60**:145–52.

Chapter 23

The management of treatment-resistant bipolar disorder

Salih Selek, Ives Cavalcante Passos, and Jair C. Soares

Definition of treatment resistance in bipolar disorder

According to the World Health Organization (WHO), bipolar disorder (BD) is among the ten leading causes of disability in young adults.[1] A significant proportion of patients with BD respond incompletely or unsatisfactorily to first-line treatments. For instance, it is known that non-response in bipolar depression is highly prevalent and occurs in 40% of patients after eight weeks of treatment with quetiapine.[2] Other first-line treatments, such as lithium, lamotrigine, olanzapine, or olanzapine-fluoxetine combination, have similar or even less favourable outcome.[2,3,4] Also, the addition of antidepressants to an ongoing treatment with mood stabilizers will be helpful in only a quarter of patients with bipolar depression.[5] How to treat this large number of refractory patients is a major challenge, since treatment-resistant BD is associated with greater morbidity, suicide attempts, as well as with extensive use of depression-related and general medical services.[6]

Consensus opinion on the classification of treatment resistance in BD has not been established yet.[7] With this caveat in mind, the most accepted definition of treatment resistance in BD is non-responsiveness to at least two adequate trials of medications within a specific episode.[8] Thereby, according to Sachs,[9] treatment-refractory mania could be defined as mania without remission despite six weeks of adequate therapy with at least two antimanic agents, while treatment-refractory bipolar depression was defined as depression without remission despite two adequate trials of standard antidepressant agents. He also defined the term treatment-refractory mood cycling, which means continued cycling despite maximal tolerated combined medications for a period of three times the average cycle length, or six months.[9] Moreover, Yatham and colleagues suggested another definition for treatment refractoriness in BD: patients who failed to respond to a trial with lithium at serum levels of 0.8 mmol/L and above for six weeks, following previous other researchers.[10] In this chapter, we will refer to treatment resistance as a failure of two adequate drug trials if not otherwise specified.[11] The main focus of this chapter is on somatic treatments including pharmacotherapy, electroconvulsive therapy (ECT), and novel therapeutic approaches. We will also review the current bipolar treatment guidelines' third- or further-line treatments although treatment resistance is not underlined in most of the guidelines.

Management of treatment-resistant mania

Review of the guidelines

Most available guidelines do not provide a working definition of treatment resistance term but Sachs[9] proposes that treatment resistance could refer to patients with bipolar disorder who failed to respond to third- and above-line treatment interventions. Herein, we will review several currently available treatment guidelines including the American Psychiatric Association (APA), the Texas Implementation of Medication Algorithms (TIMA), the British Association for Psychopharmacology (BAP), the Canadian Network for Mood and Anxiety Treatments (CANMAT), the World Federation of Societies of Biological Psychiatry (WFSBP), and the Korean Medication Algorithm for Bipolar Disorder. These guidelines were selected to reflect the scientific evidence and heterogeneity of treatment strategies globally.

APA guideline

The first APA Practice Guideline for BD was published in 1995 with only five types of medication.[12] The guideline was revised in 2002 and the work group classified its suggestions into three groups reflecting the evidence from the research. Level I indicated substantial clinical confidence whereas level III suggestions were with low clinical confidence.[13] This guideline uses the terms 'refractory' and resistance interchangeably. The task team suggests clozapine and ECT for treatment-resistant cases—the ECT with higher level of clinical confidence. Clozapine trials were rated as having lower clinical confidence.

Texas Implementation of Medication Algorithms (TIMA)

The Texas Medication Algorithm Project (TMAP) was developed in 1995 by the Texas Department of Mental Health and Mental Retardation in collaboration with Texas universities to assess the value of an algorithm-driven disease-management programme in the pharmacological management of mentally ill patients. The guideline for BD was updated in 2005.[14] Throughout this chapter, we consider the third and fourth treatment steps as indicative of therapeutic approaches for treatment-resistant BD since the algorithm is stepwise, and those stages are recommended for those patients who failed or did not respond to the first two stages, although working definitions of non-response and partial response are not clearly provided in this guideline. The algorithm suggests combinations of two drugs, including lithium, valproic acid, atypical antipsychotics, typical antipsychotics, carbamazepine, and oxcarbamazepine. The guideline also suggests not combining two antipsychotics and not using clozapine at the third stage. Before moving to the next stage, symptom-targeted add-on treatments such as clonidine for aggression and hypnotics for insomnia are recommended. At the fourth stage, for patients who did not respond to a two-drug combination, the guideline suggests the use of either ECT or clozapine or three-drug combinations.[14]

British Association of Psychopharmacology (BAP) guidelines

The first BAP guideline for BD was published in 2003[15] and revised in 2009.[16] The guideline has four evidence levels for casual relationships and treatment.[17] This consensus panel recommends clozapine or ECT for more refractory illness.[16]

The Canadian Network for Mood and Anxiety Treatments (CANMAT) and the International Society for Bipolar Disorders (ISBD) guideline

CANMAT published its first guideline for BD in 2005 and updated it several times in collaboration with the ISBD.[18] The guideline has four evidence criteria. Although the guideline does not define treatment-resistant mania, its fourth step includes treatment resistant by us according to the defined criteria above, since the first step includes general principles rather than new interventions including discontinuing antidepressants and avoiding caffeine and alcohol, instead of drugs substances of abuse.[19] The guideline offers replacing one or both agents with other first-line agents including lithium, divalproex/extended release (ER), olanzapine, risperidone, quetiapine/XR, aripiprazole, ziprasidone, asenapine, and paliperidone ER for the fourth step. The guideline also suggests considering a switch to second- or third-line options or ECT. Second-line treatments also include carbamazepine, carbamazepine ER, and haloperidol as drug monotherapy options other than ECT. In addition, third-line treatment includes chlorpromazine, clozapine, oxcarbazepine, tamoxifen, and cariprazine. In case of non-response, novel agents including zotepine, levetiracetam, phenytoin, mexiletine, omega-3 fatty acids, calcitonin, rapid tryptophan depletion, allopurinol, amisulpride, folic acid, and memantine are offered as possible therapeutic alternatives.[19]

World Federation of Societies of Biological Psychiatry (WFSBP) guidelines

The WFSBP updated its guideline for acute mania in 2009. The authors of the guideline borrowed their anxiety guideline evidence criteria that has six categories of evidence and five levels of recommendation also considering the safety and tolerability of available treatments.[20] Combinations of recommendations are also allowed. The authors offer ECT in particular for treatment-refractory mania but if the third level is accepted as treatment resistance, a combination of their first-choice treatment including aripiprazole, risperidone, valproate, and ziprasidone, and if long treatment is considered at the same time, then lithium is provided as an option for treatment-resistant mania.[21] For the further levels clozapine is also considered.

Korean Medication Algorithm for Bipolar Disorder

The Korean Medication Algorithm Project for Bipolar Disorder (KMAP-BP) began in 2001 and has since been updated several times.[22] The guideline was based upon the outcomes of a 56-item questionnaire that was used to obtain the consensus of experts, including 110 Korean psychiatrists and 38 experts for child and adolescent psychiatry. Thus, the recommendations appear to be more naturalistic rather than evidence-based. If the third stage is considered as indicative of treatment resistance, then the guideline offers one or two atypical antipsychotics combined with lithium and/or valproate.[23] In addition, ECT and benzodiazepines can be used based on the clinician's clinical evaluation at any time regardless of the level of resistance and/or severity. For further steps, clozapine combination with other mood stabilizers or antipsychotics is recommended for treatment.

As a summary, guidelines in general suggest clozapine or ECT for treatment-resistant mania. Some guidelines offer drug combinations including classical mood stabilizers and antipsychotic agents. Novel agents including omega-3 fatty acids and memantine are also suggested. A main limitation of currently available guidelines is the lack of an operating definition of treatment-resistant BD.

Specific psychopharmacological interventions

Herein, we will review some of the psychopharmacological interventions that are explored in available guidelines. Since lithium, valproic acid, second-generation antipsychotics and/or combination treatments are regarded as first- or second-line treatment, we will not discuss all of the drugs here.

Clozapine

Clozapine has been repeatedly suggested as a treatment for refractory mania.[24] Banov et al. has given clozapine to a large variety of patients, including 52 treatment-resistant bipolar patients and found better outcomes for manic patients than for patients with either unipolar or bipolar depression.[25]

Recently, a systematic review reported 15 clinical trials for treatment-resistant BD and reported that add-on treatment with clozapine was superior to treatment as usual in mania.[26] However, authors also stressed the limitations due to great heterogeneity of the trials. A Danish database study explored the real-world effectiveness of clozapine in bipolar patients and showed that clozapine reduced the number of psychiatric admissions, length of stay, polypharmacy, and hospitalization due to self-harm/suicide attempts.[27] However, the authors' 'treatment resistance' definition was based on the assumption of a more restricted use of clozapine for treatment-resistant cases of BD.

Eslicarbazepine

(S-[+]-licarbazepine), a relatively new anticonvulsant whose active metabolite is oxcarbazepine, has been tried in at least one case of refractory mania but a double-blind randomized phase II trial failed to show its efficacy in acute mania.[28]

ECT and other interventions

The use of ECT in BD dates back to the 1940s. More than 300 hospitals were using ECT at that time in the 1940s.[29] MacKinnon reported 84% recovery rates and great 'improvement' in a sample of patients with manic depressive psychosis (excited phase) after three weeks of the last ECT session.[30] Hobbs et al. (1965) compared outcomes of the 'ECT era' to ones reported for previous insulin coma, and also to ECT and neuroleptic use phases. ECT had shortened the hospital stays but the readmission rates were higher than both phases. On the other hand, use of both neuroleptics and ECT in functional psychosis had better outcomes just at the beginning of the neuroleptic age.[31] There were reports that ECT can be effective for manic patients who did not respond to drug treatments.[32] Nowadays, most guidelines offer ECT for treatment-resistant mania although clinical studies are scarce.[33] Currently, there is a re-emergence of the use of ECT for the treatment of refractory mania. Furthemore, the overall costs of a course of ECT seem lower than repeated courses of available agents.[34]

Repetitive transcranial magnetic stimulation did not show any significant efficacy for mania although evidence is rather limited. Moreover, results with other interventions including vagus nerve stimulation and magnetic seizure therapy are very few.[35,36]

Management of Treatment resistant bipolar depression

Depressive symptomatology predominates in the clinical picture of BD.[37] In addition, it is associated with significantly greater psychosocial impairment and suicidality compared to (hypo) manic episodes.[38] It is known that non-response in bipolar depression is highly prevalent, and occurs in 40% of patients after eight weeks of treatment with quetiapine for instance.[2] Other first-line treatments, such as lithium, lamotrigine, olanzapine, or olanzapine–fluoxetine combination, have similar or even less favourable outcomes.[2,3,4] Moreover, the addition of antidepressants to an ongoing treatment with mood stabilizers will be helpful in only a quarter of patients with bipolar depression.[5] More data exists regarding TRB depression. We will review guidelines' recommendations first and then look over specific treatment options.

Review of the guidelines

APA guideline

This guideline suggests the use of ECT for treatment-resistant cases. However, this guideline offers several recommendation options after second-line treatment and before ECT including add-on use of selective serotonin reuptake inhibitors (SSRIs), venlafaxine, and monoamino oxidase (MAO) inhibitors, which may be attempted before considering ECT (APA, 2002).[13] The update of this guideline reports preliminary pramipexole trials, and one of those studies was conducted in a sample with treatment-resistant bipolar depression.[39,40] More recently, Dell'Osso and Ketter reviewed the use of pramipexole in bipolar depression either as a monotherapy or adjunctive treatment. Pramipexole was used in almost all treatment-resistant cases as adjunctive therapy. Notwithstanding these authors evidenced a large effect size in reviewed trials, they suggest caution due to safety and tolerability concerns related to the use of pramipexole, including treatment-emergent affective switches, exacerbation of psychotic symptoms, and neurological side effects.[41]

Texas Implementation of Medication Algorithms (TIMA)

As previously discussed, the third and fourth steps are reffered to as interventions for treatment-resistant cases, and include combinations of two of the following medications: lithium, lamotrigine, quetiapine, or olanzapine–fluoxetine are offered in the third step of the acute treatment phase of bipolar I depression. The fourth step includes third-step combinations and valproate or carbamezapine in combination with antidepressants including all SSRIs, bupropion, or venlafaxine. If lamotrigine is used, the authors suggest adding an antimanic treatment since lamotrigine lacks significant clinical benefits for mania. ECT is recommended in the fourth step due to the limited availability of controlled data.[14]

British Association of Psychopharmacology (BAP) guidelines

As previously discussed, it is difficult to interpret treatment resistance in this guideline because it follows a different stepwise approach. However, after initial treatment, adding SSRIs and antidepressants other than tricyclic agents is the suggested course. Next-step treatment options following inadequate responses to an antidepressant trial can be referred to as an intervention for treatment-resistant bipolar disorder. This guideline refers to the BAP guideline on the use of antidepressants based on experience primarily obtained from the management of unipolar depression.[16] The unipolar depression guidelines suggest increasing the dose of the antidepressant, switching to either within- or between-classes antidepressants, or otherwise combination with quetiapine, aripiprazole, or lithium as first-line treatment options.[42] On the other hand, the guidelines for the treatment of bipolar disorder emphasize that in spite of the effectiveness of adjuvant aripiprazole for treatment-resistant depression was shown, two randomized clinical trials have failed to show the same effectiveness in bipolar depression.[43]

The Canadian Network for Mood and Anxiety Treatments (CANMAT) and the International Society for Bipolar Disorders (ISBD) guideline

As previously discussed, step four is accepted as treatment-resistant therapy options. The guideline offers different treatment pathways with different medications in previous steps. Thus, it is important to know on which medication the patient was started. Regarding the fourth step, it suggests replacing one or both agents in step three with one of the first- or second-line agents that have not been tried before. An example case would be that lithium is started initially and then will be added to with an SSRI (except paroxetine or bupropion) or will be switched to quetiapine or lamotrigine. Then if there is no response, the patient could be switched to first- or second-line treatments such as olanzapine and an SSRI (except paroxetine) or lurasidone. Paroxetine is excluded because of the low efficacy shown in several trials.[44,45] For further steps in treatment resistance, the guideline suggests olanzapine, carbamazepine, and ECT as monotherapy. ECT is also accepted as a treatment alternative but could be used as first- or second-line treatment in certain situations. For combination treatment, the guideline suggests several combinations that can be seen in Table 23.1. The guideline also suggests that novel or experimental options can be used in further steps.[19]

World Federation of Societies of Biological Psychiatry (WFSBP) guideline

This guideline does not offer a stepwise approach to treatment. The authors rate the strength of evidence and make recommendations on each treatment modality. Thus, it is difficult to extract treatment-resistance data or make assumptions as established in previous guidelines. Although the guideline mentions the preliminary lamotrigine add-on treatment's effectiveness according to Nierenberg's research, no significant difference among lamotrigine, inositol, and risperidone augmentation in

Table 23.1 Offered combination treatments by CANMAT in treatment-resistant bipolar depression

Lithium	Carbamazepine
	Pramipexole
	MAOI
	TCA
	Venlafaxine
	SSRI (except paroxetine) & lamotrigine
Divalproex	Venlafaxine
	TCA
	SSRI (except paroxetine) & lamotrigine
Quetiapine	Lamotrigine

treatment-resistant bipolar depression was found.[46,47] Nevertheless, this guideline provides an explicit indication on the use of ECT for treatment-resistant bipolar depression.[48]

Korean Medication Algorithm for Bipolar Disorder

This medication algorithm offers different treatment pathways for mild, moderate, and severe psychotic depression. However, in the third step, which can be accepted as the first line of treatment resistance, the algorithm branches are united. The authors suggest changing the mood stabilizers (valproic acid, lithium, or carbamazepine), atypical antipsychotics, or antidepressants that were not used in previous steps. For the next step, the authors suggest adding stimulants, thyroid hormone, or buspirone to the treatment. If no adequate response is obtained, the authors recommend ECT or clozapine for treatment.[23] On the other hand, according to the algorithm, ECT and benzodiazepines can be applied at any time if necessary.

The ISBD task force report on antidepressant use in BD

Pacchiarotti and colleagues[49] suggests specific treatment recommendations stepwise. Treatment-resistant bipolar I depression was defined as a failure to achieve remission (Clinical Global Impression for Bipolar Disorder <2 or Hamilton Depression Rating Scale <7) despite adequate trials of lithium (0.8 mEq/l serum levels) or combination of lamotrigine (50–200 mg/day) and ongoing mood stabilizer or full dose (≥600 mg per day) quetiapine monotherapy.[49] The authors suggest that the olanzapine-fluoxetine combination or quetiapine-lamotrigine combination as first-line treatment steps. A failure to respond to this step is regarded as treatment-resistant bipolar I depression. For refractory bipolar I depression, adjusting the olanzapine–fluoxetine dose or starting lithium and SSRI or bupropion with therapeutic doses or quetiapine antidepressant combination including SSRI and bupropion or novel agent trials are suggested. Unless remission is achieved, the term involutional bipolar I depression is applied and one full cycle of ECT is recommended for final treatment.

Pachiarotti et al.'s[49] approach also differentiates bipolar I and II depression. It suggests a similar stepwise approach to bipolar II depression. Instead of combining SSRI or bupropion in the second treatment step, add-on MAO inhibitors were suggested.[49]

Specific psychopharmacological interventions

Lurasidone

Lurasidone is a new atypical antipsychotic that has been approved by the US Food and Drug Administration (FDA) for the treatment of bipolar I depression either as monotherapy or adjunctive therapy.[50] Notwithstanding no controlled trial has been conducted to date for treatment-resistant bipolar depression, a meta-analysis compared the agents and ranked them according to their efficacy. Lurasidone was ranked better than olanzapine monotherapy and worse than quetiapine according to that study.[51] Among the ten treatments compared, lurasidone was the fourth better treatment in this study.

Clozapine

Although better outcomes in mania than depression have been shown with clozapine, several studies suggest its efficacy in treatment-resistant bipolar depression.[25] A systematic review conducted by Li et al.[26] indicates that add-on clozapine to either lithium or valproate could be effective for the management of treatment-resistant bipolar depression although evidence is somewhat limited. Treatment resistance was defined as failure to respond to two adequate trials of antidepressants. Better outcomes in lithium and clozapine combination group than valproate and clozapine combination group were observed.[26]

Ketamine

Ketamine is an N-methyl-D-aspartate NMDA receptor antagonist anaesthetic agent also used for chronic pain.[52] One of the first trials with ketamine was Diazgranados' add-on study for treatment-resistant bipolar I or II depression. Subjects included in this study were either on lithium or valproic acid. A rapid improvement in depressive symptoms after the infusion of ketamine which was maintained for up to three days after the termination of infusion was noted in this placebo-controlled, double-blind, crossover study.[53] Cusin et al. reported two cases of treatment-resistant bipolar II depression who responded to intramuscular but not to oral or intranasal ketamine in the long-term. One of them remained asymptomatic for four months and the other partially responded to ketamine for at least six months.[54] Several trials tested the efficacy of ketamine for unipolar depression Cusin et al. (2012) reported two cases of treatment-resistant bipolar II depression who responded to intramuscular but not to oral or intranasal ketamine in the long-term.[55] A Polish study investigated ketamine monotherapy for treatment-resistant bipolar depression, and found a 40% remission rate after 14 days of infusion. Moreover, the Polish study showed that responders had significantly higher prevalence rates of co-occuring alcohol use disorders and a positive family history of alcoholism, and their levels of vitamin B12 were significantly higher than in treatment non-responders.[56] Recently, Poon et al. reviewed previous studies on ketamine and suggested that the use of ketamine could be efficacious for treatment-resistant bipolar depression.[57]

Ketamine may have different effects on several symptom clusters. Diamond et al. reported subjective memory improvements with a study conducted on both unipolar and bipolar treatment-resistant patients after ketamine infusion.[58] A randomized, double-blind, placebo-controlled, crossover study found that ketamine rapidly reduces anhedonia in patients with treatment-resistant bipolar depression.[59] Ketamine has also been reported to decrease suicidality as an add-on treatment in for treatment-resistant bipolar depression.[53]

The addictive potential of ketamine has been a source of considerable concern. In fact, ketamine abuse has been reported worldwide, especially in Southeast Asia, causing gastrointestinal, lower urinary tract, and respiratory symptoms.[60] In the 36th meeting of the WHO Expert Committee on Drug Dependence, ketamine abuse was addressed as 'currently not appear to pose a sufficient public-health risk of global scale to warrant scheduling'. The committee recommended that ketamine should not be placed under international control at that time. It also suggested that countries with significant substance-related public health issues should introduce or otherwise maintain several control measures.[61] Overall, ketamine appears to be a promising agent for the acute management of treatment-resistant bipolar depression as a rapid-acting intravenous antidepressant whose effects typically last between one week to one month. However, further studies are required to evaluate its long-term efficacy.[55]

Use of antidepressants

Although several guidelines suggest adding antidepressants in the subsequent treatment steps of the management of treatment-resistant bipolar depression, the ISBD Task Force reported that there was insufficient evidence on treatment benefits of antidepressants combined to mood stabilizers. The ISBD Task Force also reported that SSRIs and bupropion may carry lower rates of treatment-emergent manic switches than tricyclic and tetracyclic antidepressants and norepinephrine-serotonin reuptake inhibitors.[62]

Complementary and alternative treatments (CATs)

An increasing number of patients are using CATs, defined as a group of diverse medical and health systems, practices, and products that are not currently considered to be part of conventional medicine.[63] Despite high usage, there is paucity of research on their efficacy in bipolar disorder. The APA's Task Force highlighted the potential benefits of omega-3 fatty acids—folate augmentation to enhance lithium's response—when added to a short-term exercise intervention (half an hour for ten days) to the medication regimen of bipolar patients.[64] A four-month, double-blind, randomized, placebo-controlled, adjunctive trial of ethyl-eicosapentanoate (EPA) 6 g/day did not show any significant effect in bipolar depression.[65]

ECT and other interventions

ECT

ECT has been used for a long time to manage bipolar depression for a long time and most available guidelines offer ECT and an effective management option for treatment-resistant bipolar depression after first-line treatment, as previously reported. Dierckx et al.'s meta-analysis reported a similar efficacy for ECT in both unipolar and bipolar depression, notwithstanding patients with bipolar depression had a history of more severe depression.[66] ECT is not offered as a first-step treatment because it is a procedure done under general anesthesia, but overall costs appear to be lower than repetitive medication trials.[34]

A recent randomized controlled trial compared the efficacy of ECT and algorithm-based pharmacological treatments. Goodwin and Jamison's treatment guideline was applied in a stepwise approach in the pharmacological arm.[67] The response rate was significantly higher in the ECT group than in the pharmacologically-treated group (73.9% versus 35.0%), but remission rates were similar between groups (34.8% versus 30.0%).

Data on maintenance ECT (mECT) are also limited. Besides several case reports indicating the efficacy of mECT, Vaidya et al. showed that mECT was effective in reducing hospitalization rates in patients with treatment-resistant bipolar depression in a retrospective study.[68] A recent German retrospective study including unipolar depression cases also showed reduced hospitalizations after mECT.[69]

Magnetic seizure therapy (MST)

This is a new treatment that integrates therapeutic aspects of ECT and transcranial magnetic stimulation (TMS), in order to achieve the efficacy of the former with the safety of the latter. However, few studies have included participants with treatment-resistant bipolar disorder in their research.[70]

Deep brain stimulation (DBS)

Use of electricity in medicine actually goes back to ancient times and Greeks used ray fish to alleviate headaches more than 2,000 years ago.[71] Thus, use of electrical stimulation by implanted stimulators has developed gradually from a long experience.[72] Although DBS has been used for several neurological conditions including Parkinson's disease and pain, only few studies suggest its use in treatment-resistant bipolar depression. Holtzheimer et al. applied subcallosal cingulate DBS to ten unipolar and seven treatment-resistant bipolar depression patients. A decrease in depressive symptoms and an increase in functionality were observed. Patients with either unipolar or bipolar depression did not relapse. Finally, the efficacy was similar in both groups in this small sample-sized study.[73] The primary brain site where DBS is applied may be related to treatment response. Based on electrophysiological studies in animal models and preliminary studies, we suggest superolateral medial forebrain bundle (sl-MFB) as the primary site for DBS because sl-MFB has more projections to the frontal cortex.[74]

Transcranial magnetic stimulation (TMS)

Most currently available TMS trials have enrolled patients with unipolar depression but one has found preliminary evidence of efficacy in treatment-resistant bipolar depression. An add-on low-frequency TMS of the right dorsolateral prefrontal cortex combined with brain navigation that allows targeting of the treatment site in 11 bipolar I and II treatment-resistant patients was found to be effective and well tolerated.[41] In addition to its small sample size, this study excluded ECT non-responsive patients, which might have interfered with the findings.

Vagus nerve stimulation (VNS)

The majority of studies have reported outcomes for either unipolar or heterogeneous samples of both bipolar and unipolar treatment-resistant depressive patients. Thus, few data are available for treatment-resistant bipolar depression. In addition, limitations of this treatment include a slow onset of antidepressant action and moderate response rates.[35]

Special conditions in treatment resistance

Mixed states

The *Diagnostic and Statistical Manual of Mental Disorders* (5th edition) (DSM-5) replaced the diagnosis of 'mixed episode' with a mixed-features specifier that can be applied to all types of affective episodes including major depression, hypomania, or mania because most patients do not fully meet the more stringent criteria for mixed episodes as defined in the DSM-IV.[75] The ISBD suggests that antidepressants should be avoided during mixed states. In addition, the ISBD suggests that lithium may have a more limited efficacy during mixed states. Data related to treatment-resistant mixed states are few. One large sample-sized study evaluated ECT's efficacy in 197 treatment-resistant mixed bipolar patients and found 41.6% response and 30.5% remission rates after treatment.[76] A recent study with 40 treatment-resistant mixed-state patients found that low-frequency repetitive transcranial magnetic stimulation (rTMS) of the right Dorsolateral Prefrontal Cortex (DLPFC) had a moderate effects in reducing depressive and manic scores. For depression rating scales, 46.6% had reduced scores more than half while for mania scores 15% had reduced scores more than half in this three-week study.[77]

Co-morbidities in treatment resistance

Substance abuse

Substance use disorders are highly prevalent among patients with BD. Approximately half of patients with bipolar disorder have substance use disorders.[78] Because most of trials exclude substance abuse, data for both routine treatment or interventions for treatment resistance are extremely limited.[15,49]

Anxiety

Although anxiety co-morbidity in bipolar patients is highly prevalent and associated with poorer prognosis, data on the association of co-occuring anxiety disorders and treatment resistance in bipolar disorder are scarce.[79] Interventions primarily targeting anxiety disorders in patients with BD are few but post hoc analyses suggest efficacy for quetiapine and the olanzapine-fluoxetine combination in treating anxiety.[80,81]

Concluding remarks

Treatment-resistant mania

Notwithstanding there is limited evidence to guide the management of treatment-resistant mania, clozapine and ECT seem to be the most efficacious therapeutic options (Figure 23.1).

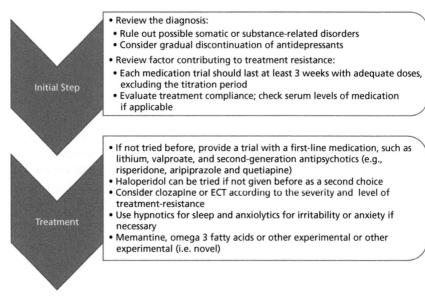

Figure 23.1 Assessment and management of treatment-resistant mania

TRB depression

Overall, due to the limited evidence base, definitive statements regarding the management of treatment-resistant depressive episodes of bipolar disorder cannot be provided. Most trials included heterogeneous samples (with participants with both unipolar and bipolar depression). Despite advances in technology and pharmacology, evidence-based interventions are lacking for treatment-resistant bipolar depression. However, ketamine appears to be a promising agent among novel treatments. ECT appears to be the foremost treatment option among those interventions. Redefining the primary sites for DBS could be a promising avenue for further investigation.

References

1. **Mathers, Colin D., Kim M. Iburg,** and **Stephen Begg.** "Adjusting for dependent comorbidity in the calculation of healthy life expectancy." *Population Health Metrics* 4.1 (2006): 1.

2. **Sienaert, Pascal, et al.** "Evidence-based treatment strategies for treatment-resistant bipolar depression: a systematic review." *Bipolar Disorders* 15.1 (2013): 61–69.

3. **Geddes, John R., Joseph R. Calabrese,** and **Guy M. Goodwin.** "Lamotrigine for treatment of bipolar depression: independent meta-analysis and meta-regression of individual patient data from five randomised trials." *The British Journal of Psychiatry* 194.1 (2009): 4–9.

4. **Sidor, Michelle M.,** and **Glenda M. MacQueen.** "Antidepressants for the acute treatment of bipolar depression: a systematic review and meta-analysis." *The Journal of clinical psychiatry* 72.2 (2010): 156–167.

5. **Perlis, Roy H., et al.** "Predictors of recurrence in bipolar disorder: primary outcomes from the Systematic Treatment Enhancement Program for Bipolar Disorder (STEP-BD)." *American Journal of Psychiatry* 163.2 (2006): 217–224.

6. **Crown, W. H., et al.** "HEALTH CARE UTILIZATION IN PATIENTS WITH TREATMENT RESISTANT DEPRESSION." *Value in Health* 4.2 (2001): 143–144.

7. **Gitlin, M.** "Treatment-resistant bipolar disorder." *Molecular psychiatry* 11.3 (2006): 227–240.

8. **Poon SH, Sim K, Sum MY, Kuswanto CN, & Baldessarini RJ.** Evidence-based options for treatment-resistant adult bipolar disorder patients, *Bipolar Disorders* 2012;**14**(6):573–84. doi: 10.1111/j.1399-5618.2012.01042.x

9. **Sachs GS.** Treatment-resistant bipolar depression, *Psychiatric Clinics of North America* 1996;**19**(2):215–36. doi: 10.1016/S0193-953X(05)70285-9

10. **Yatham LN, Calabrese JR, & Kusumakar V.** Bipolar depression: criteria for treatment selection, definition of refractoriness, and treatment options, *Bipolar Disorders* 2003;**5**(2):85–97. doi: 10.1034/j.1399–5618.2003.00019.x

11. **Sienaert P, Lambrichts L, Dols A, & De Fruyt J.** Evidence-based treatment strategies for treatment-resistant bipolar depression: a systematic review, *Bipolar Disorders* 2013;**15**(1):61–9. doi: 10.1111/bdi.12026

12. **American Psychiatric A.** *Practice Guideline for Treatment of Patients with Bipolar Disorder* (Washington, DC: American Psychiatric Association, 1995).

13. **Association, AP & Kernberg.** *American Journal of Psychiatry: Practice Guidelines for the Treatment of Patients with Bipolar Disorder* (American Psychiatric Pub, 2002).

14. **Suppes T, Dennehy EB, Hirschfeld RM, Altshuler LL, Bowden CL, Calabrese JR, Swann AC.** The Texas implementation of medication algorithms: update to the algorithms for treatment of bipolar I disorder, *Journal of Clinical Psychiatry* 2005;**66**(7):870–86.

15. **Goodwin G.** Evidence-based guidelines for treating bipolar disorder: recommendations from the British Association for Psychopharmacology, *Journal of Psychopharmacology* 2003;**17**(2):149–73.

16. **Goodwin GO.** Evidence-based guidelines for treating bipolar disorder: revised second edition—recommendations from the British Association for Psychopharmacology, *Journal of Psychopharmacology* 2009;**23**(4):346–88.

17. **Shekelle PG, Woolf SH, Eccles M, & Grimshaw J.** Clinical guidelines: developing guidelines, *British Medical Journal* 1999;**318**(7183):593.

18. **Yatham LN, Kennedy SH Schaffer A, Parikh SV, Beaulieu S, O'Donovan C, Ravindran A.** Canadian Network for Mood and Anxiety Treatments (CANMAT) and International Society for Bipolar Disorders (ISBD) collaborative update of CANMAT guidelines for the management of patients with bipolar disorder: update 2009, *Bipolar Disorders* 2009;**11**(3):225–55.

19. **Yatham LN, Kennedy SH, Parikh SV, Schaffer A, Beaulieu S, Alda M, Sharma V.** Canadian Network for Mood and Anxiety Treatments (CANMAT) and International Society for Bipolar Disorders (ISBD) collaborative update of CANMAT guidelines for the management of patients with bipolar disorder: update 2013, *Bipolar Disorders* 2013;**15**(1):1–44.

20. **Bandelow B, Zohar J, Hollander E, Kasper S, Möller H-J, Bandelow B, Möller H-J.** World Federation of Societies of Biological Psychiatry (WFSBP) guidelines for the

pharmacological treatment of anxiety, obsessive–compulsive and post-traumatic stress disorders-first revision, *World Journal of Biological Psychiatry* 2008;**9**(4):248–312.

21. **Grunze H, Vieta E, Goodwin GM, Bowden C, Licht RW, Moeller H-J, . . . Vieta E.** The World Federation of Societies of Biological Psychiatry (WFSBP) guidelines for the biological treatment of bipolar disorders: update 2009 on the treatment of acute mania, *World Journal of Biological Psychiatry* 2009;**10**(2):85–116.

22. **Shin YC, Min KJ, Yoon BH, Kim W, Jon DI, Seo JS, . . . Bahk WM.** Korean medication algorithm for bipolar disorder: second revision, *Asia-Pacific Psychiatry* 2013;**5**(4):301–8.

23. **Woo YS, Lee JG, Jeong J-H, Kim M-D, Sohn I, Shim S-H, . . . Min KJ.** Korean Medication algorithm Project for Bipolar Disorder: third revision, *Neuropsychiatric Disease and Treatment* 2015;**11**:493.

24. **Kimmel SE, Calabrese JR, Woyshville MJ, & Meltzer HY.** Clozapine in treatment-refractory mood disorders, *Journal of Clinical Psychiatry* 1994.

25. **Banov MD, Zarate CA, Jr., Tohen M, Scialabba D, Wines JD, Jr., Kolbrener M, . . . Cole JO.** Clozapine therapy in refractory affective disorders: polarity predicts response in long-term follow-up, *J Clin Psychiatry* 1994;**55**(7):295–300.

26. **Li XB, Tang YL, Wang CY, & Leon J.** Clozapine for treatment-resistant bipolar disorder: a systematic review, *Bipolar Disorders* 2015;**17**(3):235–47.

27. **Nielsen J, Kane JM, & Correll CU.** Real-world effectiveness of clozapine in patients with bipolar disorder: results from a 2-year mirror-image study, *Bipolar Disorders* 2012;**14**(8):863–9.

28. **Grunze H, Kotlik E, Costa R, Nunes T, Falcao A, Almeida L, & Soares-da-Silva P.** Assessment of the efficacy and safety of eslicarbazepine acetate in acute mania and prevention of recurrence: experience from multicentre, double-blind, randomised phase II clinical studies in patients with bipolar disorder I, *J Affect Disord* 2015;**174**:70–82. doi: 10.1016/j.jad.2014.11.013

29. **Kolb L & Vogel VH.** The use of shock therapy in 305 mental hospitals, *American Journal of Psychiatry* 1942;**99**(1):90–100.

30. **MacKinnon A.** Electric shock therapy, Can Med Assoc 1948;**58**(5):478.

31. **Hobbs GE, Wanklin J, & Ladd KB.** Changing patterns of mental hospital discharges and readmissions in the past two decades, Can Med Assoc J 1965;**93**:17–20.

32. **McCabe MS & Norris B.** ECT versus chlorpromazine in mania, Biol Psychiatry 1977;**12**(2):245–54.

33. **Neve M, Huyser J, Eshuis J, & Storosum J.** [Electroconvulsive therapy in therapy-resistant mania. A case study]. *Tijdschrift voor psychiatrie* 2006;**49**(11):851–4.

34. **Markowitz J, Brown R, Sweeney J, & Mann JJ.** Reduced length and cost of hospital stay for major depression in patients treated with ECT, *The American Journal of Psychiatry* 1987;**144**(8):1025–9.

35. **Albert U, Maina G, Aguglia A, Vitalucci A, Bogetto F, Fronda C, . . . Lanotte M.** Vagus nerve stimulation for treatment-resistant mood disorders: a long-term naturalistic study, *BMC Psychiatry* 2015;**15**:64. doi: 10.1186/s12888-015-0435-8

36. **Kaptsan A, Yaroslavsky Y, Applebaum J, Belmaker RH, & Grisaru N.** Right prefrontal TMS versus sham treatment of mania: a controlled study, Bipolar Disord 2003;**5**(1):36–9.

37. Judd LL, Akiskal HS, Schettler PJ, Endicott J, Maser J, Solomon DA, & Keller MB. The long-term natural history of the weekly symptomatic status of bipolar I disorder. *Archives of General Psychiatry* 2002;**59**(6):530-7.

38. Judd LL, Akiskal HS, Schettler PJ, Coryell W, Endicott J, Maser JD, ... Keller MB. A prospective investigation of the natural history of the long-term weekly symptomatic status of bipolar II disorder. *Archives of General Psychiatry* 2003;**60**(3):261-9.

39. Goldberg JF, Burdick KE, & Endick CJ. Preliminary randomized, double-blind, placebo-controlled trial of pramipexole added to mood stabilizers for treatment-resistant bipolar depression, Am J Psychiatry 2004;**161**(3):564-6.

40. Hirschfeld RM. *Guideline Watch: Practice Guideline for the Treatment of Patients with Bipolar Disorder* (Arlington, VA: American Psychiatric Association, 2005).

41. Dell'Osso B & Ketter TA. Assessing efficacy/effectiveness and safety/tolerability profiles of adjunctive pramipexole in bipolar depression: acute versus long-term data, *International Clinical Psychopharmacology* 2013;**28**(6):297-304.

42. Anderson I, Ferrier I, Baldwin R, Cowen P, Howard L, Lewis G, ... Scott J. Evidence-based guidelines for treating depressive disorders with antidepressants: a revision of the 2000 British Association for Psychopharmacology guidelines, *Journal of Psychopharmacology* 2008;**22**(4):343-96.

43. Thase ME, Jonas A, Khan A, Bowden CL, Wu X, McQuade RD, ... Owen R. Aripiprazole monotherapy in nonpsychotic bipolar I depression: results of 2 randomized, placebo-controlled studies, *Journal of Clinical Psychopharmacology* 2008;**28**(1):13-20.

44. McElroy SL, Weisler RH, Chang W, Olausson B, Paulsson B, Brecher M, ... Young AH. A double-blind, placebo-controlled study of quetiapine and paroxetine as monotherapy in adults with bipolar depression (EMBOLDEN II), *Journal of Clinical Psychiatry* 2010;**71**(2):163.

45. Shelton RC & Stahl SM. Risperidone and paroxetine given singly and in combination for bipolar depression, *Journal of Clinical Psychiatry* 2004;**65**(12):1715-19.

46. Frye MA, Ketter TA, Kimbrell TA, Dunn RT, Speer AM, Osuch EA, ... Post RM. A placebo-controlled study of lamotrigine and gabapentin monotherapy in refractory mood disorders, *Journal of Clinical Psychopharmacology* 2000;**20**(6):607-14.

47. Nierenberg AA, Ostacher MJ, Calabrese JR, Ketter TA, Marangell LB, Miklowitz DJ, ... Investigators S-B. Treatment-resistant bipolar depression: a STEP-BD equipoise randomized effectiveness trial of antidepressant augmentation with lamotrigine, inositol, or risperidone, *American Journal of Psychiatry* 2006;**163**(2):210-16. doi: doi:10.1176/appi.ajp.163.2.210

48. Grunze H, Vieta E, Goodwin GM, Bowden C, Licht RW, Möller H-J, & Kasper S. The World Federation of Societies of Biological Psychiatry (WFSBP) guidelines for the biological treatment of bipolar disorders: update 2010 on the treatment of acute bipolar depression, *The World Journal of Biological Psychiatry* 2010;**11**(2):81-109.

49. Pacchiarotti I, Mazzarini L, Colom F, Sanchez-Moreno J, Girardi P, Kotzalidis GD, & Vieta E. Treatment-resistant bipolar depression: towards a new definition, *Acta Psychiatrica Scandinavica* 2009;**120**(6):429-40. doi: 10.1111/j.1600-0447.2009.01471.x

50. McIntyre RS, Cha DS, Kim RD, & Mansur RB. A review of FDA-approved treatment options in bipolar depression, *CNS spectrums* 2013;**18**(s1):1–21.

51. Selle V, Schalkwijk S, Vázquez GH, & Baldessarini RJ. Treatments for acute bipolar depression: meta-analyses of placebo-controlled, monotherapy trials of anticonvulsants, lithium and antipsychotics, *Pharmacopsychiatry* 2014;**47**(02):43–52. doi: 10.1055/s-0033-1363258

52. Mathew S, Shah A, Lapidus K, Clark C, Jarun N, Ostermeyer B, & Murrough J. Ketamine for treatment-resistant unipolar depression, *CNS Drugs* 2012;**26**(3):189–204. doi: 10.2165/11599770-000000000-00000

53. Diazgranados N, Ibrahim L, Brutsche NE, Newberg A, Kronstein P, Khalife S, ... Zarate CA, Jr. A randomized add-on trial of an N-methyl-D-aspartate antagonist in treatment-resistant bipolar depression, Arch Gen Psychiatry 2010;**67**(8):793–802. doi: 10.1001/archgenpsychiatry.2010.90

54. Cusin C, Hilton GQ, Nierenberg AA, & Fava M. Long-term maintenance with intramuscular ketamine for treatment-resistant bipolar II depression, Am J Psychiatry 2012;**169**(8):868–9. doi: 10.1176/appi.ajp.2012.12020219

55. DeWilde KE, Levitch CF, Murrough JW, Mathew SJ, & Iosifescu DV. The promise of ketamine for treatment-resistant depression: current evidence and future directions, Ann N Y Acad Sci 2015;**1345**:47–58. doi: 10.1111/nyas.12646

56. Permoda-Osip A, Skibinska M, Bartkowska-Sniatkowska A, Kliwicki S, Chlopocka-Wozniak M, & Rybakowski JK. [Factors connected with efficacy of single ketamine infusion in bipolar depression], Psychiatr Pol 2014;**48**(1):35–47.

57. Poon SH, Sim K, & Baldessarini RJ. Pharmacological approaches for treatment-resistant bipolar disorder, Curr Neuropharmacol 2015;**13**(5):592–604.

58. Diamond PR, Farmery AD, Atkinson S, Haldar J, Williams N, Cowen PJ, McShane R. Ketamine infusions for treatment resistant depression: a series of 28 patients treated weekly or twice weekly in an ECT clinic, J Psychopharmacol 2014;**28**(6):536–44. doi: 10.1177/0269881114527361

59. Lally N, Nugent AC, Luckenbaugh DA, Ameli R, Roiser JP, & Zarate CA. Anti-anhedonic effect of ketamine and its neural correlates in treatment-resistant bipolar depression, Transl Psychiatry 2014;**4**:e469. doi: 10.1038/tp.2014.105

60. Xu J & Lei H. Ketamine—an update on its clinical uses and abuses, *CNS Neuroscience & Therapeutics* 2014;**20**(12), 1015–1020. doi: 10.1111/cns.12363

61. Organization WH & Dependence WECoD. *WHO Expert Committee on Drug Dependence: Thirty-sixth Report* (World Health Organization, 2015).

62. Pacchiarotti I, Bond DJ, Baldessarini RJ, Nolen WA, Grunze H, Licht RW, Vieta E. The International Society for Bipolar Disorders (ISBD) task force report on antidepressant use in bipolar disorders, *The American Journal of Psychiatry* 2013;**170**(11):1249–62. doi: 10.1176/appi.ajp.2013.13020185

63. Ernst E. Complementary medicine: where is the evidence?, *Journal of Family Practice* 2003;**52**(8):630–6.

64. Freeman MP, Fava M, Lake J, Trivedi MH, Wisner KL, & Mischoulon D. Complementary and alternative medicine in major depressive disorder: the American Psychiatric Association Task Force report, *Journal of Clinical Psychiatry* 2010;**71**(6):669.

65. **Keck PE, Jr., Mintz J, McElroy SL, Freeman MP, Suppes T, Frye MA, Post RM.** Double-blind, randomized, placebo-controlled trials of ethyl-eicosapentanoate in the treatment of bipolar depression and rapid cycling bipolar disorder, Biol Psychiatry 2006;**60**(9):1020–2. doi: 10.1016/j.biopsych.2006.03.056

66. **Dierckx B, Heijnen WT, van den Broek WW, & Birkenhäger TK.** (2012) Efficacy of electroconvulsive therapy in bipolar versus unipolar major depression: a meta-analysis. *Bipolar Disorders, 14*(2), 146–150.

67. **Goodwin FK & Jamison KR.** *Manic-depressive Illness: Bipolar Disorders and Recurrent Depression* (Oxford University Press, 2007).

68. **Vaidya NA, Mahableshwarkar AR, & Shahid R.** Continuation and maintenance ECT in treatment-resistant bipolar disorder, *The Journal of ECT* 2003;**19**(1):10–16.

69. **Post T, Kemmler G, Krassnig T, & Brugger A.** *Wirksamkeit einer EKT-Erhaltungstherapie (EEKT) bei Patienten mit therapieresistenten affektiven Störungen—Ergebnisse einer retrospektiven Datenanalyse, Neuropsychiatrie* 2015. doi: 10.1007/s40211-015-0150-1

70. **Cretaz E, Brunoni AR, & Lafer B.** *Magnetic Seizure Therapy for Unipolar and Bipolar Depression: A Systematic Review* Neural Plasticity 2015;*ID:* 521398.

71. **Finger S.** The overlooked literary path to modern electrophysiology: philosophical dialogues, novels, and travel books, Prog Brain Res 2013;**205**:3–17. doi: 10.1016/b978-0-444-63273-9.00001-0

72. **Gildenberg PL.** Evolution of neuromodulation, *Stereotactic and Functional Neurosurgery* 2005;**83**(2–3):71–9. doi: 10.1159/000086865

73. **Holtzheimer PE, Kelley ME, Gross RE,** et al. Subcallosal cingulate deep brain stimulation for treatment-resistant unipolar and bipolar depression, *Archives of General Psychiatry* 2012;**69**(2):150–8. doi: 10.1001/archgenpsychiatry.2011.1456

74. **Gálvez JF, Keser Z, Mwangi B, Ghouse AA, Fenoy AJ, Schulz PE, Soares JC.** The medial forebrain bundle as a deep brain stimulation target for treatment resistant depression: a review of published data, *Progress in Neuro-Psychopharmacology and Biological Psychiatry* 2015;**58**:59–70. doi: http://dx.doi.org/10.1016/j.pnpbp.2014.12.003

75. **Association D-AP.** *Diagnostic and Statistical Manual of Mental Disorders* 2013.

76. **Medda P, Toni C, Mariani MG, De Simone L, Mauri M, & Perugi G.** Electroconvulsive therapy in 197 patients with a severe, drug-resistant bipolar mixed state: treatment outcome and predictors of response, J Clin Psychiatry 2015. doi: 10.4088/JCP14m09181

77. **Pallanti S, Grassi G, Antonini S, Quercioli L, Salvadori E, & Hollander E.** rTMS in resistant mixed states: an exploratory study, *Journal of Affective Disorders* 2014;**15**:66–71. doi: http://dx.doi.org/10.1016/j.jad.2013.12.024

78. **Regier DA, Farmer ME, Rae DS, Locke BZ, Keith SJ, Judd LL, & Goodwin FK.** Comorbidity of mental disorders with alcohol and other drug abuse. Results from the Epidemiologic Catchment Area (ECA) Study, JAMA 1990;**264**(19):2511–18.

79. **Lee JH & Dunner DL.** The effect of anxiety disorder comorbidity on treatment resistant bipolar disorders, *Depression and Anxiety* 2008;**25**(2):91–7. doi: 10.1002/da.20279

80. **Hirschfeld RM, Weisler RH, Raines SR, & Macfadden W.** Quetiapine in the treatment of anxiety in patients with bipolar I or II depression: a secondary analysis from a randomized, double-blind, placebo-controlled study, *Journal of Clinical Psychiatry* 2006;**67**(3):355–62.

81. **Tohen M, Vieta E, Calabrese J, Ketter TA, Sachs G, Bowden C, Baker RW.** Efficacy of olanzapine and olanzapine–fluoxetine combination in the treatment of bipolar I depression, *Archives of General Psychiatry* 2003;**60**(11):1079–88.

Chapter 24

Staging and neuroprogression in bipolar disorder: treatment implications

Ives Cavalcante Passos and Flávio Kapczinski

Introduction

Bipolar disorder (BD) affects about 2% of the world's population.[1] Although there are several treatment options for the prevention and treatment of mood episodes, they are frequently suboptimal. For instance, about 37% of patients relapse into depression or mania within one year, and 60% within two years.[2] Moreover, about 40% of patients with bipolar depression are refractory to treatment. The addition of antidepressants to an ongoing treatment with mood stabilizers will be helpful in only a quarter of patients with bipolar depression.[3] It is known that although available treatments effectively reduce mood episodes symptoms, they are less effective in recovering cognition and functioning. This framework illustrates the caveats of the current treatment strategy in BD, which focuses mainly on the stabilization of acute mood episodes and prevention of recurrence while neglects illness progression and functional recovery.

Kraepelin reported that the recurrence of episodes tended to accelerate over time. He graphed mood episodes as a function of the increasingly shorter duration of euthymic periods between successive episodes.[4] Furthermore, Kraepelin recognized that psychosocial stressors often precipitated the initial episodes, but with multiple occurrences they could also occur with just the anticipation of stressors or none at all, yielding the idea of a later, more autonomous stage of illness. Finally, he reported that some subtypes of mania and depression, characterized by high levels of anxiety and irritability, ran a more difficult course and required more hospitalizations. All of these observations of faster episode recurrence, the transition from precipitated to more spontaneous episode occurrence, and illness subtypes have been widely replicated and set the stage for their incorporation into various staging models.[5,6]

It is accepted that that if not all, a substantial proportion of patients with BD present a progressive course. In this sense, the term 'neuroprogression' has been proposed as the pathological rewiring of the brain that takes place in parallel with the clinical deterioration in the course of BD.[7] However, the molecular underpinnings of neuroprogression remain poorly understood. It is reported that late-stage patients have reduced grey matter volume and maladaptive regulation of inflammatory markers.[8,9] These biological underpinnings and others reported in this chapter could develop the foundations of the neuroprogression model as a mean to explain why as the illness progresses, patients with BD are more prone to have functioning and cognitive impairment and treatment refractoriness. Given that many current treatment guidelines do not take these treatment implications that change with illness progression into account, the appreciation of such important features of BD in this chapter is key.

Based on the concept of neuroprogression and its treatment implications in BD, here we aim to review the following aspects: (a) the neurobiological underpinnings of neuroprogression in BD, (b) clinical risk factors associated to neuroprogression, and (c) treatment implications.

Neurobiological underpinnings of neuroprogression

In order to make sense of the process of cellular endangerment that seemed to take place in a portion of those with BD, Kapczinski et al.[10] adapted the concept of allostatic load. Accordingly, allostatic load driven by stress, co-morbidity, and other risk factors could lead to the progressive changes shown in BD.[10] In addition to the constitutive changes in neuroplasticity suggested earlier by Robert Post, further allostatic changes induced the pathological brain rewiring suggested by Kapczinski et al.[6] The neurobiological foundation of these twin constructs was conceptualized under the paradigm of neuroprogression to involve changes in pathways of mitochondrial dysfunction, inflammation, neurogenesis, and oxidative stress.[7] In a follow-up to his seminal article, Berk et al. suggested a balance between neuroprogression and neuroprotection as a key factor to be considered in the field of psychiatry.[7] These emerging data suggest that the concept has proven to be useful in understanding the multidimensional changes described in the context of illness progression in psychiatry.

Accordingly, on the one hand, neuroprogression seems to take place from a constitutive perspective, meaning that patients that experience multiple episodes, stress, and drugs of abuse may develop specific changes in neuronal plasticity that lead into more complex and refractory clinical presentations. These changes are likely to be related to synaptic tagging and metaplastic changes, particularly in dopaminergic neurons. On the other hand, neuroprogression has been suggested to take place from an allostatic perspective. Mechanisms of the allostatic load may explain the cumulative medical burden associated with the recurrent mood episodes and characterize the disorder as a stress-related condition. The study of the biological underpinnings of neuroprogression has the potential to identify targets for treatment and a better management of the disorder.

'Neurodegeneration vs. neuroplasticity' dualism

Bipolar patients have been shown to present several neuropathological and neuroimaging alterations in different brain structures, some of which are evident at the early stages of the illness. These appear driven by both glial and neuronal changes. For instance, post-mortem studies report reductions in neuronal density in individual cortical layers, a lower glial cell count and density, and a decrease in the number of oligodendrocytes in different brain regions,[11] which is in accordance with reports of reduced myelin staining in brain of bipolar patients.[12] Accordingly, these observed alterations in white matter microstructures are suggestive of abnormalities in axonal myelination, concordant with diffusion tensor imaging (DTI) findings of disrupted white matter connectivity in BD.[13] As the illness progresses, most likely due to shrinkage of these neural structures and alterations in markers of synaptic plasticity, more substantial alterations take place in the brain as a whole. Progressive brain atrophy has been suggested as an outcome of illness progression, which is also supported by findings of increased ventricle volumes in patients with BD and multiple episodes.[8] Also, reductions in the volume of several structures have also been reported in late-stage BD patients, including the hippocampus,[14] the prefrontal cortex,[15] the anterior cingulate,[16] and corpus callosum,[17] as well as an increase in the volume of the amygdala.[18] Functional magnetic resonance imaging (MRI) findings also report changes in activation patterns involving fronto-limbic circuitry related to different phases of the illness.[19]

Based on this evidence, white matter pathological mechanisms have been hypothesized to underlie early stage alterations, whereas grey matter loss seems to be associated with more advanced stages of the illness.[20] Given this, neurodegeneration emerged as a potential mechanism by which these alterations might be taking place in BD. A recent study has also demonstrated neurodegenerative outcomes in some cases of BD, including argyrophilic grain-type taupathy and Lewy-related alpha-synucleinopathy.[21] The most accepted hypothesis, however, states that most of the alterations may result from impairments in neuroplasticity. This results in shrinkage of brain structures by reducing neurites and intercellular connections in the neuronal network. This framework does not exclude the possibility that brain cells might also be dying to some extent, which has been suggested by studies showing increased levels of apoptotic markers in post-mortem brain from BD patients.[22] Conversely, a mechanism of 'synaptic apoptosis', which is characterized by localized apoptotic biochemical cascades in synaptic terminals, might underlie the discordance between this substantial increase in apoptotic markers seen in patients without overt corresponding neurodegeneration. It is also possible that an initial white matter pathology solely based on neuroplasticity impairments might progress to a grey matter pathology associated with neuronal apoptosis and a more substantial brain rewiring.

The search for biomarkers of neuroprogression

Several cross-sectional studies have compared the levels of biomarkers of neuroplasticity, oxidative stress, and inflammation between early and late-stage patients with BD. Regarding neuroplasticity mechanisms, brain-derived neurotrophic factor (BDNF), which is the most abundant neurotrophic factor in the adult brain and is known to induce neuroprotective effects, is reduced in acute episodes of BD.[23] Its involvement in this process was initially proposed based on a study showing that late-stage patients present decreased serum BDNF levels when compared with those at an early stage of the illness.[9] Even though post-mortem brains from BD patients display decreased BDNF levels,[22] the exact role played by this protein in BD needs to be longitudinally assessed.

Oxidative stress markers have also been studied under the concept of BD neuroprogression, and evidence points to an increase in the activities of glutathione reductase and glutathione S-transferase in late-stage patients compared with those at an early stage.[24] Further, the number of manic episodes has been associated with elevated DNA oxidation and shortened telomeres.[25] Early stage alterations include increased 3-nitrotyrosine levels[24] and protein carbonylation, which suggest that oxidative and nitrosative damage to proteins is an early event in the progression of the illness. These findings give support to initial hypotheses regarding the potential role of mitochondrial dysfunction in BD neuroprogression,[7] which has never been directly assessed in patients.

Lastly, another key mechanism thought to underlie BD neuroprogression is inflammation. Not only do patients differ from controls in the levels of several cytokines and chemokines, but those at a late-stage of illness seem to present increased levels of some chemokines, such as (C-C motif) ligand 11 (CCL11), CCL24, and C-X-C motif ligand 10 (CXCL10), and decreased levels of CXCL827. Moreover, tumour necrosis factor (TNF)-alpha and interleukin (IL)-6 may be increased in patients at both early and late stages, while IL-10 was only increased at the early stage of the illness.[9] Accordingly, a hypothetical model for the role of inflammation in BD neuroprogression suggests that recurrence of mood episodes might induce an excessive production of proinflammatory cytokines that would exceed the downregulatory capacity of the system to restore their normal levels, maintaining microglial cells in a constantly activated state. Of note, markers of neuroinflammation have been shown to be significantly upregulated in post-mortem brains from patients with BD.[26]

So far, no single biomarker with sufficient specificity and sensitivity for neuroprogression to facilitate a clinical staging approach has been identified. However, the ones that have been shown to be altered between patients at different stages inform important neurobiological aspects of illness progression and ultimately allow us to propose a hypothesis for this process.[7] Of note, clarification of the operative mechanisms underlying neuroprogression will only come from longitudinal studies assessing the same group of patients for long periods of time.

Clinical features of neuroprogression

Cognitive and functional impairment, treatment refractoriness, hospitalizations, and suicide attempts are the main clinical outcomes related to neuroprogression in BD.[7] However, not all patients with BD will present these unfavourable clinical features. Therefore, early identification of which patients will develop a neuroprogressive disorder with an unfavourable course is an important unmet challenge in BD treatment. The first step to achieving this goal is identifying the risk factors associated with neuroprogression in BD. The phenomenon of sensitization in patients with BD, in which early episodes are often triggered by psychosocial stress, but end up occurring autonomously after a sufficient number of recurrences is theorized to lead to a pernicious course of the disease. Increased number of episodes, trauma exposure, and co-morbidity with psychiatric and medical illness may further drive sensitization and cross-sensitization to other factors contributing to unfavourable outcomes.[27] Figure 24.1 presents a conceptual model that integrates risk factors and meaningful clinical outcomes related to the neuroprogression.

Longitudinal studies have shown the impact of early trauma on BD course. A study reported that those with childhood trauma presented earlier onset of BD, more co-morbid substance use, increased number of suicide attempts and manic episodes, and faster cycling pattern.[28] Another longitudinal study showed that trauma predicted severity of mood symptoms in patients with BD.[29] Also, this impact is evident as early as the first episode, with those exposed to trauma displaying poorer functional and symptomatic outcomes.[30]

Number of episodes also may have predictive value for neuroprogression in BD. A longitudinal study showed that the rate of relapse leading to hospitalization increased with the number of mood episodes.[31] Furthermore, patients with multiple episodes had functional impairment and poor quality of life.[32] Regarding the treatment approach, patients with an increased number of episodes have a worse response to lithium[33,34] and cognitive behavioural therapy (CBT). Also, a study showed that response rates with olanzapine for manic and depressive episodes were

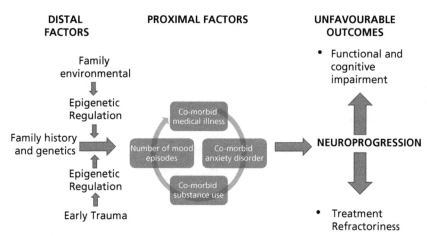

Figure 24.1 Risk factors and treatment implications associated with neuroprogression. Some patients with bipolar disorder will present an unfavourable course with functional and cognitive impairment and treatment refractoriness. Herein, we present distal and proximal factors associated with neuroprogression. The model proposed takes into account the classic psychosocial and genetic risk for bipolar disorder and integrates findings on sensitization and cross-sensitization models to explain the pernicious course associated to neuroprogression. Distal factors lead to long-term effects on gene expression and regulation. Also, distal factors may not directly lead to neuroprogression but are linked to unfavourable outcomes through the effects of proximal factors.

significantly lower among those individuals with >5 previous episodes.[35] Finally, lithium and carbamazepine, are less effective in patients with rapid cycling.[36] Of note, rapid cycling is a course specifier of BD, which is defined as at least four mood episodes during a 12-month period according to the *Diagnostic and Statistical Manual of Mental Disorders* (5th edition) (DSM-5).

Co-morbid psychiatric and other medical disorders are also associated with poor outcomes in BD. A meta-regression analysis in patients with BD showed a significant association between suicide attempts and substance use disorders.[37] Furthermore, alcohol and cannabis use in patients with BD were associated with lower remission rates, and functional impairment.[38] Co-morbid attention deficit hyperactivity disorder (ADHD) was associated with poor functioning and refractory treatment.[37] Moreover, a recent study showed evidence of cross-sensitization between number of episodes and post-traumatic stress disorder (PTSD).[39] Co-morbid PTSD was associated with functional impairment, a higher number of manic/hypomanic episodes, and earlier initiation of illicit drug use.[39] Also, it was suggested that patients with BD and co-morbid anxiety disorder have a poorer response to pharmacotherapy than patients with BD alone.

Patients with BD presented increased rates of several medical illnesses. A recent study of 440 patients with BD and three or more medical illnesses compared with 202 patients with BD and no history of medical illness, found an association with a history of anxiety disorder, rapid cycling mood episodes, and suicide attempts.[40] Notably, patients with BD are at higher risk of premature death from cardiovascular disease, diabetes, chronic obstructive pulmonary disease (COPD), influenza, or pneumonia compared with the general population.[41] These two studies validate the hypothesis of cross-sensitization between BD and other medical diseases, showing that medical co-morbidities worsen BD prognosis and vice versa. This implies the presence of common underpinning neurobiological pathways, with inflammation and oxidative stress the best established, and suggests common approaches for management and prevention of these non-communicable disorders.

Cognitive and functional impairment

BD is associated with cognitive impairment, even during euthymic periods. According to meta-analysis, specific domains of impairment include executive control, verbal learning and memory, working memory, and sustained attention.[42] However, recent studies have shown that the percentage of BD patients with clinically significant neurocognitive impairments may vary from 30% to 62%. To explain why not all patients with BD have cognitive impairment, it was reported that successive episodes might be related to a progressive neurocognitive decline. A confirmatory study found that verbal memory dysfunctions were related to the number of previous manic episodes.[43] Also, it was proposed that the trajectory of cognitive change appears to begin early in the disease process, perhaps as early as the prodrome.

A positive association between neurocognitive dysfunction and functional impairment has been shown in cross-sectional and longitudinal studies. Patients with BD may suffer from functional impairment, even when euthymic. A longitudinal study showed that almost all first-episode manic patients with BD had syndromal recovery within two years, but only one-third had functional recovery.[44] Therefore, functional and symptomatic recovery are not associated, and may need different therapeutic approaches. Moreover, it was proposed that functional impairment may be an outcome associated with the progression of the disorder. By applying latent class analysis, two subtypes of patients presenting 'good' and 'poor' functional outcome were presented.[45] Estimated verbal intelligence, number of mood episodes, level of residual depressive symptoms, and inhibitory control were the risk predictors of functional impairment in such study.[45] Of note, functional outcome was not predicted by illness duration and age of onset.[45] Furthermore, previous studies reported that co-morbid anxiety and co-morbid substance use disorders are risk factors of functional impairment.

Treatment implications

Ideally, clinical implications based in neuroprogression would be supported by longitudinal studies and treatment implications should be derived by randomized controlled trials (RCTs) with a staging approach. With those caveats in mind, we reviewed here potential clinical implication based on the longitudinal course of the disorder.[46]

Subjects at risk

Subjects at risk of BD would be the ones presenting a positive family history, exposure to childhood trauma, and some prodromal symptoms, such as anxiety and sleep disorders, minor mood disorders, and substance use disorders during adolescence. In this sense, Duffy and colleagues have proposed a chain of behavioural events based on these prodromal symptoms starting during childhood.[47] However, what is not known is whether any prophylactic benefits would be associated with mood stabilizing treatments among patients at risk.

Emerging evidence suggests that nutritional, such as omega-3, and psychosocial interventions may have the potential to prevent BD in youth at ultra-high risk. Multifamily psycho-educational groups and family focused therapy (FFT) have also shown promising results. In addition, treatment approach in youth at ultra-high risk should be based on the optimal control of environmental risk factors (substance use disorders, physical activity, nutritional status, body mass index, trauma exposure, and family dysfunction) associated with possible bipolar illness activity and progression.

Early intervention in bipolar disorder

Early intervention has the potential to prevent or minimize the functional and cognitive impairment. Using Danish registry data (n = 4714), a study reported that early intervention was associated with an increased probability of lithium response compared with patients starting lithium later.[48] This is a very interesting data and confirms results from a prior study about the lack of efficacy of lithium in patients with a history of many previous episodes.[33] Psycho-education for caregivers of patients with BD in early stages of the disease is an effective therapy to improve time to recurrence. However, psycho-education in BD was not associated with functional recovery in a clinical trial involving 239 outpatients with moderate to severe functional impairment.[49] Moreover, CBT showed effectiveness in preventing recurrence in patients with few episodes, but not in those with more than 12 previous episodes.[34] Specifically, CBT was more effective in those with less than six episodes, and it led to higher relapse rates compared with treatment as usual among patients who had more than 30 episodes.

Addressing functional impairment in severe bipolar disorder

Most severe patients with BD will require complex pharmacological therapy as well as integrated intensive psychosocial treatment approaches, including functional remediation.[49] In synthesis, the illness progression to severe BD sets the pace for a deteriorating course in which the focus of treatment shifts from the control of environmental factors and common evidence-based therapeutic interventions into an intensive model of palliative care.

Among pharmacological interventions that could improve functioning in treatment-resistant patients, clozapine has recently showed promising efficacy. A systematic review with a total sample of 1,044 patients showed that clozapine monotherapy or combined with other treatments was associated with improvement in social functioning, suicidal ideation, the number and duration of hospitalizations, and the number of psychotropic co-medications. Also, many patients with treatment-resistant BD achieved a remission or response.[50] Despite proven effectiveness in severe BD, major concerns regarding toxicity, medical co-morbidities (metabolic disturbances and cardiovascular disorders), and significant side effect profile (weight gain and sedation) continue to limit clozapine prescription.

Cognitive remediation (CR) has also been pursued as a combined intensive psychosocial intervention to address cognitive impairment in BD. CR is an intervention that is designed to remediate neurocognitive deficits and improve functioning. Although much of the focus of this treatment during the last decade has centred on schizophrenia spectrum disorders, emerging evidence suggests that CR is effective for BD. Moreover, a functional remediation programme has been recently developed meeting the specific psychosocial needs and functional disabilities encountered in severe BD.[49] Functional remediation is a neurocognitive intervention designed specifically for patients with BD, and involves neurocognitive techniques, training, psycho-education on cognition-related issues, and problem-solving within an ecological framework. In a multicentre RCT involving 239 outpatients, such novel group intervention has shown significant efficacy in improving moderate to severe functioning impairment in BD.[49] In addition, another study showed that functional remediation appears to be effective in improving psychosocial functioning in patients with BD type 2. This means that assessment of functioning levels and then clinical staging should be considered key factors to determine who can benefit from functional remediation in BD.

Conclusion

Treatment refractoriness and functional and cognitive impairment are outcomes related to neuroprogression. However, they have been largely neglected in current treatment guidelines in BD. While treatments such as lithium monotherapy, CBT, and psycho-education seem to be better suited to prevent further recurrences within patients with few episodes, complex pharmacological strategies and functional remediation might be considered in more severe patients. Of note, patients with poor clinical risk factors of a neuroprogressive disease (density of episodes, co-morbidity, and trauma exposure) should be carefully evaluated. Finally, the use of multimodal data sets coupled with multivariate pattern-recognition techniques, such as machine learning, may help to build predictive models of outcomes related to neuroprogression. These models may predict treatment response in BD, as well as of functional and cognitive impairment.

References

1. **Merikangas KR, Akiskal HS, Angst J, Greenberg PE, Hirschfeld RMA, Petukhova M**, et al. Lifetime and 12-month prevalence of bipolar spectrum disorder in the National Comorbidity Survey replication, Arch Gen Psychiatry 2007 May;**64**(5):543–52.

2. **Gitlin MJ, Swendsen J, Heller TL, and Hammen C**. Relapse and impairment in bipolar disorder, Am J Psychiatry 1995 Nov;**152**(11):1635–40.

3. **Sachs GS, Nierenberg AA, Calabrese JR, Marangell LB, Wisniewski SR, Gyulai L**, et al. Effectiveness of adjunctive antidepressant treatment for bipolar depression, N Engl J Med 2007 Apr 26;**356**(17):1711–22.

4. **Kraepelin E**. *Manic Depressive Insanity and Paranoia* (Bristol: Thoemmes Press, 1921).

5. **Passos IC, Kapczinski NS, Quevedo J, Kauer-Sant'Anna M, and Kapczinski F**. Staging models and functional outcomes in bipolar disorder: clinical implications, Curr Treat Options Psychiatry 2015 Jul 9.

6. **Kapczinski F, Dias VV, Kauer-Sant'Anna M, Frey BN, Grassi-Oliveira R, Colom F**, et al. Clinical implications of a staging model for bipolar disorders, Expert Rev Neurother 2009 Jul;**9**(7):957–66.

7. **Berk M, Kapczinski F, Andreazza AC, Dean OM, Giorlando F, Maes M**, et al. Pathways underlying neuroprogression in bipolar disorder: focus on inflammation, oxidative stress and neurotrophic factors, Neurosci Biobehav Rev 2011 Jan;**35**(3):804–17.

8. **Strakowski SM, DelBello MP, Zimmerman ME, Getz GE, Mills NP, Ret J**, et al. Ventricular and periventricular structural volumes in first- versus multiple-episode bipolar disorder, Am J Psychiatry 2002 Nov;**159**(11):1841–7.

9. **Kauer-Sant'Anna M, Kapczinski F, Andreazza AC, Bond DJ, Lam RW, Young LT**, et al. Brain-derived neurotrophic factor and inflammatory markers in patients with early- vs late-stage bipolar disorder, Int J Neuropsychopharmacol 2009 May;**12**(4):447–58.

10. **Kapczinski F, Vieta E, Andreazza AC, Frey BN, Gomes FA, Tramontina J**, et al. Allostatic load in bipolar disorder: implications for pathophysiology and treatment, Neurosci Biobehav Rev 2008 Jan;**32**(4):675–92.

11. **Rajkowska G, Halaris A**, and **Selemon LD**. Reductions in neuronal and glial density characterize the dorsolateral prefrontal cortex in bipolar disorder, Biol Psychiatry 2001 May 1;**49**(9):741–52.

12. **Regenold WT, Phatak P, Marano CM, Gearhart L, Viens CH**, and **Hisley KC**. Myelin staining of deep white matter in the dorsolateral prefrontal cortex in schizophrenia, bipolar disorder, and unipolar major depression, Psychiatry Res 2007 Jun 30;**151**(3):179–88.

13. **Lagopoulos J, Hermens DF, Hatton SN, Tobias-Webb J, Griffiths K, Naismith SL**, et al. Microstructural white matter changes in the corpus callosum of young people with bipolar disorder: a diffusion tensor imaging study, PLoS One 2013 Jan;**8**(3):e59108.

14. **Cao B, Passos IC, Mwangi B, Bauer IE, Zunta-Soares GB, Kapczinski F**, et al. Hippocampal volume and verbal memory performance in late-stage bipolar disorder, J Psychiatr Res.

15. **Mwangi B, Wu M-J, Cao B, Passos IC, Lavagnino L, Keser Z**, et al. Individualized prediction and clinical staging of bipolar disorders using neuroanatomical biomarkers, Biol Psychiatry Cogn Neurosci Neuroimaging 2016 Jan.

16. **Sassi RB, Brambilla P, Hatch JP, Nicoletti MA, Mallinger AG, Frank E**, et al. Reduced left anterior cingulate volumes in untreated bipolar patients, Biol Psychiatry 2004 Oct 1;**56**(7):467–75.

17. **Lavagnino L, Cao B, Mwangi B, Wu M-J, Sanches M, Zunta-Soares GB**, et al. Changes in the corpus callosum in women with late-stage bipolar disorder, Acta Psychiatr Scand 2015 Jan 31.

18. **Bora E, Fornito A, Yücel M**, and **Pantelis C**. Voxelwise meta-analysis of gray matter abnormalities in bipolar disorder, Biol Psychiatry 2010 Jun 1;**67**(11):1097–105.

19. **Lim CS, Baldessarini RJ, Vieta E, Yucel M, Bora E**, and **Sim K**. Longitudinal neuroimaging and neuropsychological changes in bipolar disorder patients: review of the evidence, Neurosci Biobehav Rev 2013 Mar;**37**(3):418–35.

20. **Lin A**, Reniers RLEP, and **Wood SJ**. Clinical staging in severe mental disorder: evidence from neurocognition and neuroimaging, Br J Psychiatry Suppl 2013 Jan;**54**:s11–17.

21. **Shioya A, Saito Y, Arima K, Kakuta Y, Yuzuriha T, Tanaka N**, et al. Neurodegenerative changes in patients with clinical history of bipolar disorders, Neuropathology 2015 Jun;**35**(3):245–53.

22. **Kim H-W, Rapoport SI**, and **Rao JS**. Altered expression of apoptotic factors and synaptic markers in postmortem brain from bipolar disorder patients, Neurobiol Dis 2010 Mar;**37**(3):596–603.

23. **Fernandes BS, Berk M, Turck CW, Steiner J**, and **Gonçalves C-A**. Decreased peripheral brain-derived neurotrophic factor levels are a biomarker of disease activity in major psychiatric disorders: a comparative meta-analysis, Mol Psychiatry 2014 Jul;**19**(7):750–1.

24. **Andreazza AC, Kapczinski F, Kauer-Sant'Anna M, Walz JC, Bond DJ, Gonçalves CA**, et al. 3-Nitrotyrosine and glutathione antioxidant system in patients in the early and late stages of bipolar disorder, J Psychiatry Neurosci 2009 Jul;**34**(4):263–71.

25. **Soeiro-de-Souza MG, Andreazza AC, Carvalho AF, Machado-Vieira R, Young LT**, and **Moreno RA**. Number of manic episodes is associated with elevated DNA oxidation in bipolar I disorder, Int J Neuropsychopharmacol 2013 Aug;**16**(7):1505–12.

26. **Rao JS, Harry GJ, Rapoport SI,** and **Kim HW.** Increased excitotoxicity and neuroinflammatory markers in postmortem frontal cortex from bipolar disorder patients, Mol Psychiatry 2010 Apr;**15**(4):384–92.

27. **Post RM** and **Kalivas P.** Bipolar disorder and substance misuse: pathological and therapeutic implications of their comorbidity and cross-sensitisation, Br J Psychiatry 2013 Mar;**202**(3):172–6.

28. **Leverich GS** and **Post RM.** Course of bipolar illness after history of childhood trauma, Lancet 2006 Apr 1;**367**(9516):1040–2.

29. **Gershon A, Johnson SL,** and **Miller I.** Chronic stressors and trauma: prospective influences on the course of bipolar disorder, Psychol Med 2013 Dec;**43**(12):2583–92.

30. **Daglas R, Conus P, Cotton SM, Macneil CA, Hasty MK, Kader L,** et al. The impact of past direct-personal traumatic events on 12-month outcome in first episode psychotic mania: trauma and early psychotic mania, Aust NZJ Psychiatry 2014 Nov;**48**(11):1017–24.

31. **Kessing LV, Hansen MG,** and **Andersen PK.** Course of illness in depressive and bipolar disorders. Naturalistic study, 1994–1999, Br J Psychiatry 2004 Nov;**185**:372–7.

32. **Magalhães PV, Dodd S, Nierenberg AA,** and **Berk M.** Cumulative morbidity and prognostic staging of illness in the Systematic Treatment Enhancement Program for Bipolar Disorder (STEP-BD), Aust NZJ Psychiatry 2012 Nov;**46**(11):1058–67.

33. **Swann AC, Bowden CL, Calabrese JR, Dilsaver SC,** and **Morris DD.** Differential effect of number of previous episodes of affective disorder on response to lithium or divalproex in acute mania, Am J Psychiatry 1999 Aug;**156**(8):1264–6.

34. **Scott J, Paykel E, Morriss R, Bentall R, Kinderman P, Johnson T,** et al. Cognitive-behavioural therapy for severe and recurrent bipolar disorders: randomised controlled trial, Br J Psychiatry 2006 Apr;**188**:313–20.

35. **Berk M, Brnabic A, Dodd S, Kelin K, Tohen M, Malhi GS,** et al. Does stage of illness impact treatment response in bipolar disorder? Empirical treatment data and their implication for the staging model and early intervention, Bipolar Disord 2011 Feb;**13**(1):87–98.

36. **Post RM, Fleming J,** and **Kapczinski F.** Neurobiological correlates of illness progression in the recurrent affective disorders, J Psychiatr Res 2012 May;**46**(5):561–73.

37. **Hauser M, Galling B,** and **Correll CU.** Suicidal ideation and suicide attempts in children and adolescents with bipolar disorder: a systematic review of prevalence and incidence rates, correlates, and targeted interventions, Bipolar Disord 2013 Aug;**15**(5):507–23.

38. **Bahorik AL, Newhill CE,** and **Eack SM.** Characterizing the longitudinal patterns of substance use among individuals diagnosed with serious mental illness after psychiatric hospitalization, Addiction 2013 Jul;**108**(7):1259–69.

39. **Passos IC, Jansen K, Cardoso T de A, Colpo G, Zeni C, Quevedo J,** et al. Clinical outcomes associated with comorbid posttraumatic stress disorder among patients with bipolar disorder, J Clin Psychiatry 2016;in press.

40. **Forty L, Ulanova A, Jones L, Jones I, Gordon-Smith K, Fraser C,** et al. Comorbid medical illness in bipolar disorder, Br J Psychiatry 2014 Oct 30;**205**(6):465–72.

41. **Crump C, Sundquist K, Winkleby MA,** and **Sundquist J.** Comorbidities and mortality in bipolar disorder: a Swedish national cohort study, JAMA Psychiatry 2013 Sep;**70**(9):931–9.

42. **Bora E, Yucel M,** and **Pantelis C.** Cognitive endophenotypes of bipolar disorder: a meta-analysis of neuropsychological deficits in euthymic patients and their first-degree relatives, J Affect Disord 2009 Feb;**113**(1–2):1–20.

43. Martínez-Arán A, Vieta E, Reinares M, Colom F, Torrent C, Sánchez-Moreno J, et al. Cognitive function across manic or hypomanic, depressed, and euthymic states in bipolar disorder, Am J Psychiatry 2004 Feb;161(2):262–70.

44. Tohen M, Hennen J, Zarate CM, Baldessarini RJ, Strakowski SM, Stoll AL, et al. Two-year syndromal and functional recovery in 219 cases of first-episode major affective disorder with psychotic features, Am J Psychiatry 2000 Feb;157(2):220–8.

45. Reinares M, Papachristou E, Harvey P, Mar Bonnín C, Sánchez-Moreno J, Torrent C, et al. Towards a clinical staging for bipolar disorder: defining patient subtypes based on functional outcome, J Affect Disord 2013 Jan 10;144(1–2):65–71.

46. da Costa SC, Passos IC, Lowri C, Soares JC, and Kapczinski F. Refractory bipolar disorder and neuroprogression, Prog Neuropsychopharmacol Biol Psychiatry 2015 Sep 11.

47. Duffy A, Horrocks J, Doucette S, Keown-Stoneman C, McCloskey S, and Grof P. The developmental trajectory of bipolar disorder, Br J Psychiatry 2014 Feb;204(2):122–8.

48. Kessing LV, Vradi E, and Andersen PK. Starting lithium prophylaxis early v late in bipolar disorder, Br J Psychiatry 2014 Sep;205(3):214–20.

49. Torrent C, Bonnin C del M, Martínez-Arán A, Valle J, Amann BL, González-Pinto A, et al. Efficacy of functional remediation in bipolar disorder: a multicenter randomized controlled study, Am J Psychiatry 2013 Aug 1;170(8):852–9.

50. Li X-B, Tang Y-L, Wang C-Y, and de Leon J. Clozapine for treatment-resistant bipolar disorder: a systematic review, Bipolar Disord 2014 Oct 27.

Chapter 25

Pharmacotherapy of bipolar disorder: impact on neurocognition

Vicent Balanzá-Martínez, Sofia Brissos, Maria Lacruz, and Rafael Tabarés-Seisdedos

Introduction

Neurocognitive dysfunction is currently considered a core feature of bipolar disorder (BD) for a number of reasons: (i) neurocognitive impairments across the broad domains of attention, verbal memory/learning, and executive cognition usually persist into euthymia; (ii) it is a key predictor of patients' functional outcomes; (iii) a suitable endophenotype; and (iv) a major therapeutic target.[1-3] Additional clinical and therapeutic variables may further compound these deficits, including co-morbidities and the side effects of medications.[4,5]

Clinical guidelines recommend the use of mood stabilizers and atypical antipsychotics as first-line treatments for BD.[6] The impact of these medications on neurocognition has been compared to a two-edge sword; they may help to arrest the cognitive deterioration associated with BD by means of effective relapse prevention, but may induce cognitive side effects which in turn could negatively affect patients' functional outcomes.[7] There is growing interest on the neurocognitive profile of antibipolar medications. However, this has proven to be a complex issue. Marked heterogeneous therapeutic regimens exist across patients in both clinical practice and research studies. This includes variability in medication types, doses, periods of treatment, and treatment response. Moreover, polypharmacy is the rule rather than the exception in BD, which makes particularly difficult to disentangle any specific cognitive influence of treatments that are used in combination.[4]

In this chapter, we present a critical update of the literature expanding our previous reviews.[4,8] To that end, we adopt a descriptive approach, mostly focused on human data and clinical studies specifically addressed to BD.

Lithium

Lithium remains as the cornerstone of pharmacological treatment in BD, and has also been the most investigated mood stabilizer from a neuropsychological perspective.

One of the complaints frequently reported by patients on lithium is the subjective experience of cognitive slowing. According to pioneer narrative reviews,[9,10] lithium may exert mild deleterious effects in verbal memory and psychomotor speed, while visuospatial, attentional, and executive performance are spared. Of note, patients are not always aware of these otherwise objective deficits.[9]

Its neurocognitive effects have been meta-analysed elsewhere.[11] In 326 euthymic patients with affective disorders, of whom 171 were on lithium, this agent seems to exert mild effects on immediate verbal learning and memory (effect size, ES = 0.24) and creativity (ES = 0.33), and specially a moderate (ES = 0.62) adverse effect on psychomotor speed, whereas visual memory, delayed verbal memory, attention, and executive function are spared.[11] Since less than half of the pooled sample (six studies) had a diagnosis of BD, it is not clear to what extent these results apply specifically to BD. Moreover, most of these studies used a cross-sectional design.

Longitudinal studies on the cognitive impact of long-term monotherapy with lithium suggest that evidence for detrimental effects is weak. Verbal memory remained stable over six years in a small group of BD patients, although this study did not include a control group.[12] More recently, euthymic BD patients on lithium monotherapy showed stable deficits over a two-year period in the broad domains of attention/processing speed and executive cognition, but not in verbal memory.[13]

Lithium-associated cognitive deficits might revert upon drug cessation. For instance, in a prospective, controlled study, Kocsis et al.[14] reported that deficits in psychomotor speed and verbal memory improved after a two-week lithium discontinuation. However, this remains as a controversial issue.[8]

In clinical practice, lithium intoxication is always a concern. It may be associated with neurologic and cognitive impairments, some of them being potentially persistent.[15] The incidence and severity of lithium neurotoxicity and cognitive side effects correlates with duration of lithium exposure rather than its serum concentration.[11] The evidence for sustained negative effects is equivocal[16] whereas other systematic reviews conclude that long-term treatment may be associated with neurotoxic effects, especially in combination with antipsychotics.[17] Hence, duration of lithium exposure and risk of neurotoxicity owing to its narrow therapeutic index may further worsen deleterious effects.

One-third of lithium-treated patients are *excellent lithium responders* (ELRs), as defined by complete prevention of affective episodes. Compared to healthy controls, ELRs have preserved neurocognitive functioning even after long-term duration of BD.[18] The most relevant mechanism explaining this would be the effective prevention of relapses which themselves may lead to neurocognitive deterioration. In addition, the potential neurotrophic and neuroprotective effects of lithium may also contribute.[18]

According to growing evidence from preclinical studies, these effects include potent inhibition of glycogen synthase kinase 3 (GSK-3β), increase of brain-derived neurotrophic factor (BDNF), and decreased oxidative stress and pro-inflammatory status.[19] Whether the *neurotrophic and neuroprotective* properties of lithium translate into cognitive benefits for BD patients is currently under active debate. On the one hand, several observational and case registry studies have shown that long-term treatment with lithium is associated with a lower risk for incident dementia and Alzheimer's disease among BD patients,[19] which has led researchers to suggest a potential therapeutic role of lithium in neurodegenerative disorders. On the other hand, some evidence exists in neuroimaging structural studies. A replicated finding is that chronic treatment with lithium is associated with increased total brain grey matter volume and in key neural regions involved in the regulation of mood and cognition, such as the hippocampus, amygdala, and anterior cingulate gyrus.[20] Conversely, antipsychotics and anticonvulsants are not associated with such findings.[20] Moreover, lithium might counteract the small reduction in hippocampal volume associated with BD, according to a recent meta-analysis of magnetic resonance imaging (MRI) cross-sectional studies.[21] These neurostructural changes would be mediated by the neuroprotective/neuro-trophic properties of lithium.

In sum, clinical studies have mostly favoured the neurotoxic hypothesis of lithium based on patients' cognitive complaints and cases of lithium intoxication, while the preclinical literature has largely supported the neuroprotective hypothesis.[17] Of note, none of the reviewed clinical studies were designed to test the neurocognitive effects of lithium and there is no randomized clinical trial (RCT) in this area. Therefore, equivocal evidence remains about the impact of lithium on BD patients' cognition.

Anticonvulsants

The cognitive effects of anticonvulsants or antiepileptic drugs (AEDs) have been mostly studied in patients with epilepsy and healthy subjects. Given that AEDs decrease or supress neuronal excitability, they may impair cognition, including psy-chomotor slowing, and memory and attentional deficits. Overall, these side effects are dose-related, increase with polytherapy, and revert with drug cessation.[8]

The first-generation or older AEDs — *valproic acid (valproate)* and carbamazepine — seem similarly associated with mild impairments in attentional and memory tasks. Deficits tend to improve following valproate discontinuation.[22] However, little is known about their neurocognitive impact in BD patients.

Few studies have directly compared the neurocognitive profiles of AEDs and lithium. A cross-sectional study in 159 BD patients compared the neurocognitive effects of lithium and five AEDs on tests of attention, psychomotor speed, processing speed, reaction time, cognitive flexibility, and memory.[23] Patients treated with lamo-trigine and oxcarbazepine had the best scores in the neuropsychological battery, followed by those receiving lithium, which in turn showed milder deficits than those on valproate, carbamazepine, and topiramate.[23]

In a subsequent study, euthymic patients treated only with lithium (n = 17) or only with valproate (n = 11) had similar global cognition.[24] Relative to healthy controls (n = 29), both clinical groups were similarly impaired on immediate verbal memory. The results of this study are limited by its small sample size. In addition, a recent non-randomized study concluded that lithium, but not other mood stabilizers, might be associated with better decision-making abilities, measured by the Iowa Gambling Task, during euthymia.[25]

A subanalysis of the STOP-EM study compared euthymic patients recently recovered from a first episode of mania treated with either lithium (n = 34) or valproate (n = 38) to matched healthy controls (n = 40). Overall, both clinical groups performed similarly on the domains of processing speed, attention, verbal memory, non-verbal memory, and executive functioning. However, treatment with valproate, and not lithium, was associated with working memory deficits early in the course of BD.[26] However, 80% of both clinical groups were receiving combination treatment with antipsychotics, which have also been associated with potential cognitive impairment.

Collectively, the literature suggests that treatment with valproate would be associated with worse neurocognition than treatment with lithium in BD. However, in these non-randomized studies, patients received medications under naturalistic conditions; therefore, a selective pre-treatment bias cannot be completely ruled out.

Even less is known about the neurocognitive effects of *carbamazepine* in BD. In a cross-sectional study during euthymia,[27] patients on carbamazepine (n = 18), patients on lithium (n = 18), medication-free patients (n = 12), and healthy controls (n = 15) had a similar performance on all neuropsychological tests.

Regarding the new-generation AEDs, *lamotrigine* has clearly demonstrated a better cognitive profile than the older AEDs in healthy and epileptic populations. Indeed, cognitive disturbances associated with lamotrigine are infrequent and probably transient.[4,8] Lamotrigine is indicated for the prophylaxis of BD with predominantly depressive episodes and is also the new AED with more studies specifically focused on BD. Post-hoc analysis of two clinical trials suggest that open-label lamotrigine may be associated with better self-reported cognitive scores in BD-I patients.[28,29] In a naturalistic study of euthymic BD patients, those treated with lamotrigine (n = 15) showed significantly better phonemic verbal fluency and a trend on immediate verbal memory compared with patients receiving carbamazepine or valproate (n = 18).[30] Conversely, groups did not differ on measures of attention, working memory, and executive functioning. However, findings may be biased by small sample size and overrepresentation of BD type II patients, who are more prone to depressive episodes. Finally, paediatric BD patients showed significant improvements in working memory and verbal memory, but not in attention, after 14-week treatment with lamotrigine.[31]

Topiramate is currently not considered as a first-line option for BD but in clinical practice it is used to treat co-morbid conditions, such as addictions or eating disorders. Neurocognitive disturbances associated with topiramate in epilepsy patients include psychomotor slowing, impaired attention and concentration, and especially word-finding (verbal fluency) difficulties.[4,8] In BD, topiramate has been also associated with the greatest cognitive impairment, similar to those observed with the older AEDs valproate and carbamazepine.[23]

In sum, research examining the neurocognitive profile of AEDs specifically focused on BD has grown in recent years. The cognitive adverse effects of AEDs seem to increase with polytherapy and high doses. Older AEDs are associated with a worse cognitive profile than the new ones, with the exception of topiramate. Of note, lamotrigine might improve, rather than impair, cognition in BD. However, there is no RCT in this area, hence prospective RCTs are warranted to confirm these findings and establish recommendations about the cognitive effects of AEDs in BD. In addition, extrapolating data from the epilepsy literature into BD is problematic because epilepsy is associated with cognitive deficits and doses of AEDs used in BD are typically lower than those used to treat epilepsy.[4]

Antipsychotics

Antipsychotics, especially atypical or second-generation antipsychotics (SGAs), have been increasingly prescribed for the acute and maintenance management of BD.[32] Echoing the schizophrenia literature at that time, an early review[33] suggested that the use of SGAs might convey neurocognitive advantages over conventional or first-generation antipsychotics (FGAs) in BD, as well. This issue has received less attention than in schizophrenia and remains a matter of debate. In a naturalistic study of euthymic patients,[34] treatment with risperidone was associated with better performance on the Trail Making Test-part B, a measure of executive attention, compared with conventional antipsychotics. In two subsequent reviews about the neurocognitive profile of antibipolar medications,[4,8] we summarized some preliminary data cautioning against optimism. In several observational studies, antipsychotic usage has been associated with deficits in verbal fluency, verbal learning and memory, working memory, and executive functions in BD subjects.[35–37] Moreover, discontinuation of antipsychotics was associated with improved cognition in a 12-month follow-up of recent-onset BD patients.[38]

Recent meta-analyses of observational studies have examined the potential confounding effects of medications on neuropsychological status during euthymia.[1,39] Based on post-hoc analysis, antipsychotic use was associated with higher magnitude of impairment on psychomotor speed and omission errors, a measure of sustained attention.[39] Given that psychomotor slowing was in turn associated with worse performance on other speeded information-processing tasks, antipsychotics might indirectly contribute to several neurocognitive deficits in BD. However, it is important to keep in mind that these results might be confounded by history of psychotic symptoms in BD leading to antipsychotic prescription.[4] In a more recent mega-analysis, mixed model regressions were used to examine potential medication effects on neurocognition during euthymia.[1] Lithium, anticonvulsants, or antidepressants had no effect on performance on any of the 11 outcome measures. However, treatment with antipsychotics was associated with worse performance on verbal learning only.

On the other hand, head-to-head comparative studies may reveal neurocognitive differences among SGAs. For instance, Torrent and colleagues[40] compared four groups of euthymic BD patients treated with quetiapine (n = 12), olanzapine (n = 26), risperidone (n = 30) or drug-free (n = 16), and healthy controls (n = 35). A complex pattern of results emerged, but findings became non-significant after adjustment for 'history of psychotic symptoms'. Compared with the other two SGAs, quetiapine seems to be less associated with deficits in measures of verbal memory. The authors concluded that RCTs are warranted to give a definite answer to this key issue.

A double-blind crossover RCT compared the acute neurocognitive effects of low-dose risperidone and quetiapine in clinically stable BD patients. Quetiapine was associated with more somnolence, worse global cognition, and more immediate cognitive side effects on psychomotor speed, attention, and working memory.[41] Moreover, a recent, six-week, placebo-controlled RCT examined quetiapine extended release (XR) adjunctive to mood stabilizers in non-acute BD-I or BD-II patients.[42] Those receiving placebo, but not those treated with quetiapine XR, showed significant improvements on tasks of sustained attention, psychomotor speed, and motor function, as well as in performance-based functioning. According to the authors, the anticholinergic and antihistaminergic properties of quetiapine as well as associated increased somnolence may explain the lack of improvement. However, the small sample size (n = 23) and the absence of a control group limit the generalization of these findings.

In sum, compared with lithium and AEDs, relatively few clinical studies have examined the neurocognitive effects of antipsychotics in BD. However, the quality of the evidence is better since RCTs in this area have been confined to antipsychotics. Current research suggests that antipsychotics may have some detrimental impact on psychomotor speed, verbal memory/learning, and possibly executive cognition. It is not yet clear whether SGAs confer more cognitive benefits than conventional antipsychotics in BD, and the issue as a whole remains as controversial due to limited and inconsistent data.

Other medications

Regarding *antidepressants*, selective serotonin reuptake inhibitors (SSRIs) generally do not induce major cognitive side effects, whereas trycyclic antidepressants may impair cognition, especially verbal learning and memory, due to their anticholinergic effects.[4,8] However, to our knowledge, no study has examined the cognitive effects of antidepressants specifically in BD.

Benzodiazepines are generally not recommended as pharmacological treatment in BD. In clinical practice, however, their use is often continued from the acute to the remitted phase. Their use has been shown to impair attention, psychomotor speed, and memory (for a review, see Stewart).[43] Even at low dosages, GABAergic agonists, including benzodiazepines and hypnotics such as zolpidem, have been associated with impaired visuospatial working memory during euthymia.[44] Interestingly, this deficit was independent of deficits in attention or psychomotor speed, and the use of other medications, such as lithium, AEDs, and antipsychotics.

Anticholinergic antiparkinsonian medications are mostly used to treat or prevent extrapyramidal symptoms associated with antipsychotics. These drugs are well known to induce several side effects, including cognitive dysfunction and even delirium. In schizophrenia, the use of anticholinergics has been associated with deficits in verbal memory/learning, attention, working memory, and executive function (for a recent review, see Ogino et al.).[45]

Overall summary

The role of medications upon neurocognition in BD is controversial. Inconsistent results are likely the consequence of heterogeneous clinical samples, mood states, neuropsychological tests administered, and complex medication regimens. Whereas combination treatment is the most common pharmacological approach for BD in clinical practice, polypharmacy is not common in research samples. Moreover, antipsychotics and AEDs represent miscellaneous groups of medications with likely diverging neurocognitive profiles. There are a plethora of methodological limitations in this field (see as follows).

Emerging evidence can be summarized as follows. First, most antibipolar medications may be associated with potential cognitive side effects and this risk may increase with high doses and polytherapy. Second, lithium treatment has been associated with negative effects on verbal memory and psychomotor speed. Third, lamotrigine seems to have a better cognitive profile than the first-generation AEDs carbamazepine and valproate, and topiramate. Fourth, antipsychotic use may exert a negative impact on several cognitive functions. Fifth, the cognitive profile of other medications, such as antidepressants, have not been suitably examined in BD.

According to a recent meta-analysis,[1] medications did not show any significant effect on performance on most neuropsychological tests during euthymia. Compared with any medication, drug-free status was associated with improved performance only on two measures of verbal learning and memory.[1] Moreover, non-medicated euthymic patients showed better cognitive performance than did patients on SGAs such as risperidone, olanzapine, and quetiapine.[40] In this line, antipsychotic-free BD patients performed similarly to healthy controls across a broad neuropsychological battery.[36]

Hence, the neurocognitive dysfunction associated with BD may be at least in part iatrogenic in origin. Indeed, polypharmacy may be detrimental for cognitive functioning. The few studies examining polypharmacy suggest that side effects may be more frequent compared to monotherapy (for a review of polypharmacy and non-medicated patients, the reader is referred to Dias et al.).[8] Nevertheless, medication is clearly not the only potential source of cognitive dysfunction in BD since similar, yet milder, deficits have also been described in non-medicated patients and unaffected relatives of BD patients.[46]

Recommendations for future research studies

Several methodological flaws limit the generalization of the current findings. There is a relative dearth of RCTs specifically designed to examine the neurocognitive effects of antibipolar medications. Indeed, most are naturalistic, cross-sectional, small-sample studies. Non-randomized studies do not allow conclusions about causality and small sample size increase the likelihood of type II error and lack sufficient statistical power to detect neuropsychological differences, especially if subtle. Moreover, most studies have attempted to control the potential influence of medications by means of post-hoc analyses, and hence the evidence is indirect.

In addition, results from studies with healthy individuals might not be extrapolated onto clinical groups, and the same holds true when inferring data from patients with epilepsy and schizophrenia treated with AEDs and antipsychotics, respectively. Moreover, findings from patients stabilized on monotherapy might not be extrapolated to the broader group of BD patients on polytherapy and the generalizability of data from unmedicated patients is also limited.[4]

In this section, we suggest several potentially profitable directions to move the field forward, expanding previous recommendations.[4] First, large, adequately powered RCTs are critically needed to better understand this key issue. Ideally, they should include head-to-head comparisons of antibipolar medications. Second, the inclusion of formal neuropsychological assessments as part of future clinical trials of medications in BD has been recently endorsed by an expert panel.[2] Third, measures of social functioning and quality of life should also be used to further explore the potential benefits of antibipolar medications on this important targets. Fourth, observational follow-up studies are also essential to better establish the contribution of medications to cognitive functioning in real-world patients with BD. To control for practice effects, either alternate forms of neuropsychological tests or a parallel group of healthy subjects should be considered. Fifth, studies of unmedicated patients should differentiate between drug-naïve and drug-free patients in order to examine whether past treatments make any difference in the long-term. Sixth, with some exceptions (eg Pavuluri et al.),[31] there is a dearth of data about the neurocognitive effects of medications at the extremes of the cycle life, namely paediatric or geriatric BD. Seventh, most BD patients present with medical co-morbidities (eg hypertension, diabetes, metabolic syndrome) and/or psychiatric co-morbidities (eg addictive and anxiety disorders), which have been independently associated with cognitive dysfunction.[5] Although complex, future studies should take into account the neurocognitive effects of these conditions and those of the medications used to treat them. Finally, pharmacogenetics will help to identify polymorphisms of susceptibility for cognitive side effects which in turn may allow the prescription of more customized therapies in clinical practice.

Recommendations for clinical practice

From a clinical perspective, *side effects* of medications such as cognitive difficulties are among the major reasons for patients' non-adherence or partial adherence. The management of cognitive side effects of mood stabilizers may be challenging in clinical practice.[47,48] Most adverse effects are usually transient or dose-related and can be managed by optimizing drug doses to the lowest effective dose.[48] Whenever cognitive dysfunction is suspected to be induced by lithium or AEDs, serum levels should be checked, and clinicians should consider a dosage reduction when possible.

Clinical or subclinical *hypothyroidism* is a common adverse effect of lithium that may negatively impact BD patients' cognition, but this has been virtually ignored.[47] Cognitive improvement has been reported after addition of low doses of L-thyroxine, even in the absence of hypothyroidism.[49] A recent, pilot study found that euthymic patients with subclinical hypothyroidism treated with thyroid hormone showed a pervasive cognitive impairment compared to euthyroid patients.[50]

Clinicians should be also aware of the neurocognitive side effects associated with medications with *anticholinergic* properties and *benzodiazepines*, which may offset the potential cognitive benefits of other medications.[45] Elderly patients are especially sensitive to these negative effects due to the physiological changes associated with aging. In clinical practice, judicious use of these medications, regular monitoring of side effects, re-evaluating their continuous use, and timely discontinuation whenever possible are recommended.[44,45] Due to their anticholinergic effects, the use of tricyclic antidepressants should be carefully balanced against their therapeutic efficacy.

Psychoeducation usually deals with information on side effects and their management.[47] Patients are also encouraged to report side effects when clinicians adopt an open attitude. However, subjective complaints do not always correspond to objective cognitive deficits, so patients should be reassured in order to enhance adherence to medication. Performing a formal *neurocognitive assessment* should be considered before prescribing medications with the potential to impair cognition, and may be warranted in cases of abrupt cognitive decline that does not correlate with changes in medication regimen.[8]

Finally, no specific antibipolar medication has shown clear cognitive advantages over others. The development of cognitive-enhancing agents in major psychiatric disorders is gaining traction. In the absence of approved pro-cognitive medications, clinicians should consider the use of medications with neutral cognitive profiles. Moreover, functional remediation and cognitive rehabilitation therapies have demonstrated efficacy in BD. These psychological approaches merit further development and generalization in clinical practice in order to benefit patients' neurocognitive and social functioning. It is envisioned that future developments will also consider multimodal approaches, encompassing pharmacotherapies, psychological therapies, and lifestyle interventions, including aerobic exercise and diet/nutrition.[51]

References

1. Bourne C, Aydemir Ö, Balanzá-Martínez V, Bora E, Brissos S, Cavanagh JTO, et al. Neuropsychological testing of cognitive impairment in euthymic bipolar disorder: an individual patient data meta-analysis, Acta Psychiatr Scand 2013;**128**(3):149–62.

2. Burdick KE, Ketter TA, Goldberg JF, and Calabrese JR. Assessing cognitive function in bipolar disorder: challenges and recommendations for clinical trial design, J Clin Psychiatry 2015;**76**(3):e342–50.

3. Martínez-Arán A and Vieta E. Cognition as a target in schizophrenia, bipolar disorder and depression, Eur Neuropsychopharmacol 2015;**25**(2):151–7.

4. Balanzá-Martínez V, Selva G, Martínez-Arán A, Prickaerts J, Salazar J, González-Pinto A, Vieta E, and Tabarés-Seisdedos R. Neurocognition in bipolar disorders—a closer look at comorbidities and medications, Eur J Pharmacol 2010;**626**(1):87–96.

5. Balanzá-Martínez V, Crespo-Facorro B, González-Pinto A, and Vieta E. Bipolar disorder comorbid with alcohol use disorder: focus on neurocognitive correlates, Front Physiol 2015;**6**:108.

6. Yatham LN, Kennedy SH, Parikh SV, Schaffer A, Beaulieu S, Alda M, et al. Canadian Network for Mood and Anxiety Treatments (CANMAT) and International Society for Bipolar Disorders (ISBD) collaborative update of CANMAT guidelines for the management of patients with bipolar disorder: update 2013, Bipolar Disord 2013;**15**(1):1–44.

7. Vieta E. The influence of medications on neurocognition in bipolar disorder, Acta Psychiatr Scand 2009;**120**(6):414–15.

8. Dias VV, Balanzá-Martinez V, Soeiro-de-Souza MG, Moreno RA, Figueira ML, Machado-Vieira R, and Vieta E. Pharmacological approaches in bipolar disorders and their impact on cognition: a critical overview, Acta Psychiatr Scand 2012;**126**(5):315–31.

9. Honig A, Arts BM, Ponds RW, and Riedel WJ. Lithium induced cognitive side effects in bipolar disorder: a qualitative analysis and implications for daily practice, Int Clin Psychopharmacol 1999;**14**(3):167–71.

10. Pachet AK and Wisniewski AM. The effects of lithium on cognition: an updated review, *Psychopharmacology* 2003;**170**(3):225–34.

11. Wingo AP, Wingo TS, Harvey PD, and Baldessarini RJ. Effects of lithium on cognitive performance: a meta-analysis, J Clin Psychiatry 2009;**70**(11):1588–1597.

12. Engelsmann F, Katz J, Ghadirian AM, and Schachter D. Lithium and memory: a long-term follow-up study, J Clin Psychopharmacol 1988;**8**(3):207–12.

13. Mur M, Portella MJ, Martínez-Arán A, Pifarré, J, and Vieta E. Neuropsychological profile in bipolar disorder: a preliminary study of monotherapy lithium-treated euthymic bipolar patients evaluated at a 2-year interval, Acta Psychiatr Scand 2008;**118**(5):373–81.

14. Kocsis JH, Shaw ED, Stokes PE, Wilner P, Elliot AS, Sikes C, et al. Neuropsychologic effects of lithium discontinuation, J Clin Psychopharmacol 1993;**13**(4):268–75.

15. Ivkovic A and Stern TA. Lithium-induced neurotoxicity: clinical presentations, pathophysiology, and treatment, *Psychosomatics* 2014;**55**(3):296–302.

16. Tsaltas E, Kontis D, Boulougouris V, and Papadimitriou GN. Lithium and cognitive enhancement: leave it or take it?, *Psychopharmacology (Berlin)* 2009;**202**(1–3):457–76.

17. Fountoulakis KN, Vieta E, Bouras C, Notaridis G, Giannakopoulos P, Kaprinis G, and Akiskal H. A systematic review of existing data on long-term lithium therapy: neuroprotective or neurotoxic?, Int J Neuropsychopharmacol 2008;**11**(2):269–87.

18. Rybakowski JK. Response to lithium in bipolar disorder: clinical and genetic findings, ACS Chem Neurosci 2014;**5**(6):413–21.

19. Diniz BS, Machado-Vieira R, and Forlenza OV. Lithium and neuroprotection: translational evidence and implications for the treatment of neuropsychiatric disorders, Neuropsychiatr Dis Treat 2013;**9**:493–500.

20. Hafeman DM, Chang KD, Garrett AS, Sanders EM, and Phillips ML. Effects of medication on neuroimaging findings in bipolar disorder: an updated review, Bipolar Disord 2012;**14**(4):375–410.

21. Otten M and Meeter M. Hippocampal structure and function in individuals with bipolar disorder: a systematic review, J Affect Disord 2015;**174**:113–25.

22. Hommet C, Mondon K, deToffol B, and Constans T. Reversible cognitive and neurological symptoms during valproic acid therapy, J Am Geriatr Soc 2007;**55**(4):628.

23. Gualtieri CT and Johnson LG. Comparative neurocognitive effects of 5 psychotropic anticonvulsants and lithium, Med Gen Med 2006;**8**(3):46.

24. Senturk V, Goker C, Bilgic A, Olmez S, Tugcu H, Oncu B, and Atbasoglu EC. Impaired verbal memory and otherwise spared cognition in remitted bipolar patients on monotherapy with lithium or valproate, Bipolar Disord 2007;**9**(Suppl 1):136–44.

25. Adida M, Jollant F, Clark L, Guillaume S, Goodwin GM, Azorin JM, and Courtet P. Lithium might be associated with better decision-making performance in euthymic bipolar patients, Eur Neuropsychopharmacol 2015;**25**(6):788–97.

26. Muralidharan K, Kozicky JM, Bücker J, Silveira LE, Torres IJ, and Yatham LN. Are cognitive deficits similar in remitted early bipolar I disorder patients treated with

lithium or valproate? Data from the STOP-EM study, Eur Neuropsychopharmacol 2015;**25**(2):223–30.

27. **Joffe RT, Macdonald C, and Kutcher S**. Lack of differential cognitive effects of lithium and carbamazepine in bipolar affective disorder, J Clin Psychopharmacol 1988;**8**(6):425–8.

28. **Khan A, Ginsberg LD, Asnis GM, Goodwin FK, Davis KH, Krishnan AA, and Adams BE**. Effect of lamotrigine on cognitive complaints in patients with bipolar I disorder, J Clin Psychiatry 2004;**65**(11):1483–90.

29. **Kaye NS, Graham J, Roberts J, Thompson T, and Nanry K**. Effect of open-label lamotrigine as monotherapy and adjunctive therapy on the self-assessed cognitive function scores of patients with bipolar I disorder, J Clin Psychopharmacol 2007;**27**(4):387–91.

30. **Daban C, Martínez-Arán A, Torrent C, Sánchez-Moreno J, Goikolea JM, Benabarre A, Comes M, Colom F, and Vieta E**. Cognitive functioning in bipolar patients receiving lamotrigine: preliminary results, J Clin Psychopharmacol 2006;**26**(2):178–81.

31. **Pavuluri MN, Passarotti AM, Mohammed T, Carbray JA, and Sweeney JA**. Enhanced working and verbal memory after lamotrigine treatment in pediatric bipolar disorder, Bipolar Disord 2010;**12**(2):213–20.

32. **Pillarella J, Higashi A, Alexander GC, and Conti R**. Trends in use of second-generation antipsychotics for treatment of bipolar disorder in the United States, 1998–2009, Psychiatr Serv 2012;**63**(1):83–6.

33. **MacQueen G and Young T**. Cognitive effects of atypical antipsychotics: focus on bipolar spectrum disorders, Bipolar Disord 2003;**5**(Suppl 2):53–61.

34. **Reinares M, Martinez-Aran A, Colom F, Benabarre A, Salamero M, and Vieta E**. [*Efectos a largo plazo del tratamiento con risperidona versus neurolépticos convencionales en el rendimiento neuropsicológico de pacientes bipolares eutímicos*], Actas Esp Psiquiatr 2000;**28**:231–8.

35. **Frangou S, Donaldson S, Hadjulis M, Landau S, and Goldstein LH**. The Maudsley Bipolar Disorder Project: executive dysfunction in bipolar disorder I and its clinical correlates, Biol Psychiatry 2005;**58**(11):859–64.

36. **Jamrozinski K, Gruber O, Kemmer C, Falkai P, and Scherk H**. Neurocognitive functions in euthymic bipolar patients, Acta Psychiatr Scand 2009;**119**(5):365–74.

37. **Kozicky JM, Torres IJ, Silveira LE, Bond DJ, Lam RW, and Yatham LN**. Cognitive change in the year after a first manic episode: association between clinical outcome and cognitive performance early in the course of bipolar I disorder, J Clin Psychiatry 2014;**75**(6):e587–93.

38. **Torres IJ, Kozicky J, Popuri S, Bond DJ, Honer WG, Lam RW, and Yatham LN**. 12-month longitudinal cognitive functioning in patients recently diagnosed with bipolar disorder, Bipolar Disord 2014;**16**(2):159–71.

39. **Bora E, Yucel M, and Pantelis C**. Cognitive endophenotypes of bipolar disorder: a meta-analysis of neuropsychological deficits in euthymic patients and their first-degree relatives, J Affect Disord 2009;**113**(1–2):1–20.

40. **Torrent C, Martinez-Aran A, Daban C, Amann B, Balanza-Martinez V, Bonnin CM, et al**. Effects of atypical antipsychotics on neurocognition in euthymic bipolar patients, Compr Psychiatry 2011;**52**(6):613–22.

41. **Harvey PD, Hassman H, Mao L, Gharabawi GM, Mahmoud RA, and Engelhart LM**. Cognitive functioning and acute sedative effects of risperidone and quetiapine in patients

with stable bipolar I disorder: a randomized, double-blind, crossover study, J Clin Psychiatry 2007;**68**(8):1186–94.

42. **Rakofsky JJ, Dunlop BW, Beyer JL, Oliver AM, Mansson EE, Sancheti MT, and Harvey PD**. Cognitive effects of quetiapine XR in patients with euthymic bipolar disorder, J Clin Psychopharmacol 2014;**34**(3):383–5.

43. **Stewart SA**. The effects of benzodiazepines on cognition, J Clin Psychiatry 2005;**66**(Suppl 2):9–13.

44. **Pan Y-J, Hsieh MH, and Liu S-K**. Visuospatial working memory deficits in remitted patients with bipolar disorder: susceptibility to the effects of GABAergic agonists, Bipolar Disord 2011;**13**(4):365–76.

45. **Ogino S, Miyamoto S, Miyake N, and Yamaguchi N**. Benefits and limits of anticholinergic use in schizophrenia: focusing on its effect on cognitive function, Psychiatr Clin Neurosci 2014;**68**(1):37–49.

46. **Balanzá-Martínez V, Rubio C, Selva-Vera G, Martínez-Aran A, Sánchez-Moreno J, Salazar–Fraile J**, et al. Neurocognitive endophenotypes (endophenocognitypes) from studies of relatives of bipolar disorder subjects: a systematic review, Neurosci Biobehav Rev 2008;**32**(8):1426–38.

47. **Dols A, Sienaert P, van Gerven H, Schouws S, Stevens A, Kupka R, and Stek ML**. The prevalence and management of side effects of lithium and anticonvulsants as mood stabilizers in bipolar disorder from a clinical perspective: a review, Int Clin Psychopharmacol 2013;**28**(6):287–96.

48. **Murru A, Popovic D, Pacchiarotti I, Hidalgo D, León-Caballero J, and Vieta E**. Management of adverse effects of mood stabilizers, Curr Psychiatry Rep 2015;**17**(8):603.

49. **Tremont G and Stern RA**. Use of thyroid hormone to diminish the cognitive side effects of psychiatric treatment, Psychopharmacol Bull 1997;**33**(2):273–80.

50. **Martino DJ and Strejilevich SA**. Subclinical hypothyroidism and neurocognitive functioning in bipolar disorder, J Psychiatr Res 2015;**61**:166–7.

51. **Sarris J, Logan AC, Akbaraly TN, Amminger P, Balanzá-Martínez V, Freeman MP**, et al. Nutritional medicine as mainstream in psychiatry, *The Lancet Psychiatry* 2015;**2**(3):271–74.

Chapter 26

Cognitive enhancement in bipolar disorder: current evidence and methodological considerations

Kamilla W. Miskowiak and Lars V. Kessing

Cognitive dysfunction as an emerging treatment target

Cognitive dysfunction is common in bipolar disorder (BD) and occurs across several cognitive domains including verbal memory, sustained attention, and executive function.[1] These non-specific cognitive deficits persist after clinical remission from affective episodes and are not reversed by antipsychotic or mood-stabilizing treatments.[1] The profile of cognitive deficits in BD is similar to the non-specific cognitive dysfunction in schizophrenia and unipolar depression,[2,3] although the degree of the deficits in BD is less pronounced than in schizophrenia and greater than in unipolar depression.[4,5] This highlights cognitive dysfunction is an important illness dimension in psychiatric disorders that transcends traditional diagnostic boundaries.[6]

Trait-related cognitive dysfunction in BD has been observed already at illness onset and is more severe at late illness stages,[7] suggesting that is reflects both genetic abnormalities and neurotoxic effects of affective episodes. Although the 'cognitive neuroprogression hypothesis' remains controversial, some emerging findings support the hypothesis, including (i) meta-analytical evidence for more pronounced cognitive dysfunction in BD patients with a history of psychosis,[8] (ii) demonstration of progressive grey matter volume reduction with longer illness duration,[9] and (iii) observation of a positive correlation between the number of affective episodes and risk of dementia.[10]

Persistent neurocognitive deficits contribute to occupational and psychosocial disability.[11] Unemployment rates among BD patients are substantially higher than in the general population,[12] and two-thirds of patients experience a moderate to severe impact of the illness on their occupational capacity.[13] Together with residual depressive symptoms, the persistent cognitive dysfunction in BD is among the strongest contributors to patients' functional disability.[14] Nevertheless, there are no reliably efficacious treatments for cognitive dysfunction in BD. Current pharmacological treatments may, in fact, have cognitive side-effects due to anticholinergic, extrapyramidal, sedative, and/or blunting effects.[15] Cognitive dysfunction is therefore emerging as a potential treatment target to improve patients' functional recovery and quality of life.

The first part of the chapter systematically reviews the current evidence from randomized controlled trials (RCTs) or open studies that explore the efficacy of novel pharmacological and psychological treatments for cognitive dysfunction in BD. The second part discusses some key methodological challenges in this emerging field and highlights some methodological perspectives that may improve success rates of future cognition trials.

Current evidence for new targets

The neurobiological underpinnings of the cognitive deficits in BD remain elusive. However, emerging evidence indicates an association between cognitive dysfunction and a wide range of changes in neurotrophin levels, neurogenesis, metabolism, neurotransmitters (including acetylcholine, dopamine, and glutamate), inflammation, oxidative stress and cortisol in BD. Within the last decade, a series of studies have therefore been conducted to investigate the efficacy of compounds that act on some or multiple of these pathways and may thereby exert neuroprotective effects. Tables 26.1–26.3 display the characteristics of the identified randomized, controlled, or open-label cognition trials in BD. Seventeen studies of new pharmacological treatments were identified: two were open-label,[15,16,17] were randomized and placebo-controlled, and, of these, improvement of cognition was the primary treatment aim in 12 trials. In addition, five studies investigated the effects of new psychological interventions for cognitive dysfunction in BD;[18,19,20,21,22] three[19,21,22] were randomized and controlled, and, of these, improvement of cognition was the primary treatment aim in two trials.[19,21] Only five drug trials[23,24,25,26,27] and two psychological intervention trials[19,21] specified one or two cognition measure(s) as the primary outcome. Overall, the sample size of the trials were small; three studies had ≤10 participants per group, 12 studies included 12–34 participants per group, and only one multicentre study (of functional remediation with cognition as the secondary outcome measure) had a large sample with 77–82 participants per group (see Tables 26.1–26.3). Taken together, there is a scarcity of studies of which only half (11 of 22) specified cognition as the primary treatment target and which generally had small to moderate sample sizes.

Candidate pharmacological compounds

Mifepristone—one of the first trials targeting cognition in BD was a proof-of-concept study by Young and colleagues (2004) of the corticosteroid receptor antagonist mifepristone.[27] The study was inspired by evidence that hyper-cortisolaemia in BD may exacerbate patients' neurocognitive dysfunction. Nineteen BD patients with current depression were given mifepristone (600 mg/day) or placebo for one week in a placebo-controlled, cross-over design. A beneficial effect of mifepristone was observed on spatial working memory but not on verbal memory (co-primary outcomes) or on any of the secondary cognition outcomes (see Table 26.1). This effect

Table 26.1 Main characteristics of pharmacological interventions with cognition as the primary target (studies sorted chronologically)

Treatment	Author	Patients	Randomized	Double-blind	Screening for cognitive impairment	Main finding	Cognitive outcome measures
Mifepristone	Young et al. (2004) *Ref.id*[27]	Mifepristone = 19, placebo = 19 (cross-over design, ie a total of 19 patients) (BD with depression)	√	√	–	Mifepristone improved spatial working memory. However, group-comparisons revealed no significant effects on measures of verbal memory (co-primary outcomes) or the secondary cognition outcomes.	**Primary outcomes:** Spatial Working Memory (CANTAB) and the Rey Auditory Verbal Learning Test. **Secondary outcomes:** the Wechsler forward and backward digit span test, the Spatial Span Test, Pattern Recognition Test and Spatial Recognition tests from the CANTAB, verbal fluency test, Wechsler Adult Intelligence Scale digit symbol subtest, and a computerized continuous performance task (a total of 13 cognition outcomes).
	Gallagher et al. (2005) *Ref.id*[23]	Mifepristone = 19, placebo = 19 (cross-over design, ie a total of 19 patients) (BD with depression)	√	√	–	Mifepristone produced no cognitive improvement on any of the cognition outcomes.	**Primary outcomes:** Spatial Working Memory (CANTAB) and the Rey Auditory Verbal Learning Test. **Secondary outcomes:** the Wechsler forward and backward digit span test, the Spatial Span Test, Pattern Recognition Test and Spatial Recognition tests from the CANTAB, verbal fluency test, Wechsler Adult Intelligence Scale digit symbol subtest, and a computerized continuous performance task (a total of 13 cognition outcomes).

(continued)

Table 26.1 Continued

Treatment	Author	Patients	Randomized	Double-blind	Screening for cognitive impairment	Main finding	Cognitive outcome measures
	Watson et al. (2012) Ref.id.[26]	Mifepristone = 30, placebo = 30 (BD with depression)	√	√	–	Mifepristone produced significant improvement of spatial working memory compared with placebo six weeks after treatment, but not immediately after treatment completion (day 21). However, group-comparisons revealed no significant effects on the remaining cognition outcomes.	**Primary outcome:** Spatial Working Memory (CANTAB). **Secondary outcomes:** The Rey Auditory Verbal Learning Test, the Wechsler forward and backward digit span test, the Spatial Span Test, Pattern Recognition Test and Spatial Recognition tests from the CANTAB, verbal fluency test, Wechsler Adult Intelligence Scale digit symbol subtest, and a computerized continuous performance task (13 outcomes).
Galantamine	Matthews et al. (2008) Ref.id.[17]	Galantamine = 9, No galantamine = 8 (BD, UD, SZA with depression)	–	–	–	Galantamine had no effect on the primary cognition outcome (MMSE total scores). However, exploratory analyses (post-treatment between-group comparisons with adjustment for baseline performance) showed that galantamine produced a slight reduction in ECT-related side-effects on sub-scores of memory and abstract reasoning.	**Primary cognition outcome not defined.** Mini-Mental-State-Examination 3MS (4 items and 1 total score; 5 measures)

Study	Sample				Results	Outcomes
Ghaemi et al. (2009) Ref.id.[29]	Galantamine = 10, Placebo = 6 (BD in remission)	√	√	–	Galantamine improved verbal memory from baseline to after treatment, but not processing speed. The opposite pattern was seen with placebo. None of the other cognitive outcomes showed any effects of galantamine.	**Primary cognition outcome not defined.** California Verbal Learning Test, the Delis-Kaplan Executive Functioning System Trail Making and Verbal Fluency tests (number scanning, number sequencing, letter sequencing, and letter-number alternation), both the letter and category fluency examinations, the Wisconsin Card Sorting Test (categories completed, total errors and preservative responses) (ten outcomes)
Iosifescu et al. (2009) Ref.id.[16]	Galantamine = 19 (BD in remission)	–	–	Subjective criteria (patient reports)	Galantamine improved attention and verbal memory, but not executive function.	**Primary cognition outcome not defined.** The California Verbal Learning Test (scores for trial 1 and trials 1–5), Conner's Continuous Performance Test commission errors, Wisconsin Card Sorting Test (total errors and failure to maintain set) (five outcomes)

(continued)

Table 26.1 Continued

Treatment	Author	Patients	Randomized	Double-blind	Screening for cognitive impairment	Main finding	Cognitive outcome measures
	Matthews et al. (2013) *Ref.id.*[28]	Galantamine = 12, Placebo = 18 (BD, UD, SZA with depression)	√	√	–	Galantamine improved one measure of delayed memory at discharge compared with the control group.	**Primary cognition outcome not defined.** Repeatable Battery for the Assessment of Neuropsychological Status (RBANS): tests within five domains: immediate and delayed memory, visuospatial skills, attention and language); Mini Mental Status Examination 3MS; Wechsler Abbreviated Scale of Intelligence (vocabulary, matrix reasoning) (11 outcomes)
N-acetyl cysteine	Dean et al. (2012) *Ref.id.*[30]	NAC = 21, Placebo = 25 (BD with depression)	√	√	–	NAC produced no cognitive improvement in comparison with placebo	**Primary cognition outcome not defined.** Digit span, word learning, Trail Making Test A and B, verbal fluency (six outcomes)
Pramipexole	Burdick et al. (2012) *Ref.id.*[31]	Pramipexole = 24, Placebo = 21 (BD patients in partial remission)	√	√	–	Pramipexole produced no cognitive improvement compared with placebo.	**Primary cognition outcome not defined.** Stroop, Trail Making Test A and B, Digits forward, Digits backward, d2 test of attention, HVLT, verbal fluency, Digit Symbol Test (11 outcomes)

386

Insulin	McIntyre et al. (2013) *Ref.id.*[24]	Intranasal insulin = 34, Placebo = 28 (BD in remission)	√	–	The study revealed no beneficial effect of insulin on the primary cognition outcomes. Improvement was observed on one secondary outcome, Trail Making Test B.	**Primary outcomes:** California Verbal Learning Test and Process Dissociation Tasks. **Secondary outcomes:** the Trail Making Test A and B, the Digit Symbol Substitution Test, the Controlled Oral Word Association Test (Letter and Category Fluency), the Visual Backward Masking Test, the Shipley Institute of Living–Abstraction Test, the Continuous Visual Memory Test, and the Cognitive Failures Questionnaire (ten neuropsychological outcomes).
Withania somnifera	Chengappa et al. (2013) *Ref.id.*[32]	Withania somnifera = 24, Placebo = 29 (BD in remission)	√	–	Compared to placebo, withania somnifera improved performance on three measures: digit span backward, Flanker neutral response time, and the Penn Emotional Acuity Test. No effects were seen on the remaining cognitive measures.	**Primary cognition outcome not defined.** Set shifting Test, Strategic Target Detection Test, Flanker Test, Auditory Digit Span forward and backward, Word List Memory, Finger Tapping Test, Penn Emotional Acuity Test (20 outcomes).

(continued)

Table 26.1 Continued

Treatment	Author	Patients	Randomized	Double-blind	Screening for cognitive impairment	Main finding	Cognitive outcome measures
Erytrophoietin	Miskowiak et al. (2014) Ref.id.[25]	EPO = 23, Placebo = 20 (BD in partial remission)	√	√	Subjective criteria (CPFQ score)	There was only a trend towards improvement in RAVLT total recall but there was a significant improvement in EPO vs. saline-treated participants in sustained attention and facial expression recognition (happy faces), and measures of attention and executive function (tertiary outcomes). Improvement was seen on 8 of the 15 measures.	**Primary outcome:** Rey Auditory Verbal Learning Test (total recall); **Secondary outcomes:** Rapid Visual Processing (CANTAB), the facial expression recognition task from the Emotional Test Battery; tertiary: Trail Making A and B, verbal fluency, WAIS-III letter-number sequencing, the Repeatable Battery for the Assessment of Neuropsychological Status (RBANS) digit span and coding tests (15 outcomes).

List of abbreviations: CPFQ—Cognitive and Physical Functioning Questionnaire; BD—bipolar disorder; UD—unipolar disorder; SZA—schizoaffective disorder; ST—standard treatment; Ref. id.—reference ID.

survived Bonferroni correction for multiple testing across the primary outcome measures. However, in a follow-up replication study mifepristone failed to produce any cognitive improvement in symptomatic BD patients.[23] The authors also conducted an RCT in a larger sample of 60 depressed BD patients,[26] which revealed mifepristone-associated spatial working memory improvement (the primary study outcome) six weeks but not immediately after treatment completion. No effects were observed on any of the secondary cognition tests spanning memory, attention, and psychomotor speed at any time point. Although these trials had selected one primary or two co-primary cognition outcomes a priori, their mixed findings provide only preliminary evidence for efficacy of mifepristone on spatial working memory.

Galantatine—another line of research focused on galantamine, a compound with dual mechanisms of action on the cholinergic system. The first trial was an open-label study of the effects of galantamine in a mixed sample of patients with BD, unipolar disorder (UD) and schizoaffective disorder (SZA) during electroconvulsive treatment (ECT).[17] No beneficial effect of galantamine (4 mg bid throughout ECT) was found on overall cognitive function, but exploratory analysis revealed a minor benefit of galantamine on subtests of memory and abstract reasoning after treatment completion (see Table 26.1). The authors therefore conducted an RCT of galantamine (N = 12) versus placebo (N = 18) in a sample of BD, UD, and SZA patients undergoing ECT.[28] Galantamine improved one measure of memory function but had no effects on the seven additional cognitive outcomes. The efficacy of galantamine on cognition was also investigated in a double-blind, placebo-controlled trial of remitted BD patients.[29] Cognitive change over a three-month treatment period examined for galantamine (N = 10) and placebo- (N = 6) treated patients. The galantamine group showed verbal memory improvement but slowed psychomotor speed and no improvement in attention or executive function. Further, four-month galantamine treatment (8–24 mg/day) was associated with improvement of attention and verbal memory but not of executive function in an open-label proof-of-concept trial.[16] None of these four studies[16,17,28,29] had defined a primary cognition outcome a priori, and the observed effects would therefore not have survived Bonferroni correction for the 5–11 cognition measures in the trials. In addition, one trial had no placebo-control and two trials used suboptimal statistical analyses with no adjustment for learning effects over time. Taken together the findings of the galantamine studies must therefore be considered preliminary.

N-acetyl cysteine—n-acetyl cysteine is another candidate compound that has been examined as a candidate compound to target cognitive dysfunction in BD based on evidence for its beneficial effects on antioxidant status, glutamate transmission, inflammation and neurogenesis, and efficacy for depressive symptoms in BD.[30] However, an RCT of n-acetyl cysteine (2,000 mg/day) (N = 21) versus placebo (N = 25) over six months revealed no effects on cognition.

Pramipexole—given convergent evidence for a role of dopaminergic dysfunction in cognitive dysfunction in BD, an RCT was conducted to investigate the cognitive effects of eight weeks administration of the dopamine agonist pramipexole (N = 24) or placebo (N = 21) to partially remitted BD patients.[31] The trial found no effects of pramipexole over placebo treatment on cognition. Post-hoc exploratory analyses in the subgroup of *euthymic* patients showed beneficial effects of pramipexole (N = 19) over placebo (N = 16) on psychomotor speed and working memory, although these effects would have not survived Bonferroni correction for multiple testing given the lack of an a priori defined cognition outcome.

Insulin—insulin dysregulation is thought to be involved in neurocognitive dysfunction and intranasal insulin administration improves cognition in patients with mild cognitive impairment. McIntyre and colleagues therefore conducted an RCT to evaluate the effect of eight weeks intranasal insulin (N = 24) versus placebo (N = 28) on cognitive dysfunction in 62 euthymic BD patients.[24] The study revealed no beneficial effect of intranasal insulin on the primary cognition outcomes (see Table 26.1). Cognitive improvement was observed in the insulin group on a secondary measure of executive function. However, this effect occurred in the absence of changes in the additional secondary measures of attention, psychomotor speed, memory and executive function, and would have rendered non-significant with Bonferroni correction.

Withania somnifera—another interesting study investigated the potential pro-cognitive effects of withania somnifera, a herbal medicine with antioxidant, neuro-protective, and memory-enhancing activity.[32] Fifty-three euthymic BD patients were randomized to receive eight weeks of daily withania somnifera (500 mg/d) (n = 24) or placebo (n = 29) as add-on to their mood-stabilizing treatment. Primary outcomes were changes in measures of attention and executive function, and verbal and visuos-patial memory post-treatment. Compared with placebo, withania somnifera extract improved performance on three cognitive tests: a test of working memory, a measure of reaction time, and a measure of social cognition. These effects should, however, be interpreted with caution since no primary cognition outcome was defined and the effects would therefore not have survived Bonferroni correction for the 20 cognition measures.

Erythropoietin—erythropoietin (EPO) has recently emerged as a candidate treat-ment for cognitive deficits in neuropsychiatric disorders. Endogenous brain-derived EPO mediates neuroprotection and plays a key role in cognition and systemically administered EPO has neuroprotective and neurotrophic actions in preclinical models of neuropsychiatric disease and improves cognition through direct neuro-biological actions.[33] Encouraged by this evidence, our group set up an RCT of eight weeks of weekly EPO (40,000 IU) (N = 23) versus saline (N = 20) administration to partially remitted BD patients.[25] The trial revealed only a trend toward improvement of verbal memory (primary outcome) in response to EPO versus placebo. However, EPO improved sustained attention and social cognition (secondary outcomes), and several measures of executive function and working memory (tertiary outcomes) (see Table 26.1). In particular, EPO-associated improvement was observed on eight of the 15 cognition outcomes, and the EPO-associated improvement of sustained attention survived Bonferroni correction. Notably, the effects of EPO were unrelated to changes in mood and persisted after normalization of red blood cells, indicat-ing a mechanism beyond red cell regulation such as modulation of neuroplasticity and neurogenesis. Despite the absence of significant improvement in the primary outcome, the substantial effects of EPO across the secondary and tertiary cognition outcomes were encouraging and deserve to be further investigated.

Pregnenolone—pregnenolone is a precursor of the glucocorticoids, mineralocorticoids, progestogens, androgens, estrogens, and neuroactive steroids and improves cognition in rodents. In an RCT, Osuji and colleagues (2010) therefore investigated whether eight weeks' pregnenolone supplementation (100 mg/day) (N = 29) versus placebo (N = 31) would improve mood and cognition in a group of symptomatic BD and UD patients with a history of substance use disorder.[34] There were no effects of prenenolone on memory and executive function. However, it should be noted that the study was not for investigation of the cognitive effects of prenenolone since improvement of cognition was a secondary aim and cognition was only measured with one memory test and two executive function tests.

Citicoline—the dietary supplement citicoline is a precursor for the synthesis of phosphatidylcholine (a key component of cell membranes), and has been shown to decrease cell-membrane breakdown during ischaemic or hypoxia conditions, reduce glutamate-mediated injury, and improve cognition in preclinical studies. An RCT therefore examined the effects of 12 weeks citicoline (N = 23; 500–2,000 mg/day) versus placebo (N = 21) on verbal memory and mood symptoms in symptomatic BD or SZA patients with cocaine dependence.[35] Citicoline improved one measure of verbal memory, which survived Bonferroni correction for the number of memory measures. However, a follow-up RCT of 12 weeks' citicoline (2,000mg/day) (N = 28) or placebo (N = 20) treatment of depressed BD or UD patients with methamphetamine dependence[36] showed no treatment-associated memory improvement in comparison to placebo.

Ketamine—the NMDA-receptor antagonist ketamine has fast-acting antidepressant properties and was investigated for its potential to mitigate cognitive side effects of ECT in a mixed sample of patients with BD or UD with non-psychotic depression.[37] Depressed patients in ECT were randomized to receive ketamine (0.5 mg/kg) (N = 22) or saline (N = 24) in addition to thiopentone during anaesthesia for ECT. No beneficial effects of ketamine were observed on cognitive outcome of ECT. An RCT of anaesthesia with ketamine (N = 21) versus methohexital (N = 17) also revealed no protective effects of ketamine on cognition.[38]

Potential psychological interventions

A small number of studies investigated new *psychological* treatments for cognitive and psychosocial impairments in BD. These studies were inspired by the robust effects of cognitive remediation (CR) on cognitive and psychosocial function in schizophrenia.[39] Four trials in BD have investigated CR (18–21), while one trial examined functional remediation (FR).[22] Although both CR and FR involve cognitive training, compensation techniques, and coping strategies to overcome cognitive difficulties in daily settings, the relative foci since this is pluralis of these interventions differ. While CR emphasizes computerized training of cognitive functions and compensational skills, FR is more focused on psychosocial skills training.[22]

Cognitive Remediation—the first CR trial was conducted by Naismith and colleagues (2008) and was a preliminary proof-of-concept study of a mixed sample of two BD and 14 UD patients allocated to ten weeks of twice-weekly group-based

Table 26.2 Main characteristics of studies of pharmacological candidate treatments targeting both depressive symptoms and cognition

Treatment	Author	Patients	Randomized	Double-blind	Screening for cognitive impairment	Main finding	Cognitive outcome measures
Pregnenolone	Osuji et al. (2010) Ref.Id.[34]	Pregnenolone = 29, Placebo = 31 (BD, UD with depression)	√	√	–	Pregnonone produced no cognitive improvement.	**Primary cognition outcome not defined.** Rey Auditory Verbal Learning Test, Trail Making Test, and Stroop Test.
Citicoline	Brown et al. (2007) Ref.Id.[35]	Citicoline = 23, Placebo = 21 (BD, SZA in depressed or mixed mood states)	√	√	–	Citicoline improved recall of the alternative list, but produced no change in total recall across the learning trials or in delayed recall.	**Primary cognition outcome not defined.** Rey Auditory Verbal Learning Test (subscales measuring total words recalled over five trials, recall after a 30-minute delay, and recall on an alternative word list) (three memory measures)

	Study	Sample				Outcome	Cognitive tests
	Brown et al. (2012) *Ref.id.*[36]	Citicoline = 28, Placebo = 20 (BD, UD with depression)	√	√	–	Citicoline produced no memory improvement.	Hopkins Auditory Verbal Learning Test
Ketamine	Loo et al. (2012) *Ref.id.*[37]	Ketamine = 22, Placebo = 24 (BD, UD with depression)	√	√	–	The addition of ketamine to thiopentone during anaesthesia for ECT did not decrease cognitive impairment.	**Primary cognition outcome not defined.** CFT; HVLT; COWAT; SDMT; Wood cock Johnson Cross-Out Test; AMI-SF; NART
	Rasmussen et al. (2014) *Ref.id.*[38]	Ketamine = 21, Methohexital = 17 (BD, UD with non-psychotic depression)	√	√	–	Ketamine did not reduce the cognitive side effects of ECT.	Mini-Mental-State-Examination (MMSE)

CR (N = 8) or wait list control (N = 8).[21] The intervention involved group-based computerized training tailored to each patient's strengths and weaknesses. The study revealed CR-related improvement in memory encoding and retention, the primary cognition outcomes. No improvement was observed across the secondary outcomes spanning attention, psychomotor speed, and executive function. However, no Bonferroni corrections should be conducted given a prior selection of memory as the primary outcome and the trial can therefore be regarded as positive. Another research group investigated the effects of three-month CR in an open trial with 18 BD patients and no control group.[18] The programme consisted of 14 sessions, with weekly sessions from weeks 1–12 followed by two bi-weekly sessions. Three consecutive modules consisting of each four sessions were delivered, focusing on: (i) mood monitoring and treatment of residual symptoms; (ii) organization, planning, and time management; and (iii) attention and memory training. The study revealed improvement in an *observer*-based measure of executive function (a secondary treatment aim). Based on this preliminary evidence, our group conducted an RCT of 12 weeks group-based CR (N = 18) versus standard treatment (N = 22) in partially remitted BD patients[19]. The sessions were divided into four consecutive modules: sessions 1–2 involved *education* about the nature of cognitive function and dysfunction in BD, sessions 3–5 focused on computerized *training* of attention and *compensation* techniques, sessions 6–8 addressed learning and memory, and sessions 9–12 targeted executive function. The study revealed no effects of CR on the primary or secondary cognition outcomes. CR improved subjective mental sharpness, quality of life, and a measure of executive function, but these were merely tertiary outcomes and the effects would not have survived Bonferroni correction. Although the trial turned out to have suboptimal statistical power for the primary outcome analysis, calculation of the 95% confidence interval for the effects of CR showed that it was highly unlikely that a larger sample size would have rendered any beneficial effects. More intensive, individual treatment and a longer duration may thus be necessary. Notably, the negative finding may also be related the absence of *objective* neuropsychological deficits in our sample despite patients' *subjective* cognitive complaints.

Functional Remediation—FR was investigated by Torrent and colleagues in a multicentre RCT of 239 euthymic BD patients. Patients were allocated to 21 weeks of FR (N = 77), psychoeducation (N = 82), or treatment as usual (N = 80).[22] The FR programme involved weekly sessions addressing attention, memory, and executive function with emphasis on patients' functioning in their daily life settings. Although FR improved psychosocial function compared with treatment as usual (primary outcome), there were no cognitive benefits of FR over psychoeducation or treatment as usual (secondary outcomes). Post-hoc analyses revealed FR-associated verbal memory improvement in a subgroup of patients with cognitive deficits, although this effect would not have survived Bonferroni correction for the 24 secondary cognition outcomes.[40]

In conclusion, the intensive research efforts into novel pharmacological or psychological treatments for cognitive dysfunction in BD have so far produced disappointing results. Trials investigating the efficacy of n-acetyl cysteine, pregnolone, ketamine, and pramipexole and two RCTs of the psychological interventions CR and FR demonstrated no cognitive improvement. Studies of mifepristone, galantamine, insulin, EPO, withania somnifera, and citicoline as well as a small CR trial[21] revealed improvement of either a single or a subset of cognition measures, which in all but three cases[21,25,27] would have rendered non-significant if subjected to Bonferroni corrections. Among the most promising pharmacological treatments for cognitive dysfunction is EPO, but the evidence is still only preliminary. Nevertheless, the field evolves rapidly with several ongoing studies of novel treatments such as modafinil, lurasidone, memantine, GLP-1 agonists, and new cognitive training programmes. There is, therefore, hope that new efficacious treatments will be identified in the near future. Notwithstanding, the field is marked by a number of methodological challenges that need to be addressed to improve the success rates of future cognition trials.

Methodological challenges

There are two potential explanations for the lack of efficacious treatments for cognitive dysfunction in BD: that the investigated treatments are not effective or that efficacy of some of these treatments was masked by methodological problems. In particular, the study design has proved to be pivotal for the results of these trials.[31,41] It is therefore problematic that there is no existing consensus or guidelines for the design of cognition trials, including (i) whether the trials should screen for cognitive impairment—and if so, whether the criteria should be *subjective* or *objective*—or (ii) which cognition measures for *tracking* treatment effects should be defined a priori to study start. Other unresolved questions are whether participants should be euthymic or can have current mood symptoms, how concomitant medication should be managed, whether the interventions should target certain BD illness stages, and what statistical methods should be employed. The absence of a clear consensus regarding these issues is a serious limitation that must be addressed to advance the field. This section provides an in-depth discussion of questions (i) and (ii) and touches briefly on the additional issues. See also the preliminary recommendations by Burdick and colleagues.[41]

Additional (i): screening for cognitive impairment

Eighteen trials employed no screening for cognitive dysfunction, four trials used *subjective* criteria, and no trials used *objective* criteria for cognitive impairment (see Tables 26.1–26.3). In schizophrenia trials, there is no need to screen for cognitive impairment since almost patients display severe non-specific cognitive deficits with effect sizes >1.[42] In contrast, patients with BD show less severe deficits (1) and 40–60% may be relatively 'cognitively intact'.[43] This introduces a great risk of including BD patients with no cognitive dysfunction in trials that target cognition. This will inevitably increase the risk of type II error, ie *not* detecting potential treatment efficacy.[31,40] Indeed, secondary analysis of our EPO trial data revealed that the patients with memory dysfunction at baseline had 126 times greater chances of achieving a clinically relevant treatment-related memory improvement than patients

Table 26.3 Main characteristics of psychological interventions

Treatment	Author	Patients	Cognition as primary/ secondary aim	Randomized	Double-blind	Screening for cognitive impairment	Main finding	Cognitive outcome measures
Cognitive remediation	Naismith et al. (2008) Ref.id.[21]	Cognitive Training = 8, ST = 8 (UD and BD in partial remission)	Primary	√	√	–	Cognitive training improved memory encoding and retention but produced no change in measures of attention, psychomotor speed or executive function.	**Primary outcomes:** Rey Auditory Verbal Learning Test total recall and delayed recall; **Secondary outcomes:** Trail Making Test A and B, Rey Complex Figure, Controlled Word Associations Test (verbal and semantic fluency) (seven outcomes)
	Dechersbach et al. (2010) Ref.id.[18]	Cognitive Remediation = 18 (BD in partial remission)	Secondary	–	–	–	Improvement from pre- to post-treatment in observer-based ratings of executive function, but not in measures of apathy or disinhibition.	**Primary cognition outcome not defined.** Executive functioning (ie planning and problem-solving) in daily life was assessed using the Frontal Systems Behaviour Rating Scale, which includes three subscales: apathy, disinhibition, and executive dysfunction.

Study	Sample	Design				Results	Measures
Meusel et al. (2014) *Ref.id.*[20]	Cognitive Remediation = 38 (BD, UD in partial remission)	Primary	—	—	—	Cognitive remediation produced a slight improvement in working memory but not in verbal memory or any of the remaining cognitive tests that were part of a comprehensive test battery (details on this test battery not provided)	**Primary cognition outcome not defined.** Hopkins Verbal Learning Test Revised, WAIS-R Backward digit span and a series of additional unspecified cognitive tests (data provided on the number of tests)
Demant et al. (2015) *Ref.id.*[19]	Cognitive Remediation = 18, ST = 22 (BD in remission)	Primary	√	√	Subjective criteria according to the CPFQ	Cognitive remediation produced no cognitive improvement in comparison with ST.	**Primary outcomes:** Rey Auditory Verbal Learning Test total recall; **Secondary outcomes:** Trail Making Test B, Rapid Visual Processing (CANTAB); Tertiary outcomes: RBANS coding and digit span; Delayed Match to Sample and Spatial Working Memory (CANTAB), WAIS-III letter-number sequencing, verbal fluency, Trail Making Test A, Facial Expression Recognition from the Emotional Test Battery (23 outcomes)

(continued)

Table 26.3 Continued

Treatment	Author	Patients	Cognition as primary/ secondary aim	Randomized	Double-blind	Screening for cognitive impairment	Main finding	Cognitive outcome measures
Functional remediation	Torrent et al. (2015) *Ref.id.*[22]	Functional remediation = 77, psychoeducation = 82, ST = 80 (BD in remission)	Secondary	√	√	Subjective criteria according to the CPFQ	Functional remediation produced no cognitive improvement.	**Primary cognition outcome not defined since cognition was only the secondary treatment target.** WAIS-III digit-symbol coding and symbol search, verbal fluency, Computerized Wisconsin Card Sorting Test, the Stroop Colour-Word Interference Test, the phonemic (F-A-S) and categorical (animal naming) components of the Controlled Oral Word Association Test, Trail Making Test A and B, the Rey-Osterrieth Complex Figure, California Verbal Learning Test, WAIS-III Logical Memory Scale, WAIS-III: arithmetic, digits forward and backward, and letter-number sequencing, Continuous Performance Test-II, version 5 (24 outcomes)

with 'intact' baseline memory.[44] Systematic screening for cognitive impairment in participants for trials that target cognition could therefore improve the success rates of these trials. However, the question still remains how we best screen for cognitive impairment: can we rely on patients' *subjective* cognitive complaints—or are *objective* neuropsychological tools necessary?

The use of *subjective* screening criteria has several advantages: first, it is important for recruitment purposes that the patients *experience* cognitive difficulties to be motivated for taking part in the study. Second, it is easy to simply ask patients whether they experience cognitive difficulties or use a self-report questionnaire. Nevertheless, a key disadvantage is the weak or absent correlation between subjective and objective measures of cognitive function.[45,46] This may be explained by an above normal pre-morbid cognitive capacity. Hence, if patients had better than normal cognitive capacity before illness onset, then objective tests are unlikely to pick up the cognitive decline *after* illness onset, at which point their performance is merely within normal range. The subjective measures may be better at capturing these patients' cognitive decline in home and work settings, consistent with our observation that subjective cognitive difficulties are more closely associated with socio-occupational impairment than objective cognitive deficits.[45,46] However, this cannot fully account for the phenomenon, since improvement in objective cognitive performance is not always accompanied by decreased subjective cognitive difficulties.[25] Other factors, such as depressive symptoms, are therefore likely to play a role in the poor correlation between objective and subjective cognitive function, as demonstrated in several of our studies.[45,46] Subjective cognitive difficulties may therefore not be an assay of cognition per se, which highlights the need for *objective* neuropsychological screening tools. The benefits of this would be detection of measurable, objective deficits (in comparison with norms) that provide scope for cognitive improvement and avoid ceiling effects. Indeed, we found that it was patients' objective rather than subjective cognitive impairment at baseline that predicted EPO treatment success.[44] Together with the preliminary findings from the studies by Burdick and colleagues[31] and Bonnin and colleagues,[40] these findings indicate that future screening for *objective* cognitive impairment likely to improve the success rates in trials targeting cognition. Nevertheless, objective criteria should not stand alone; patients should also have subjective cognitive complaints and/or socio-occupational impairment to ensure that the treatment is clinically meaningful and patients are motivated to comply with the study requirements.

Given the lack of short, feasible screening tools for cognitive dysfunction in BD, we investigated two new brief and feasible screening instruments to detect objective cognitive deficits in BD: one subjective, the Cognitive Complaints in Bipolar Disorder Rating Assessment (COBRA), and one objective: the Screen for Cognitive Impairment in Psychiatry (SCIP).[46] The SCIP had highest sensitivity and specificity for cognitive impairment (84% and 87%, respectively). We therefore recommend the use of an *objective* neuropsychological screening tool in BD such as the SCIP to verify that patients with cognitive complaints also display measurable cognitive dysfunction before their inclusion in cognition trials.[46]

Additional (ii): selection of outcomes for tracking treatment efficacy

It is a key question how we best track treatment-associated changes in cognition. One could argue that a treatment is only clinically meaningful if patients *experience* cognitive improvement. However, the poor correlation between objective and subjective measures of cognition[25] indicates that patients may be unable to correctly assess their own cognitive capacity. Objective cognition measures are therefore essential to directly measure treatment-induced changes in cognition. Accordingly, all the identified trials of novel candidate treatments for cognitive dysfunction in BD but one[18] used objective neuropsychological tests for investigating treatment-associated changes in cognition. Cognitive dysfunction has been shown to contribute to socio-occupational impairment, independent of affective symptoms.[47] Nevertheless, neuropsychological function is often regarded as a 'technical' outcome that has little in common with patients' functional capacity, which may be a more *clinically relevant* primary outcome. Nevertheless, multiple factors contribute to patients' socio-occupational functioning. Hence, to determine if the candidate treatment actually exerts *pro-cognitive* effects, it is necessary to select an objective cognition measure as primary outcome. To determine the functional implications of any cognitive improvement, a functional measure should be included as a co-primary or secondary outcome. Notably, it is likely that the functional improvement takes *longer* to emerge. A sequential approach could therefore be implemented with inclusion of functional capacity as a co-primary or secondary outcome at an additional follow-up assessment three to six months after trial completion.

It is unresolved whether treatment-associated effects on cognition should be tracked with a *single* or *multiple* cognition outcomes. The majority of studies have investigated multiple cognition outcomes with no a priori defined hierarchy (primary, secondary, tertiary; see Tables 26.1–26.3). These trials face the challenge of Bonferroni corrections for multiple testing, which should be applied to minimize the risk of type 1 error. Indeed, the majority of these trials would have rendered non-significant results with Bonferroni corrections. Such selective outcome reporting has in fact turned out to be a common problem in clinical trials. This is addressed in the CONSORT (Consolidated Standards for Reporting Trials) statement, a now widely implemented guideline for reporting RCTs. To adhere to the CONSORT criteria, cognition trials must prioritize the cognition measures into primary, secondary, and tertiary outcomes and specifically state the primary time for these endpoint assessments. If the primary outcome turns out negative at the primary assessment time, the trial must be deemed overall negative. This predetermined priority between outcomes in clinical trials can thus safeguard against post-hoc distortive claims. Another advantage is that Bonferroni correction should only be applied within each outcome level; ie if a single primary outcome measure is selected, the statistical threshold for detection of a treatment-related effect is typically $P = 0.05$ even if the study has multiple secondary outcomes, whereas selection of two co-primary outcomes would involve reduction of the alpha-level to $P = 0.05/2 = 0.025$). This approach has been used by only a subset of cognition trials to date[19,21,23,24,25,26,27] but its implementation is critical for future studies.

There is a lack of consensus on which neuropsychological measures to use as primary outcomes in cognition trials in BD and whether the primary outcome should be a single neuropsychological test (or subtest measure) or a cognitive composite score that summarizes performance across several cognitive domains. The MATRICS Consensus Cognitive Battery (MCCB) was developed as a standard test battery for trials in schizophrenia, with the primary outcome being change in a MCCB composite score. Although no such consensus battery has yet been developed for BD, the primary outcomes measure(s) in such battery should include more difficult neuropsychological tests that are sensitive to the cognitive deficits in BD and relatively unaffected by mood symptoms. Further, non-specific cognitive dysfunction in BD speaks for implementation of a global cognitive composite score as primary outcome. Given the heterogeneity of cognitive deficits in BD, the global composite score may by summarizing the changes across domains be a more robust measure than a single cognition test. A global composite score would also be more likely to pick up small cumulative treatment effects across several cognitive domains. This could help resolve the difficulty with predicting which single cognitive domains are targeted by novel candidate treatments based on their pharmacological profile and effects in preclinical studies. This challenge can be illustrated by our EPO trial, in which our pre-specified choice of verbal memory over sustained attention as primary outcome was arbitrary.[25] At the time of hypothesis generation, there was equal evidence for trait-related deficits in verbal memory and sustained attention in BD, and we had found proof-of-concept evidence for EPO-related improvement of both cognitive domains. A lesson learnt was that a broader cognitive composite score would have been more informative and sensitive primary outcome.[25] The cognitive deficits should be stable and prevalent over a time period, eg a month, before inclusion in the RCT, although such an inclusion criterion would decrease study participation rates.

Additional methodological challenges

Affective state—affective symptoms impact on cognitive performance. Trials that include patients in symptomatic illness states and demonstrate improvement of both cognition and affective symptoms are therefore unable to rule out pseudo-specificity. Affective symptoms may also mask potential efficacy of a cognitive enhancement intervention as demonstrated in the pramipexole study.[31] Nevertheless, *sub-syndromal* affective symptoms should be allowed for two reasons; first, inclusion of only patients in full remission would render a rather unrepresentative patient sample and thereby limit the generalizability of the findings. Second, such strict criteria would reduce enrolment feasibility. We therefore recommend that trials recruit patients who are in partial or full remission and are stable for mood symptoms and that affective symptoms assessed during the study are controlled for in the outcome analyses, similar to the approach in our EPO trial.[25]

Role of concomitant medication—treatments that target cognition in BD must be given as add-on to patients' usual medication for both ethical reasons and the intervention to be representative of the actual clinical practice. However, these medications may be associated with adverse actions on cognition.[15] This may confound cognitive outcomes by potentially masking or enhancing effects of the investigational compound.[41] One way to tackle this is to ensure that patients' concomitant medication is within the recommended dose range (for lithium and antipsychotics, in particular) from at least two weeks before trial start and that this medication is carefully recorded and kept stable throughout the trial. Post-hoc analyses should be conducted to explore any potential interaction effects of patients' medication and the investigational compound.

Staging—BD is thought to involve 'clinical staging', a progression from prodromal (at-risk) to more severe and resistant presentations. The idea is based on the observation that treatment response is generally better when introduced early in the course of illness[48] and assumes that earlier stages require simpler treatment interventions.[49] In line with the staging model, it is conceivable that the effect of the interventions for cognitive dysfunction may differ between disease states. Inclusion of a heterogeneous group of patients at different stages of their illness could therefore mask pro-cognitive effects of a particular intervention (especially in trials with small sample sizes). Given the greater success rate of pro-cognitive treatment of patients with more severe cognitive deficits, as demonstrated in our EPO trial,[44] interventions targeting cognition may be more beneficial at *later* illness stages, which are generally associated with more cognitive and functional impairment. On the other hand, cognitive dysfunction during later stages may be more treatment resistant and be accompanied by extensive functional disability, which could have been prevented by early treatment of cognitive dysfunction. Nevertheless, there is no evidence for such stage-specific effects on response to pro-cognitive treatment and future studies of this issue are therefore warranted.

Statistical methods—there is general agreement in RCTs that intention-to-treat (ITT) analyses should be implemented to prevent bias caused by the loss of participants, which could disrupt the baseline equivalence established by random assignment. However, ITT is poorly defined and involves several approaches handling missing data in longitudinal trials: a widely used strategy is the last observation carried forward (LOCF) method. This involves imputation of the missing values with the last observed value, assuming that the outcomes would not have changed from the last observed value. Although LOCF minimizes the number of participants eliminated from the analysis, it has been criticized for giving a biased estimate of the treatment effect and underestimating the variability of the estimated result, particularly if there is a large amount of missing data. Recommended alternatives for handling missing data are multiple imputation or mixed models, which are more robust and take account of missing values and inter-individual changes during the trial course. These methods are increasingly used in clinical research because of their availability in many statistical software packages. Nevertheless, there are no universal standards, as the most appropriate method handling missing data for a particular trial depends on its goals, endpoints, and context.

Future directions for treatment development

In addition to methodological challenges in clinical cognition studies, drug-screening strategies are faced by another more fundamental difficulty: the absence of sensitive biomarkers for detecting and refining therapeutic-like action of novel candidate treatments in experimental medicine (phase 1 and 2) clinical trials. Drug screening, therefore, typically involves use of animal models to test the efficacy of novel compounds. If beneficial effects are seen in these models, the compound is moved directly into clinical efficacy trials in patient populations. However, in animal studies it is difficult to model the genetic, developmental, and environmental factors that contribute to cognitive dysfunction in psychiatric disorders.[6] Discovery of pro-cognitive effects of a new compound in animal models therefore provides poor prediction of its efficacy in patients.[6] Most drug-discovery programmes have not used a brain 'circuit-based' approach and hence had no information on whether the compounds modulated the target neural circuit of interest. The failure of many of these programmes may, therefore, be due to the drugs not effectively modulating the key neural circuits that underlie the observed cognitive deficits. Future clinical research should therefore identify a 'circuit-based' neuroimaging biomarker model, which can help identify key neurobiological targets of cognitive enhancement and guide the development of new mechanism compounds. The implementation of such circuit-based biomarker model in future drug development could become a conceptually important middle step between investigation of novel compounds in animal models and large-scale clinical efficacy trials.[50]

Chances of detecting efficacy of new interventions for cognitive dysfunction in BD may also be increased by a *multilevel approach*; rather than targeting cognition with one single treatment modality, future trials should also investigate the effects of *combined* pharmacological and psychological treatment for cognitive dysfunction. Indeed, it is likely that the combination of pharmacological and psychological/behavioural interventions can produce synergistic effects on brain function that translate into more robust cognitive efficacy than either treatment modality alone.

Conclusion

Cognitive dysfunction in BD is a new emerging treatment target. Over the past decade, a series of clinical trials of novel candidate treatments have been conducted. Overall, the results of these research efforts are disappointing. This may be due to either lack of efficacy of the investigated treatments or the critical methodological challenges in this relatively new field. A key issue is the absence of consensus regarding the need for and methods to screen for cognitive impairment in BD and regarding the choice of primary outcome measure(s) to assess treatment efficacy. We suggest that screening for cognitive impairment is critical for trials that target cognition and should involve use of an objective neuropsychological test battery. We also recommend that the primary outcome measure of treatment effects is defined as a global cognitive composite score of tests that are sensitive for cognitive dysfunction in BD. Socio-occupational function should be included as co-primary or secondary outcome. In addition, participants in these trials should be in full or partial remission, concomitant medication should be within the recommended doses and kept stable throughout the trials, and statistical methods should include mixed models or similar ways to take account of missing values and inter-individual changes during the trial period. A strategy that may improve the success rates of future cognition trials is the implementation a neuroimaging 'circuit-based' biomarker model as a middle step between preclinical studies and clinical-efficacy studies. A promising strategy to increase success rates of these trials is also to *combine* different treatment modalities into a multilevel approach, which may produce synergistic robust efficacy on cognitive dysfunction in BD.

References

1. Bourne C, Aydemir O, Balanza-Martinez V, Bora E, Brissos S, Cavanagh JT, et al. Neuropsychological testing of cognitive impairment in euthymic bipolar disorder: an individual patient data meta-analysis, Acta Psychiatr Scand 2013 Sep;128(3):149–62.

2. Barch DM. Neuropsychological abnormalities in schizophrenia and major mood disorders: similarities and differences, Curr Psychiatry Rep 2009 Aug;11(4):313–19.

3. Rund BR, Sundet K, Asbjornsen A, Egeland J, Landro NI, Lund A, et al. Neuropsychological test profiles in schizophrenia and non-psychotic depression, Acta Psychiatr Scand 2006 Apr;113(4):350–9.

4. Reichenberg A, Harvey PD, Bowie CR, Mojtabai R, Rabinowitz J, Heaton RK, et al. Neuropsychological function and dysfunction in schizophrenia and psychotic affective disorders, Schizophr Bull 2009 Sep;35(5):1022–9.

5. Schretlen DJ, Cascella NG, Meyer SM, Kingery LR, Testa SM, Munro CA, et al. Neuropsychological functioning in bipolar disorder and schizophrenia, Biol Psychiatry 2007 Jul 15;62(2):179–86.

6. Millan MJ, Agid Y, Brune M, Bullmore ET, Carter CS, Clayton NS, et al. Cognitive dysfunction in psychiatric disorders: characteristics, causes and the quest for improved therapy, Nat Rev Drug Discov 2012 Feb;11(2):141–68.

7. Rosa AR, Magalhaes PV, Czepielewski L, Sulzbach MV, Goi PD, Vieta E, et al. Clinical staging in bipolar disorder: focus on cognition and functioning, J Clin Psychiatry 2014 May;75(5):e450–6.

8. Bora E, Yucel M, and Pantelis C. Neurocognitive markers of psychosis in bipolar disorder: a meta-analytic study, J Affect Disord 2010 Dec;127(1–3):1–9.

9. Gildengers AG, Chung KH, Huang SH, Begley A, Aizenstein HJ, and Tsai SY. Neuroprogressive effects of lifetime illness duration in older adults with bipolar disorder, Bipolar Disord 2014 Sep;16(6):617–23.

10. Kessing LV and Andersen PK. Does the risk of developing dementia increase with the number of episodes in patients with depressive disorder and in patients with bipolar disorder?, J Neurol Neurosurg Psychiatry 2004 Dec;75(12):1662–6.

11. Torrent C, Martinez-Aran A, del Mar BC, Reinares M, Daban C, Sole B, et al. Long-term outcome of cognitive impairment in bipolar disorder, J Clin Psychiatry 2012 Jul;73(7):e899–e905.

12. Kogan JN, Otto MW, Bauer MS, Dennehy EB, Miklowitz DJ, Zhang HW, et al. Demographic and diagnostic characteristics of the first 1000 patients enrolled in the Systematic Treatment Enhancement Program for Bipolar Disorder (STEP-BD), Bipolar Disord 2004 Dec;6(6):460–9.

13. **Suppes T, Leverich GS, Keck PE, Nolen WA, Denicoff KD, Altshuler LL,** et al. The Stanley Foundation Bipolar Treatment Outcome Network. II. Demographics and illness characteristics of the first 261 patients, J Affect Disord 2001 Dec;**67**(1–3):45–59.

14. **Bonnin CM, Martinez-Aran A, Torrent C, Pacchiarotti I, Rosa AR, Franco C,** et al. Clinical and neurocognitive predictors of functional outcome in bipolar euthymic patients: a long-term, follow-up study, J Affect Disord 2010 Feb;**121**(1–2):156–60.

15. **Dias VV, Balanza-Martinez V, Soeiro-de-Souza MG, Moreno RA, Figueira ML, Machado-Vieira R,** et al. Pharmacological approaches in bipolar disorders and the impact on cognition: a critical overview, Acta Psychiatr Scand 2012 Nov;**126**(5):315–31.

16. **Iosifescu DV, Moore CM, Deckersbach T, Tilley CA, Ostacher MJ, Sachs GS,** et al. Galantamine-ER for cognitive dysfunction in bipolar disorder and correlation with hippocampal neuronal viability: a proof-of-concept study, CNS Neurosci Ther 2009;**15**(4):309–19.

17. **Matthews JD, Blais M, Park L, Welch C, Baity M, Murakami J,** et al. The impact of galantamine on cognition and mood during electroconvulsive therapy: a pilot study, J Psychiatr Res 2008 Jun;**42**(7):526–31.

18. **Deckersbach T, Nierenberg AA, Kessler R, Lund HG, Ametrano RM, Sachs G,** et al. RESEARCH: Cognitive rehabilitation for bipolar disorder: an open trial for employed patients with residual depressive symptoms, CNS Neurosci Ther 2010 Oct;**16**(5):298–307.

19. **Demant KM, Vinberg M, Kessing LV,** and **Miskowiak KW.** Effects of short-term cognitive remediation on cognitive dysfunction in partially or fully remitted individuals with bipolar disorder: results of a randomised controlled trial, PLoS One 2015;**10**(6):e0127955.

20. **Meusel LA, Hall GB, Fougere P, McKinnon MC,** and **MacQueen GM.** Neural correlates of cognitive remediation in patients with mood disorders, Psychiatry Res 2013 Nov 30;**214**(2):142–52.

21. **Naismith SL, Redoblado-Hodge MA, Lewis SJ, Scott EM,** and **Hickie IB.** Cognitive training in affective disorders improves memory: a preliminary study using the NEAR approach, J Affect Disord 2010 Mar;**121**(3):258–62.

22. **Torrent C, Bonnin CM, Martinez-Aran A, Valle J, Amann BL, Gonzalez-Pinto A,** et al. Efficacy of functional remediation in bipolar disorder: a multicenter randomized controlled study, Am J Psychiatry 2013 Aug;**170**(8):852–9.

23. **Gallagher P, Watson S, Smith MS, Ferrier IN,** and **Young AH.** Effects of adjunctive mifepristone (RU-486) administration on neurocognitive function and symptoms in schizophrenia, Biol Psychiatry 2005 Jan 15;**57**(2):155–61.

24. **McIntyre RS, Soczynska JK, Woldeyohannes HO, Miranda A, Vaccarino A, Macqueen G,** et al. A randomized, double-blind, controlled trial evaluating the effect of intranasal insulin on neurocognitive function in euthymic patients with bipolar disorder, Bipolar Disord 2012 Nov;**14**(7):697–706.

25. **Miskowiak KW, Ehrenreich H, Christensen EM, Kessing LV,** and **Vinberg M.** Recombinant human erythropoietin to target cognitive dysfunction in bipolar disorder: a double-blind, randomized, placebo-controlled phase 2 trial, J Clin Psychiatry 2014 Jul 8.

26. **Watson S, Gallagher P, Porter RJ, Smith MS, Herron LJ, Bulmer S,** et al. A randomized trial to examine the effect of mifepristone on neuropsychological performance and mood in patients with bipolar depression, Biol Psychiatry 2012 Dec 1;**72**(11):943–9.

27. **Young AH, Gallagher P, Watson S, Del-Estal D, Owen BM**, and **Ferrier IN**. Improvements in neurocognitive function and mood following adjunctive treatment with mifepristone (RU-486) in bipolar disorder, *Neuropsychopharmacology* 2004 Aug;**29**(8):1538–45.

28. **Matthews JD, Siefert CJ, Blais MA, Park LT, Siefert CJ, Welch CA**, et al. A double-blind, placebo-controlled study of the impact of galantamine on anterograde memory impairment during electroconvulsive therapy, J ECT 2013 Sep;**29**(3):170–8.

29. **Ghaemi SN, Gilmer WS, Dunn RT, Hanlon RE, Kemp DE, Bauer AD**, et al. A double-blind, placebo-controlled pilot study of galantamine to improve cognitive dysfunction in minimally symptomatic bipolar disorder, J Clin Psychopharmacol 2009 Jun;**29**(3):291–5.

30. **Dean OM, Bush AI, Copolov DL, Kohlmann K, Jeavons S, Schapkaitz I**, et al. Effects of N-acetyl cysteine on cognitive function in bipolar disorder, Psychiatry Clin Neurosci 2012 Oct;**66**(6):514–17.

31. **Burdick KE, Braga RJ, Nnadi CU, Shaya Y, Stearns WH**, and **Malhotra AK**. Placebo-controlled adjunctive trial of pramipexole in patients with bipolar disorder: targeting cognitive dysfunction, J Clin Psychiatry 2012 Jan;**73**(1):103–12.

32. **Chengappa KN, Bowie CR, Schlicht PJ, Fleet D, Brar JS**, and **Jindal R**. Randomized placebo-controlled adjunctive study of an extract of withania somnifera for cognitive dysfunction in bipolar disorder, J Clin Psychiatry 2013 Nov;**74**(11):1076–83.

33. **Miskowiak KW, Vinberg M, Harmer CJ, Ehrenreich H**, and **Kessing LV**. Erythropoietin: a candidate treatment for mood symptoms and memory dysfunction in depression, *Psychopharmacology (Berlin)* 2012 Feb;**219**(3):687–98.

34. **Osuji IJ, Vera-Bolanos E, Carmody TJ**, and **Brown ES**. Pregnenolone for cognition and mood in dual diagnosis patients, Psychiatry Res 2010 Jul 30;**178**(2):309–12.

35. **Brown ES, Gorman AR**, and **Hynan LS**. A randomized, placebo-controlled trial of citicoline add-on therapy in outpatients with bipolar disorder and cocaine dependence, J Clin Psychopharmacol 2007 Oct;**27**(5):498–502.

36. **Brown ES** and **Gabrielson B**. A randomized, double-blind, placebo-controlled trial of citicoline for bipolar and unipolar depression and methamphetamine dependence, J Affect Disord 2012 Dec 20;**143**(1–3):257–60.

37. **Loo CK, Katalinic N, Garfield JB, Sainsbury K, Hadzi-Pavlovic D**, and **Mac-Pherson R**. Neuropsychological and mood effects of ketamine in electroconvulsive therapy: a randomised controlled trial, J Affect Disord 2012 Dec 15;**142**(1–3):233–40.

38. **Rasmussen KG, Kung S, Lapid MI, Oesterle TS, Geske JR, Nuttall GA**, et al. A randomized comparison of ketamine versus methohexital anesthesia in electroconvulsive therapy, Psychiatry Res 2014 Feb 28;**215**(2):362–5.

39. **Wykes T, Huddy V, Cellard C, McGurk SR**, and **Czobor P**. A meta-analysis of cognitive remediation for schizophrenia: methodology and effect sizes, Am J Psychiatry 2011 May;**168**(5):472–85.

40. **Bonnin CM, Reinares M, Martinez-Aran A, Balanza-Martinez V, Sole B, Torrent C**, et al. Effects of functional remediation on neurocognitively impaired bipolar patients: enhancement of verbal memory, Psychol Med 2015 Sep 21;1–11.

41. **Burdick KE, Ketter TA, Goldberg JF**, and **Calabrese JR**. Assessing cognitive function in bipolar disorder: challenges and recommendations for clinical trial design, J Clin Psychiatry 2015 Mar;**76**(3):e342–50.

42. Schaefer J, Giangrande E, Weinberger DR, and Dickinson D. The global cognitive impairment in schizophrenia: consistent over decades and around the world, Schizophr Res 2013 Oct;150(1):42–50.

43. Burdick KE, Russo M, Frangou S, Mahon K, Braga RJ, Shanahan M, et al. Empirical evidence for discrete neurocognitive subgroups in bipolar disorder: clinical implications, Psychol Med 2014 Oct;44(14):3083–96.

44. Miskowiak KW, Rush AJ, Gerds TA, Vinberg M, and Kessing LV. Predictors of treatment success in cognition trials—secondary analyses of a randomized, controlled trial of erythropoietin treatment in mood disorder, in preparation 2015.

45. Demant KM, Vinberg M, Kessing LV, and Miskowiak KW. Assessment of subjective and objective cognitive function in bipolar disorder: correlations, predictors and the relation to psychosocial function, Psychiatry Res 2015 Sep 30;229(1–2):565–71.

46. Jensen JH, Støttrup MM, Nayberg E, Knorr U, Ullum H, Purdon SE, et al. Optimising screening for cognitive dysfunction in bipolar disorder: validation and evaluation of objective and subjective tools, J Affect Disord 2015;187(10):19.

47. Mur M, Portella MJ, Martinez-Aran A, Pifarre J, and Vieta E. Influence of clinical and neuropsychological variables on the psychosocial and occupational outcome of remitted bipolar patients, *Psychopathology* 2009;42(3):148–56.

48. Kessing LV, Vradi E, and Andersen PK. Starting lithium prophylaxis early v late in bipolar disorder, Br J Psychiatry 2014 Sep;205(3):214–20.

49. Vieta E, Reinares M, and Rosa AR. Staging bipolar disorder, Neurotox Res 2011 Feb;19(2):279–85.

50. Nathan PJ, Phan KL, Harmer CJ, Mehta MA, and Bullmore ET. Increasing pharmacological knowledge about human neurological and psychiatric disorders through functional neuroimaging and its application in drug discovery, Curr Opin Pharmacol 2014 Feb;14:54–61.

Chapter 27

The role of electroconvulsive therapy in the treatment of bipolar disorder

Roumen Milev

Introduction

Bipolar disorder (BD) is a common condition associated with significant burden. It is a complex disorder presenting with alternating episodes of mania and depression, and periods of remission. The treatment of BD is also complicated, and many patients do not achieve full remission, despite availability of numerous effective therapeutic approaches.[48,49] In this chapter we review the use of electroconvulsive therapy (ECT) in BD, including bipolar mania, bipolar depression, and mixed states. We review the efficacy and tolerability of ECT, in relation to electrode placements, stimulus parameters etc. Unfortunately, there is a paucity of research in this area and the existing literature consists mainly of case reports, case series, and retrospective chart reviews. Prospective and randomized controlled trials are rare.

Brief overview of ECT

ECT is a well-established treatment for psychiatric disorders, introduced in the 1930s and in use since then. ECT induces generalized tonic–clonic seizure by the electrical current applied on the scalp. The brain seizure produces depolarization and repolarization of neurons, changes in the neuronal sensitivity, and also affects brain neurotransmitters. Newer data suggests that ECT stimulates the production of neurotrophic factors (ie brain-derived neurotrophic factor—BDNF), which would stimulate neuroplasticity in certain areas of the brain (eg hippocampus and olfactory bulb). ECT has undergone significant modifications and changes over the years. ECT is delivered by a team of trained physicians, nurses, and other health professionals. Short lasting general anaesthesia is applied and partial muscular paralysis is achieved prior to the actual treatment.

Stimulus parameters

Several parameters of the electrical stimulus could be modified in the ECT device and are set in advance by the psychiatrist. These include the width of the electrical pulse measured in milliseconds (ms), usually a brief pulse of 1–2 ms or, more recently, an ultra-brief pulse with width of 0.25–0.5 ms. Frequency refers to how many pulses per second are delivered and is measured in hertz (Hz). Duration of the electrical stimulus is usually set to between half a second and up to 8 seconds or more. The electrical current is measured in amperes (A) and is usually 0.5–0.9 A. The total amount of electrical charge is measured in coulombs (C), and depends on a combination of the above four parameters. The usual ECT stimulus delivers of a charge from very few up to 500–600 millicoulombs (mC) in devices in North America and up to 1000 mC or more for devices throughout the rest of the world.

Electrode placements

The stimulating electrodes are positioned on the head and could be placed symmetrically on both sides in a so-called bilateral placement. Most common bilateral placements are bi-temporal (BT) when the electrodes are placed over the temporal lobes and bi-frontal (BF) when the electrodes are positioned over the frontal lobes. Rarely, asymmetrical bilateral positions have also been used. Electrodes could be positioned also unilaterally over only one hemisphere of the brain, usually over the non-dominant hemisphere, which for most people is the right hemisphere—right unilateral (RUL) placement.

Seizure threshold

The minimal amount of electrical charge, which could induce a seizure, is known as seizure threshold. It varies significantly between people and is usually higher in older people and in men. Seizure threshold is affected by psychotropic medication, eg antiepileptic medications increase the seizure threshold. Seizure threshold also varies with different placements of the electrodes. The seizure threshold also seems to increase after a series of ECT treatments. Once the seizure threshold is determined, usual settings of 1.5 to 2 times seizure threshold charge is used in bi-lateral treatments and 5, 6, or even 8 times the seizures thresholds for unilateral treatment (suprathreshold). The length of the seizure induced is usually monitored by two-channel electroencephalography (EEG) and by observed tonic and clonic muscular twitches in the limbs, torso, or face of the patients. A number of vital signs such as oxygen saturation, heart rate and electrocardiogram (ECG), blood pressure, etc are monitored before, during, and after the treatment. Treatments are usually given between two and three times per week and an acute treatment course typically consists of six to 15 treatments or more.

Efficacy, safety, and tolerability

ECT is one of the most efficacious treatment methods in psychiatry and for depressive disorders response rates could reach 70–80% and remission rates of 40–50% or higher. ECT is one of the safest treatments with mortality rates of 1 per 73,440 treatments or less, approximating the mortality of general anaesthesia. More frequently reported side effects include mild to moderate headaches, muscular pain, nausea, somnolence, and impairment of cognitive function. Retrograde and anterograde amnesia are common, but usually short-lived, and impairment of autobiographical memory is less common but of significant concern.

ECT in BD

ECT has been and continues to be used in patients with BD. Different studies examine a variety of different treatment methods, electrode positioning, stimuli intensity, and patient populations, which makes comparisons and evidence-based decisions quite difficult. Table 27.1 summarizes all randomized trials in BD. Loo et al.[20] conducted one of the best systematic reviews of the literature of the physical treatments for BD including ECT. In 2011, Versiani et al.[44] conducted a systematic review of the literature of the use of ECT in BD. They had found a total of 51 articles Of them reporting efficacy and safety of ECT in BD with 10 or more subjects. which 28 were in mania, 9 in depression, 10 in bipolar depression versus unipolar depression, and 4 in mixed states. Most of the trials were small, quite often retrospective studies, and they found only three controlled studies for mania comparing ECT versus sham ECT, versus lithium or versus lithium and haloperidol and they did not find any controlled studies for bipolar depression. The authors concluded that the lack of scientific evidence contrasts with the widely held positive view by physicians of the efficacy and tolerability of ECT in BD, including bipolar depression, and suggested that future studies need to be done.

Thirthalli, Prasad, and Gangedhar[39] conducted a narrative review of the literature about the use of ECT in BD. They concluded that 'the response to ECT is impressive in mania, depression and in mixed affective states'. They also found some preliminary evidence about benefits of maintenance ECT in BD. However, they also found that most of the literature on efficacy and adverse effects comes from case series, retrospective reports, and open trials with very few controlled trials. The concurrent use of lithium and antiepileptics along with ECT is common in clinical practice and appears to be largely safe, although one should be mindful about the lithium levels. The use of suprathreshold unilateral ECT and BF placement may have some benefits over other methods. Another more recent review of the literature of brain stimulation techniques for BDs (Oldani et al.)[30] came to very similar conclusions (Table 27.1).

Black et al.[6] conducted a chart review of all patients treated with ECT in a 12-year period in a university hospital medical centre. They identified 368 unipolar depression patients, 55 bipolar depressed patients, and 37 manic patients. Manic patients required a lower number of treatments and received, on average, six treatments while both unipolar and bipolar depressed patients received, on average, nine treatments. They found that 78.4% of patients with mania had marked improvement while 69.8% and 69.1% were rated as markedly improved in the unipolar and bipolar depression, respectively. The conclusion of the authors was that ECT was an effective treatment for mania, and unipolar and bipolar depression.

Virit et al.[45] examined attitudes towards ECT in both patients with BDs and their relatives. They found that although the patients and relatives believed that they had not received adequate information about ECT, both groups were quite satisfied with the treatment and found it beneficial and maintained a positive attitude towards its use.

Table 27.1 Summary of randomized trials of ECT in BD patients

Author	Diagnosis	Treatment evaluated	n	Result	Cognition
Hiremani RM et al.[16] (2008)	Bipolar mania	BF vs BT ECT	BF n = 17 BT n = 19	YMRS BF respond faster	No difference
Mohan TSP et al.[28] (2009)	Bipolar mania	BT ECT at ST vs at 2.5 x ST	ST n = 26 2.5 x ST n = 24	No difference	No difference
Schoeyen HK et al.[33] (2014)	Treatment-resistant bipolar depression	RUL ECT vs algorithm-based pharmacotherapy	RUL n = 36 Pharmacotherapy n = 30	Response— RUL>pharmacotherapy Remission—no difference	No difference in general cognition, reduced autobiographical consistency in ECT group
Sikdar S et al.[36] (1994)	Bipolar mania	BT ECT + CPZ vs sham ECT + CPZ	ECT n = 15 Sham n = 15	ECT + CPZ faster and better improvement	Not reported
Barekatain M et al.[4] (2008)	Bipolar mania	BT 1 x ST vs BF 1.5 x ST	BT n = 14 BF n = 14	Similar efficacy between two groups	Better cognitive outcome in BF group

ECT—electroconvulsive therapy; BF—bi-frontal; BT—bi-temporal; YMRS—Young Mania Rating Scale; ST—seizure threshold; RUL—right unilateral; CPZ—chlorpromasine

Use of ECT for acute bipolar mania

ECT is a very efficacious treatment in acute manic episodes and has been used as a first-line treatment in the past (eg Perris and d'Elia[32], McCabe[22]). Greenblatt et al.,[14] in one of the first chart reviews, compared ECT with a variety of antidepressants in patients admitted to three state hospitals in the Boston area at the time, treated with ECT, imipramine, fentazin, isocarboxazid, and placebo. The diagnostic population of mixed patients consisted of 'psychoneurotics, manic depressives, involutionals, schizophrenic reactions, schizoaffective types' and a mixed category of character disorders with depression. The authors reported 76% of marked improvement in the ECT group as compared with 28–50% for the different antidepressants or placebo groups. For a good review of the older literature, see Mukherjee et al.[29] Although recognized as effective treatment for BD, ECT has been gradually replaced by the increased use of antipsychotics and mood stabilizers for these purposes. Indeed, the Canadian Network for Mood and Anxiety Treatments (CANMAT) Guidelines for the Treatment of BDs (Yatham et al.),[48,49] the use of ECT for acute manic episodes, is recommended as a second-line treatment approach. In a commentary, Fink[13] also strongly recommends the use of ECT in manic episodes in BD. de Macedo-Soares et al.[11] descried a case series of six patients with treatment-resistant BD and were treated with 12 sessions of bilateral ECT delivered three times a week. All six patients responded well to the treatment, four of them in manic or mixed episodes, and two in depressive episodes.

Efficacy and placement of electrodes

Black et al.[5] conducted a chart review of 438 patients hospitalized with bipolar mania over a 12-year period. The authors compared patients treated with ECT versus lithium versus neither of the two, further subdividing the lithium-treated group to adequate and inadequate based on lithium levels recorded. They found that significantly greater percentage (78%) of patients who received ECT had marked improvement compared with those who received either adequate or inadequate lithium treatment (62% and 56% respectively) or neither treatment (37%) and concluded that ECT was demonstrated to be an effective treatment for mania. In a retrospective chart review, Thirthalli et al.[38] compared 23 patients with mania who received threshold bilateral ECT with 37 manic patients who received suprathreshold (at two times seizure threshold) bilateral ECT and determined that, on average, patients who received threshold level needed two more ECT sessions had about ten more days as inpatients compared with the suprathreshold bilateral ECT, confirming similar findings by Black et al.[6] These findings were not replicated in one of the very few randomized controlled trials of ECT in acute mania. Mohan et al.[28] compared bilateral treatments given at seizure threshold versus 2.5 times seizure threshold in patients with acute mania combined with antipsychotics. They reported significant improvement as measured by clinical global impression in 92.3% of the patients receiving threshold ECT and 91.7% in the patients given suprathreshold ECT with also very similar remission rates of approximately 88% for both groups. There were no major differences between the two groups in the time for improvement and number of ECT given and also both interventions were equally safe.

In a double-blind, randomized controlled study, Hiremani et al.[16] compared the short-term efficacy of BF versus BT ECT in acute mania patients. Thirty-six inpatients with mania were randomly assigned to receive either BF or BT ECT. The authors reported that the patients in the BF ECT group showed faster improvement compared with the BT ECT group and that, by the end of the study period, 87.5% of the subjects in the BF group and 72.2% of the subjects in the BT ECT group had met the response criteria. There was no difference in the cognitive side effects between the two groups. Sikdar et al.[36] conducted a randomized, double-blind, controlled study of 30 patients who received chlorpromazine 600 mg together with ECT or chlorpromazine with sham ECT in acute mania. ECT in combination with chlorpromazine was significantly better and 12 out of the 15 patients had recovered completely by the end of the treatment.[8] In the sham ECT group, patients required a much higher dose of antipsychotic medication and recovered in a much slower fashion. Small et al.[37] randomly assigned 34 hospitalized manic patients to treatment of an average series of nine bilateral ECT sessions, followed by maintenance by lithium versus lithium carbonate alone. They found that the ECT patients had higher improvement rates during the first eight weeks and this was especially true of patients with mixed symptoms of mania and depression. After the initial eight weeks and during the follow-up period, there were no significant differences between the two groups including rate of relapse, recurrence, and re-hospitalization. Barekatain et al.[4] compared BF versus BT ECT in severe manic patients. They enrolled 28 patients with severe mania admitted to university hospital to a double-blind, randomized trial to receive moderate-dose BF or low-dose BT ECT. All patients received at least six sessions of ECT. Both groups did not differ in the primary outcome and all completers showed a good response to ECT with a very good or marked clinical improvement of manic symptoms defined as a reduction of more than 50% of their Young Mania Rating Scale (YMRS) scores. The cognitive side-effect evaluation (as determined by mini-mental state evaluation) showed statistically significant worse outcomes with BT treatment compared with BF.

One important issue to be discussed is the concomitant use of lithium salts that are commonly used in patients with BD and ECT. In a retrospective study, Volpe et al.[47] describes 90 patients who were treated concurrently with lithium and ECT. The authors could not find any evidence of negative outcome in terms of side effects or several unfavourable outcomes in this group, compared to the patients who received ECT without lithium.

There is very little evidence to support continuation and maintenance ECT in refractory mania and only case reports have been described (eg see Tsao et al.,[41] Sienaert and Peuskens[34]).

In summary, ECT for acute mania has been commonly used in clinical practice for decades, but there is little good-quality research to support it. Both BF and BT positioning seem to be effective, the latter arguably associated with more cognitive side effects.

ECT in mixed states

Valenti et al.[42] conducted a systematic review of the literature on treatment of mixed states in BD with ECT. They found only three prospective trials with more than five patients per trial. The combined number of patients with mixed episodes from the three studies was 58. The response rate reported in these studies varied between 56 and 100%. Minnai et al.[27] reported a case series of 14 patients with rapid cycling BD (types I and II) where maintenance ECT was very effective. They found that males and bipolar II patients did better. In a prospective study of ECT in medication non-responsive patients with mixed mania and bipolar depression, Ciapparelli et al.[9] followed 41 patients with bipolar I disorder with mixed mania and 23 patients with bipolar I depression, who were consecutively assigned to ECT treatments. They found significant improvements in both groups, on the Montgomery-Åsberg Depression Rating Scale (MADRS), the Clinical Global Impression (CGI), and the Brief Psychiatric Rating Scale (BPRS). They also observed that the mixed mania group exhibited a more rapid and marked response as well as a greater reduction in suicidal ideation. In their study, the response to ECT was not influenced by presence of delusions. Medda et al.[23,26] compared the response and remission rates in patients with bipolar I disorder, resistant to pharmacological treatment, who were subsequently treated with ECT. Ninety-six patients were included in a prospective naturalistic study, with 46 of them with bipolar depression and 50 with mixed states. The response rates were 69.6% for bipolar depression and 66% for mixed states, with remission rates of 26.1% and 30.0%, respectively.

ECT in bipolar depression

Most of the older and many of the newer studies of ECT in depression include patients with major depressive disorder (unipolar) and bipolar depression in the same trials. In a retrospective chart review, Abrams et al.[1] compared the responses of 28 unipolar depressed patients to 15 bipolar depressed patients (interestingly, there were no men in the bipolar group) and found no significant difference between the responses of patients in both groups.

Penland and Ostroff[31] reported a case series of nine patients with bipolar depression who were treated with ECT concurrently with up-titration of lamotrigine. Of the nine patients, five were men, four had BD type I and four with BD type II, and one was schizoaffective. All nine patients did achieve remission and the use of lamotrigine was deemed safe and did not interfere with routine ECT practice, hence allowing for transition to maintenance pharmacotherapy.

Hallam, Smith, and Berk[15] reviewed the difference between subjective and objective assessment of ECT outcomes in patients with bipolar and unipolar depression. This was a naturalistic file audit of 787 consecutive inpatients admitted to a private psychiatric clinic. One hundred and six of them received ECT as part of their treatment with an average of four treatments. Seventy-three had major depressive disorder and 33 had bipolar depression. Outcome was rated as significantly improved by both physicians and nurses in both groups of patients. Patients rated their outcome using the Depression, Anxiety, and Stress Scale (DASS). Interestingly, the authors found significant reduction of the scores for depression, anxiety, and stress in the group with major depressive disorder but no such reduction in the patients with bipolar depression. The authors concluded that patients with bipolar depression seemed to have a poor subjective response to ECT, compared with patients with unipolar depression.

A very important study was completed and published recently by Schoeyen et al.[33] To our knowledge, this is the first and only randomized, controlled trial that examines ECT versus algorithm-based pharmacological treatment in treatment-resistant bipolar depression. The design of the Norwegian study was described previously (Kessler et al.).[17] It was a prospective randomized, controlled, multicentre, six-week acute treatment trial with seven clinical assessments, with a planned extension follow-up visit at 26 weeks or until remission of a maximum of 52 weeks, comparing patients from seven study centres, across Norway, all of them being acute psychiatric departments. The study was not sponsored by industry. A total of 73 bipolar depression patients were recruited between April 2008 and May 2011. They were adults aged 18 and over who fulfilled the criteria for treatment-resistant depression in BD. The cut-off for inclusion in the study was a score of the MADRS of at least 25 at baseline. ECT was delivered at three sessions per week for up to six weeks, with a total of up to 18 treatments using RUL brief pulse stimulation and was compared with the control group, which used algorithm-based pharmacological treatment. This report only covers the first six-week acute trial. The results of the long-term extension of the study will be reported separately at a later stage. Patients were 26–79 years old, currently depressed with a MADRS score of 25 or more, fulfilling the criteria for BD type 1 or 2. The treatment resistance was determined by the participating clinicians and was defined by a lack of response to two trials in patients' lifetime using antidepressants or mood stabilizers with documented efficiency in bipolar depression. They were lithium, lamotrigine, quetiapine, or olanzapine for at least six weeks or cessation of treatment due to side effect. The main outcome measure was the change of MADRS score. The RUL placement followed the d'Elia method, and a pulse width of 0.5 ms was used. The seizure thresholds were determined by an aged-based gender-adjusted method. The algorithm-based pharmacology treatment followed the treatment algorithm for bipolar depression of Goodwin and Jamieson with pharmacotherapy protocol chosen for each patient before the randomization, taking into account the patient's medication history. Both the patient and treating psychiatrist were not blinded to the treatment modality, but the MADRS interviews were audiotaped and rated by blinded raters.

In this study, ECT was significantly more effective than the pharmacological treatment with mean MADRS score at six weeks 6.6 points lower in the ECT group (statistically significant difference). The other important difference was the fact that the ECT group's MADRS scores changed much faster and the time to response was much quicker. At the end of the six-week treatment period, response rates were higher in the ECT group (73.9%) than in the pharmacological group (35%). The remission rate was not significantly different between the two groups—34.8% versus 30%, respectively. The authors believed that the reason for the lower remission rate was not due to the unilateral placement of the electrode as opposed to bilateral, but most likely to selection of patients with a low potential for remission.

This study had some limitations acknowledged by the authors, specifically the fact that neither treating psychiatrists nor patients were blinded to the treatment modality, which might have biased the outcome. The relatively small study group and high dropout rates also limited the statistical power of the analysis and might have been a source for type 2 errors. Another limitation pointed out by the authors was the fact that the most severely depressed patients were not included because of their inability to give informed consent or that their treating psychiatrists' opinion was that they were in urgent need of ECT and hence not enrolled in the study. In a commentary about the study, Tohen and Abbott[40] questioned whether the patients were a truly treatment-resistant group due to the fact that the requirement was failure of two therapeutic trials in the lifetime of the patients, rather than in the current episode. Another limitation pointed out was the fact that the pharmacological treatment algorithm, although being a state of the art in 2007 when the study was designed and initiated, would currently not be considered standard as newer treatment for bipolar depression including combination of olanzapine and fluoxetine or lurasidone in monotherapy or in combination were apparently not included as first-line treatment. Not withstanding all these limitations, we need to point out that this is the first randomized, controlled trial comparing ECT with pharmacological treatment in a very important patient group with serious unmet needs. The long-term data for the continuation phase of the study will be forthcoming and is expected to answer some specific questions about continuation ECT.

One of the hotly debated topics has been the use antiepileptic medication as mood stabilizers in patients with BDs and what their effects have been on ECT in terms of seizure threshold, efficacy of ECT treatments, etc. In an attempt to shed light on the issue, Virupaksha et al.[46] conducted retrospective patient-records analysis for all consecutive non-epileptic BD patients referred for ECT in a two-year period to an academic psychiatric hospital. They have found 79 patients who were on antiepileptic medication during their ECT and 122 patients who were not on antiepileptic medication during their ECT treatment. They have confirmed that both groups achieved similar improvement at the end of the ECT course; however, patients who were on antiepileptic medication had significantly higher seizure threshold, higher incidence of failure to obtain seizures, and shorter duration of motor seizures. Even more, patients on antiepileptic medication had received a significantly higher number of ECT treatments (mean 7.9 + 3.0) than the patients who were not on antiepileptic medication (mean 6.3 + 2.1). They also had longer hospitalizations. Even when the authors controlled for the effects of duration of illness, gender, drug treatment, and presence of co-morbidity, the differences in outcome remained significant.

Switch to mania

In 94 patients with depression treated with ECT, Lewis and Nasrallah[19] reported 6.4% switch to mania. Andrade et al.[2] reported that 4 out of 32 patients (12.5%) with 'endogenous depression' according to the research diagnostic criteria (RDC) switch to mania during the ECT treatment. In all cases, the mania subsided spontaneously within two to five days. In a retrospective chart review of 100 inpatients treated with ECT for bipolar depression types 1 or 2, Bost-Baxter et al.[7] found that overall switch to hypomania or mania was 24.8%. These switches were not correlated with diagnosis, concurrent antidepressant medication, use of an antimanic medication, or history of rapid cycling. In the subset of patients who were not taking antimanic medication during ECT, switch was associated with receiving a higher number of ECT treatments. Stopping ECT and initiating medication was reported in approximately half of the patients. Zavorotnyy et al.[50] presented a case report of a 66-year-old woman with bipolar depression with a 35-year history of BD. ECT was initiated because of lack of response to medication. During the course of ECT, she developed frequent mood fluctuations fulfilling the criteria of ultra-rapid cycling. These symptoms were treated with lithium successfully and ECT was continued.

Maintenance therapy

Sienaert and Peuskens[34] reported a case of a 53-year-old woman with a 31-year history of recurrent manic and depressive episodes, with poor response to medication. She achieved remission after a course of 12 treatments and continued with ECT treatments at weekly intervals for the next 37 months. Following discontinuation of the continuous ECT, she relapsed with a severe manic episode. Restarting ECT resulted in a rapid remission. During her treatment she showed no signs of cognitive impairment. Medda et al.[24] followed 50 patients with bipolar depression[36] or mixed episode[14] naturalistically after responding to a course of ECT for a period of 20 to 146 weeks. They observed that the rate of relapse was quite low, but was correlated to a longer length of the depressed episode.

Comparisons between unipolar and bipolar depression

Dierckx et al.[12] conducted a meta-analysis (including reports until June 2010) comparing ECT efficacy in bipolar depression versus unipolar depression. They included six studies in their meta-analysis, five of them were prospective, and one was chart review with a total number of 790 patients with unipolar depression and 316 patients with bipolar depression. They found that the overall remission rates were very similar with 50.9% achieving remission in the unipolar depression versus 53.2% in the bipolar depression group. Bailine et al.[3] compared the response and remission rates of patients with unipolar depression versus patients with bipolar depression. They conducted a randomized, double-masked, multicentred, National Institute of Mental Health (NIMH)-funded, controlled trial in 2002–2006. Patients were randomly assigned to BF, BT, or RUL treatment. Both bi-lateral treatments were set at 1.5 times seizure threshold and the RUL used six times seizure threshold. They enrolled 170 unipolar depressed patients and 50 bipolar patients. Both unipolar and bipolar patients had a very similar response (78.8% vs 80.0%, respectively) and remission (unipolar depression 61.2%, bipolar depression 64%) rates, which allowed the authors to conclude that ECT is equally effective in both conditions.

Speed of improvement

In an interesting attempt to determine the speed of improvement, Daly et al.[10] conducted combined analysis of the data from three separate double-blind treatment protocols comparing patients with unipolar and bipolar depression. Although the protocols were very different in design, patients were randomly assigned to be in two different treatment arms comparing, in general, RUL with bilateral ECT treatments. A total of 162 patients with unipolar depression and 66 patients with bipolar depression were included in the analysis. Patients with bipolar depression seemed to respond quicker and received significantly fewer ECT treatments compared with unipolar patients. This was true for both bipolar I and bipolar II patients. The more rapid response of patients with bipolar depression compared with unipolar depression was also shown by Sienaert et al.[35] who conducted a randomized trial comparing ultra-brief pulse BF ECT at 1.5 times seizure threshold versus unilateral ECT at six times seizures threshold. From the 64 patients enrolled in the trial, 13 had bipolar depression. The rates of response to the treatment were similar at 84.6% for bipolar patients and 76.4% for unipolar depression. The speed of response was faster in the bipolar depression group and they also had significantly fewer treatments needed to achieve remission. Somewhat different results were reported by Medda et al.[25] who explored predictors of response to ECT of patients who were resistant to pharmacological treatments. In 208 depressed patients, the majority of whom were with bipolar depression (76 bipolar I and 101 bipolar II), they found that having BD predicted a worse outcome to ECT treatment.

Use in youth

There have been occasional case reports for use of ECT for BDs in children and youth (eg see Carr et al.[8]). Kutcher et al.[18] described ECT treatments of 16 youth with treatment-resistant BD, eight of them in acute manic state, and eight of them in acute depressive state. The authors found that ECT was generally quite effective and well tolerated. There was significant reduction of the length of stay to the inpatient unit compared with patients with similar illness characteristics, but refused to have ECT treatments.

Cognitive impairment

MacQueen et al.[21] conducted comprehensive cognitive assessments in two groups of patients with BD and compared them with a control group of healthy volunteers. The two bipolar patients groups had similar past illness history burden, but one group never received ECT and the other did. They found that compared with healthy subjects, patients had verbal learning and memory deficits. Patients who had received ECT in the past had further impairment in a variety of learning and memory tests when compared with patients with no past history of ECT. As this was a retrospective non-controlled study, the authors pointed out that it was possible that the patients with history of ECT treatments might have had a more severe illness and hence might have had more cognitive deficits to start with. In a prospective study of

83 patients with depression (13 of them with bipolar depression) treated with ECT, van Waarde et al.[43] found that the cognitive outcome was better in patients with bipolar depression as opposed to the unipolar depression.

Conclusion

As previously discussed, the use of ECT in people with BDs is common and widespread in clinical practice. There is proven efficacy, with high response and remission rates in both acute mania and depression. ECT seems to be effective also in mixed states. There is some evidence for usefulness in maintenance therapy and in youth. Placement of electrodes and stimulus intensity need additional studies. ECT seems to be well tolerated and side-effect profile is well established. Unfortunately, the overall quality of research and available evidence is relatively low. Good-quality prospective randomized controlled studies are urgently needed to address numerous unanswered questions, as outlined before. This seems to be the common conclusion of virtually every one of the numerous reviews of the literature conducted.

References

1. **Abrams R** and **Taylor MA**. Unipolar and bipolar depressive illness: phenomenology and response to electroconvulsive therapy, Arch Gen Psychiatry 1974;**30**(3):320–1.

2. **Andrade C, Gangadhar B, Swaminath G**, and **Channabasavanna S**. Mania as a side effect of electroconvulsive therapy, J ECT 1988;**4**(1):81–3.

3. **Bailine S, Fink M, Knapp R, Petrides G, Husain M, Rasmussen K**, et al. Electroconvulsive therapy is equally effective in unipolar and bipolar depression, Acta Psychiatr Scand 2010;**121**(6):431–6.

4. **Barekatain M, Jahangard L, Haghighi M**, and **Ranjkesh F**. Bifrontal versus bitemporal electroconvulsive therapy in severe manic patients, J ECT 2008 Sep;**24**(3):199–202.

5. **Black DW, Winokur G**, and **Nasrallah A**. Treatment of mania: a naturalistic study of electroconvulsive therapy versus lithium in 438 patients, J Clin Psychiatry 1987.

6. **Black DW, Winokur G**, and **Nasrallah A**. ECT in unipolar and bipolar disorders: a naturalistic evaluation of 460 patients, J ECT 1986;**2**(4):231–8.

7. **Bost-Baxter E, Reti IM**, and **Payne JL**. ECT in bipolar disorder: incidence of switch from depression to hypomania or mania, J Depress Anxiety 2012;**1**(5):1–5.

8. **Carr V, Dorrington C, Schrader G**, and **Wale J**. The use of ECT for mania in childhood bipolar disorder, Br J Psychiatry 1983 Oct;**143**:411–15.

9. **Ciapparelli A, Dell'Osso L, Tundo A, Pini S, Chiavacci MC, Di Sacco I**, et al. Electroconvulsive therapy in medication-nonresponsive patients with mixed mania and bipolar depression, J Clin Psychiatry 2001 Jul;**62**(7):552–5.

10. **Daly JJ, Prudic J, Devanand D, Nobler MS, Lisanby SH, Peyser S**, et al. ECT in bipolar and unipolar depression: differences in speed of response, Bipolar Disord 2001;**3**(2):95–104.

11. **de Macedo-Soares MB, Moreno RA, Rigonatti SP**, and **Lafer B**. Efficacy of electroconvulsive therapy in treatment-resistant bipolar disorder: a case series, J ECT 2005;**21**(1):31–4.

12. Dierckx B, Heijnen WT, van den Broek, Walter W, and Birkenhäger TK. Efficacy of electroconvulsive therapy in bipolar versus unipolar major depression: a meta-analysis, Bipolar Disord 2012;14(2):146–50.

13. Fink M. ECT in therapy-resistant mania: does it have a place? Bipolar Disord 2006;8(3):307–9.

14. Greenblatt M, Grosser GH, and Wechsler H. Differential response of hospitalized depressed patients to somatic therapy, Am J Psychiatry 1964;120(10):935–43.

15. Hallam K, Smith D, and Berk M. Differences between subjective and objective assessments of the utility of electroconvulsive therapy in patients with bipolar and unipolar depression, J Affect Disord 2009;112(1):212–18.

16. Hiremani RM, Thirthalli J, Tharayil BS, and Gangadhar BN. Double-blind randomized controlled study comparing short-term efficacy of bifrontal and bitemporal electroconvulsive therapy in acute mania, Bipolar Disord 2008;10(6):701–7.

17. Kessler U, Vaaler AE, Schoyen H, Oedegaard KJ, Bergsholm P, Andreassen OA, et al. The study protocol of the Norwegian randomized controlled trial of electroconvulsive therapy in treatment resistant depression in bipolar disorder, BMC Psychiatry 2010 Feb 23;10:16-244X-10–16.

18. Kutcher S and Robertson HA. Electroconvulsive therapy in treatment-resistant bipolar youth, J Child Adolesc Psychopharmacol 1995;5(3):167–75.

19. Lewis DA and Nasrallah HA. Mania associated with electroconvulsive therapy, J Clin Psychiatry 1986.

20. Loo C, Katalinic N, Mitchell PB, and Greenberg B. Physical treatments for bipolar disorder: a review of electroconvulsive therapy, stereotactic surgery and other brain stimulation techniques, J Affect Disord 2011;132(1):1–13.

21. MacQueen G, Parkin C, Marriott M, Begin H, and Hasey G. The long-term impact of treatment with electroconvulsive therapy on discrete memory systems in patients with bipolar disorder, J Psychiatry Neurosci 2007 Jul;32(4):241–9.

22. McCabe MS. ECT treatment of mania: a controlled study, Am J Psychiatry 1976.

23. Medda P, Perugi G, Zanello S, Ciuffa M, and Cassano G. Response to ECT in bipolar I, bipolar II and unipolar depression, J Affect Disord 2009;118(1):55–9.

24. Medda P, Mauri M, Fratta S, Ciaponi B, Miniati M, Toni C, et al. Long-term naturalistic follow-up of patients with bipolar depression and mixed state treated with electroconvulsive therapy, J ECT 2013 Sep;29(3):179–88.

25. Medda P, Mauri M, Toni C, Mariani MG, Rizzato S, Miniati M, et al. Predictors of remission in 208 drug-resistant depressive patients treated with electroconvulsive therapy, J ECT 2014 Dec;30(4):292–7.

26. Medda P, Perugi G, Zanello S, Ciuffa M, Rizzato S, and Cassano GB. Comparative response to electroconvulsive therapy in medication-resistant bipolar I patients with depression and mixed state, J ECT 2010 Jun;26(2):82–6.

27. Minnai GP, Salis PG, Oppo R, Loche AP, Scano F, and Tondo L. Effectiveness of maintenance electroconvulsive therapy in rapid-cycling bipolar disorder, J ECT 2011 Jun;27(2):123–6.

28. Mohan TSP, Tharyan P, Alexander J, and Raveendran NS. Effects of stimulus intensity on the efficacy and safety of twice-weekly, bilateral electroconvulsive therapy (ECT) combined with antipsychotics in acute mania: a randomised controlled trial, Bipolar Disord 2009;11(2):126–34.

29. **Mukherjee S, Sackeim HA**, and **Schnur DB**. Electroconvulsive therapy of acute manic episodes: a review of 50 years' experience, Am J Psychiatry 1994 Feb;**151**(2):169–76.

30. **Oldani L, Altamura AC, Abdelghani M**, and **Young AH**. Brain stimulation treatments in bipolar disorder: a review of the current literature, *The World Journal of Biological Psychiatry* **2014**(0):1–13.

31. **Penland HR** and **Ostroff RB**. Combined use of lamotrigine and electroconvulsive therapy in bipolar depression: a case series, J ECT 2006;**22**(2):142–7.

32. **Perris C** and **d'Elia G**. A study of bipolar (manic-depressive) and unipolar recurrent depressive psychoses. IX. therapy and prognosis, Acta Psychiatr Scand 1966;**194**(Suppl):153–71.

33. **Schoeyen HK, Kessler U, Andreassen OA, Auestad BH, Bergsholm P, Malt UF**, et al. Treatment-resistant bipolar depression: a randomized controlled trial of electroconvulsive therapy versus algorithm-based pharmacological treatment, Am J Psychiatry 2014;**172**(1):41–51.

34. **Sienaert P** and **Peuskens J**. Electroconvulsive therapy: an effective therapy of medication-resistant bipolar disorder, Bipolar Disord 2006;**8**(3):304–6.

35. **Sienaert P, Vansteelandt K, Demyttenaere K**, and **Peuskens J**. Ultra-brief pulse ECT in bipolar and unipolar depressive disorder: differences in speed of response, Bipolar Disord 2009;**11**(4):418–24.

36. **Sikdar S, Kulhara P, Avasthi A**, and **Singh H**. Combined chlorpromazine and electroconvulsive therapy in mania, Br J Psychiatry 1994 Jun;**164**(6):806–10.

37. **Small JG, Klapper MH, Kellams JJ, Miller MJ, Milstein V, Sharpley PH**, et al. Electroconvulsive treatment compared with lithium in the management of manic states, Arch Gen Psychiatry 1988;**45**(8):727–32.

38. **Thirthalli J, Kumar CN, Bangalore RP**, and **Gangadhar BN**. Speed of response to threshold and suprathreshold bilateral ECT in depression, mania and schizophrenia, J Affect Disord 2009;**117**(1):104–7.

39. **Thirthalli J, Prasad MK**, and **Gangadhar BN**. Electroconvulsive therapy (ECT) in bipolar disorder: a narrative review of literature, *Asian Journal of Psychiatry* 2012;**5**(1):11–17.

40. **Tohen M** and **Abbott CC**. Use of electroconvulsive therapy in bipolar depression, Am J Psychiatry 2014;**172**(1):3–5.

41. **Tsao CI, Jain S, Gibson RH, Guedet PJ**, and **Lehrmann JA**. Maintenance ECT for recurrent medication-refractory mania, J ECT 2004;**20**(2):118–19.

42. **Valentí M, Benabarre A, García-Amador M, Molina O, Bernardo M**, and **Vieta E**. Electroconvulsive therapy in the treatment of mixed states in bipolar disorder, *European Psychiatry* 2008;**23**(1):53–6.

43. **van Waarde JA, van Oudheusden LJ, Heslinga OB, Verwey B, van der Mast RC**, and **Giltay E**. Patient, treatment, and anatomical predictors of outcome in electroconvulsive therapy: a prospective study, J ECT 2013 Jun;**29**(2):113–21.

44. **Versiani M, Cheniaux E**, and **Landeira-Fernandez J**. Efficacy and safety of electroconvulsive therapy in the treatment of bipolar disorder: a systematic review, J ECT 2011 Jun;**27**(2):153–64.

45. **Virit O, Ayar D, Savas HA, Yumru M**, and **Selek S**. Patients' and their relatives' attitudes toward electroconvulsive therapy in bipolar disorder, J ECT 2007 Dec;**23**(4):255–9.

46. **Virupaksha HS, Shashidhara B, Thirthalli J, Kumar CN,** and **Gangadhar BN.** Comparison of electroconvulsive therapy (ECT) with or without anti-epileptic drugs in bipolar disorder, J Affect Disord 2010;**127**(1):66–70.

47. **Volpe FM** and **Tavares AR.** Lithium plus ECT for mania in 90 cases: safety issues, J Neuropsychiatry Clin Neurosci 2012;**24**(4):E33.

48. **Yatham LN, Kennedy SH, O'Donovan C, Parikh S, MacQueen G, McIntyre R,** et al. Canadian Network for Mood and Anxiety Treatments (CANMAT) guidelines for the management of patients with bipolar disorder: consensus and controversies, Bipolar Disord 2005;**7**(Suppl):5.

49. **Yatham LN, Kennedy SH, Parikh SV, Schaffer A, Beaulieu S, Alda M,** et al. Canadian Network for Mood and Anxiety Treatments (CANMAT) and International Society for Bipolar Disorders (ISBD) collaborative update of CANMAT guidelines for the management of patients with bipolar disorder: update 2013, Bipolar Disord 2013;**15**(1):1–44.

50. **Zavorotnyy M, Diemer J, Patzelt J, Behnken A,** and **Zwanzger P.** Occurrence of ultra-rapid cycling during electroconvulsive therapy in bipolar depression, *World Journal of Biological Psychiatry* 2009;**10**(4):987–90.

Chapter 28

Neuromodulatory approaches for bipolar disorder: current evidences and future perspectives

Andre Russowsky Brunoni,
Bernardo de Sampaio Pereira Júnior,
and Izio Klein

Introduction

Several pharmacological options for the treatment of bipolar disorder (BD) have been developed over the past half-century, but treatment resistance remains a frequent and challenging clinical issue. The treatment of bipolar depression is limited to a few efficacious pharmacological agents, which may prevent some significant adverse effects, such as cognitive impairment[1] and metabolic side effects, leading to elevated rates of non-adherence and treatment discontinuation.[2] Different consensus guidelines remarkably diverge regarding first-line treatments for bipolar depression: while some recommend only lithium, lamotrigine, and quetiapine as a first-line treatments, others allow the use of antidepressant drugs, which should be used in association with mood stabilizers due to the risk of treatment-emergent (hypo)mania, and other anticonvulsants and antipsychotics. For refractory BD, the available level I evidence is very scarce, with only five studies exploring this issue hitherto.[3] Considering novel therapies, in two controlled trials, ketamine was superior to placebo but clinical effects were short-lived; in addition, ketamine is not routinely administered orally; pramipexole was barely superior to placebo in one controlled trial; and three other drug trials were not significant versus placebo.[4] This reinforces the need for novel and more efficacious treatments for refractory bipolar depression, such as brain stimulation techniques.

Neuromodulation

The first description of the use of brain stimulation approaches dates back to ancient times. In his *Compositiones medicae*, Scribonius Largus (1–50 AD), a Roman physician, described the use of the 'torpedo fish' for the treatment of headache and gout. However, the investigation of the therapeutic use of electric stimulation was only possible after the introduction of the voltaic pile in the 1800s by Alessandro Volta. After him, Giovani Aldini performed experiments using the voltaic pile to stimulate biological tissues.[5]

In the first half of the twentieth century, several forms of brain stimulation were introduced. For instance, electroconvulsive therapy (ECT) was introduced in Italy, by Ugo Cerletti, in 1938. After World War II, its use was widespread to Europe and the United States (US). However, in the last decades of the twentieth century, with the advent and dissemination of psychopharmacology, techniques on brain stimulation remained in the background of clinical practice. In 1985, Anthony Barker et al. developed a device which was able to modify brain activity by means of electromagnetic induction; transcranial magnetic stimulation (TMS) was initially developed with the purpose of being used solely as a diagnostic tool. In 1995, the first 'proof of concept' studies conducted in patients with severe depression using repetitive magnetic pulses were carried out. Despite the initial enthusiasm, concerns about the safety of this technique emerged. Thus, there were several conferences to discuss the safety of this tool, as in 1998 and 2008. In 2008, the technique has gained regulatory approval in the US for the treatment of depression, after the completion of approximately 40 clinical trials.

In the twenty-first century, the evolution of non-invasive brain stimulation has been substantial. In the last decade, there was a reappraisal of transcranial direct current stimulation (tDCS). In 2000, Nitsche and Paulus showed that tDCS was capable of altering cortical excitability and those effects were dependent on polarity—'anodal' increased motor cortex excitability, whereas 'cathodal' decreased it. In the invasive brain stimulation field, the use of vagus nerve stimulation, cortical stimulation, and deep brain stimulation have shown positive results. We hereby provide a brief overview of the techniques discussed in this chapter. ECT is discussed elsewhere (Chapter 27).

Neuromodulatory approaches

Repetitive transcranial magnetic stimulation (rTMS)

TMS uses the principle of electromagnetic induction to promote targeted changes in excitability in the brain.[6] When applied transiently, the effects last only a few minutes; however, when applied repetitively, rTMS (repetitive TMS) can modulate cortical excitability for several minutes beyond the train of stimulation.[7] There are two types of rTMS commonly used for the treatment of depressive disorders: (i) low-frequency rTMS (<1Hz) that is applied over the right dorsolateral prefrontal cortex (DLPFC) to induce a decrease in cortical excitability and (ii) high-frequency rTMS (>5Hz) that is applied on the left DLPFC to increase cortical excitability. Both approaches induce neuroplastic changes in targeted areas—in fact, it has been suggested that high-frequency rTMS is associated with long-term potentiation (LTP) and low-frequency rTMS with long-term depression (LTD).[8] Chen and colleagues[9] used a protocol (0.1 Hz for 15 minutes) similar to the one that induced LTD in cortical slice preparations to stimulate the motor cortex of volunteers, showing a decrease in motor-evoked potential that lasted for several minutes, in an LTD-like phenomenon; while a TMS/electroencephalography (EEG) study showed LTP-like changes in EEG activity after high-frequency (5Hz) rTMS.[10] However, there is an important inter-individual variability related to these effects, ie subjects might respond differently to high- compared to low-frequency rTMS according to other factors such as baseline cortical activity.[11] Thus, it has been hypothesized that high-frequency TMS acts by increasing activity in the left DLPFC area, thus ameliorating depressive symptoms. Low-frequency rTMS, on the other hand, might act by modifying interhemispheric imbalance—ie, as major depressive disorder (MDD) might be associated with an imbalance in prefrontal cortex activity, decreasing the right DLPFC activity 'releases' left DLPFC, which was being inhibited via transcallosal connections.[12] The same rationale used for unipolar depression is commonly extrapolated to bipolar depression. This theoretical framework is less clear for mania, although some researchers advocate that low frequency rTMS over the left or high frequency rTMS over the right DLPFC may be useful approaches for these cases, as we discuss as follows.

rTMS has been tested for several neurological and psychiatric conditions, but none has had the same number of studies and positive results than unipolar depression. In fact, rTMS has been approved for use in Brazil, Canada, Israel, and some European countries, and, also in the US for the treatment of unipolar depression.

Loo and colleagues[13] reviewed all published rTMS trials for side effects. They found that rTMS is a treatment virtually absent of serious side effects: in fact, only 16 patients presented seizures—most of them having prior neurological disorders or using parameters outside of recommended guidelines. In addition, they showed that rTMS does not induce cognitive impairments; and on the other hand, some studies showed that active groups presented cognitive improvement compared to sham. In addition, it has been shown that rTMS may transiently increase the auditory threshold, thus wearing earplugs is recommended. Common side effects also include headaches and facial pain due to muscular twitches that readily respond to oral analgesia. Lastly, rates of treatment-emergent (ie, during or after rTMS treatment) manic/hypomanic switches seem to be low; a meta-analysis showed that risk rates did not differ for active (0.84%) and sham (0.73%) groups.[14] However, 9 out of 13 patients who presented treatment-emergent mania/hypomania had bipolar depression.

Several variables should be considered when delivering rTMS treatment, such as site of stimulation, frequency of trains, intensity of stimulus, frequency of sessions, and duration of treatment. Regarding left versus right stimulation, accumulating evidence favours the former as more studies were performed stimulating the left DLPFC.[15] However, 1 Hz rTMS seems to be better tolerated[16] and might be an interesting approach in selected cases. Regarding the frequency of trains, most low-frequency protocols use 1 Hz or less, whereas pivotal and more recent studies have employed a frequency of 10 Hz.[17-20] Notwithstanding, the intensity of stimulus (indexed to the motor threshold—MT) may vary 80–120% MT, more recent studies have favoured intensities >100%, when compared with initial trials that used intensities <100%.[21] rTMS is usually delivered daily during weekdays (ie five sessions per week) although other studies used different protocols such as three times a week or two times per day.[22]. Finally, several studies have shown that a large number of sessions is associated with a better response.[21,23] Nevertheless, this number can range from 10 to 30 sessions (ie 2–6 weeks, as sessions are not usually delivered during weekends).

Deep repetitive transcranial magnetic stimulation (dTMS)

'Deep' TMS is a neuromodulation technique that shares, at its core, the same principles of rTMS. The difference between the two is the extent of the magnetic field applied in the patient's brain. To this end, dTMS uses various types of coils, the H-coil being the most studied one, with the most consistent evidence regarding efficacy and safety. The figure-of-eight coil used in rTMS produces a magnetic field that can reach 2.5–3 cm; while the H-coil can generate magnetic fields with a depth of up to 6 cm from the scalp.

Currently, dTMS has been tested in the management of treatment-resistant unipolar depression, auditory hallucinations, and negative symptoms in schizophrenia, and also for bipolar depression, and the H-coil was recently approved for use in clinical settings for the treatment of depressive episodes by the Food and Drug Administration (FDA).

Transcranial direct current stimulation (tDCS)

tDCS is a new therapeutic intervention that has shown fast progress in recent years and appears to be a promising technique in the treatment of various neuropsychiatric disorders. The studies involving the application of electrical currents to modulate brain responses were intensified in the 1970s, but decreased by the time that more psychopharmacological agents became available. A renewed interest in tDCS started in 2000. This technique consists of applying a continuous and direct low-intensity electrical current in the brain through electrodes placed in specified positions on the scalp. It was shown that, with the use of adequate doses, electrodes, and equipment, a significant amount of electrical current reaches neural networks, leading to neuromodulation. The most standardized protocol of this therapeutic method uses two surface electrodes—one serving as a cathode and the other as an anode. It is believed that the anode exerts an excitatory effect on the applied region, depolarizing nearby neurons, while the cathode has an inhibitory effect by hyperpolarizing neurons in this region. Therefore, the anode is typically placed over the area of the brain where an increase in neuronal activity is desired, while the cathode is positioned over the area that where the activity should be decreased; but one or the other could be placed in an extra-encephalic site, if only one effect is desired.

Currently, clinical trials have shown that the technique might be an effective treatment for MDD. Furthermore, some translational studies have demonstrated the therapeutic potential of this method; for example, in reducing nicotine craving for cigarettes, improving the cognitive performance of aged people with Alzheimer's disease, and reducing pain in patients with fibromyalgia.

Invasive brain-stimulation techniques

The two main invasive brain-stimulation techniques are deep brain stimulation (DBS) and vagus nerve stimulation (VNS). VNS was developed relatively in the 1990s and works by having an electrode attached from a pacemaker implanted on the left side of the chest to the left vagus nerve in the neck.[24,25] Although its mechanism of action remains elusive, it has been suggested that impulses from the vagus nerve are transmitted to the following regions: locus ceruleus, raphe nuclei, and nucleus tractus soliarious, which then projects to other regions of the brain, ultimately affecting the limbic system. Therefore, this may be a less focal method of electrical stimulation. In fact, the lack of focality of this technique might be associated with the limited clinical results and might favour the use of other techniques such as rTMS or DBS. In addition, it might also be used in combination with another focal method of brain stimulation. Finally, VNS is used intermittently with trains of stimulation 24 hours per day.[26,27] VNS is FDA-approved for treating chronic or refractory depression in patients not showing an adequate response after four antidepressant treatments. In a recent systematic review, Daban and colleagues[28] could only identify one randomized clinical study, the others being open-label studies and series of cases; ie, studies of lower methodological quality. In fact, the only blinded trial was inconclusive. Therefore, VNS may be seen as a new promising form of treatment; however, the current evidence supporting its use is still limited.

DBS was first developed in the 1950s and was initially used for treatment of chronic pain. When using DBS, electrodes connected to pulse generators (IPG) are implanted in specific brain areas. DBS is the most invasive therapy option for treatment-resistant depression. It was observed in preliminary studies that in these patients the subgenual region of the cingulate region (Broadmann area 25) is overactive—providing a rationale for implantation of deep brain stimulation devices with the aim of reducing this increased activity as stimulation in DBS has the goal to interrupt local activity. Mayberg et al. investigated the use of DBS in six patients with treatment-resistant depression; specifically, such patients had failed in four different medication strategies and five of six to ECT.[29] After six months of treatment, four responded to DBS and three had full or almost full remission of depressive symptoms; while two patients had to have their DBS devices removed due to persistent infections.[29] Because the data is still scarce with this condition, several questions then need to be addressed, such as: whether DBS might be the long-term solution to patients who respond to non-invasive brain stimulation or whether it will be possible to develop portable techniques of non-invasive brain stimulation. Another important question is how to localize the optimal site of stimulation—and whether neuroimaging is enough to localize such area as it may vary across patients.

To the best of our knowledge, there are no randomized clinical trials that investigated the efficacy of VNS or DBS recruiting only patients with BD.

The use of neuromodulation techniques in treatment of bipolar disorder

Depressive episodes

Although the efficacy of rTMS in the treatment of unipolar depression is supported by a consistent level of evidence,[30] its efficacy as a therapeutic tool for bipolar depression remains unclear. Most studies with rTMS in depression included mixed populations with both unipolar and bipolar depression, without reporting outcomes for these disorders in separation. Its effectiveness, so far, has been tested in a few studies that enrolled small samples. In treatment-resistant bipolar depression, patients often take complex medication regimens, with an elevated risk of troublesome adverse reactions, and a heightened risk of dangerous drug–drug interactions. Thus, a higher likelihood of treatment withdrawal is anticipated. In this context, rTMS has been investigated.

The first clinical trial of bipolar depression was conducted with 20 patients randomly assigned to placebo or active rTMS, with results favouring the active group. However, a similar study with the same design did not replicate these initial findings.[31]

Nahas et al.,[32] in other similar study with 23 patients, showed no effectiveness of the technique. The study also used scales for the assessment of mania, and no treatment-emergent affective switches were verified. Tamas et al.[33] conducted a small study with five patients diagnosed with bipolar type I who were depressed, without current use of antidepressants, but with the retention of other drugs such as lithium, risperidone, valproate, among others. The study had low methodological rigour, but demonstrated positive results after six weeks of follow-up. No treatment-emergent affective switches were observed.

A recent open study enrolled 11 participants with treatment-resistant bipolar depression. The authors found an improvement in depressive symptoms with low-frequency rTMS on the right DLPFC. The same group also reported that a sustained remission during a one-year follow-up[34] (Table 28.1).

Deep TMS

Despite some limitations (small sample sizes, concomitant use of medications, and no sham group), a study conducted by Harel et al., with 19 patients diagnosed with bipolar depression, found response and remission rates of 63.2% (12/19) and 52.6% (10/19), respectively.[35]

In a recent study with a mixed sample (ie participants with either bipolar or unipolar depression), 24 drug-resistant patients were evaluated in a 12-month follow-up period with maintenance dTMS. All the participants underwent daily dTMS sessions for four weeks and, after the first dTMS cycle, a significant reduction in Hamilton Depression Rating Scale (HDRS) scores was observed in all participants. This study indicates that maintenance treatment with dTMS for bipolar patients may be a useful therapeutic alternative.[36]

tDCS

The use of tDCS in bipolar depression was not sufficiently investigated, with a single open-label study comparing the efficacy of tDCS in patients with unipolar depression versus patients with bipolar depression. Overall, tDCS was equally effective for both conditions. Another open study evaluated a sample of unipolar and bipolar patients for three months. However, this trial did not report results for participants with bipolar depression separately.[37]

There are four stand-alone case reports in the literature[38–41] and some reports in randomized clinical trials of induction of mania or hypomania following treatment with tDCS. Most of these episodes resolved spontaneously, with tDCS withheld for

Table 28.1 The efficacy of rTMS in the treatment of depressive episodes in bipolar disorder

Authors	N	Study design	Stimulation site	Frequency	Stimulation parameters	Results	Comments
Dolberg et al., 2002	20	RCT	N/A	N/A	N/A	Real rTMS significantly superior to sham rTMS	Low methodological rigour
Nahas et al., 2003	23	RCT	Left DLPFC	5 Hz	110% of MT, 1,600 stimuli/day, for 10 days	No effectiveness of the technique	Low number of total stimuli
Tamas et al., 2007	5	Open-label	Right DLPFC	1 Hz	95% of MT, 100 stimuli/day, for 8 days	Positive results after six weeks of follow-up	Low methodological rigour
Dell'Osso et al., 2009	11	Open-label	Right DLPFC	1 Hz	110% of MT, 300 stimuli/day, for 15 days	HAM-D score reduction of ≥50% compared to baseline (p < 0.0001)	Patients with treatment-resistant bipolar depression

N: number of patients; ND: not described in the paper; RCT: randomized control trial; DLPFC: dorsolateral prefrontal cortex; MT: motor threshold; HAM-D: Hamilton Depression Rating Scale a few days, or with small dose adjustments/introduction of a new antimanic drug, although one of these cases was a full-blown manic episode with psychotic features.[41]

It is difficult to estimate the precise frequency of this adverse effect or, even, if it is a direct consequence tDCS or if these case reports rather represent a consequence of the natural course of the underlying BD. In addition, data other brain stimulation therapies indicate that having a diagnosis of BD place a patient with a higher risk of manic/hypomanic switches after tDCS. Therefore, the same recommendations of care for patients with unipolar depression may be extrapolated when using tDCS as an antidepressant treatment—ie, careful observation of the patients' clinical outcomes throughout treatment. Furthermore, patients should be carefully assessed for history of (hypo)manic episodes and history of switching into mania with past antidepressant treatments, as these factors may point to a higher risk of manic switches with tDCS. In these patients, concurrent treatment with mood-stabilizer medications during the tDCS treatment course should be considered.

Finally, Pereira-Junior et al. conducted a pilot, double-blind, study in which five patients with bipolar depression received active tDCS. The response and remission rates were 40% (two patients) and 20% (one patient), respectively. The average rate of improvement was 30%, similar to most tDCS studies in unipolar depression. The small number of patients and the lack of a sham control were significant limitations.[42]

Manic episodes

TMS

Five clinical trials using rTMS have been published hitherto. All these studies have in common their enrolment of small sample sizes and the concomitant use of mood stabilizers among participants. Still, most studies have been open, with only two randomized and sham-controlled designs. Therefore, the studies conducted so far have low methodological quality and were essentially exploratory.

The first study was conducted in 1998 by Grisaru et al. In this study, 'partially' double-blinded (the study had an initial stage which was not blinded) using 20 Hz (2 s-long sequences, 20 sequences per day, for ten consecutive days), 16 manic patients were randomized to receive stimulation on the right or the left prefrontal cortices, and 'right stimulation' was more effective in lowering manic symptoms (although stimulation was also effective to the left).[43] A few years later, the same group performed a randomized, double-blind, sham-controlled trial, for patients with mania.[44] The results showed no difference between active and sham groups.

In 2004, two open studies using high-frequency stimulation in the right prefrontal cortex in patients with mania were reported in the literature, with favourable outcomes for this type of intervention. Saba et al. has carried out fast rTMS (five trains of 15 s, 80% of the motor threshold, 10 Hz) over the right DLPFC. They were evaluated using the Mania Assessment Scale (MAS) and the Clinical Global Impression (CGI) scale at baseline and at day 14, with a significant improvement at endpoint.[45] Michael et al. enrolled nine patients in a pharmacological add-on and open-label trial. The treatment lasted four weeks and a sustained reduction in Bech-Rafaelsen Mania Rating Scale (BRMAS) scale scores, which was observed in all patients.[46]

Table 28.2 The efficacy of rTMS in the treatment of manic episodes in bipolar disorder

Authors	N	Study design	Stimulation site	Frequency	Stimulation parameters	Results	Comments
Grisaru et al., 1998	16	'Partially' double-blinded	Right and left DLPFC (randomized)	20 Hz	80% of MT, 800 stimuli/day, for 10 days	Stimulation of right DLPFC was more effective than left	Study had an initial stage not blinded, small sample size and the concomitant use of mood stabilizers
Kaptsan et al., 2003	25	RCT	Right DLPFC	20 Hz	80% of MT, 800 stimuli/day, for 10 days	No effectiveness of the technique	Study used circular coil, and the concomitant use of mood stabilizers
Saba et al., 2004	8	Open-label	Right DLPFC	10 Hz	80% of MT, 750 stimuli/day, for 10 days	All patients except one showed clinical improvement	Small sample size
Michael et al., 2004	9	Open-label	Right DLPFC	20 Hz	80% of MT, 800 stimuli/day, for 16 days	Sustained reduction of manic symptoms was observed in all patients	Small sample size
Praharaj et al., 2009	41	RCT	Right DLPFC	20 Hz	110% of MT, 800 Stimuli/day, for 10 days	Reduction of manic symptoms in 72% in the active group (in CGI-S, p = 0.016)	concomitant use of mood stabilizers

N: number of patients; RCT: randomized control trial; DLPFC: dorsolateral prefrontal cortex; MT: motor threshold; CGI-S: Clinical Global Impression Scale

In 2009, Praharaj et al., in a randomized, placebo-controlled, double-blind trial, studied the efficacy of rTMS at high frequency (20 Hz, 110% of motor threshold, 20 sequences, 10 s between sequences) in the right DLPFC in 41 manic patients. There was a reduction of manic symptoms in 72% in the active stimulation group versus 43% in the control group, which was statistically significant[47] (see Table 28.2).

tDCS

tDCS has been reported as a possible trigger of mania when used in bipolar patients.[40,48] However, the administration of this technique in combination with effective treatments for bipolar mania may be safe, as reported in Schestatsky et al.[49] In this case report, five sessions of anodal tDCS were applied over the right DLPFC in a patient with an acute manic episode. There was improvement in agitation and manic symptoms, respectively measured by Nursing Observational Scale for In-patient Evaluation (NOISE) and Young Mania Rating Scale (YOUNG) scales.

Concluding remarks

Neuromodulatory approaches may play an increasing role in the treatment of BD. These approaches may improve adherence to treatment due to the relatively low rates of adverse effects presented by those methods. In addition, these strategies carry a lower risk of possible drug interactions. This is an area of increasing research interest. Nevertheless, evidence remains limited, and thus these methods should not be formally recommended for the routine care of BD.[50] Therefore, the field awaits the conduction of well-designed and adequately powered randomized controlled trials.

References

1. **Henin A, Mick E, Biederman J**, et al. Is psychopharmacologic treatment associated with neuropsychological deficits in bipolar youth?, J Clin Psychiatry 2009;**70**:1178–85.

2. **Velligan DI, Weiden PJ, Sajatovic M**, et al. The expert consensus guideline series: adherence problems in patients with serious and persistent mental illness, J Clin Psychiatry 2009;**70**(Suppl 4):1–46; quiz 7–8.

3. **Tondo L, Vazquez GH**, and **Baldessarini RJ**. Options for pharmacological treatment of refractory bipolar depression, Curr Psychiatry Rep 2014;**16**:431.

4. **Sienaert P, Lambrichts L, Dols A**, and **De Fruyt J**. Evidence-based treatment strategies for treatment-resistant bipolar depression: a systematic review, Bipolar Disord 2013;**15**:61–9.

5. **Zago S, Ferrucci R, Fregni F**, and **Priori A**. Bartholow, Sciamanna, Alberti: pioneers in the electrical stimulation of the exposed human cerebral cortex, *Neuroscientist* 2008;**14**:521–8.

6. **Fregni F** and **Pascual-Leone A**. Technology insight: noninvasive brain stimulation in neurology-perspectives on the therapeutic potential of rTMS and tDCS, Nat Clin Pract Neurol 2007;**3**:383–93.

7. **Pascual-Leone A, Tarazona F, Keenan J, Tormos JM, Hamilton R**, and **Catala MD**. Transcranial magnetic stimulation and neuroplasticity, *Neuropsychologia* 1999;**37**:207–17.

8. **Ilic TV** and **Ziemann U**. Exploring motor cortical plasticity using transcranial magnetic stimulation in humans, Ann NY Acad Sci 2005;**1048**:175–84.

9. **Chen R, Classen J, Gerloff C**, et al. Depression of motor cortex excitability by low-frequency transcranial magnetic stimulation, *Neurology* 1997;**48**:1398–1403.

10. **Esser SK, Huber R, Massimini M, Peterson MJ, Ferrarelli F**, and **Tononi G**. A direct demonstration of cortical LTP in humans: a combined TMS/EEG study, Brain Res Bull 2006;**69**:86–94.

11. **Fregni F, Boggio PS, Valle AC**, et al. Homeostatic effects of plasma valproate levels on corticospinal excitability changes induced by 1 Hz rTMS in patients with juvenile myoclonic epilepsy, Clin Neurophysiol 2006;**117**:1217–27.

12. **Steele JD, Currie J, Lawrie SM**, and **Reid I**. Prefrontal cortical functional abnormality in major depressive disorder: a stereotactic meta-analysis, J Affect Disord 2007;**101**:1–11.

13. **Loo CK, McFarquhar TF**, and **Mitchell PB**. A review of the safety of repetitive transcranial magnetic stimulation as a clinical treatment for depression, Int J Neuropsychopharmacol 2008;**11**:131–47.

14. **Xia G, Gajwani P, Muzina DJ**, et al. Treatment-emergent mania in unipolar and bipolar depression: focus on repetitive transcranial magnetic stimulation, Int J Neuropsychopharmacol 2008;**11**:119–30.

15. **Schutter DJ**. Antidepressant efficacy of high-frequency transcranial magnetic stimulation over the left dorsolateral prefrontal cortex in double-blind sham-controlled designs: a meta-analysis, Psychol Med 2009;**39**:65–75.

16. **Wassermann EM**. Risk and safety of repetitive transcranial magnetic stimulation: report and suggested guidelines from the International Workshop on the Safety of Repetitive Transcranial Magnetic Stimulation, 5–7 June 1996, Electroencephalogr Clin Neurophysiol 1998;**108**:1–16.

17. **O'Reardon JP, Cristancho P, Pilania P, Bapatla KB, Chuai S**, and **Peshek AD**. Patients with a major depressive episode responding to treatment with repetitive transcranial magnetic stimulation (rTMS) are resistant to the effects of rapid tryptophan depletion, Depress Anxiety 2007;**24**:537–44.

18. **Mogg A, Pluck G, Eranti SV**, et al. A randomized controlled trial with 4-month follow-up of adjunctive repetitive transcranial magnetic stimulation of the left prefrontal cortex for depression, Psychol Med 2008;**38**:323–33.

19. **Loo CK, Mitchell PB, McFarquhar TF, Malhi GS**, and **Sachdev PS**. A sham-controlled trial of the efficacy and safety of twice-daily rTMS in major depression, Psychol Med 2007;**37**:341–9.

20. **Herwig U, Fallgatter AJ, Hoppner J**, et al. Antidepressant effects of augmentative transcranial magnetic stimulation: randomised multicentre trial, Br J Psychiatry 2007;**191**:441–8.

21. **Schutter DJ**. Antidepressant efficacy of high-frequency transcranial magnetic stimulation over the left dorsolateral prefrontal cortex in double-blind sham-controlled designs: a meta-analysis, Psychol Med 2008:1–11.

22. **Brunoni A** and **Fregni F**. Improving the design of non-invasive brain stimulation trials, in press.

23. **Lisanby SH, Husain MM, Rosenquist PB**, et al. Daily left prefrontal repetitive transcranial magnetic stimulation in the acute treatment of major depression: clinical predictors of outcome in a multisite, randomized controlled clinical trial, *Neuropsychopharmacology* 2009;**34**:522–34.

24. **Lamberg L**. Interest surging in electroconvulsive and other brain stimulation therapies, JAMA 2007;**298**:1147–9.

25. Approval Letter: VNS therapy system—P970003s050. Food and Drug Administration, 2005. Available at http://www.fda.gov/cdrh/PDF/p970003s050a.pdf.

26. **Dumitriu D CK, Alterman R**, and **Mathew S**. Neurostimulatory therapeutics in management of treatment-resistant depression with focus on deep brain stimulation, Mount Sinai J of Med 2008;**75**:263–75.

27. **Marangell LB MM, Jurdi RA**, and **Zboyan H**. Neurostimulation therapies in depression: a review of new modalities, Acta Psychiatr Scand 2007;**116**:174–81.

28. **Daban C, Martinez-Aran A, Cruz N**, and **Vieta E**. Safety and efficacy of vagus nerve stimulation in treatment-resistant depression. A systematic review, J Affect Disord 2008;**110**:1–15.

29. **Mayberg HS LA, Voon V**, et al. Deep brain stimulation for treatment-resistant depression, Neuron 2005;**45**:651–60.

30. **Lefaucheur JP, Andre-Obadia N, Antal A**, et al. Evidence-based guidelines on the therapeutic use of repetitive transcranial magnetic stimulation (rTMS), Clin Neurophysiol 2014;**125**:2150–206.

31. **Dolberg OT, Dannon PN, Schreiber S**, and **Grunhaus L**. Transcranial magnetic stimulation in patients with bipolar depression: a double blind, controlled study, Bipolar Disord 2002;**4**(Suppl 1):94–5.

32. **Nahas Z, Kozel FA, Li X, Anderson B**, and **George MS**. Left prefrontal transcranial magnetic stimulation (TMS) treatment of depression in bipolar affective disorder: a pilot study of acute safety and efficacy, Bipolar Disord 2003;**5**:40–7.

33. **Tamas RL, Menkes D**, and **El-Mallakh RS**. Stimulating research: a prospective, randomized, double-blind, sham-controlled study of slow transcranial magnetic stimulation in depressed bipolar patients, J Neuropsychiatry Clin Neurosci 2007;**19**:198–9.

34. **Dell'Osso B, Mundo E, D'Urso N**, et al. Augmentative repetitive navigated transcranial magnetic stimulation (rTMS) in drug-resistant bipolar depression, Bipolar Disord 2009;**11**:76–81.

35. **Harel EV, Rabany L, Deutsch L, Bloch Y, Zangen A**, and **Levkovitz Y**. H-coil repetitive transcranial magnetic stimulation for treatment resistant major depressive disorder: an 18-week continuation safety and feasibility study, *The World Journal of Biological Psychiatry: the Official Journal of the World Federation of Societies of Biological Psychiatry* 2012.

36. **Rapinesi C, Bersani FS, Kotzalidis GD**, et al. Maintenance deep transcranial magnetic stimulation sessions are associated with reduced depressive relapses in patients with unipolar or bipolar depression, Front Neurol 2015;**6**:16.

37. **Dell'osso B, Zanoni S, Ferrucci R**, et al. Transcranial direct current stimulation for the outpatient treatment of poor-responder depressed patients, *European Psychiatry: the Journal of the Association of European Psychiatrists* 2012;**27**:513–17.

38. **Arul-Anandam AP, Loo C**, and **Mitchell P**. Induction of hypomanic episode with transcranial direct current stimulation, J ECT 2010;**26**:68–9.

39. **Baccaro A, Brunoni AR, Bensenor IM**, and **Fregni F**. Hypomanic episode in unipolar depression during transcranial direct current stimulation, Acta Neuropsychiatrica 2010;**22**:316–18.

40. Galvez V, Alonzo A, Martin D, Mitchell PB, Sachdev P, and Loo CK. Hypomania induction in a patient with bipolar II disorder by transcranial direct current stimulation (tDCS), J ECT 2011;**27**:256–8.

41. Brunoni AR, Valiengo L, Zanao T, de Oliveira JF, Bensenor IM, and Fregni F. Manic psychosis after sertraline and transcranial direct-current stimulation, *The Journal of Neuropsychiatry and Clinical Neurosciences* 2011;**23**:E4–5.

42. Pereira Junior Bde S, Tortella G, Lafer B, et al. The bipolar depression electrical treatment trial (BETTER): design, rationale, and objectives of a randomized, sham-controlled trial and data from the pilot study phase, Neural Plast 2015;**2015**:684025.

43. Grisaru N, Chudakov B, Yaroslavsky Y, and Belmaker RH. Transcranial magnetic stimulation in mania: a controlled stud, Am J Psychiatry 1998;**155**:1608–10.

44. Kaptsan A, Yaroslavsky Y, Applebaum J, Belmaker RH, and Grisaru N. Right prefrontal TMS versus sham treatment of mania: a controlled study, Bipolar Disord 2003;**5**:36–9.

45. Saba G, Rocamora JF, Kalalou K, et al. Repetitive transcranial magnetic stimulation as an add-on therapy in the treatment of mania: a case series of eight patients, Psychiatry Res 2004;**128**:199–202.

46. Michael N and Erfurth A. Treatment of bipolar mania with right prefrontal rapid transcranial magnetic stimulation, J Affect Disord 2004;**78**:253–7.

47. Praharaj SK, Ram D, and Arora M. Efficacy of high frequency (rapid) suprathreshold repetitive transcranial magnetic stimulation of right prefrontal cortex in bipolar mania: a randomized sham controlled study, J Affect Disord 2009;**117**:146–50.

48. Loo CK, Alonzo A, Martin D, Mitchell PB, Galvez V, and Sachdev P. Transcranial direct current stimulation for depression: 3-week, randomised, sham-controlled trial, Br J Psychiatry 2012;**200**:52–9.

49. Schestatsky P, Janovik N, Lobato MI, et al. Rapid therapeutic response to anodal tDCS of right dorsolateral prefrontal cortex in acute mania, Brain Stimul 2013;**6**:701–3.

50. Holtzheimer PE, 3rd, Kosel M, and Schlaepfer T. Brain stimulation therapies for neuropsychiatric disease, Handb Clin Neurol 2012;**106**:681–95.

Chapter 29

The role of complementary and alternative therapies for the management of bipolar disorder

Arun V. Ravindran and Tricia L. da Silva

Introduction

Despite many advances in pharmacological and psychological treatments for bipolar disorder (BD), a significant proportion of patients do not achieve remission with treatment, and many experience intolerable adverse events that interfere with drug compliance.[1] Perhaps as a result of these limitations, many patients are turning to complementary and alternative medicine (CAM) therapies. CAM therapies are defined as a group of diverse medical and health systems, practices and products that are not currently considered to be part of conventional medicine.[2,3] These therapies—which include herbal remedies, nutraceuticals, physical therapies, as well as mindfulness-based practices—have gained a marked increase in popularity over the years.[4] Studies have shown that about 50% of patients with various chronic conditions in both developed and non-developed countries use CAM therapies, and approximately 40% of BD patients reportedly use some form of alternative treatment.[4,5]

CAM therapies are often perceived by users to be as effective as conventional pharmacotherapy, but better tolerated and safer.[1,2] Being in control of the treatment and not requiring a physician's prescription add to the perceived benefits. However, careful evaluation of the risks and benefits of the available forms of CAM therapies is relatively limited in BD.[2] This chapter will attempt to provide an evidence-based review of the safety and efficacy of commonly used CAM therapies in BD.

CAM therapies used in bipolar disorder

Physical therapies

Physical therapies encompass physical practices such as aerobic exercise and yoga, and biological treatments such as chronotherapeutics and acupuncture. While popular culture perceives most physical therapies as aids to improve physical fitness and relieve stress, some (eg light therapy) are proven to benefit mood.[1] Evidence on the benefits of exercise, acupuncture and chronotherapies in BD are discussed as follows and summarized in Table 29.1.

Exercise

Studies have shown that physical exercise improves mood and anxiety in normal populations.[6] It has also been recommended as a useful and well-tolerated intervention in major depressive disorder (MDD).[3,6,7] The mechanisms mediating the benefit of exercise on mood are not fully understood but, in general, it is believed to modulate synaptic connections and signalling pathways, improving the efficiency, plasticity, and adaptability of the brain.[6]

The benefit of exercise specifically for BD has not been well studied. One small randomized controlled trial (RCT) found significant improvements in depression in medicated patients with both unipolar and bipolar illness assigned to a walking programme[6] and similar positive results were reported in unipolar and bipolar depression in an open trial of aerobic training as add-on to psychotropics.[7] However, a retrospective study reported a modest decrease in depression and anxiety symptoms but no change in clinical condition among medicated BD participants compared to non-participants.[8] Nonetheless, it should be reiterated that several large meta-analyses confirm the benefits of exercise for unipolar depression, and it is also recommended by several guidelines.[3] The significant overlap of symptoms and aetiological factors between the two subtypes and the high likelihood of the inclusion of depressive patients with 'hidden' or undiagnosed bipolarity in unipolar depression studies[9] would suggest that many bipolar patients are likely to benefit from exercise during the depressive and recovery phases.

With medical clearance and supervision when appropriate, exercise is generally thought of as a healthy and beneficial practice with no significant negative effects. However, plasma lithium levels can be affected by exercise and should be monitored carefully in bipolar patients.[10]

In conclusion, while the evidence for the benefit of exercise as add-on to pharmacotherapy in bipolar depression remains preliminary, its confirmed benefit in unipolar depression would support its use in BD and would recommend more systematic evaluations in the future.

Acupuncture

Acupuncture is a traditional Chinese medicine practice in which fine needles are inserted into the skin at specific body points (acupoints) to produce therapeutic benefits in a variety of medical conditions, including pain disorders.[1,11] Although the mechanisms mediating the benefit of acupuncture are not fully elucidated, increased turnover of endorphins and monoaminergic neurotransmitters such as serotonin and norepinephrine has been proposed.[11]

While a significant number of RCTs, systematic reviews, and meta-analyses on the efficacy of acupuncture in unipolar depression have been conducted, these studies have yielded contradictory results.[1] The mixed findings have been at least partly

Table 29.1 Evidence for physical therapies for bipolar disorder

Study	Type	Sample size	Duration	Agent	Comparator	Co-medications	Efficacy results[†]
Exercise							
Dimeo et al., 2001	Open trial	n = 7 (UD = 7; BD = 5)	10 days	Aerobic training programme	None	Ongoing treatment with psychotropics	Significant improvement in depression with aerobic training in the total sample (p = 0.006)
Knubben et al., 2006	RCT	n = 38 (UD = 21; BD = 7)	10 days	Walking (n = 20)	Low-intensity stretching and relaxation (n = 18)	Ongoing treatment with lithium and/or antidepressants, or no treatment*.	Significant better improvement in depression with exercise in the total sample (p = 0.01).
Ng et al., 2007	Retrospective cohort study	n = 98	24 months	Voluntary walking group (n = 24)	Non-participants (n = 74)	Not specified.	Significantly better improvement in depression in walking group (p = 0.005).
Acupuncture							
Dennehy et al., 2009	RCT	Hypomania patients (n = 20), depressed patients (n = 26)	Hypomania group, 12 weeks depression group, 8 weeks	Targeted acupuncture (hypomania patients, n = 10) (depressed patients, n = 13)	Sham acupuncture (hypomania patients, n = 10) (depressed patients, n = 13)	Ongoing treatment with lithium, anticonvulsants, antidepressants, antipsychotics and/or benzodiazepines.	No group differences; both groups showed similar improvement in depression and mania.

Study	Design	n	Intervention	Comparator	Concomitant treatment	Outcome
Hu, 1996	Case report	n = 1	Acupuncture	None	Ongoing treatment with psychotropics	Significant improvement in mania with acupuncture. No p-value reported.
Kurland, 1976	Case series	n = 3 (BD = 2, schizophrenia = 1)	Acupuncture	ECT	Ongoing treatment with psychotropics	Significantly better improvement in depression with ECT, but acupuncture better tolerated. No p-values reported.
Total Sleep Deprivation (TSD)						
Benedetti et al., 2001a	RCT	n = 28	TSD + amineptine (n = 14)	TSD + placebo (n = 14)	None	No group differences; both groups showed similar improvements in depression.
Benedetti et al., 2001b	Open trial	n = 30	TSD + SPA	Pre-treatment condition	Ongoing treatment with lithium or no treatment*	Significant improvement in depression with TSD + SPA when combined with lithium (p = 0.04). No improvement in unmedicated patients.

(continued)

Table 29.1 Continued

Study	Type	Sample size	Duration	Agent	Comparator	Co-medications	Efficacy results[†]
Benedetti et al., 2005	Open trial	n = 60	3 cycles[a]	TSD + BLT	Pre-treatment condition	Ongoing treatment with lithium and/or antidepressants, or no treatment*.	Significant improvement in depression with TSD + BLT (p = 0.0138).
Benedetti et al., 2007	Open trial	n = 39	3 cycles[a]	TSD + BLT	Pre-treatment condition	Ongoing treatment with mood stabilizers and antidepressants, or no treatment*.	Significant improvement in depression with TSD + BLT (p<0.001)
Benedetti et al., 2009	Open trial	n = 19	3 cycles[a]	TSD + BLT	Pre-treatment condition	Ongoing treatment with lithium.	Significant improvement with TSD + BLT (p<0.00001)
Benedetti et al., 2014	Open trial	n = 141	3 cycles[a]	TSD + BLT	Pre-treatment condition	Ongoing treatment with lithium.	Significant improvement in depression with TSD + BLT (p<00001).
Colombo et al., 2000	RCT	n = 115	3 cycles[a]	TSD + BLT (2,500 lux) (n = 42)	TSD + dim light (150 lux) (n = 38) OR TSD + ambient light (80 lux) (n = 35)	Ongoing treatment with lithium or no treatment*.	Significantly better improvement in depression with TSD + BLT (p = 0.015)

Study	Design	n	Duration	Treatment	Pre-treatment condition	Adjunctive treatment	Results
Wu et al., 2009	RCT	n = 49	4 days (1 night of TSD followed by 3 days of BLT and SPA)	TST + BLT + SPA	Pre-treatment condition	Ongoing treatment with antidepressants and/or mood stabilizers.	Significant improvement in depression with TSD + BLT + SPA (p = 0.02).

Bright Light Therapy (BLT)

Study	Design	n	Duration	Treatment	Pre-treatment condition	Adjunctive treatment	Results
Dauphinais et al., 2012	RCT	n = 38	8 weeks	BLT (7,000 lux) (n = 18)	Negative air ions (n = 20)	Ongoing treatment with mood stabilizers.	No group differences; no change in depression or mania in either group.
Krauss et al., 1991	Open trial	Bipolar depressed patients (n = 6), healthy controls (n = 7)	3 weeks of sequential treatment	BLT (2,500 lux) from 6–8AM and from 6–8PM for 2 weeks (all patients and controls, n = 13)	Dim light (300 lux) for 1 week (all patients and controls, n = 13)	None	Significantly better improvement in depression with BLT (p<0.05).
Leibenluft et al, 1995	Case series	n = 9	13 weeks	BLT (10,000 lux) for 1 hour in the morning (n = 5), midday (n = 5), or evening (n = 3)	Pre-treatment condition	Ongoing treatment with lithium, antipsychotics, mood stabilizers and/or anxiolytics.	20% decrease in days hypomanic and/or depressed in 3 subjects in the midday BLT group. No p-values reported.
Papatheodorou & Kutcher, 1993	Case series	n = 7	1 week	BLT (10,000 lux) for 45–60 minutes 7–9AM and 7–9PM	Pre-treatment condition	Ongoing treatment with lithium, antipsychotics and/or mood stabilizers.	Significant improvement in depression with BLT (p<0.005).

(continued)

Table 29.1 Continued

Study	Type	Sample size	Duration	Agent	Comparator	Co-medications	Efficacy results[†]
Sit et al., 2007	Case series	n = 9	4 weeks of sequential treatment	BLT (7,000 lux) for 15–45 minutes in the morning (n = 4) or midday (n = 5) for 2 weeks (all subjects, n = 9)	Red light (50 lux) for 2 weeks (all subjects, n = 9)	Ongoing treatment with lithium, antipsychotics and/or anxiolytics.	Improvement in depression and/or mania in one woman in the morning BLT group and four women in the midday BLT group. No p-values reported.
Dark Therapy							
Barbini et al., 2005	Open trial	n = 32	3 days	Dark therapy (14 hrs/day)	Pre-treatment condition	Ongoing treatment with mood stabilizers and lithium.	Significant decrease in mania with dark therapy (p<0.00001).
Henriksen et al., 2014	Case study	n = 1	6 days	Blue-light blocking lenses	Clear-lensed glasses	Ongoing treatment with lithium and anti-delirium treatment.	Rapid and sustained decline in mania with blue-light blocking lenses . No p-values reported.

Study	Type	n	Duration	Intervention	Comparison	Ongoing treatment	Results
Wehr et al., 1998	Case study	n = 1	21 months	Bed rest in the dark (10–14 hrs/day)	Pre-treatment condition	Ongoing treatment with antidepressants and mood stabilizers.	Stabilization of sleep and mood observed after 3 months of dark rest. No p-values reported.
Wirz-Justice et al., 1999	Case study	n = 1	3 months	Bed rest in the dark (10–14 hrs/day) + BLT added after 4 weeks of dark therapy	Pre-treatment condition	Ongoing treatment with valproate.	Immediate cessation of rapid cycling upon initiation of dark rest, and gradual improvements in depression after addition of BLT. No p-values reported.

Abbreviations: BD = bipolar disorder; BLT = bright light therapy; SPA = sleep phase advance; TSD = total sleep deprivation; RCT = randomized controlled trial; UD = unipolar depression

† Significant, p≤0.05

* If patients were not already taking psychotropic medications, they were not administered any pharmacological treatment for the study

ª One cycle of sleep deprivation = one night of sleep deprivation followed by one recovery night attributed to the difficulty in 'masking' the placebo condition, with the result that even 'sham' treatments have been postulated to produce benefits.

There are no large RCTs or meta-analyses published on the use of acupuncture for BD. An early case series found ECT more effective than acupuncture as augmentation to psychotropics for bipolar depression, but acupuncture was better tolerated.[12] A later case report found acupuncture add-on effective for treating mania.[13] A more recent small RCT in bipolar depression found that both targeted acupuncture (ie acupoints specific to symptoms) and sham acupuncture (ie acupoints off the acupuncture meridian), as add-on to pharmacotherapy, improved mood.[11]

Acupuncture is usually well tolerated, with mostly mild adverse events reported.[1] These include bleeding, pain, and bruising at needling points, as well as non-specific drowsiness, fatigue, and headache.[14] Very rarely, more serious adverse events such as seizures, pneumothorax, and temporary neuropathy have been noted.[14]

Thus, there is currently little evidence for the benefit of acupuncture in bipolar depression. However, this conclusion is based on a review of English-language literature only, and it is likely that a larger publication base may exist in Chinese languages, which may provide more definitive findings.

Chronotherapeutics

Chronotherapy is the use of interventions, such as modulation of sleep–wake cycles and exposure to environmental light and darkness, to favourably influence illnesses whose symptoms include altered circadian rhythms.[15] The rationale for using chronotherapeutics in BD is that patients with BD or those at high risk of developing BD have abnormal sleep patterns and circadian rhythm disturbances.[16] The three main forms evaluated in BD include total sleep deprivation, bright light therapy, and dark therapy.

Total sleep deprivation

Total sleep deprivation (TSD), as the name implies, is an intervention in which subjects are deprived of sleep for variable lengths of time, usually for 36 hours, by extending the daytime wake through the night and until the evening of the day after.[17] A TSD cycle consists of one night of TSD followed by a night of recovery sleep. A substantial body of literature confirms that sleep deprivation leads to significant reduction of depressive symptoms, even comparable to that observed with antidepressant medications.[3,17]

The antidepressant effects of sleep deprivation are believed to involve a number of mechanisms, including potentiation of serotonergic, noradrenergic and dopaminergic signalling; increases in thyroid hormones; functional and metabolic changes in the ventral/anterior cingulate cortex and medial prefrontal cortex; and increased fronto-limbic connectivity.[1,17]

While the literature on the benefit of sleep deprivation is more extensive in treatment-resistant unipolar depression, a number of RCTs and open trials in bipolar depression confirm the immediate benefit of TSD, either alone or most often in combination with mood stabilizing medications.[18-20] However, one major drawback is the occurrence of rebound depression, in particular when TSD is used alone.[20]

To counter this phenomenon, many studies have attempted to use TSD with other interventions to maintain the benefit. In BD, studies have shown that antidepressant effects achieved with TSD can be enhanced and/or sustained when it is used in combination with medications and/or non-pharmacological interventions, such as sleep phase advance (SPA) or bright light therapy (BLT).[19-21] Of note, the combination of TSD and BLT has been noted to produce immediate and effective alleviation of depressive and suicidal symptoms in subjects with bipolar depression resistant to medications.[22,23]

Adverse events associated with TSD therapy include excessive daytime sleepiness, fatigue, deficits in cognitive function, and switch from depression to hypomania/mania (though such switches are reported to be relatively uncommon).[17] Of note, the rate of switch from depression to hypomania/mania with TSD is similar to rates reported with conventional antidepressants or placebo.[24]

Thus, TSD has good evidence for benefit in bipolar depression, either as monotherapy or in combination with medications and/or light therapy. The challenge of sustaining its benefit and the practical considerations of application outside a hospital setting limit its wider use.

Bright light therapy

BLT is a procedure in which subjects are exposed to an artificial source of bright light.[25] BLT has been shown to be very effective in the treatment of seasonal affective disorder (SAD), where it is recommended as the first-line intervention.[3] Several RCTs also support its efficacy as an augmentation to antidepressants in unipolar depression.[1,3]

BLT is proposed to exert its therapeutic effect through modulation of the suprachiasmatic nuclei (SCN) to influence the neurophysiological and biochemical processes governed by the SCN.[26] These include favourable circadian cycle phase shifts, increase in daytime serum serotonin, and suppression of daytime melatonin secretion, among others.[26]

The significant overlap of symptoms between SAD and bipolar depression, including the common presence of reversed neurovegetative symptoms, such as increased appetite, weight gain, and hypersomnia, as well as fatigue, has led to the speculation that BLT may benefit bipolar depression.[27] However, the benefits of BLT have not been well evaluated in BD. The published literature consists mostly of small open trials and case series which report that, in comparison to dim light, daily exposure to a bright light at high intensities results in further attenuation of depressive symptoms in BD patients already on a stable medication regimen.[28-30] In contrast, an RCT with medicated BD patients found no difference between BLT or placebo as add-on treatment and the results were attributed to a high placebo response.[25]

Adverse events associated with BLT are few, mostly benign, and short-term, and include nausea, headache, eyestrain, irritability, and fatigue.[28-30] However, some reports document precipitation of hypomania,[31,32] and there is some indication that the likelihood of such occurrences increases when BLT is used in the morning or evening.[28,30]

In conclusion, currently there is insufficient evidence to recommend BLT for bipolar depression. However, given its benefits in MDD, more research in BD may be of clinical value.

Dark therapy

In dark therapy, patients are deprived of light for a number of hours, usually by lengthening patients' bedtime to approximately 14 hours and, thus, it could be conceived as being the opposite of sleep deprivation.[33] It is hypothesized that creating an environment in which exposure to light is shortened and bedtime is extended may promote sleep and synchronization of sleep–wake cycles with the day–night cycles, and subsequently, stabilize mood in BD patients in the hypomanic/manic phase.[34]

The very preliminary evidence supporting the benefit of dark therapy in mania comes from two early case reports[34,35] and one small open trial,[36] but has not been further substantiated. It is of note that in all three reports, dark therapy was used as an add-on to mood stabilizers and antipsychotic medications.

More recently, one case report has noted benefits with the use of amber-tinted glasses as add-on to pharmacotherapy in the management of mania.[37] Such glasses are purported to create a 'virtual darkness' by blocking blue wavelengths of light, to which retinal photoreceptors involved in light entrainment of the SCN are sensitive.[33] Since these blue-light blocking glasses reduce light exposure without enforcing complete darkness, they may represent a more pragmatic delivery of dark therapy.[33,37]

No significant adverse events were reported for dark therapy or blue-light blocking lenses in the literature. However, blue-light blocking lenses may trigger phase-advance and worsen seasonal depression.[33] Moreover, given that exposure to blue wavelengths of light is thought to improve cognitive performance, blocking them may, at least in theory, impair cognition.[33]

Thus, dark therapy and blue-light blocking lenses remain experimental interventions for mania that need significant evaluation before use.

Nutraceuticals

Nutraceuticals (also known as dietary supplements) are concentrated forms of naturally occurring substances, such as vitamins and minerals. They are categorized as natural health products that can be used without a prescription, and they are popularly used for nutritional and health support, both individually and in combination with standard pharmaceutical medications.[1] Reports on the efficacy of common nutraceuticals used as complementary therapies in BD, such as omega-3 fatty acids, folate, inositol, magnesium, and choline, are discussed as follows and summarized in Table 29.2.

Omega-3 fatty acids

Omega-3 fatty acids (ω-3 FAs) are essential fatty acids, commonly found in oily fish and seafood, which have garnered popularity as a health supplement for their cardiovascular benefits.[38] They also have reasonable evidence for benefit in unipolar depression.[3] The initial interest in a potential preventative role for ω-3 FAs in BD came from

Table 29.2 Evidence for nutraceuticals for bipolar disorder

Study	Type	Sample size	Duration	Agent	Comparator	Co-medications	Efficacy results[†]
Omega-3 Fatty Acids							
Chiu et al., 2005	RCT	n = 14	4 weeks	4.4 g/day EPA + 2.4 g/day DHA (n = 7)	Placebo (n = 7)	Ongoing treatment with valproate; use of lorazepam allowed	No group differences; both groups showed similar improvement in mania.
Frangou et al., 2006	RCT	n = 75	12 weeks	1 g/day EPA (n = 24), 2 g/day EPA (n = 26)	Placebo (n = 26)	Ongoing treatment with mood stabilizers, antidepressants, antipsychotics and/or benzodiazepines, or no treatment*.	Significantly better improvement in depression with EPA, regardless of dose (p<0.04).
Frangou et al., 2007	RCT	n = 14	12 weeks	2 g/day EPA (n = 7)	Placebo (n = 7)	Ongoing treatment with lithium.	No group differences; no change in depression in either group.
Keck et al., 2006	RCT	n = 116	16 weeks	6 g/day EPA (n = 61)	Placebo (n = 55)	Ongoing treatment with mood stabilizers.	No group differences; no change in depression or mania in either group.
Osher et al., 2005	Open trial	n = 12	Up to 6 months	1.5–2.0 g/day EPA	Pre-treatment condition	Ongoing treatment with mood stabilizers and antidepressants.	Significant (≥50%) improvement in depression with EPA. No p-values reported.

(continued)

Table 29.2 Continued

Study	Type	Sample size	Duration	Agent	Comparator	Co-medications	Efficacy results[†]
Murphy et al., 2012	RCT	n = 45	16 weeks	2 g/day cytidine + 3 g/day EPA + 2 g/day DHA (n = 15)	Placebo + 3 g/day EPA + 2 g/day DHA (n = 15) OR Placebo + placebo (n = 15)	Ongoing treatment with mood stabilizers, anticonvulsants, antipsychotics, antidepressants or anxiolytics.	No group differences; both groups showed similar improvement in depression and mania.
Stoll et al., 1999	RCT	n = 30	16 weeks	6.2 g/day EPA + 3.4 g/day DHA (n = 14)	Placebo (olive oil) (n = 16)	Ongoing treatment with mood stabilizers, antipsychotics and/or antidepressants, or no treatment*.	Significantly better improvement in depression with omega-3 fatty acids (p<0.002).
Folate							
Behdazi et al., 2009	RCT	n = 88	3 weeks	Valproate + 3 mg folic acid (n = 44)	Valproate + placebo (n = 44)	None	Significantly better improvement in mania with valproate + folic acid (p<0.005).
Coppen et al., 1986	RCT	n = 75	52 weeks	Lithium + 200 µg folic acid (n = 42)	Lithium + placebo (n = 33)	None	No group differences; no change in depression in either group.
Inositol							
Chengappa et al., 2000	RCT	n = 24	6 weeks	12 g inositol (n = 12)	Placebo (n = 12)	Ongoing treatment with lithium, valproate or carbamazepine.	No group differences; both groups showed similar improvement in depression.

Evins et al., 2006	RCT	n = 17	950 mg inositol (n = 9)	Placebo (n = 8)	Lithium or valproate	Highly variable response to inositol. Two subjects had worsening of depression, three subjects had no response, and four subjects had improvement. No p-values reported.
Nirenberg et al., 2006	RCT	n = 65	10-25 g inositol (n = 23)	Risperidone (n = 21) or Lamotrigine (n = 21)	Ongoing treatment with antidepressants.	Significantly better improvement in depression with lamotrigine ($p<0.05$). No group differences for mania.
Magnesium (Mg)						
Giannini et al., 2000	RCT	n = 20	Verapamil + 375 mg Mg (n = 10)	Verapamil + placebo (n = 10)	None	Significant improvement in mania with verapamil + Mg ($p<0.0015$).
Heiden et al., 1999	Case report series	n = 10	Intravenous infusions of Mg at 2.44± 0.34 mmol/l	Pre-treatment condition	Ongoing treatment with lithium, haloperidol or clonazepam.	Marked improvement in manic symptoms for seven patients with Mg infusion. No p-values reported.

(continued)

Table 29.2 Continued

Study	Type	Sample size	Duration	Agent	Comparator	Co-medications	Efficacy results[†]
Choline							
Brown et al., 2007	RCT	n = 44	12 weeks	500–2000 mg/day citicoline (n = 23)	Placebo (n = 21)	Ongoing treatment with lithium, anticonvulsants, antidepressants, antipsychotics, hypnotics or anxiolytics.	No group differences; no change in depression or mania in either group.
Brown & Gabrielson, 2012	RCT	n = 48	12 weeks	2000 mg citicoline (n = 28)	Placebo (n = 20)	Ongoing treatment with lithium, anticonvulsants, antidepressants, antipsychotics or sedative or anxiolytics.	Significantly better improvement in depression with citicoline (p = 0.05).
Lyoo et al., 2003	RCT	n = 8	12 weeks	50 mg/kg/day choline bitartrate (n = 4)	Placebo (n = 4)	Ongoing treatment with lithium, benzodiazepines and/or neuroleptics.	No group differences; no change in depression or mania in either group.
Stoll et al., 1996	Case report series	n = 6	1 month	780 mg choline bitartrate	Pre-treatment condition	Ongoing treatment with mood stabilizers, antidepressants and/or antipsychotics.	Five patients had a substantial reduction in manic symptoms with choline, and four patients had marked reductions in all mood symptoms. No p-values reported.

N-acetylcysteine (NAC)

Berk et al., 2008	RCT	n = 75	6 months	2 g NAC (n = 38)	Placebo (n = 37)	Ongoing treatment with mood stabilizers, antidepressants and/or antipsychotics	Significantly better improvement in depression with NAC (p = 0.002). No group differences for mania; both groups improved comparably. No group differences in time to mood episode.
Berk et al., 2011	Open trial	n = 156	2 months	2 g NAC	Pre-treatment condition	Ongoing treatment with psychotropics	Significantly better improvement in depression (p<0.001) and mania (p<0.05) with NAC.
Beck et al., 2012	RCT (continuation of Berk. et al., 2011)	n = 149	6 months	2 g NAC (n = 76)	Placebo (n = 73)	Ongoing treatment with psychotropics	No group differences in time to mood episode.

EM Power Plus (EMP+)

Kaplan et al., 2000	Case series	n = 11	6 months	EMP+ (32 capsules)	Pre-treatment condition	Ongoing treatment with mood stabilizers, antipsychotics and/or antidepressants.	Significant improvement in depression (p<0.01) and mania (p<0.01) with EMP+; medication use reduced by >50% (p<0.01).

(continued)

Table 29.2 Continued

Study	Type	Sample size	Duration	Agent	Comparator	Co-medications	Efficacy results[†]
Popper, 2001	Case series	n = 22	Up to 6–9 months	EMP+ (32 capsules)	Pre-treatment condition	Ongoing treatment with psychotropics or no treatment*.	Clinically significant improvement in 45% of patients with EMP+; 73% of medicated patients discontinued psychotropics. No p-values reported.
Simmons, 2003	Case series	n = 19	Up to 13 months	EMP+ (32 capsules)	Pre-treatment condition	Ongoing treatment with psychotropics or no treatment*.	Clinically significant improvement in 63% of patients with EMP+; 69% of medicated patients discontinued psychotropics. No p-values reported.

Abbreviations: DHA = docosahexaenoic acid; EMP+ = EM Power Plus; EPA = eicosapentanoate acid; Mg = magnesium; NAC = N-acetylcysteine; RCT = randomized controlled trial

[†] Significant, p≤0.05

* If patients were not already taking psychotropic medications, they were not administered any pharmacological treatment for the study

the observation that consumption of fish and seafood (which is considered to be a measure of ω-3 FA intake) was inversely correlated with the prevalence of BD.[39] The mood-stabilizing effects of ω-3 FAs is suggested to be related to their incorporation into membrane phospholipids, which in turn leads to dampening of signal transduction pathways, similar to the action of mood stabilizers.[40,41]

Several studies have assessed the benefits of ω-3 FA as add-on to conventional pharmacotherapy in BD, with conflicting findings. While two placebo-controlled RCTs[40,41] and an open trial[42] found daily intake of ω-3 FA supplements to be associated with significant improvements in depression and lower relapse rates in patients with BD, several other RCTs reported no benefits either in depression or mania.[43-46] Meta-analysis of these same studies, however, found a significant positive effect of ω-3 FAs on bipolar depression.[38,47,48] In interpreting this finding, it should be noted that the meta-analyses were not conducted on raw data from included studies, but rather the authors calculated effect sizes based only on the published data from those studies. Also, the data from Frangou et al.,[40] in which two doses of eicosapentaenoic acid (EPA) were tested, were separated by dose and re-analysed as two separate studies in two of the meta-analyses.[47,48] Thus, their results should be interpreted with caution. Another meta-analysis similarly found ω-3 FAs effective as augmentation for bipolar depression, but this was based on analysis of only one study[40] as the other studies compiled did not provide raw data for evaluation; methodological quality across the studies was also highly variable.[38]

The conflicting results reported also may be attributed, at least in part, to differences in dose range and compositions of ω-3 FAs used in the studies, eg EPA alone,[40,44,45] or differing ratios of EPA to docosahexaenoic acid (DHA).[41,43] Formulations with higher levels of EPA (using a 2:1 or 3:1 ratio of EPA to DHA) have been noted to be more effective in unipolar depression.[3] However, findings for similar formulations or EPA alone in BD have been equivocal, precluding any recommendations on formulation or dosage.

ω-3 FA supplements are consistently reported to be safe and well tolerated, and the occurrence of adverse events (eg diarrhoea, fatigue, etc) is similar to that with placebo.[40,45] An added benefit for their use in BD is the low likelihood of the hypomanic or manic switches often noted with antidepressant therapy.

On balance, there appears to be at least preliminary evidence for the benefit of ω-3 FA supplements in bipolar depression, with caveats. Their efficacy in unipolar depression and good tolerability encourage more systematic evaluations in BD.

Folate

Folate belongs to a family of water-soluble B vitamins that have vital roles in cellular activity, immune and nervous system functioning, and neurochemical mechanisms that influence cognitive performance and mood.[49] Low plasma, serum or red blood cell folate concentrations have been associated with mood disorders such as major depression and BD, suggesting that folate supplements may be beneficial in the management of mood.[49] Small systematic reviews have also reported folate to be effective as an augmenting agent in unipolar depression.[1]

The efficacy of folate as an add-on to pharmacotherapy for BD, however, has not been studied extensively, and available data are mixed. An early RCT found no differences between folic acid or placebo augmentation in improving bipolar depression.[50] However, a more recent RCT found that folic acid add-on resulted in significant decreases in manic symptoms.[49]

These studies did not report any adverse effects associated with folate add-on to pharmacotherapy, but as a caution, other literature indicates that high folic acid doses are associated with increased depression, sleep difficulties, irritability, hyperactivity, and malaise.[1]

In conclusion, the evidence for the benefit of folate in BD remains very preliminary. More data is needed for a better evaluation of its potential as a treatment strategy.

Inositol

Inositol is a precursor of the phosphatidyl inositol (PI) cycle second messenger system, which is a signal transduction system associated with the activity of various neurotransmitter systems.[51] An association with BD was suggested by the observation that cerebrospinal fluid and frontal cortex of BD patients had reduced levels of inositol.[52]

The efficacy of inositol as an add-on treatment for BD has been studied in a few RCTs, with conflicting results. While two RCTs found no benefits to inositol supplementation of mood stabilizers for bipolar depression,[51,53] the third reported that it improved depression in some patients but worsened symptoms in others.[54]

Reported adverse events with inositol include loose stools or diarrhoea, moderately severe hand tremors, and non-specific headaches;[51] as well as increased agitation and suicidal ideation, leading to hospitalization.[54]

In summary, the generally negative evidence would preclude the use of inositol as add-on in the treatment of BD.

Magnesium

Magnesium (Mg) is an essential mineral nutrient with roles in energy metabolism, neurotransmitter synthesis and signalling, and nerve conduction, among others.[55] Its deficiency is believed to negatively affect mood in the general population.[56] Mg modulates the signalling of neurotransmitters and receptors involved in mood disorders by blocking calcium influx and non-competitively antagonizing N-methyl-D-aspartate (NMDA) channels, similar to the action of mood stabilizers.[55]

The only data on the use of Mg in depressive disorders is as add-on in the treatment of mania. One case series reported marked improvement in mania in severe, treatment-resistant patients following Mg infusion as add-on to pharmacotherapy;[55] and one small RCT reported that the combination of Mg and verapamil was more effective in reducing manic symptoms than verapamil treatment alone.[57]

Adverse events associated with intravenous Mg infusions include bradycardia and sensation of burning in the veins, both of which can be resolved by decreasing Mg concentrations.[55] High doses of oral Mg can also lead to diarrhoea.[55]

Altogether, there is very preliminary but encouraging evidence on the antimanic effects of Mg. More research is needed to elucidate its efficacy and safety profile in BD.

Choline

Choline is an essential dietary amino acid involved in structural integrity and signalling of cell membranes, cholinergic neurotransmission, muscle function, and lipid transport from the liver.[58] Altered balance of adrenergic and cholinergic neurotransmitter systems has been proposed in the aetiology of BD, and changes in measures of choline metabolism have been reported in BD patients.[59]

Choline has been evaluated mostly in BD, with little data in unipolar depression. Therapeutically, an early case series reported that choline bitartate as adjunct to psychotropics was more effective than placebo in reducing manic symptoms.[60] However, a small RCT found no difference between choline and placebo as add-on to existing medications for BD depression or mania.[61] More recently, two RCTs examined the effect of citicoline—a naturally occurring, over-the-counter nutritional supplement that is metabolized into cytidine and choline—on mood regulation in BD, with mixed results.[62,63] One study reported that citicoline and placebo as augmentation to psychotropics had similar effects on depressive or manic symptoms,[62] while the other found citicoline add-on superior to placebo in improving bipolar depression.[63]

Both choline and citicoline appear to be well tolerated. The infrequent adverse events include insomnia, fishy breath, and gastrointestinal symptoms.[60,63]

On balance, there is insufficient evidence for the efficacy of choline and citicoline in BD, precluding any recommendations.

N-acetylcysteine

N-acetylcysteine (NAC) derives from the amino acid, cysteine, which is the precursor of the chief brain antioxidant, glutathione.[64] Higher oxidative stress, which is implicated in the pathophysiology of depression, is linked to impaired glutathione metabolism; however, NAC administration increases blood and brain glutathione levels.[64] NAC is also associated with enhanced neurogenesis, similar to the effects of antidepressants and mood stabilizers, as well as modulation of glutamate and dopamine and reversal of mitochondrial dysfunction, which have both been implicated in BD.[64,65]

Very sparse data for NAC in unipolar depression has had mixed results,[66] but though also preliminary, findings in BD have been more positive. A small maintenance treatment RCT found NAC add-on to pharmacotherapy superior to placebo in improving bipolar depression, but not mania, and there were no group differences in time to mood episode.[67] A subsequent two-phase maintenance RCT by the same researchers found adjunctive NAC beneficial for bipolar depression and mania in the open-label phase,[68] but there was no difference from placebo in time to depressive or manic relapse in the double-blind phase.[64]

NAC was generally been well tolerated in published trials. Animal studies also suggest that NAC add-on may prevent lithium-induced renal dysfunction.[65] Common side effects include gastrointestinal symptoms, headache, joint pain, and muscle spasms, but the overall frequency of adverse events is similar to that with placebo.[66,67]

To summarize, there is preliminary evidence of benefit of NAC in bipolar depression. Its tolerability and potential to mitigate mood-stabilizer side effects encourage further exploration of its benefits in BD.

EM Power Plus

EM Power Plus (EMP+) is a proprietary nutritional supplement made up of 36 chelated trace vitamins and minerals. It is thought to influence mood through correction of nutritional deficiencies that may contribute to metabolic dysfunction.[69]

Data in unipolar depression is lacking, but there is some evidence for the benefit for EMP+ in BD, albeit only from case reports. EMP+ augmentation was associated with improved bipolar depression and mania, and reduced or discontinued use of psychotropic medications, in three case series.[69-71] However, two cases of hypomanic switch, and resumption of medications by some patients after post-study symptom recurrence, were also reported in one of these case series.[71] It is also of note that a placebo-controlled RCT of EMP+ was discontinued due to recruitment challenges, large expectancy effects and inconclusive results.[72]

EMP+ showed good tolerability in the published studies. A systematic review also found EMP+ more tolerable than psychiatric medications, with no reported toxicity, and mild headache and transient gastrointestional symptoms the most common side effects reported.[73] However, as noted previously, there is potential risk of manic switch in some patients.[71]

Overall, there is insufficient evidence to recommend the use of EMP+ in BD.

Herbal products

Herbal remedies are non-prescription, natural health products derived from plants and plant extracts, such as leaves, flowers, roots, bark, and berries.[1] Although herbal remedies are frequently used to support general wellness or manage symptoms associated with physical or mental stress, published evidence for their efficacy and safety in BD is limited.[1] Most publications on herbal remedies used in BD relate to St John's Wort and Free and Easy Wanderer Plus, a Chinese herbal formulation. They are discussed as follows and summarized in Table 29.3.

St John's Wort

St John's Wort (SJW) is a flowering plant that has become a popular form of treatment for mood and anxiety disorders within the last decade. While its mechanism of action is not fully understood, active ingredients found in SJW—hypericin and hyperforin, among others—have been noted as having antidepressant effects and actions similar to monoamine oxidase inhibitors (MAOIs) and selective serotonin reuptake inhibitors (SSRIs).[74]

While there is substantial evidence for the efficacy of SJW for unipolar depression from RCTs and meta-analyses,[3] its benefits in BD have only been evaluated in case

Table 29.3 Evidence for herbal remedies for bipolar disorder

Study	Type	Sample size	Duration	Agent	Comparator	Co-medication	Efficacy results[†]
St John's Wort (SJW)							
Moses & Mallinger, 2000	Case series	n = 3	Variable. 2 + weeks.	SJW	Pre-treatment condition	Ongoing treatment with mood stabilizers and/or antidepressants.	Improvement in depression with SJW, bordering on manic switch. No p-values reported.
Stevinson & Ernst, 2004	Case series	n = 17	Variable	SJW	Pre-treatment condition	Ongoing treatment with mood stabilizers, antipsychotics and/or sedative/anxiolytics.	Changes in mood, bordering on manic switch or psychotic induction, with SJW. No p-values reported.
Free and Easy Wanderer Plus (FEWP)							
Zhang et al., 2007a	RCT	n = 235	12 weeks	CBZ + 36 mg FEWP (n = 89)	CBZ (n = 88) or Placebo (n = 44)	If needed, benzodiazepines.	Significantly greater improvement in depression with CBZ + FEWP (p = 0.032). Both CBZ groups improved mania comparably, and were superior to placebo alone (p<0.05).

(continued)

Table 29.3 Continued

Study	Type	Sample size	Duration	Agent	Comparator	Co-medication	Efficacy results[†]
Zhang et al., 2007b	RCT	Study 1 (continuation of Zhang et al., 2007a): n = 188 Study 2: n = 149 (UD = 85; BD = 62)	Study 1: 26 weeks Study 2: 12 weeks	Study 1: CBZ + 36 mg FEWP (n = 89) Study 2: FEWP alone (n = 86)	Study 1: CBZ + placebo (n = 88) Study 2: Placebo alone (n = 63)	Both studies: if needed, benzodiazepines and/or anticholinergic agents.	Study 1: Significantly lower discontinuation due to relapse with CBZ + FEWP (p = 0.009). No group differences in continued improvement. Study 2: Significantly greater improvement in unipolar (p = 0.007) and bipolar depression (p = 0.03) with FEWP alone.

Abbreviations: BD = bipolar disorder; CBZ = carbamazepine; FEWP = Free and Easy Wanderer Plus; RCT = randomized controlled trial; SJW = St John's Wort; UD = unipolar depression

[†] Significant, p≤0.05

reports. Many of these reports found no evidence of benefit for SJW in BD, and some reported manic switches with its use.[75,76]

There are reported drug interactions with SJW, including with antiretrovirals, immunosuppressants, antihistamines, anticoagulants, and antidepressants.[77] This adds to the caution needed for its use, particularly in older patients, who may be more susceptible to mania with SJW use due to age-related decreases in drug metabolism or increases in central nervous system (CNS) drug sensitivity.[2]

In conclusion, there is currently little data to support the use of SJW in BD. However, the notable benefits reported with SJW in unipolar depression would encourage its further investigation in BD in larger, controlled studies.

Free and Easy Wanderer Plus

Free and Easy Wanderer Plus (FEWP) is a Chinese herbal compound that has been most associated in traditional Chinese medicine with the treatment of depression.[78] Though primarily used in China, either on its own or in conjunction with conventional antidepressants, FEWP has also been utilized in Europe and North America to relieve symptoms like irritability, premenstrual tension, and menopausal syndromes.[78] Its mechanisms of action may involve the regulation of various neurotransmitters and neuromodulators, including but not limited to, central gamma-aminobutyric acid (GABA), monoamine receptors and cytokine activity, similar to the action of antidepressants.[79] Moreover, animal studies have shown that Chaihu, a key ingredient within FEWP, can increase norepinephrine and dopamine levels in the brain.[80]

FEWP has been extensively studied in unipolar depression, though mostly in China, where large meta-analyses have reported its efficacy as an augmentation agent.[78] However, the literature on FEWP for BD is limited. Two large RCTs reported that FEWP add-on to carbamezepine resulted in significant improvements in bipolar depression[81] and lower discontinuation due to relapse than placebo augmentation.[82] Another RCT found FEWP monotherapy superior to placebo in improving both unipolar and bipolar depression.[82]

As an added benefit, FEWP counteracts some of the adverse events associated with the mood stabilizer, carbamazepine, improving its tolerability.[81] However, FEWP does have its own adverse effects, such as constipation, fatigue, dry mouth, tachycardia, insomnia, somnolence, dizziness, and headache,[78] though incidence of such effects has been reported to be similar or lower than with placebo.[81,82]

To summarize, FEWP has reasonable data for benefit in BD. However, the evidence base consists mostly of studies published in Chinese languages.[81] Further studies in non-Chinese populations may provide more credible basis for clinical use.

Conclusion

CAM therapies are often seen as more naturalistic interventions compared with conventional pharmacotherapy by many patients with medical and psychiatric illnesses, including those with BD. However, the overall body of research on their benefit remains relatively limited for BD.

Among the CAM therapies, sleep deprivation has good evidence for benefit in bipolar depression, but has practical limitations for its use. Other interventions that have preliminary evidence or potential benefit include exercise, BLT, ω-3 fatty acids, NAC, and FEWP. There are also more novel and experimental therapies, such as dark therapy and magnesium, and therapies with currently negative evidence in BD that still warrant further exploration due to their proven efficacy in unipolar depression, such as SJW.

As with studies investigating CAM therapies in other conditions, those reported with bipolar subjects have significant methodological deficits. These include small sample sizes, lack of control groups, contradictory and/or preliminary results, and/or failure to replicate results, highlighting the need for better-quality investigations to evaluate both efficacy and safety. Future research on CAM modalities used in BD should also attempt to elucidate dosage and treatment duration requirements, as well as, in the case of nutraceuticals and herbal remedies, any potential interactions with pharmacotherapies used in BD.

Given the sparse data, methodological weaknesses of studies, and limited clinical experience with these agents, most CAMs can only be recommended for use in BD after standard primary interventions such as antidepressants and mood stabilizers. It is also recommended that they always be used under medical supervision and with caution.

References

1. **Ravindran AV** and **da Silva TL**. Complementary and alternative therapies as add-on to pharmacotherapy for mood and anxiety disorders: a systematic review, J Affect Disord 2013;**150**:707–19.

2. **Andreescu C, Mulsant BH**, and **Emanuel JE**. Complementary and alternative medicine in the treatment of bipolar disorder—a review of the evidence, J Affect Disord 2008;**110**:16–26.

3. **Ravindran AV, Balneaves LG, Faulkner G, Ortiz A, McIntosh D, Morehouse RL, Ravindran L, Yatham LN, Kennedy SH, Lam RW, MacQueen GM, Milev RV, Parikh SV; CANMAT Depression Work Group**. Canadian Network for Mood and Anxiety Treatments (CANMAT) 2016 Clinical Guidelines for the Management of Adults with Major Depressive Disorder: Section 5. Complementary and Alternative Medicine Treatments. Can J Psychiatry 2016;**61**:576–87.

4. **Eisenberg DM, Davis RB, Ettner SL, Appel S, Wilkey S, Van Rompay M**, and **Kessler RC**. Trends in alternative medicine use in the United States, 1990–1997: results of a follow-up national survey, JAMA 1998;**280**:1569–75.

5. **Strejilevich SA, Sarmiento MJ, Scapola M, Gil L, Martino DJ, Gil JF**, and **Gomez-Restrepo C**. Complementary and alternative medicines usage in bipolar patients from Argentina and Colombia: associations with satisfaction and adherence to treatment, J Affect Disord 2013;**149**:393–7.

6. **Knubben K, Reischies FM, Adli M, Schlattmann P, Bauer M**, and **Dimeo F**. A randomized, controlled study on the effects of a short-term endurance training programme in patients with major depression, Br J Sports Med 2007;**41**:29–33.

7. **Dimeo F, Bauer M, Varahram I, Proest G**, and **Halter U**. Benefits from aerobic exercise in patients with major depression: a pilot stud,. Br J Sports Med 2001;**35**:114–17.

8. **Ng F, Dodd S,** and **Berk M.** The effects of physical activity in the acute treatment of bipolar disorder: a pilot study, J Affect Disorder 2007;**01**:259–62.

9. **Correa R, Akiskal H, Gilmer W, Nierenberg AA, Trivedi M,** and **Zisook S.** Is unrecognized bipolar disorder a frequent contributor to apparent treatment resistant depression?, J Affect Disord 2010;**127**:10–18.

10. **Wright KA, Everson-Hock ES,** and **Taylor AH.** The effects of physical activity on physical and mental health among individuals with bipolar disorder: a systematic review, Ment Heal and Phys Act 2009;**2**:86–94.

11. **Dennehy EB, Schnyer R, Bernstein IH, Gonzalez R, Shivakumar G, Kelly DI, Snow DE, Sureddi S,** and **Suppes T.** The safety, acceptability, and effectiveness of acupuncture as an adjunctive treatment for acute symptoms in bipolar disorder, J Clin Psychiatry 2009;**0**:897–905.

12. **Kurland HD.** ECT and Acu-EST in the treatment of depression, Am J Chin Med (Gard City NY) 1976;**4**:289–92.

13. **Hu J.** Acupuncture treatment of manic psychosis, J Tradit Chin Med 1996;**16**: 238–40.

14. **White A.** A cumulative review of the range and incidence of significant adverse events associated with acupuncture, Acupunt Med 2004;**22**:122–33.

15. **Bellivier F, Geoffroy PA, Etain B,** and **Scott J.** Sleep- and circadian rhythm-associated pathways as therapeutic targets in bipolar disorder, Expert Opin Ther Targets 2015;**19**:747–63.

16. **Gonzalez R.** The relationship between bipolar disorder and biological rhythms, J Clin Psychiatry 2014;**75**:e323–31

17. **Benedetti F** and **Colombo C.** Sleep deprivation in mood disorders, *Neuropsychobiology* 2011;**64**:141–51.

18. **Benedetti F, Campori E, Barbini B, Fulgosi MC,** and **Colombo C.** Dopaminergic augmentation of sleep deprivation effects in bipolar depression, Psychiatry Res 2001a;**104**:239–46.

19. **Benedetti F, Barbini B, Campori E, Fulgosi MC, Pontiggia A,** and **Colombo C.** Sleep phase advance and lithium to sustain the antidepressant effect of total sleep deprivation in bipolar depression: new findings supporting the internal coincidence model?, J Psychiatr Res 2001b;**35**:323–9.

20. **Colombo C, Lucca A, Benedetti F, Barbini B, Campori E,** and **Smeraldi E.** Total sleep deprivation combined with lithium and light therapy in the treatment of bipolar depression: replication of main effects and interaction, Psychiatry Res 2000;**95**:43–53.

21. **Wu JC, Kelsoe JR, Schachat C, Bunney BG, DeModena A, Golshan S, Gillin JC, Potkin SG,** and **Bunney W.** Rapid and sustained antidepressant response with sleep deprivation and chronotherapy in bipolar disorder, Biol Psychiatry 2009;**66**:298–301.

22. **Benedetti F, Barbini B, Fulgosi MC, Colombo C, Dallaspezia S, Pontiggia A,** and **Smeraldi E.** Combined total sleep deprivation and light therapy in the treatment of drug-resistant bipolar depression: acute response and long-term remission rates, J Clin Psychiatry 2005;**66**:1535–40.

23. **Benedetti F, Riccaboni R, Locatelli C, Poletti S, Dallaspezia S,** and **Colombo C.** Rapid treatment response of suicidal symptoms to lithium, sleep deprivation, and light therapy (chronotherapeutics) in drug-resistant bipolar depression, J Clin Psychiatry 2014;**75**:133–40.

24. Colombo C, Benedetti F, Barbini B, Campori E, and Smeraldi E. Rate of switch from depression into mania after therapeutic sleep deprivation in bipolar depression, Psychiatry Res 1999;**86**:267–70.

25. Dauphinais DR, Rosenthal JZ, Terman M, DiFebo HM, Tuggle C, and Rosenthal NE. Controlled trial of safety and efficacy of bright light therapy vs negative air ions in patients with bipolar depression, Psych Res 2012;**196**:57–61.

26. Oldham MA and Ciraulo DA. Bright light therapy for depression: a review of its effects on chronobiology and the autonomic nervous system, Chronobiol Int 2014;**31**:305–19.

27. Roecklein KA, Rohan KJ, and Postolache TT. Is seasonal affective disorder a bipolar variant?, Curr Psychiatr 2010;**9**:42–54.

28. Leibenluft E, Turner EH, Feldman-Naim S, Schwartz PJ, Wehr TA, and Rosenthal NE. Light therapy in patients with rapid cycling bipolar disorder: preliminary results, Psychopharmacol Bull 1995;**31**:705–10.

29. Papatheodorou G and Kutcher S. The effect of adjunctive light therapy on ameliorating breakthrough depressive symptoms in adolescent-onset bipolar disorder, J Psychiatry Neurosci 1993;**20**:226–32.

30. Sit D, Wisner KL, Hanusa BH, Stull S, and Terman M. Light therapy for bipolar disorder: a case series in women, Bipolar Disord 2007;**9**:918–27.

31. Chan PK, Lam RW, and Perry KF. Mania precipitated by light therapy for patients with SAD, J Clin Psychiatry 1994;**55**:454.

32. Kripke DF. Timing of phototherapy and occurrence of mania, Biol Psychiatry 1991;**29**:1156.

33. Phelps J. Dark therapy for bipolar disorder using amber lenses for blue light blockade, Med Hypotheses 2008;**70**:224–9.

34. Wehr TA, Turner EH, Shimada JM, Lowe CH, Barker C, and Leibenluft E. Treatment of rapidly cycling bipolar patient by using extended bed rest and darkness to stabilize the timing and duration of sleep, Biol Psychiatry 1998;**43**:822–8.

35. Wirz-Justice A, Quinto C, Cajochen C, Werth E, and Hock C. A rapid-cycling bipolar patient treated with long nights, bedrest, and light, Biol Psychiatry 1999;**45**:1075–7.

36. Barbini B, Benedetti F, Colombo C, Dotoli D, Bernasconi A, Cigala-Fulgosi M, and Smeraldi E. Dark therapy for mania: a pilot study, Bipolar Disord 2005;**7**:98–101.

37. Henriksen TEG, Skrede S, Fasmer OB, Hamre B, Gronli J, and Lund A. Blocking blue light during mania—markedly increased regularity of sleep and rapid improvement of symptoms: a case report, Bipolar Disord 2014;**16**:894–8.

38. Montgomery P and Richardson AJ. Omega-3 fatty acids for bipolar disorder, Cochrane Database Syst Rev 2008;**2**:CD005169.

39. Noaghiul S and Hibbeln JR. Cross-national comparisons of seafood consumption and rates of bipolar disorders, Am J Psychiatry 2003;**160**:2222–7.

40. Frangou S, Lewis M, and McCrone P. Efficacy of ethyl-eicosapentanoic acid in bipolar depression: randomized double-blind placebo-controlled study, B J Psychiatry 2006;**188**:46–50.

41. Stoll AL, Severus WE, Freeman MP, Rueter S, Zboyan HA, Diamong E, Cress KK, and Marangell LB. Omega 3 fatty acids in bipolar disorder—a preliminary double-blind, placebo-controlled trial, Arch Gen Psychiatry 1999;**56**:407–12.

42. Osher Y, Bersudsky Y,and Belmaker RH. Omega-3 eicosapentaenoic acid in bipolar depression: report of a small open-label study, J Clin Psychiatry 2005;**66**:726–9.

43. **Chiu CC, Huang SY, Chen CC**, and **Su KP**. Omega-3 fatty acids are more beneficial in the depressive phase than in the manic phase in patients with bipolar I disorder, J Clin Psychiatry 2003;**66**:1613–14.

44. **Frangou S, Lewis M, Wollard J**, and **Simmons A**. Preliminary in vivo evidence of increased N-acetyl-aspartate following eicosapentanoic acid treatment in patients with bipolar disorder, J Psychopharmacol 2007;**21**:435–9.

45. **Keck PE Jr, Mintz J, McElroy SL, Freeman MP, Suppes T, Frye MA, Altshuler LL, Kupka R, Nolen WA, Leverich GS, Denicoff KD, Grunze H, Duan N**, and **Post RM**. Double-blind, randomized, placebo-controlled trials of ethyl-eicopentanoate in the treatment of bipolar depression and rapid cycling bipolar disorder, Biol Psychiatry 2006;**60**:1020–2.

46. **Murphy BL, Stoll AL, Harris PQ, Ravichandran C, Babb SM, Carlezon WA**, and **Cohen BM**. Omega-3 fatty acid treatment, with or without cytidine, fails to show therapeutic properties in bipolar disorder—a double-blind, randomized add-on clinical trial, J Clin Psychopharmacol 2012;**32**:699–703.

47. **Grosso G, Pajak A, Marventano S, Castellano S, Galvano F, Bucolo C, Drago F**, and **Caraci, F**. Role of omega-3 fatty acids in the treatment of depressive disorders: a comprehensive meta-analysis of randomized clinical trials, PLoS ONE 2014;**9**:e96905. doi: 10.1371/journal.pone.0096905

48. **Sarris J, Mischoulon D**, and **Schweitzer I**. Omega-3 for bipolar disorder: meta-analyses of use in mania and bipolar depression, J Clin Psychiatry 2012;**73**:81–6.

49. **Behzadi A, Omrani Z, Chalian M, Asadi S**, and **Ghadiri M**. Folic acid efficacy as an alternative drug added to sodium valproate in the treatment of acute phase of mania in bipolar disorder: a double-blind randomized controlled trial, Acta Psychiatr Scand 2009;**120**:441–5.

50. **Coppen A, Chaudhry S**, and **Swade C**. Folic acid enhances lithium prophylaxis, J Affect Disord 1986;**10**:9–13.

51. **Chengappa KNR, Levine J, Gershon S, Mallinger AG, Hardan A, Vagnucci A, Pollock B, Luther J, Buttenfield J, Verfaille S**, and **Kupfer DJ**. Inositol as an add-on treatment for bipolar depression, Bipolar Disord 2000;**2**:47–55.

52. **Levine J, Kurtzman L, Rappoport A Zimmerman J, Bersudsky Y, Shapiro J, Belmaker RH**, and **Agam H**. Inositol does not predict antidepressant response to inositol. Short communication, J Neural Transm 1996;**103**:1457–62.

53. **Nierenberg AA, Ostacher MJ, Calabrese JR, Ketter TA, Marangell LB, Miklowtz DJ, Miyahara S**, and **Bauer MS**. Treatment-resistant bipolar depression: a STEP-BD equipoise randomized effectiveness trial of antidepressant augmentation with lamotrigine, inositol, or risperidone, Am J Psychiatry 2006;**162**:210–16.

54. **Evins AE, Demopulos C, Yovel I, Culhane M, Ogutha J, Grandin LD, Nierenberg AA**, and **Sachs GS**. Inositol augmentation of lithium or valproate for bipolar depression, Bipolar Disord 2006;**8**:168–74.

55. **Heiden A, Frey R, Presslich O, Blasbichler T, Smetana R**, and **Kasper S**. Treatment of severer mania with intravenous magnesium sulphate as a supplementary therapy, Psychiatry Res 1999;**89**:239–46.

56. **Schimatschek HF** and **Rempis R**. Prevalence of hypomanesemia in an unselected German population of 16,000 individuals, Magnes Res 2001;**14**:283–90.

57. **Giannini AJ, Nakoneczie AM, Melemis SM, Ventresco J**, and **Condon M**. Magnesium oxide augmentation of verapamil maintenance therapy in mania, Psychiatry Res 2000;**93**:83–7.

58. **Zeisel H.** Choline: critical role during fetal development and dietary requirements in adults, Annu Rev Nutr 2006;**26**:229–50.

59. **Moore CM, Breeze JL, Gruber SA, Babb SM, Frederick B, Villafuerte RA, Stoll AL, Hennen J, Yurgelun-Todd DA, Cohen BM,** and **Renshaw PF.** Choline, myo-inositol and mood in bipolar disorder: a proton magnetic resonance spectroscopic imaging study of the anterior cingulate cortex, Bipolar Disord 2000;**2**:207–16.

60. **Stoll AL, Sachs GS, Cohen BM, Lafer B, Christensen JD,** and **Renshaw PF.** Choline in the treatment of rapid-cycling bipolar disorder, Biol Psychiatry 1996;**40**:382–8.

61. **Lyoo IK, Demopoulos CM, Hirashima F, Ahn KH,** and **Renshaw PF.** Oral choline decreases brain purine levels in lithium-treated subjects with rapid-cycling bipolar disorder: a double-blind trial using proton and lithium magnetic resonance spectroscopy, Bipolar Disord 2003;**5**:300–6.

62. **Brown ES, Gorman AR,** and **Hynan LS.** A randomized, placebo-controlled trial of citicoline add-on therapy in outpatients with bipolar disorder and cocaine dependence, J Clin Psychopharmacol 2007;**27**:498–502.

63. **Brown ES** and **Gabrielson B.** A randomized, double-blind, placebo-controlled trial of citicoline for bipolar and unipolar depression and methamphetamine dependence, J Affect Disord 2012;**143**:257–60.

64. **Berk M, Dean OM, Cotton SM, Gama CS, Kapczinski F, Fernandes B, Kohlmann K, Jeavons S, Hewitt K, Moss K, Allwang C, Schapkaitz I, Cobb H, Bush AI, Dodd S,** and **Malhi GS.** Maintenance N-acetyl cysteine treatment for bipolar disorder: a double-blind randomized placebo controlled trial, BMC Med 2012;**14**:91.

65. **Dean O, Giorlando F,** and **Berk M.** N-acetylcysteine in psychiatry: current therapeutic evidences and potential mechanisms of action, J Psychiatry Neurosci 2011;**36**:78–86.

66. **Berk M, Dean OM, Cotton SM, Jeavons S, Tanious M, Kohlmann K, Hewitt K, Moss K, Allwang C, Schapkaitz I, Robbins J, Cobb H, Ng F, Dodd S, Bush AI,** and **Malhi GS.** The efficacy of adjunctive N-acetylcysteine in major depressive disorder: a double-blind, randomized, placebo-controlled trial, J Clin Psychiatry 2014;**75**:628–36.

67. **Berk M, Copolov DL, Dean O, Lu K, Jeavons S, Schapkaitz I, Anderson-Hunt M,** and **Bush AI.** N-acetyl cysteine for depressive symptoms in bipolar disorder—a double-blind randomized placebo-controlled trial, Biol Psychiatry 2008;**64**:468–75.

68. **Berk M, Dean O, Cotton SM, Gama CS, Kapczinski F, Fernandes BS, Kohlmann K, Jeavons S, Hewitt K, Allwang C, Cobb H, Bush AI, Schapkaitz I, Dodd S,** and **Malhi GS.** The efficacy of N-acetylcysteine as an adjunctive treatment in bipolar depression: an open label trial, J Affect Disord 2011;**135**:389–94.

69. **Kaplan B, Simpson J, Ferre R, Gorman CP, McMullen DM,** and **Crawford SG.** Effective mood stabilization with a chelated mineral supplement: an open-label trial in bipolar disorder, J Clin Psychiatry 2001;**62**:936–44.

70. **Popper CW.** Do vitamins or minerals (apart from lithium) have mood-stabilizing effects?, J Clin Psychiatry 2001;**62**:933–5.

71. **Simmons M.** Nutritional approach to bipolar disorder, J Clin Psychiatry 2003;**64**:338.

72. **ClinicalTrials.gov. Clinical Trial of a Nutritional Supplement in Adults with Bipolar Disorder.** Investigators: Kaplan BJ and Goldstein E. Study registered in April 2005, updated to September 2012. Available at: http://www.clinicaltrials.gov/ct/show/ NCT00109577?order=1 (last accessed 3 November 2015).

73. **Simpson JS, Crawford SG, Goldstein ET, Field C, Burgess E,** and **Kaplan BJ.** Systematic review of safety and tolerability of a complex micronutrient formula used in mental health, BMC Psychiatry 2011;**11**:62.

74. **Schmidt M** and **Butterweck V**. The mechanisms of action of St. John's Wort: an update, Wien Med Wochenschr 2015;**165**:229–35.

75. **Moses EL** and **Mallinger AG**. St John's Wort: three cases of possible mania induction, J Clin Psychopharmacol 2000;**20**:115–17.

76. **Stevinson C** and **Ernst E**. Can St. John's Wort trigger psychoses?, Int J Clin Pharmacol Ther 2004;**42**:473–80.

77. **Golan DE, Tashjian AH, Armstrong EJ,** and **Armstrong AW**. *Principles of Pharmacology: the Pathophysiologic Basis of Drug Therapy* (New York, NY: Lippincott, Williams and Wilkins, 2007), 49–62.

78. **Qin F, Wu X, Tang Y, Huang Q, Zhang Z,** and **Yuan JH**. Meta-analysis of randomized controlled trials to assess the effectiveness and safety of free and easy wanderer plus, a polyherbal preparation for depressive disorders, J Psychiatr Res 2011;**45**:1518–24.

79. **Wang T** and **Qin F**. Effect of Chinese herbal medicine xiaoyao powder on monoamine neurotransmitters in hippocampus of rats with postpartum depression, Zhong Xi Yi Jie He Xue Bao 2010;**8**:1075–9.

80. **Zhang H** and **Gao XF**. Effect of radix bupleuri on the monoamine neurotransmitters in the brains of rats with liver-qi stagnation, Chin J Neuroimmunol Neurol 2006;**13**:180–2.

81. **Zhang Z, Kang W, Tan Q, Li Q, Gao C, Zhang F, Wang H, Ma X, Chen C, Wang W, Guo Li, Zhang Y, Yang X,** and **Yang G**. Adjunctive herbal medicine with carbamazepine for bipolar disorders: a double-blind, randomized, placebo-controlled study, J Psychiatr Res 2007a;**41**:360–9.

82. **Zhang Z, Kang W, Li Q,** and **Tan Q**. The beneficial effects of the herbal medicine Free and Easy Wanderer Plus (FEWP) for mood disorders: double-blind, placebo-controlled studies, J Psychiatr Res 2007b;**41**:828–36.

Chapter 30

Novel therapeutic targets for bipolar disorder

Ioline D. Henter and Rodrigo Machado-Vieira

Introduction

Currently available therapeutic interventions are insufficient for many patients with bipolar disorder (BD), particularly for those suffering from bipolar depression. In contrast to the manic phase of the illness where a fairly large variety of effective treatments are available—most notably antipsychotic and antiepileptic agents—in bipolar depression effective therapeutics are scarce. For instance, a large, 26-week study funded by the National Institute of Mental Health (NIMH) found no benefit to antidepressant use for patients with BD-I or BD-II depression.[1] Furthermore, when currently available therapeutics for depression—both for major depressive disorder (MDD) and BD—do work, they are associated with a delayed onset of action of several weeks; this latency period significantly increases risk of suicide and self-harm and is a key public health issue. Because the long-term course of BD is dominated by recurrent depressive episodes and lingering depressive symptoms rather than hypomanic/manic episodes, this is especially worrisome.

Surprisingly, to date, no agent has been developed specifically to treat BD. Thus, there is an urgent need to evaluate the efficacy and safety of novel therapeutics for BD. Indeed, recent clinical evidence suggests that rapid antidepressant effects are achievable in humans. This lends an additional urgency to the development of new treatments for bipolar depression that target alternative neurobiological systems, particularly for those subgroups of patients who do not respond to any currently available pharmacological agents. New therapeutics could significantly lower morbidity and mortality for both MDD and BD and, commensurately, minimize or prevent disruption to personal, family, and occupational life and functioning as well as lower risk of suicide.

This chapter reviews some of the striking recent advances in the development of novel, rapid-acting medications for bipolar depression in particular, and highlights specific new compounds and targets with antidepressant efficacy (see Table 30.1). In addition, we present data for some targets drawn largely from MDD studies, but that we consider particularly relevant for future drug development in BD. Promising drug targets include the glutamatergic system, the cholinergic system, the melatonergic system, the glucocorticoid system, the arachidonic acid (AA) cascade, and oxidative

Table 30.1 Putative drug targets and agents for the treatment of bipolar depression

Drug target	Drug/dose	Population	Study design	Results	Presumptive mechanism	Side effects
Glutamate release and AMPA receptor. Non-competitive NMDA antagonism	Riluzole 100–200 mg/day	MDD, BD-D	OL, DB, PC	In OL BD-D and MDD, riluzole significantly decreased MADRS scores. In DB, PC it was not superior to placebo	Inhibitor of glutamate release, enhancer of AMPA trafficking and expression of glutamate reuptake transporters	Fatigue, decreased salivation, reduced sleep, nausea, weight loss, and blurred vision
NMDA antagonist	Ketamine 0.5 mg/kg/day	MDD, BD-D	OL, DB, PC	Highly effective in the first three days vs placebo in single-infusion and repeated studies	NMDA antagonism, AMPA throughput NMDA, increase in mTOR and BDNF pathway activity with neuroplasticity/synaptogenesis	Usually mild and transient. Most common are transient perceptual disturbances, dissociation, dizziness, nausea, and mild increases in blood pressure and heart rate. Long-term may induce tachyphylaxis?
Low-affinity, non-competitive NMDA antagonist (use-dependent)	Memantine 10–20 mg/day	MDD, BD-D	OL, DB, PC	Improvement in cognition and mood symptoms as add-on at four weeks (but not eight weeks)	Use-dependent NMDA antagonist, increase BDNF	Mild CNS and gastrointestinal side effects
Cholinergic (and NMDA?)	Scopolamine hydrobromide infusion 2–3–4.0 µg/kg	MDD, BD-D	DB, PC	Significant reductions in MADRS scores comparing endpoint with baseline; no manic switches	Antimuscarinic	Dry mouth, blurred vision, lightheadedness, dizziness, and hypotension; cognitive dysfunction?, euphoria similar to placebo
Cholinergic	Biperiden 12 mg/day	MDD, BD-D	OL	Significant reductions in HAM-D scores	Antimuscarinic	Similar to scopolamine

(continued)

Table 30.1 Continued

Drug target	Drug/dose	Population	Study design	Results	Presumptive mechanism	Side effects
Melatonin and Serotonergic (5-HT2C)	Agomelatine 25 mg/day	MDD, BD-D	OL, DB, PC	Meta-analysis involving 20 trials and 7,460 subjects found that agomelatine was superior to placebo	Agonist of melatonin MT$_1$ and MT$_2$ receptors and 5-HT2C antagonist	Dizziness, changes in liver function tests, and abdominal pain in more than 1%. No sexual dysfunction
Glucocorticoid synthesis (anti-glucocorticoid)	Metyrapone 2,000–4,000 mg/day	MDD, BD-D	OL, DB, PC	Superior to placebo as add-on	Inhibitor of GC synthesis	Not specified
Glucocorticoid synthesis (anti-glucocorticoid)	Ketoconazole 400–800 mg/day	MDD, BD-D	OL	No significant improvement, lack of controlled studies in BD-D	Inhibitor of GC synthesis	Nausea and constipation
GR antagonist	Mifepristone 600–1,200 mg	MDD, BD-D	OL, DB, PC	Statistically significant improvement in MADRS and cognition	GR II antagonist	No dropouts due to side effects and no manic switches
Arachidonic acid metabolism	Celecoxib 400 mg/day	MDD, BD-D	DB, PC, add-on	Celecoxib was more effective than placebo (only short-term)	COX-2 inhibitor	Well tolerated, dropped out because of rash
Oxidative stress and bioenergetics	Creatine 3-5 g/day	MDD, BD-D	OL	Significant improvement in depressive symptoms for MDD patients. Both BD-D patients developed hypomania/mania	Brain energy homeostasis	Mild adverse events: nausea and constipation. Risk of hypomania/mania
Oxidative stress and bioenergetics	N-acetyl cisteine (NAC) 1–3 g/day	MDD, BD-D	OL, DB, PC	Significant improvement, long delay to respond	Increase antioxidant glutathione levels	Very few: diarrhoea, abdominal pain, and headache

Abbreviations: AMPA—α-amino-3-hydroxyl-5-methyl-4-isoxazoleproprionic acid; BD-D—bipolar disorder, depressive episode; BDNF—brain-derived neurotrophic factor; COX—cyclooxygenase; DB—double blind; GC—glucocorticoid; GR—glucocorticoid receptor; HAM-D—Hamilton Depression Rating Scale; MADRS—Montgomery-Åsberg depression rating scale; MDD—major depressive disorder; NMDA—N-methyl-D-aspartate; OL—open label; PC—placebo-controlled stress and bioenergetics. An exhaustive review of both the clinical and preclinical evidence for these promising agents is beyond the scope of this chapter. Thus, we present clinical evidence wherever possible.

The glutamatergic system

Glutamate is the most abundant excitatory neurotransmitter in the mammalian brain, and approximately one-third of neurons in the central nervous system (CNS) use glutamate. In combination with other excitatory neurotransmitters, glutamate plays a key role in neuroplasticity, learning, and memory.[2] Furthermore, altered glutamatergic regulation is directly involved in the altered neuroplasticity and cellular resilience observed in BD. Glutamate receptor subtypes include the ionotropic and metabotropic glutamate receptors (mGluRs); both types of receptors have a wide range of effects, enzymes, downstream targets, and proposed biological models. This complexity is a key reason why some glutamatergic modulators treat mood disorders so effectively (eg, lamotrigine, ketamine) while others appear not to work (eg, memantine).

Ionotropic receptors

Three classes of ionotropic glutamate receptors have been identified based on their affinity for exogenous ligands: N-methyl-D-aspartate (NMDA), α-amino-3-hydroxyl-5-methyl-4-isoxazoleproprionic acid (AMPA), and kainate (KA). NMDA receptors have the highest affinity for glutamate.

NMDA

Preclinical evidence strongly suggests that the glutamatergic system in general—and NMDA receptors in particular—is involved in the pathophysiology of mood disorders and the mechanism of action of antidepressants.[3] Specifically, most of the evidence pertaining to the pathophysiology of mood disorders supports the presence of increased glutamate levels and activity in the brain and periphery. Some researchers have hypothesized that NMDA could even represent a convergent mechanistic target for the antidepressant action of conventional antidepressants and mood stabilizers as well as novel experimental therapeutics, precisely because chronic treatment with various classes of antidepressant agents affects NMDA receptor function (predominantly via antagonism).[3] Chronic and acute conventional antidepressants have also widely been reported to directly target NMDA receptors and dampen the presynaptic glutamate release induced by acute stress or under physiological circumstances. In addition, NMDA receptor antagonists have broadly been found to induce antidepressant-like effects in several animal models. Relatedly, enhanced glutamate levels and fewer hippocampal NMDA receptors were observed in post-mortem studies of individuals with mood disorders.[2]

AMPA

AMPA receptors play a key role in learning and memory and mediate the fast component of excitatory neurotransmission. Positive modulators of AMPA receptors, also known as AMPAkines, are allosteric effectors of the receptors. They have been extensively studied in recent years due to their potential use as a treatment for various diseases. AMPAkines are involved in activity-dependent regulation of synaptic strength and behavioural plasticity, and have been found to decrease receptor desensitization and/or deactivation rates. In preclinical studies, the rapid antidepressant effects of ketamine appeared to involve AMPA receptor activation. Increased glutamatergic activity seems key to this effect, given that AMPA receptor antagonists blocked ketamine's antidepressant effects in preclinical studies.[4] Thus, ketamine appears to exert its rapid antidepressant-like effects by enhancing AMPA relative to NMDA throughput in critical neuronal circuits and molecular pathways and targets.

Preclinical studies found that these agents exhibit antidepressant-like efficacy,[5] and several AMPA antagonists are being developed to treat MDD. These include the AMPA agonist farampator (CX-691/ORG 2448); ORG-26576, an AMPA receptor positive allosteric modulator; older AMPAkines such as levetiracetam; and more potent compounds such as coluracetam (BCI-540). While some of these agents demonstrated preliminary antidepressant efficacy in preclinical studies, they did not show promising results in initial clinical studies and thus have not been subsequently explored in the treatment of BD. As a result, they will not be discussed further in this chapter.

Metabotropic glutamate receptors (mGluRs)

mGluRs are G protein-coupled receptors that modulate glutamate levels. They are located presynaptically at glutamatergic synapses and their activation decreases neurotransmitter release, thereby limiting excitotoxic damage. Eight different classes of mGluRs have been identified and subcategorized into three subtypes based on their amino acid homology, binding properties, and activation/inhibition of second messenger/signal transduction cascades. The Group 1 metabotropic receptors—mGluR1 and mGluR5—are generally stimulatory. The Group 2 metabotropic receptors—mGluR2 and mGluR3—as well as the Group 3 metabotropic receptors—mGluR4-8—share major sequence homology (~70%) and generally inhibit glutamatergic neurotransmission. These receptors are located presynaptically at glutamatergic synapses and their activation lowers glutamate release and excitotoxic damage.

A number of mGluR2/3 antagonists and negative allosteric modulators have demonstrated antidepressant-like efficacy in preclinical models of depression (reviewed by Chaki and colleagues[6]), associated with enhanced presynaptic glutamate release. The mGluR5s are also physically and physiologically interconnected with AMPA and NMDA receptors and regulate synaptic plasticity.

Non-selective/non-competitive NMDA receptor antagonists

Ketamine

Ketamine is a non-competitive NMDA receptor antagonist that binds within the ion channel and blocks the influx of diverse ions only when the channel is open after activation.

Single-dose ketamine studies

Initial studies in this area were conducted in individuals with MDD. The first pilot study showed improvement in individuals with MDD or bipolar depression 72 hours after ketamine infusion.[7] A subsequent double-blind, placebo-controlled, crossover study found that a single ketamine infusion (0.5 mg/kg for 40 minutes) had rapid (two hours) antidepressant effects in subjects with treatment-resistant MDD.[8] In that study, more than 70% of patients responded to ketamine at 24 hours post-infusion, and 35% had a relative sustained response one week post-infusion. These rapid and robust antidepressant effects were replicated in another single-blind, non-counter-balanced design study of 10 patients with treatment-resistant depression.[9] One of the major potential limitations of these three studies, however, was the possible inadequacy of an inert (saline) placebo. To address this, another study used the short-acting benzodiazepine midazolam as a psychoactive placebo to mimic ketamine's sedative and anxiolytic effects.[10] Consistent with other clinical trials in MDD, the study found that subanaesthetic-dose ketamine infusion (0.5mg/kg x 40 minutes) was more effective than placebo 24 hours post-infusion (response rates were 64% and 28%, respectively, in subjects randomized to ketamine and midazolam).

Building on this work, other placebo-controlled studies found that ketamine, used adjunctively with lithium or valproate monotherapy, also has rapid antidepressant efficacy in patients with treatment-resistant bipolar depression. In the first study, 18 treatment-resistant subjects with bipolar depression maintained on therapeutic levels of mood stabilizers received a single subanaesthetic dose of ketamine; the patients experienced a rapid (within 40 minutes) and relatively sustained (up to three days) antidepressant response. Maximal antidepressant response was observed two days after infusion.[11] A confirmatory study using an identical design (n = 15) in bipolar depression showed similar results.[12] A recent, larger, single open-label study (n = 42) of ketamine as adjunctive therapy to mood stabilizers in patients with bipolar depression confirmed these previous results.[13] It should also be noted that ketamine seems safe for use in individuals with bipolar depression and has very low risk (similar to placebo) of inducing hypo/mania.[14]

Repeated-dose ketamine studies

Although the rapid antidepressant effect size of ketamine is large in patients with mood disorders, these antidepressant effects are also transient in most patients. Thus, repeated dosing strategies may offer more sustained antidepressant benefits. One preliminary study explored the safety, tolerability, and efficacy of repeated-dose ketamine in treatment-resistant depression.[15] Over a 12-day period, 10 unmedicated patients with treatment-resistant depression were given six open-label subanaesthetic dose (0.5 mg/kg x 40 minutes) ketamine infusions, resulting in antidepressant efficacy and a mild, transient side effect profile. Another study of 24 medication-free patients with treatment-resistant depression (including the initial 10 in the sample from aan het Rot and colleagues)[15] again administered six infusions over a 12-day period and found an antidepressant response rate of 70.8%.[16] These patients were then followed naturalistically (which allowed for traditional antidepressant treatment) over the next 83 days. The mean time to relapse was 18 days, but in about 30%

of responders, antidepressant response was maintained until the end of the naturalistic observation.

Another repeated subanaesthetic-dose (0.3 mg/kg over 100 minutes) ketamine study examined the effects of an open-label infusion in 10 patients with treatment-resistant depression. Patients received infusions twice weekly for two weeks until the subject had either received four total infusions or their symptoms remitted;[17] at the end of the study, six subjects had received the maximum number of doses (four), and three and five patients were responders and remitters, respectively; there were two non-responders. The patients were then monitored for four weeks after the test phase; 50% of the responders achieved remission while another two patients retained their initial symptom remission.

The only study to look at this issue in patients with bipolar depression administered repeated doses of ketamine to 28 medicated treatment-resistant patients with either MDD or bipolar depression. Patients received a standard dose (0.5 mg/kg × 40 minutes) of ketamine weekly or bi-weekly over three weeks for a total of three or six infusions, respectively.[18] Response was observed in 29% of all patients (n = 8), and no cognitive impairment was noted over time.

Finally, one case report described a 44-year-old patient with treatment-resistant MDD who received more than 40 ketamine infusions over several months. This patient showed initial improvement of depressive symptoms and no cognitive deficits; however, lack of improvement was observed over time, suggesting the presence of tachyphylaxis (Blier et al. 2012).[19]

Antisuicidal effects

Studies have also found that, in addition to its antidepressant and anxiolytic effects, ketamine has rapid-onset antisuicidal properties in depressed patients. In one study, 33 patients with treatment-resistant depression received a single open-label infusion of ketamine (0.5mg/kg); measures of suicidal ideation decreased within 40 minutes of infusion, an effect that was maintained for up to four hours post-infusion.[20] Other studies of patients with treatment-resistant depression found that ketamine infusion reduced both explicit suicidal ideation and implicit suicidal thinking.[21] Another study evaluated 14 acutely suicidal patients in a psychiatric emergency room and found that open-label, intravenous ketamine (0.2 mg/kg intravenous ketamine, administered over one to two minutes) had rapid antisuicidal and antidepressant efficacy.[22]

As regards bipolar depression in particular, a recent study evaluated improvement of suicidality in 108 patients with treatment-resistant MDD or bipolar depression who received a single, standard-dose infusion of ketamine and found rapid improvements in suicidal ideation compared with placebo.[23]

Other non-selective/non-competitive NMDA receptor antagonists

Memantine

Memantine is a low-trapping, non-competitive NMDA antagonist that was found to have antidepressant-like effects in preclinical models.[24] In clinical studies, an eight-week, randomized, placebo-controlled investigation of subjects with bipolar depression who had previously not responded to lamotrigine found that escalating-dose memantine had superior antidepressant improvement compared with placebo at four weeks; however, efficacy was not maintained at endpoint (eight weeks).[25] Interestingly, memantine monotherapy (20–50 mg/day) also had antimanic effects in a three-week, open-label trial of 33 subjects with acute mania.[26]

Dextromethorphan

The cough suppressant dextromethorphan, a derivate of morphine with sedative and dissociative properties, is a non-selective, non-competitive NMDA receptor antagonist. Other molecular mechanisms are also present in its mechanism of action, including serotonin transporters, calcium channels, sigma receptors, and muscarinic sites. In animal models, dextromethorphan exerted antidepressant-like effects similar to those observed with both conventional (eg, imipramine) and rapid-acting antidepressants (eg, ketamine).[27] Dextromethorphan was studied in a randomized, placebo-controlled trial as add-on therapy to valproic acid in BD; no significant group differences were seen between groups as assessed by mean Young Mania Rating Scale (YMRS) scores and Hamilton Rating Scale for Depression (HAM-D) scores.[28] Another retrospective chart review of 22 patients with either BD-II or BD not otherwise specified (BD-NOS) found that adding 20 mg dextromethorphan and 10 mg quinidine (a cytochrome 2D6 inhibitor) once or twice daily to the current medication regimen significantly improved Clinical Global Impression (CGI) scale scores.[29] This dextromethorphan–quinidine combination—Nuedexta—is approved for the treatment of pseudobulbar affect, and is now being studied for treatment-resistant depression (NCT01882829). One case report found that Nuedexta had anti-depressant effects in a single depressed patient with emotional lability.[30]

mGluR antagonists

To achieve efficacy, presynaptic mGluR2 agonists seem to reduce excessive glutamate release, while mGluR2/3 antagonists seem to enhance synaptic glutamate levels, commensurately boosting AMPA receptor transmission and firing rates and extracellular monoamine levels. Several mGluR2/3 antagonists, as well as the negative allosteric modulator RO4995819, were found to have antidepressant-like efficacy in rodent models of depression (reviewed by Chaki and colleagues[6]). The safety and tolerability of mGluR2/3 modulators have also been studied in healthy volunteers (NCT01547703 and NCT01546051). Though animal studies suggest that this class of glutamate modulators might display clinical utility for treating both depressive and manic episodes, mGluR2/3 modulators have not yet shown convincing results in clinical trials for mood disorders. Specifically, RG1578 (an mGluR2 negative allosteric modulator) was tested clinically; despite positive preliminary findings, final results were disappointing.[31]

The mGluR5s are expressed pre- and post-synaptically and are involved in AMPA receptor internalization, a key mechanism for modulating synaptic plasticity. mGluR5s are also physically and physiologically interconnected with NMDA receptors. In diverse behavioural models, several mGluR5 antagonists were found to have antidepressant-like effects.[6] Among the mGluR5 antagonists recently tested in clinical trials for treatment-resistant MDD are AZD2066 and the mGluR5 negative allosteric modulator basimglurant (RO4917523).[32] Basimglurant, in particular, has shown promising results in two clinical trials (NCT00809562, NCT01437657). In a nine-week, double-blind, placebo-controlled study of 333 individuals with treatment-resistant MDD, basimglurant (0.5 mg or 1.5/day adjunctive to ongoing treatment with selective serotonin reuptake inhibitors (SSRIs) or serotonin-noradrenaline reuptake inhibitors (SNRIs)) had significant antidepressant effects;[32] further studies are underway. In contrast, AZD2066 (12–18 mg/day for six weeks as monotherapy) was no more effective in patients with MDD than placebo and the SNRI duloxetine (NCT01145755). Studies evaluating the potent and selective mGluR5 antagonist fenobam were discontinued because of psychostimulant effects.[33]

Glutamatergic modulators that act indirectly to alter glutamate release

Riluzole

Riluzole, which is Food and Drug Administration (FDA)-approved for the treatment of amyotrophic lateral sclerosis, increases glutamate reuptake and neurotrophic factor synthesis. In initial open-label clinical trials, riluzole induced antidepressant effects and was well tolerated in patients with either treatment-resistant MDD or bipolar depression.[34,35] In the bipolar depression trial, riluzole (100–200 mg/day for six weeks) was evaluated in 14 subjects as add-on therapy to lithium.[35] There was a significant treatment effect, and no switch into hypo/mania was observed.

In patients with MDD, one study found that riluzole (50 mg/twice daily) led to a 36% decrease in HAM-D scores after one week of treatment.[36] However, another four-week, placebo-controlled, double-blind study of 42 patients with treatment-resistant MDD who had initially received a single ketamine infusion found that riluzole (100–200 mg/day) had no antidepressant effects.[37] Another study found a similar lack of efficacy when riluzole was used as an augmentation strategy,[38] suggesting that additional controlled trials are needed to clarify its potential efficacy.

The cholinergic system

The adrenergic–cholinergic balance hypothesis of BD was first proposed more than 40 years ago; depression was postulated to be associated with high cholinergic compared with adrenergic activity, while mania was proposed to be associated with hypocholinergia and increased adrenergic signalling. Interestingly, muscarinic agonists have demonstrated robust antimanic effects consistent enough to induce depressive switch.[39] Elevated muscarinic sensitivity has also been associated with depressive-like behaviours reversed by antimuscarinic agents.[40]

Evidence supports cholinergic system dysregulation in BD and, indeed, one study linked 19 cholinergic genes and BD.[41] In addition, a post-mortem study described lower M_2 and M_3 receptor binding in the frontal cortex of subjects with BD,[42] and a positron emission tomography (PET) imaging study observed reduced M_2 receptor binding in the anterior cingulate cortex of subjects with BD.[43] Cholinergic hyperactivity was also found to worsen depressive symptoms in subjects with MDD. Increased sensitivity to cholinergic activity based on neuroendocrine and pupillary responses was described in individuals with depression,[44] which was found to be blunted during manic episodes.[45] Interestingly, lithium and valproate normalized pupillary responses associated with their antimanic efficacy.[45] Finally, a single-photon emission computed tomography (SPECT) study found a decrease in β_2 nicotinic receptor availability in individuals with bipolar depression compared to both euthymic and control subjects.[46]

Controlled pilot studies with the acetylcholinesterase inhibitor physostigmine found that single or multiple intravenous injections of this agent rapidly but transiently decreased manic symptoms.[47] Similar investigations with the cholinesterase inhibitor donepezil in manic episodes obtained mixed results.[48] Another early study also found that the anticholinergic agent biperiden had antidepressant effects in 10 severely depressed inpatients.[49]

In this context, several randomized, double-blind, placebo-controlled studies have been conducted with intravenous doses of the anticholinergic agent scopolamine as add-on or monotherapy in subjects with bipolar depression or MDD.[50,51,52] Scopolamine is a muscarinic receptor antagonist that acts at all muscarinic receptor subtypes (M_1–M_5) with comparatively equivalent potency. In a placebo-controlled, double-blind, crossover, pilot study of patients with MDD (n = 9) and bipolar depression (n = 9), a rapid and robust antidepressant and anxiolytic response to scopolamine was observed, especially with a dose of 4 ug/Kg (compared with 2 or 3 ug/Kg).[53] Interestingly, scopolamine's antidepressant effects persisted for two weeks, and repeated dosing provided additional benefit and extended response. Limitations to the use of this agent include anticholinergic side effects and the risk of psychosis at higher doses, both of which may limit its broad clinical use.

The melatonergic system

Melatonin is a pineal gland neurohormone that regulates circadian-related and sleep-related responses. The key target for melatonin is the suprachiasmatic nucleus (SCN), which is implicated in diverse biological functions such as circadian rhythms, mood, behaviour, sleep regulation, and adipokine levels. It also has immunomodulatory, antioxidant, neuroprotective, and additional chronobiological effects.[54]

The two melatonin receptors (MT_1 and MT_2) are high affinity G_i/G_0 protein-coupled receptors with elevated expression in the brain. Individuals with BD were found to display circadian rhythm abnormalities and changes in sleep patterns during depressive and manic episodes. These abnormalities include circadian preference for evening,[55] sleep–wake irregularities, and abnormal actimetric parameters.[56] Furthermore, supersensitivity to melatonin suppression by light has been observed in subjects with BD, monozygotic twins discordant for BD, and the non-affected offspring of BD probands, though the findings were not confirmed in a similar study evaluating euthymic BD subjects.[57] In addition, variations in the melatonin biosynthesis pathway have been shown in BD. For instance, subjects with BD display altered melatonin suppression in response to light, suggesting a genetic trait marker in BD.[57] A polymorphism in *GPR50* (H9, melatonin-related receptor) was also associated with increased risk of BD, but this finding was not subsequently replicated.[58,59]

While no controlled studies of exogenous melatonin have been published in BD, lithium and valproate were found to lower melatonin light sensitivity in healthy volunteers,[60,61] with mixed results in subjects with BD.[62,63] In addition, adjunctive use of melatonin agonists to treat sleep disorders in patients with BD was found to improve their metabolic profile.[64]

With regard to specific therapeutics, adjunctive use of ramelteon—a selective MT_1 and MT_2 receptor agonist—was effective in maintaining mood stabilization (8 mg/day, 23 weeks double-blind, n = 83) in BD patients in euthymia who were also experiencing sleep disturbances.[65]

Agomelatine is a melatonin MT_1 and MT_2 receptor agonist and a 5-HT(2C) receptor antagonist.[66] In three controlled, large, multicentre clinical trials in MDD, agomelatine was more effective than placebo and well tolerated.[67,68,69] In bipolar depression, a recent six-week trial with agomelatine (25 mg/day, n = 21) found that 81% of patients had substantial antidepressant response at study endpoint, and 47% showed response during the first week of treatment.[70] There were no dropouts secondary to adverse events. In a 24-week, placebo-controlled, double-blind, randomized trial in MDD, agomelatine was more effective than placebo, and a significantly lower relapse rate was observed with agomelatine (n = 133) than placebo (n = 174) during a six-month extension phase.[71] Finally, a recent meta-analysis of 20 trials involving 7,460 subjects found that agomelatine improved depressive symptoms significantly more than placebo and was as effective as other antidepressants.[72] Further studies are required to confirm these promising preliminary findings.

The glucocorticoid system

Dysfunction of the hypothalamic-pituitary adrenal (HPA) axis has been associated with BD. For instance, hypercortisolemia may be central to the etiopathogenesis of both depressive symptoms and the neurocognitive deficits observed in BD. Thus, attempts to normalize the effects of cortisol, which may potentially restore HPA axis integrity, have been the focus of recent research. Interestingly, glucocorticoids acutely increase glutamate release in the prefrontal cortex and amygdala. The anti-glucocorticoid agents studied in the treatment of mood disorders include cortisol synthesis inhibitors (aminoglutethimide, ketoconazole, and metyrapone) and corticosteroid receptor antagonists (mifepristone), as well as dehydroepiandrosterone (DHEA) (reviewed in Quiroz et al.[73]). Only a few of these compounds have been tested in bipolar depression.

The non-selective, synthetic, glucocorticoid receptor antagonist mifepristone (RU-486) was found to have antidepressant and antipsychotic effects in individuals with psychotic depression.[74] Specifically, inpatients with psychotic depression and HAM-D21 scores of 18 or greater who received 600 or 1,200 mg/day RU-486 showed significant decreases in their Brief Psychiatric Rating Scale (BPRS) and HAM-D21 scores.[74] In drug-free subjects with psychotic depression, a seven-day treatment with mifepristone followed by treatment as usual was both efficacious and well tolerated.[75] In a six-week, pilot study of individuals with treatment-resistant bipolar depression, mifepristone (600 mg/day) improved depressive symptoms and cognition over placebo.[76] Interestingly, cognitive improvement was inversely associated with basal cortisol levels, supporting the presence of an anti-glucocorticoid effect. However, at least one letter to the editor found that RU-486 had no antidepressant efficacy in psychotic depression.[77] Taken together, the evidence suggests that RU-486 has predominantly short-term benefits during acute depressive episodes; nevertheless, long-term treatment could be associated with significant side effects that have yet to be properly assessed.

Inhibitors of glucocorticoid synthesis—a class that includes ketoconazole and metyrapone—are expected to potentiate the efficacy of antidepressants and, indeed, these agents had antidepressant effects in clinical and preclinical studies.[73] In a double-blind, randomized, controlled trial in MDD, metyrapone was superior to placebo as add-on therapy and accelerated the onset of antidepressant action.[78] A recent large, placebo-controlled, randomized, multicentre study from the United Kingdom evaluating metyrapone augmentation in treatment-resistant depression was completed, but results are not yet available (NCT01375920).

Similarly, add-on treatment with ketoconazole (up to 800 mg/day) was investigated in six patients with treatment-resistant BD.[79] A significant improvement in depressive symptoms was observed in three patients who received at least 400 mg/day, with no induction of manic symptoms; ketoconazole also decreased cortisol levels. One study that evaluated the five trials conducted with ketoconazole in nonpsychotic depression (either MDD or BD) found a significant difference in favour of treatment (summarized by Gallagher and colleagues[80]). However, the relative risk for drug interactions of this agent may limit its chronic use in mood disorders.

In the search for effective novel antidepressants, trials have also examined corticotropin releasing factor (CRF); glucocorticoid receptor antagonists; neuropeptides such as neurokinin 1 (NK1); vasopressin; orexin antagonists; and DHEA. This work has been conducted almost exclusively in MDD patients. Despite promising preclinical evidence, clinical results have been mixed and largely disappointing[31] and will not be discussed further in this chapter.

The arachidonic acid (AA) signalling cascade

The AA signalling pathway has been implicated in the pathophysiology and therapeutics of mood disorders. Strong evidence links the pathophysiology of depression with cytokine dysregulation,[81] and the AA pathway is a key modulator of several brain second messenger pathways associated with, among other effects, the release of AA and cyclooxygenase (COX)-mediated generation of eicosanoid metabolites such as thromboxanes and prostaglandins.

In a six-week study of individuals with MDD, the COX-2 inhibitor celecoxib (400 mg/day adjunctive to reboxetine) was more effective than placebo.[82] Another placebo-controlled study of 37 subjects with MDD examined celecoxib (400 mg/day as add-on therapy to fluoxetine) and found that it significantly decreased depression scores compared to placebo.[83] An eight-week study of 30 first-episode women with MDD similarly found that celecoxib (200 mg/day as add-on therapy to sertraline) elicited a greater antidepressant response than placebo.[84] In bipolar depression specifically, a six-week, double-blind, placebo-controlled study of celecoxib in bipolar depression (400 mg/day adjunctive to mood stabilizers) found that celecoxib demonstrated superior antidepressant effects only during the first week of treatment.[85] It should be noted, however, that the ability of celecoxib to enter the blood–brain barrier remains uncertain. In addition, higher risk of adverse cardiovascular adverse effects may limit the long-term use of selective COX-2 inhibitors.

Interestingly, a recent 12-week, randomized, placebo-controlled study (n = 60) evaluated the tumour necrosis factor antagonist infliximab (5 mg/kg infusion) at baseline, two weeks, and four weeks in patients with MDD; no efficacy compared to placebo was observed.[86]

Oxidative stress and bioenergetics

Creatine

Creatine is a non-essential dietary element and precursor of phosphocreatine (PCr); it plays a key role in brain energy homeostasis. When energy is required, PCr is converted to creatine, which increases intracellular concentrations of adenosine triphosphate (ATP). Hippocampal changes in brain creatine kinase, which phosphorylates creatine, have been observed in post-mortem BD studies.[87,88] Lower hippocampal and prefrontal cortex creatine kinase mRNA expression have also been described in post-mortem BD.[89] Interestingly, creatine supplementation alters brain high-energy phosphate metabolism and may be a novel approach for treating BD. One open-label study evaluating 3–5 mg/day of creatine monohydrate as adjunctive treatment in patients with either MDD or bipolar depression found that this agent significantly improved depressive symptoms.[90] Nevertheless, two patients with bipolar depression had a transient switch to hypo/mania. Creatine also improved depressive symptoms in co-morbid depression and fibromyalgia.[91]

N-acetyl cysteine (NAC)

Levels of glutathione—which is the most abundant antioxidant protein in the brain—are known to be altered in individuals with BD.[92] N-acetylcysteine (NAC) is a precursor of glutathione and increases its levels. NAC is thought to enhance glial cystine uptake and increase glial cystine levels via a cystine-glutamate antiporter that induces glutamate release into the extracellular space.

A number of controlled and uncontrolled studies have investigated NAC for the treatment of both acute episodes and maintenance in BD. The first placebo-controlled, randomized, double-blind investigation in BD evaluating NAC (n = 75; 1 g/twice daily added on to treatment) found that NAC displayed superior antidepressant efficacy compared with placebo, showing moderate to high effect sizes on measures of depression, quality of life, and functionality scores.[93] The authors suggested that NAC's efficacy might be due to its ability to decrease oxidative stress during mood episodes. In another analysis of 14 subjects with BD-II, improvement of depressive and manic symptoms was more consistent in those receiving NAC than in the placebo group.[94] Similarly, a large, eight-week, open-label trial of 149 patients with bipolar depression showed that adjunctive use of NAC significantly improved depression rating scale scores, overall functioning, and quality of life.[95] Thus, NAC appears to improve symptoms during mood episodes; however, this agent does not appear to alter the frequency of cycling or mood stability. In addition, in a large, 12-week, randomized, controlled, add-on trial (n = 252) of patients with MDD, those receiving NAC showed antidepressant improvement compared with the placebo group.[96]

Cytidine

Cytidine is a pyrimidine component of RNA that regulates dysfunctional neuronal-glial glutamate cycling and affects mitochondrial function, cerebral phospholipid metabolism, and catecholamine synthesis. In bipolar depression, the therapeutic role of cytidine was evaluated in a 12-week, placebo-controlled investigation of 35 subjects with bipolar depression who received cytidine as add-on therapy to valproate; depressive symptoms for those receiving cytidine remitted more rapidly—within the first week. This effect was mediated by a decrease in cerebral glutamate and/or glutamine levels assessed via proton magnetic resonance spectroscopy (MRS) at baseline and two, four, and 12 weeks after oral cytidine administration.[97] The authors speculated that cytidine supplementation may be effective in bipolar depression by directly modulating brain glutamate/glutamine levels.

Translating novel targets into new, improved, rapid-acting antidepressants

As previously discussed, promising systems for the development of new, improved therapeutics for BD—and bipolar depression in particular—include (1) the glutamatergic system, (2) the cholinergic system, (3) the melatonergic system, (4) the glucocorticoid system, (5) the AA cascade, and (6) oxidative stress and bioenergetics (see Figure 30.1). None of these new pharmacological approaches are FDA-approved for BD. Though a good number of placebo-controlled studies have been carried out—particularly with regard to glutamatergic agents—most of the studies to date comprise case reports, case series, or early proof-of-concept studies, most with relatively small samples. Nevertheless, because these findings mostly originate from proof-of-concept studies, they are likely to be relevant to future directions in drug development for BD.

As the previously discussed review has underscored, to date the most promising novel targets for achieving rapid antidepressant effects are the ionotropic glutamate receptors. Moving forward towards the goal of personalized medicine will require health professionals to identify potential responders a priori. Towards this end, the search for the unique biosignatures of rapid-acting antidepressants—those whose validity have been tested in larger samples—will require the clear evaluation of drug kinetics, ability to pass through the blood–brain barrier, and information regarding brain distribution. In the future, it is possible that trials using enriched samples may

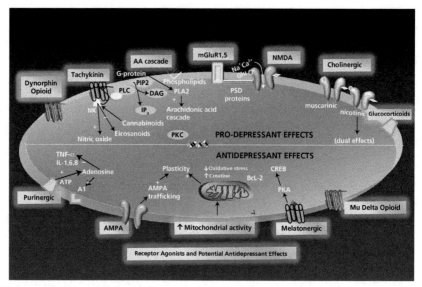

Figure 30.1 Putative therapeutic targets for mood disorders. The glutamatergic system (AMPA receptors, NMDA receptors, and mGluRs), the cholinergic system, the melatonergic system, the glucocorticoid system, the arachidonic acid (AA) cascade, and oxidative stress and bioenergetics are all promising targets for the development of novel therapeutics for the treatment of bipolar depression. Other targets in mood disorders include mitochondrial activity, the opioid system, the purinergic system, and the tachykinin neuropeptide system.

be more efficient, given that participants would more likely receive the potentially most effective agent available based on their biomarker signatures. As we define our next steps in psychiatric research, it will be critical to fully understand the true clinical utility of this novel treatment approach and the key aspects of this concept for public health. Questions crucial to future investigations include: (1) Should treatments be of long or short duration? (2) Should an agent be used adjunctively or as monotherapy? (3) What is the best route of administration? (4) Should an agent be tested in treatment-resistant cases only? And (5) Should particular diagnostic subtypes be emphasized in research? Relatedly, the novel hypothesis that some receptor-specific antagonists could be effective in very specific, well-defined subpopulations based on their biological profile and clinical dimensions is an important paradigm shift in the field of psychiatric research. Specifically, the recent shift toward RDoC symptom clusters may emphasize the potential validity of such studies and ultimately allow us to identify subgroups of patients with glutamate dysfunction-based depressive episodes, and to treat them more efficiently and effectively.

Continued exploration of new, rapid-acting antidepressant agents holds considerable promise for developing novel and urgently-needed treatments for bipolar depression. Currently available antidepressants take weeks to achieve their full effects, which leaves patients particularly vulnerable to devastating symptoms and elevated risk of self-harm. Thus, novel therapeutics that could exert rapid and sustained antidepressant effects within hours or even days could have a substantial beneficial impact on patients' quality of life as well as public health. In the same vein, novel therapeutics could benefit the large proportion of patients who do not respond to currently available therapies. As this chapter has underscored, the novel avenues for research and new agents discussed are revolutionizing the field of psychiatric research, challenging old paradigms and current limitations, and bringing hope to those who must live with these devastating disorders.

Disclosures and role of funding source

Funding for this work was supported by the Intramural Research Program at the National Institute of Mental Health, National Institutes of Health (IRP-NIMH-NIH; ZIA MH002927). The authors have no conflicts of interest to disclose, financial or otherwise.

References

1. Sachs GS, Nierenberg AA, Calabrese JR, Marangell LB, Wisniewski SR, Gyulai L, Friedman ES, Bowden CL, Fossey MD, Ostacher MJ, Ketter TA, Patel J, Hauser P, and Rapport D. Effectiveness of adjunctive antidepressant treatment for bipolar depression, N Engl J Med 2007;**356**:1711–22.

2. Machado-Vieira R, Manji HK, and Zarate CA. The role of the tripartite glutamatergic synapse in the pathophysiology and therapeutics of mood disorders, Neuroscientist 2009;**15**(5):525–39.

3. Skolnick P. Modulation of glutamate receptors: strategies for the development of novel antidepressants, Amino Acids 2002;**23**(1–3):153–9.

4. Duman RS, Li N, Liu RJ, Duric V, and Aghajanian GK. Signaling pathways underlying the rapid antidepressant actions of ketamine, Neuropharmacology 2012;**62**:35–41.

5. Bleakman D, Alt A, and Witkin JM. AMPA receptors in the therapeutic management of depression, CNS Neurol Disord Drug Targets 2007;**6**:117–26.

6. Chaki S, Ago Y, Palucha-Paniewiera A, Matrisciano F, and Pilc A. mGlu2/3 and mGlu5 receptors: potential targets for novel antidepressants, Neuropharmacology 2013;**66**:40–52.

7. Berman RM, Cappiello A, Anand A, Oren DA, Heninger GR, Charney DS, and Krystal JH. Antidepressant effects of ketamine in depressed patients, Biol Psychiatry 2000;**47**(4):351–4.

8. Zarate CA, Jr, Singh JB, Carlson PJ, Brutsche NE, Ameli R, Luckenbaugh DA, Charney DS, and Manji HK. A randomized trial of an N-methyl-D-aspartate antagonist in treatment-resistant major depression, Arch Gen Psychiatry 2006;**63**(8):856–64.

9. Valentine GW, Mason GF, Gomez R, Fasula M, Watzl J, Pittman B, Krystal JH, and Sanacora G. The antidepressant effect of ketamine is not associated with changes in occipital amino acid neurotransmitter content as measured by [(1)H]-MRS, Psychiatry Res 2011;**191**(2):122–7.

10. Murrough JW, Iosifescu DV, Chang LC, Al Jurdi RK, Green CE, Perez AM, Iqbal S, Pillemer S, Foulkes A, Shah A, Charney DS, and Mathew SJ. Antidepressant efficacy of ketamine in treatment-resistant major depression: a two-site randomized controlled trial, Am J Psychiatry 2013a;**170**(10):1134–42.

11. Diazgranados N, Ibrahim L, Brutsche N, Newberg A, Kronstein P, Khalife S, Kammerer WA, Quezado Z, Luckenbaugh DA, Salvadore G, Machado-Vieira R, Manji HK, and Zarate CA. A randomized add-on trial of an N-methyl-D-aspartate antagonist in treatment-resistant bipolar depression, Arch Gen Psychiatry 2010a;67:793–802.

12. Zarate CA, Brutsche N, Ibrahim L, Franco-Chaves J, Diazgranados N, Cravchick A, Selter J, Marquardt C, Liberty V, and Luckenbaugh DA. Replication of ketamine's antidepressant efficacy in bipolar depression: a randomized controlled add-on trial, Biol Psychiatry 2012;71:939–46.

13. Permoda-Osip A, Kisielewski J, Bartkowska-Sniatkowska A, and Rybakowski JK. Single ketamine infusion and neurocognitive performance in bipolar depression, Pharmacopsychiatry 2015;48:78–9.

14. Niciu MJ, Luckenbaugh D, Ionescu DF, Mathews D, Richards EM, and Zarate CA. Subanesthetic dose ketamine does not induce an affective switch in three independent samples of treatment-resistant major depression, Biol Psychiatry 2013;74:e23–4.

15. aan het Rot M, Collins KA, Murrough JW, Perez AM, Reich DL, Charney DS, and Mathew SJ. Safety and efficacy of repeated-dose intravenous ketamine for treatment-resistant depression, Biol Psychiatry 2010;67(2):139–45.

16. Murrough JW, Perez AM, Pillemer S, Stern J, Parides MK, aan het Rot M, Collins KA, Mathew SJ, Charney DS, and Iosifescu DV. Rapid and longer-term antidepressant effects of repeated ketamine infusions in treatment-resistant major depression, Biol Psychiatry 2013b;74(4):250–6.

17. Rasmussen KG, Lineberry TW, Galardy CW, Kung S, Lapid MI, Palmer BA, Ritter MJ, Schak KM, Sola CL, Hanson AJ, and Frye MA. Serial infusions of low-dose ketamine for major depression, J Psychopharmacol 2013;27(5):444–50.

18. Diamond PR, Farmery AD, Atkinson S, Haldar J, Williams N, Cowen PJ, Geddes JR, and McShane R. Ketamine infusions for treatment resistant depression: a series of 28 patients treated weekly or twice weekly in an ECT clinic, J Psychopharmacol 2014;28(6):536–44.

19. Blier P, Zigman D, and Blier J. On the safety and benefits of repeated intravenous injections of ketamine for depression, Biol Psychiatry 2012;72(4):e11–12.

20. DiazGranados N, Ibrahim LA, Brutsche NE, Ameli R, Henter ID, Luckenbaugh DA, Machado-Vieira R, and Zarate CA, Jr. Rapid resolution of suicidal ideation after a single infusion of an N-methyl-D-aspartate antagonist in patients with treatment-resistant major depressive disorder, J Clin Psychiatry 2010b;71(12):1605–11.

21. Price RB, Iosifescu DV, Murrough JW, Chang LC, Al Jurdi RK, Iqbal SZ, Soleimani L, Charney DS, Foulkes AL, and Mathew SJ. Effects of ketamine on explicit and implicit suicidal cognition: a randomized controlled trial in treatment-resistant depression, Depress Anxiety 2014;31(4):335–43.

22. Larkin GL and Beautrais AL. A preliminary naturalistic study of low-dose ketamine for depression and suicide ideation in the emergency department, Int J Neuropsychopharmacol 2011;1–5.

23. Ballard ED, Ionescu DF, Vande Voort JL, Niciu MJ, Richards EM, Luckenbaugh DA, Brutsche NE, Ameli R, Furey ML, and Zarate CA, Jr. Improvement in suicidal ideation after ketamine infusion: relationship to reductions in depression and anxiety, J Psychiatr Res 2014;58:161–6.

24. Rogoz Z, Skuza G, Maj J, and Danysz W. Synergistic effect of uncompetitive NMDA receptor antagonists and antidepressant drugs in the forced swimming test in rats, Neuropharmacology 2002;42:1024–30.

25. **Anand A, Gunn AD, Barkay G, Karne HS, Nurnberger JI, Mathew SJ, and Ghosh S.** Early antidepressant effect of memantine during augmentation of lamotrigine inadequate response in bipolar depression: a double-blind, randomized, placebo-controlled trial, Bipolar Disord 2012;**14**(1):64–70.

26. **Keck PE, Jr, Hsu KS, Papadakis K, and Russo J, Jr.** Memantine efficacy and safety in patients with acute mania associated with bipolar I disorder: a pilot evaluation, Clin Neuropharmacol 2009;**32**:199–204.

27. **Nguyen L and Matsumoto RR.** Involvement of AMPA receptors in the antidepressant-like effects of dextromethorphan in mice, Behav Brain Res 2015;**295**:26–34.

28. **Lee SY, Chen SL, Chang YH, Chen SH, Chu CH, Huang SY, Tzeng NS, Wang CL, Lee IH, Yeh TL, Yang YK, and Lu RB.** The DRD2/ANKK1 gene is associated with response to add-on dextromethorphan treatment in bipolar disorder, J Affect Disord 2012;**138**:295–300.

29. **Kelly TF and Lieberman DZ.** The utility of the combination of dextromethorphan and quinidine in the treatment of bipolar II and bipolar NOS, J Affect Disord 2014;**167**:333–5.

30. **Messias E and Everett B.** Dextromethorphan and quinidine combination in emotional lability associated with depression: a case report, Prim Care Companion CNS Disord 2012;**14**:PCC.12I01400.

31. **Dale E, Bang-Andersen B, and Sanchez C.** Emerging mechanisms and treatments for depression beyond SSRIs and SNRIs, Biochem Pharmacol 2015;**95**:81–97.

32. **Quiroz J, Tamburri P, Deptula D, Banken L, Beyer U, Fontoura P, and Santarelli L.** The efficacy and safety of basimglurant as adjunctive therapy in major depression: a randomized, double-blind, placebo controlled study, Neuropsychopharmacology 2014;**39**:S376–7.

33. **Palucha A and Pilc A.** Metabotropic glutamate receptor ligands as possible anxiolytic and antidepressant drugs, Pharmacol Ther 2007;**115**:116–47.

34. **Zarate CA, Payne JL, Quiroz J, Sporn J, Denicoff KK, Luckenbaugh D, Charney DS, and Manji HK.** An open-label trial of riluzole in patients with treatment-resistant major depression, Am J Psychiatry 2004;**161**(1):171–4.

35. **Zarate CA, Quiroz JA, Singh JB, Denicoff KD, De Jesus G, Luckenbaugh DA, Charney DS, and Manji HK.** An open-label trial of the glutamate-modulating agent riluzole in combination with lithium for the treatment of bipolar depression, Biol Psychiatry 2005;**57**(4):430–2.

36. **Sanacora G, Kendell SF, Levin Y, Simen AA, Fenton LR, Coric V, and Krystal JH.** Preliminary evidence of riluzole efficacy in antidepressant-treated patients with residual depressive symptoms, Biol Psychiatry 2007;**61**(6):822–5.

37. **Ibrahim L, Diazgranados N, Franco-Chaves J, Brutsche N, Henter ID, Kronstein P, Moaddel R, Wainer I, Luckenbaugh DA, Manji HK, and Zarate CA.** Course of improvement in depressive symptoms to a single intravenous infusion of ketamine vs add-on riluzole: results from a 4-week, double-blind, placebo-controlled study, Neuropsychopharmacology 2012;**37**:1526–33.

38. **Mathew SJ, Murrough JW, aan het Rot M, Collins KA, Reich DL, and Charney DS.** Riluzole for relapse prevention following intravenous ketamine in treatment-resistant depression: a pilot randomized, placebo-controlled continuation trial, Int J Neuropsychopharmacol 2010;**13**(1):71–82.

39. **Overstreet DH, Russell RW, Hay DA, and Crocker AD**. Selective breeding for increased cholinergic function: biometrical genetic analysis of muscarinic responses, Neuropsychopharmacology 1992;7:197–204.

40. **Gao ZG and Jacobson KA**. Allosteric modulation and functional selectivity of G protein-coupled receptors, Drug Discov Today Technol 2013;10:e237–43.

41. **Shi J, Hattori E, Zou H, Badner JA, Christian SL, Gershon ES, and Liu C**. No evidence for association between 19 cholinergic genes and bipolar disorder, Am J Med Genet B Neuropsychiatr Genet 2007;144:715–23.

42. **Gibbons AS, Scarr E, McLean C, Sundram S, and Dean B**. Decreased muscarinic receptor binding in the frontal cortex of bipolar disorder and major depressive disorder subjects, J Affect Disord 2009;116:184–91.

43. **Cannon DM, Carson RE, Nugent AC, Eckelman WC, Kiesewetter DO, Williams J, Rollis D, Drevets M, Gandhi S, Solorio G, and Drevets WC**. Reduced muscarinic type 2 receptor binding in subjects with bipolar disorder, Arch Gen Psychiatry 2006;63:741–7.

44. **Dilsaver SC**. Pathophysiology of 'cholinoceptor supersensitivity' in affective disorders, Biol Psychiatry 1986;21:813–29.

45. **Sokolski KN and DeMet EM**. Cholinergic sensitivity predicts severity of mania, Psychiatry Res 2000;95:195–200.

46. **Hannestad JO, Cosgrove KP, Dellagioia NF, Perkins E, Bois F, Bhagwagar Z, Seibyl JP, McClure-Begley TD, Picciotto MR, and Esterlis I**. Changes in the cholinergic system between bipolar depression and euthymia as measured with [I]5IA single photon emission computed tomography, Biol Psychiatry 2013;74:768–76.

47. **Khouzam HR and Kissmeyer PM**. Physostigmine temporarily and dramatically reversing acute mania, Gen Hosp Psychiatry 1996;18:203–4.

48. **Eden Evins A, Demopulos C, Nierenberg A, Culhane MA, Eisner L, and Sachs GS**. A double-blind, placebo-controlled trial of adjunctive donepezil in treatment-resistant mania, Bipolar Disord 2006;8:75–80.

49. **Kasper S, Moises HW, and Beckmann H**. The anticholinergic biperiden in depressive disorders, Pharmacopsychiatria 1981;14:195–8.

50. **Drevets WC, Zarate CAJ, and Furey ML**. Antidepressant effects of the muscarinic cholinergic receptor antagonist scopolamine: a review, Biol Psychiatry 2013;73:1156–63.

51. **Jaffe RJ, Novakovic V, and Peselow ED**. Scopolamine as an antidepressant: a systematic review, Clin Neuropharmacol 2013;36:24–6.

52. **Khajavi D, Farokhnia M, Modabbernia A, Ashrafi M, Abbasi SH, Tabrizi M, and Akhondzadeh S**. Oral scopolamine augmentation in moderate to severe major depressive disorder: a randomized, double-blind, placebo-controlled study, J Clin Psychiatry 2012;73:1428–33.

53. **Furey ML and Drevets WC**. Antidepressant efficacy of the antimuscarinic drug scopolamine: a randomized, placebo-controlled clinical trial, Arch Gen Psychiatry 2006;63:1121–9.

54. **Pacchierotti C, Iapichino S, Bossini L, Pieraccini F, and Castrogiovanni P**. Melatonin in psychiatric disorders: a review on the melatonin involvement in psychiatry, Front Neuroendocrinol 2001;22:18–32.

55. **Ahn YM, Chang J, Joo YH, Kim SC, and Lee KY**. Chronotype distribution in bipolar I disorder and schizophrenia in a Korean sample, Bipolar Disord 2008;10:271–5.

56. **Millar A, Espie CA, and Scott J**. The sleep of remitted bipolar outpatients: a controlled naturalistic study using actigraphy, J Affect Disord 2004;80:145–53.

57. **Hallam KT, Olver JS**, and **Norman TR**. Melatonin sensitivity to light in monozygotic twins discordant for bipolar I disorder, Aust N Z J Psychiatry 2005c;**39**(10):947.

58. **Alaerts M, Venken T, Lenaerts AS, De Zutter S, Norrback KF, Adolfsson R**, and **Del-Favero J**. Lack of association of an insertion/deletion polymorphism in the G protein-coupled receptor 50 with bipolar disorder in a Northern Swedish population, Psychiatr Genet 2006;**16**(6):235–6.

59. **Thomson PA, Wray NR, Thomson AM, Dunbar DR, Grassie MA, Condie A, Walker MT, Smith DJ, Pulford DJ, Muir W, Blackwood DH**, and **Porteous DJ**. Sex-specific association between bipolar affective disorder in women and GPR50, an X-linked orphan G protein-coupled receptor, Mol Psychiatry 2005;**10**(5):470–8.

60. **Hallam KT, Olver JS, Horgan JE, McGrath C**, and **Norman TR**. Low doses of lithium carbonate reduce melatonin light sensitivity in healthy volunteers, Int J Neuropsychopharmacol 2005a;**8**:255–9.

61. **Hallam KT, Olver JS**, and **Norman TR**. Effect of sodium valproate on nocturnal melatonin sensitivity to light in healthy volunteers, Neuropsychopharmacology 2005b;**30**:1400–4.

62. **Bersani G** and **Garavani A**. Melatonin add-on in manic patients with treatment-resistant insomnia, Biol Psychiatry 2000;**24**:185–91.

63. **Leibenluft E, Feldman-Naim S, Turner EH, Wehr TA**, and **Rosenthal NE**. Effects of exogenous melatonin administration and withdrawal in five patients with rapid-cycling bipolar disorder, J Clin Psychiatry 1997;**58**:383–8.

64. **Romo-Nava F, Alvarez-Icaza Gonzalez D, Fresan-Orellana A, Saracco Alvarez R, Becerra-Palars C, Moreno J, Ontiveros Uribe MP, Berlanga C, Heinze G**, and **Buijs RM**. Melatonin attenuates antipsychotic metabolic effects: an eight-week randomized, double-blind, parallel-group, placebo-controlled clinical trial, Bipolar Disord 2014;**16**:410–21.

65. **Norris ER, Burke K, Correll JR, Zemanek KJ, Lerman J, Primelo RA**, and **Kaufmann MW**. A double-blind, randomized, placebo-controlled trial of adjunctive ramelteon for the treatment of insomnia and mood stability in patients with euthymic bipolar disorder, J Affect Disord 2013;**144**:141–7.

66. **Bourin M** and **Prica C**. Melatonin receptor agonist agomelatine: a new drug for treating unipolar depression, Curr Pharm Des 2009;**15**:1675–82.

67. **Kennedy SH** and **Emsley R**. Placebo-controlled trial of agomelatine in the treatment of major depressive disorder, Eur Neuropsychopharmacol 2006;**16**(2):93–100.

68. **Loo H, Hale A**, and **D'Haenen H**. Determination of the dose of agomelatine, a melatoninergic agonist and selective 5-HT(2C) antagonist, in the treatment of major depressive disorder: a placebo-controlled dose range study, Int Clin Psychopharmacol 2002;**17**(5):239–47.

69. **Montgomery SA** and **Kasper S**. Severe depression and antidepressants: focus on a pooled analysis of placebo-controlled studies on agomelatine, Int Clin Psychopharmacol 2007;**22**(5):283–91.

70. **Calabrese JR, Guelfi JD**, and **Perdrizet-Chevalier C**. Agomelatine adjunctive therapy for acute bipolar depression: preliminary open data, Bipolar Disord 2007;**9**:628–35.

71. **Goodwin GM, Emsley R, Rembry S, Rouillon F**, and **Agomelatine Study Group**. Agomelatine prevents relapse in patients with major depressive disorder without evidence of a discontinuation syndrome: a 24-week randomized, double-blind, placebo-controlled trial, J Clin Psychiatry 2009;**70**:1128–37.

72. Taylor D, Sparshatt A, Varma S, and Olofinjana O. Antidepressant efficacy of agomelatine: meta-analysis of published and unpublished studies, BMJ 2014;**348**:g1888.

73. Quiroz JA, Singh J, Gould TD, Denicoff KD, Zarate CA, Jr, and Manji HK. Emerging experimental therapeutics for bipolar disorder: clues from the molecular pathophysiology, Mol Psychiatry 2004;**9**:756–76.

74. Belanoff JK, Rothschild AJ, Cassidy F, DeBattista C, Baulieu EE, Schold C, Schatzberg AF. An open label trial of C-1073 (mifepristone) for psychotic major depression, Biol Psychiatry 2002;**52**(5):386–92.

75. DeBattista C, Belanoff J, Glass S, Khan A, Horne RL, Blasey C, Carpenter LL, and Alva G. Mifepristone versus placebo in the treatment of psychosis in patients with psychotic major depression, Biol Psychiatry 2006;**60**(12):1343–9.

76. Young AH, Gallagher P, Watson S, Del-Estal D, Owen BM, and Ferrier IN. Improvements in neurocognitive function and mood following adjunctive treatment with mifepristone (RU-486) in bipolar disorder, Neuropsychopharmacology 2004;**29**:1538–45.

77. Carroll BJ and Rubin RT. Mifepristone in psychotic depression?, Biol Psychiatry 2008;**63**(1):e1; author reply e3.

78. Jahn H, Schick M, Kiefer F, Kellner M, Yassouridis A, and Wiedemann K. Metyrapone as additive treatment in major depression: a double-blind and placebo-controlled trial, Arch Gen Psychiatry 2004;**61**(12):1235–44.

79. Brown ES, Bobadilla L, and Rush AJ. Ketoconazole in bipolar patients with depressive symptoms: a case series and literature review, Bipolar Disord 2001;**3**:23–9.

80. Gallagher P, Malik N, Newham J, Young AH, Ferrier IN, and Mackin P. Antiglucocorticoid treatments for mood disorders, Cochrane Database Syst Rev 2008;Jan 23(1):CD005168.

81. Khairova R, Machado-Vieira R, Du J, and Manji HK. A potential role for pro-inflammatory cytokines in regulating synaptic plasticity in major depressive disorder, Int J Neuropsychomarmacol 2009;**12**:561–78.

82. Muller N, Schwarz MJ, Dehning S, Douhe A, Cerovecki A, Goldstein-Muller B, Spellmann I, Hetzel G, Maino K, Kleindienst N, Moller HJ, Arolt V, and Riedel M. The cyclooxygenase-2 inhibitor celecoxib has therapeutic effects in major depression: results of a double-blind, randomized, placebo controlled, add-on pilot study to reboxetine, Mol Psychiatry 2006;**11**(7):680–4.

83. Akhondzadeh S, Jafari S, Raisi F, Nasehi AA, Ghoreishi A, Salehi B, Mohebbi-Rasa S, Raznahan M, and Kamalipour A. Clinical trial of adjunctive celecoxib treatment in patients with major depression: a double blind and placebo controlled trial, Depress Anxiety 2009;**26**:607–11.

84. Majd M, Hashemian F, Hosseini SM, Vahdat Shariatpanahi M, and Sharifi A. A randomized double-blind, placebo-controlled trial of celecoxib augmentation of sertraline in treatment of drug-naive depressed women: a pilot study, Iran J Pharm Res 2015;**14**:891–9.

85. Nery FG, Monkul ES, Hatch JP, Fonseca M, Zunta-Soares GB, Frey BN, Bowden CL, and Soares JC. Celecoxib as an adjunct in the treatment of depressive or mixed episodes of bipolar disorder: a double-blind, randomized, placebo-controlled study, Hum Psychopharmacol 2008;**23**(2):87–94.

86. Raison CL, Rutherford RE, Woolwine BJ, Shuo C, Schettler P, Drake DF, Haroon E, and Miller AH. A randomized controlled trial of the tumor necrosis factor antagonist

infliximab for treatment-resistant depression: the role of baseline inflammatory biomarkers, JAMA 2013;**70**(1):31–41.

87. **Streck EL, Amboni G, Scaini G, Di-Pietro PB, Rezin GT, Valvassori SS, Luz G, Kapczinski F,** and **Quevedo J.** Brain creatine kinase activity in an animal model of mania, Life Sci 2008;**82**(7–8):424–9.

88. **Segal M, Avital A, Drobot M, Lukanin A, Derevenski A, Sandbank S,** and **Weizman A.** CK levels in unmedicated bipolar patients, Eur Neuropsychopharmacol 2007;**17**(12):763–7.

89. **MacDonald ML, Naydenov A, Chu M, Matzilevich D,** and **Konradi C.** Decrease in creatine kinase messenger RNA expression in the hippocampus and dorsolateral prefrontal cortex in bipolar disorder, Bipolar Disord 2006;**8**(3):255–64.

90. **Roitman S, Green T, Osher Y, Karni N,** and **Levine J.** Creatine monohydrate in resistant depression: a preliminary study, Bipolar Disord 2007;**9**(7):754–8.

91. **Amital D, Vishne T, Rubinow A,** and **Levine J.** Observed effects of creatine monohydrate in a patient with depression and fibromyalgia, Am J Psychiatry 2006;**163**:1840–1.

92. **Andreazza AC, Cassini C, Rosa AR, Leite MC, de Almeida LM, Nardin P, Cunha AB, Cereser KM, Santin A, Gottfried C, Salvador M, Kapczinski F,** and **Goncalves CA.** Serum S100B and antioxidant enzymes in bipolar patients, J Psychiatr Res 2007;**41**(6):523–9.

93. **Berk M, Copolov DL, Dean O, Lu K, Jeavons S, Schapkaitz I, Anderson-Hunt M,** and **Bush AI.** N-acetyl cysteine for depressive symptoms in bipolar disorder—a double-blind randomized placebo-controlled trial, Biol Psychiatry 2008;**64**(6):468–75.

94. **Magalhaes PV, Dean OM, Bush AI, Copolov DL, Malhi GS, Kohlmann K, Jeavons S, Schapkaitz I, Anderson-Hung M,** and **Berk M.** N-acetyl cysteine add-on treatment for bipolar II disorder: a subgroup analysis of a randomized placebo-controlled trial, J Affect Disord 2011;**129**:317–20.

95. **Berk M, Dean O, Cotton SM, Gama CS, Kapczinski F, Fernandes BS, Kohlmann K, Jeavons S, Hewitt K, Allwang C, Cobb H, Bush AI, Schapkaitz I, Dodd S,** and **Malhi GS.** The efficacy of N-acetylcysteine as an adjunctive treatment in bipolar depression: an open label trial, J Affect Disord 2011;**135**(1–3):389–94.

96. **Berk M, Dean OM, Cotton SM, Jeavons S, Tanious M, Kohlmann K,** and **Hewitt K.** The efficacy of adjunctive N-acetylcysteine in major depressive disorder: a double-blind, randomized, placebo-controlled trial, J Clin Psychiatry 2014;**75**:628–36.

97. **Yoon SJ, Lyoo IK, Haws C, Kim TS, Cohen BM,** and **Renshaw PF.** Decreased glutamate/ glutamine levels may mediate cytidine's efficacy in treating bipolar depression: a longitudinal proton magnetic resonance spectroscopy study, Neuropsychopharmacology 2009;**34**(7):1810–18.

Chapter 31

The treatment of bipolar disorder in the era of personalized medicine: myth or promise?

Chiara Fabbri and Alessandro Serretti

Introduction

Bipolar disorder (BD) is a chronic disease characterized by the alternation of periods of (hypo)mania and depression, resulting in high personal and socio-economic burden in terms of poor quality of life, increased rates of suicide, direct and indirect costs.[1] The rate of suicide (0.4%) among patients with bipolar disorder is more than 20 times greater than in the general population.[2] Importantly, an adequate treatment may allow for long-term remission and good functioning in the majority of patients, but the lack of reliable and reproducible markers for guiding drug choice makes often difficult the identification of the most effective treatment(s). Limited treatment efficacy and side effects often due to polypharmacy contribute to treatment non-adherence. Indeed, it has been reported that more than 75% of patients take their medication less than 75% of the time.[2] Thus, the development of tailored BD treatments that can be applied in clinical settings is a priority in order to improve the prognosis of the disease.

BD shows one of highest genetic predisposition among psychiatric disorders and the heritability index is estimated to be 0.85.[3] Genetics accounts for 20–95% of variability in CNS drug disposition and pharmacodynamics,[4] supporting the hypothesis that treatment efficacy in BD may be significantly affected by genetic variants. Thus, candidate gene studies before and most recently genome-wide association studies (GWAS) have been performed to identify the polymorphisms involved in the modulation of both response and medication side effects. Candidate gene studies are based on the investigation of a limited number of polymorphisms in a limited number of genes that are considered to be possibly involved in the modulation of the phenotype of interest (given the results of molecular, cellular, and animal studies). The investigated genes are those involved in drug mechanisms of action (pharmacodynamics) or drug metabolism (pharmacokinetics). Candidate gene association studies were the first to be performed since the success they were able to achieve in the discovery of genes involved in Mendelian (ie monogenic) diseases. On the other hand, they are not as much as decisive for complex traits, ie when a high number of polymorphisms with small effect size affect the phenotype, as in the case of interest. For complex phenotypes indeed, only few variants were demonstrated to have a medium–large effect size (for example, the HLA-B*1502 allele for carbamazepine-induced Stevens–Johnson syndrome, see 'Other mood stabilizers'). GWAS are able to provide hundreds of thousands of single nucleotide polymorphisms (SNPs) throughout the whole genome and the most recent platforms provide more than 900K SNPs. The number of available SNPs can be further increased thanks to imputation (a process that is based on the deduction of non-available genotypes on the basis of the regional linkage disequilibrium (LD) among SNPs). GWAS overcame the need of any a priori selection of SNPs and opened the way to multimarker analyses, such as pathway analysis (ie the comparison of significance in polymorphisms within a molecular pathway to the null hypothesis or to a random pathway) and polygenic risk models. Anyway, available results mainly pertain to individual polymorphisms association analysis, which are hypothesized to entail poor replication of findings due to issues of sample heterogeneity.[5] Particularly, ancestry stratification and different genotyping rates are supposed to contribute to the poor replication of results across different GWAS, as well as to the non-exciting results of each of the published GWAS. The discovery potential of GWAS could be completely exploited after the overcoming of their current methodological limitations, including the implementation of adequate methods for multiple testing correction (the high number of markers tested but their incomplete independence due to LD are often overlooked), the recruitment of samples with adequate size, and the adequate covering of genetic variation.

The present chapter aims to provide a critical overview of the pharmacogenetic findings that have or may have clinical applications for the treatment of BD in the next future. A summary of the main GWAS findings is also provided since the relevance of this kind of study for the advancement of research in the field. An overview of the recommended or most promising genetic tests for BD treatments is provided in Table 31.1.

Mood stabilizers

Lithium

Lithium is a commonly prescribed mood stabilizer for the treatment of BD, greatly decreasing suicide risk and BD symptoms during acute mania, depression, and maintenance. However, it is not effective in 30–50% of patients with classic mania and 60–70% of patients with mixed mania.[6] On the other hand, optimal lithium response (total prevention of recurrences) is observed in about one-third of BD patients.[7] Specific clinical features are associated with excellent lithium response (BD type I without mood-incongruent delusions and without co-morbidity, non-rapid cycling course, and bipolar family history), suggesting that this group of patients may represent a specific endophenotype of the disease (ie with particular genetic characteristics). Only the genetics of lithium efficacy is discussed in the present chapter given the absence/paucity of pharmacogenetics studies investigating lithium-induced side effects.

Table 31.1 Recommended or promising genotyping test for clinical application in BD treatment in the near future. For references refer to the main text. ADRs = adverse drug reactions

Gene	Polymorphism(s)	Drug/drug class	Phenotype	Level of evidence
HLA-B	HLA-B*1502	Carbamazep ne	Stevens–Johnson syndrome	Recommended in Asian ancestry
POLG	A467T, W748S	Valproate	Liver toxicity	Recommended in children/adolescents
CPS1	rs1047891	Valproate	Hyperammonaemia	Recommended in case of suspected urea cycle disorder
CYP2D6	Partially or totally inactive alleles (poor metabolizers)	Polypharmacy or treatment with some antipsychotics or antidepressants	Overall risk of ADRs	High evidence, already included in several drug labelling
BDNF, SLC6A4, DRD1, GSK3B	rs6265, 5-HTTLPR, −48 A/G, −50T/C, −1727A/T	Lithium	Response	Promising, but consistent replication needed
HLA-DQB1	6672G>C	Clozapine	Agranulocytosis	Probably will be recommended in the near future
HTR2C	−759C/T	Antipsychotics	Metabolic ADRs	Promising
MC4R	rs489693	Antipsychotics	Metabolic ADRs	Promising
Leptin	−2548A/G	Antipsychotics	Metabolic ADRs	Promising
CNR1	rs806378, rs1049353	Antipsychotics	Metabolic ADRs	Promising
DRD2	rs1800497	Antipsychotics	Tardive dyskinesia	Promising
HTR2A	102CC, −1438GG	Antipsychotics	Tardive dyskinesia	Promising
CYP2D6	Partially or totally inactive alleles	Antipsychotics	Tardive dyskinesia	Promising
HSPG2	rs2445142	Antipsychotics	Tardive dyskinesia	Promising
ZFPM2	rs12678719	Antipsychotics	Parkinsonism	Promising

Candidate gene association studies

The genes most consistently associated with lithium response are involved in synaptic plasticity (BDNF and NTRK2), serotonergic (SLC6A4) and dopaminergic (DRD1) neurotransmission, and second messenger cascades (GSK3B).

Brain-derived neurotrophic factor (BDNF) is involved in neuronal proliferation and synaptic plasticity and neurotrophic tyrosine kinase receptor type 2 (NTRK2) codes for one of the BDNF receptors. The rs6265 (196G/A or Val66Met) SNP within the BDNF gene is of particular interest since its functional effect. Indeed, the Met allele has been reported to affect intracellular trafficking and reduce the secretion of the protein. In mice, the Met/Met genotype shows impaired survival of newly born cells in the dentate gyrus and the Met allele was associated with poorer episodic memory, abnormal hippocampal activation, and metabolism in humans.[8] Pharmacogenetic studies of lithium response have suggested that the Met allele or the heterozygote genotype may have better response compared to the Val/Val homozygote, despite with no complete agreement.[9] This finding can be interpreted in line with the effect observed by pharmacogenetic studies of antidepressant response and the biological explanation is suggested by animal studies showing that too high BDNF levels may have a detrimental effect on mood.[8] The association of NTRK2 SNPs with lithium efficacy was less investigated than BDNF and independent replication is needed, but an association was found particularly in patients with euphoric mania and higher suicidality.[7]

The functional promoter insertion/deletion polymorphism (5-HTTLPR) of the serotonin transporter gene (SLC6A4) gene has been particularly investigated by pharmacogenetic studies since the 16-repeat long (L) allele is associated with a twice basal SERT expression compared to the 14-repeat short (S) allele.[8] The S allele has been associated with a predisposition to affective disorders, both bipolar and unipolar, and with prophylactic lithium non-response, despite not all studies confirming this result.[7] Interestingly, an interaction of 5-HTTLPR with BDNF rs6265 was found; indeed, in subjects carrying the S allele and the Val/Val genotype a 70% probability of lithium non-response was reported.[7]

Glycogen synthase kinase 3 beta (GSK3B) gene codes for a serine-threonine kinase regulating signalling cascades involved in neuronal development and survival, circadian cycle regulation, and it is inhibited by lithium. Two SNPs in the promoter of the gene (50T/C and 1727A/T) were associated with lithium response by two independent studies.[9] Further, the GSK3B gene was demonstrated to interact with the NR1D1 gene, coding for a transcription factor involved in the regulation of the circadian cycle and associated with prophylactic lithium response by two studies.[7]

The dopamine receptor D1 (DRD1) is the most abundant dopamine receptor in the central nervous system (CNS) and basically the bipolar 'dysregulation' concept postulates dopaminergic hyperactivity in mania and hypoactivity in depression. Two previous pharmacogenetic studies reported that the promoter—48 A/G SNP within this gene may be a modulator of lithium prophylactic efficacy.[7]

GWAS

A previous suggestive (non-genome-wide significant) association between the prevention of recurrence during lithium treatment and a region spanning the GRIA2 (glutamate receptor, ionotropic AMPA 2) and ACCN5 (acid sensing (proton gated) ion channel family member 5) genes was reported.[10] GRIA2 was found to be down-regulated by chronic lithium treatment in a human neuronal cell line. Further, hip-pocampal glutamate concentrations were demonstrated to be increased in euthymic chronically lithium-treated patients relative to healthy comparison subjects by a magnetic resonance spectroscopy study.[10] The possible association between ACCN5 and lithium efficacy was not replicated by other studies, but a gene of the same family (ACCN1) was the top finding of another GWAS investigating long-term lithium response.[11] ACCN1 is mainly permeable to Na+ and to a lesser extent to Li+ and K+ and it is largely expressed in neurons. Cation channels belonging to this family were shown to affect hippocampal-dependent long-term potentiation and spatial memory, as well as psychiatric diseases.[11]

The GWAS studies cited above were performed on subjects of Caucasian ancestry, while another one was carried out on Han Chinese descent patients. Highly genome-wide significant findings were reported by this study within the GADL1 gene, which product has still unknown physiological function.[12] Given the high significance of the findings reported by this GWAS, several others tried to replicate the results in independent samples by using several methodologies, but all of them failed to dem-onstrate any significant signal within the gene.[13]

Finally, previously published GWAS data were re-analysed through a pathway-analysis approach comparing clock genes with random control genes. Circadian rhythm abnormalities are, indeed, central features of BD and the study demon-strated enrichment of clock genes in association with lithium response, involving particularly the CRY1, NR1D1, GLUL, HIST1H1C, and EMP2 genes.[14]

Peripheral biomarkers

Several plasma or serum biomarkers were investigated as predictors of lithium effi-cacy, in both terms of gene expression and protein levels. The most promising bio-markers are molecules belonging to the group of pro-inflammatory cytokines and the insulin-growth factor 1 (IGF-1).

IGF-1 is a member of a family of hormones involved in growth and development and it may affect brain function by either local tissue expression or by peripheral cir-culating peptides crossing the blood–brain barrier. Peripheral IGF-1 mediates neu-rotrophic and antidepressant effects, whereas this effect is inhibited by anti-IGF-1 antiserum in a mice neurodegeneration model.[15] Genome-wide mRNA expression profiles of lymphoblastoid cell lines (LCLs) from BD patients showed that IGF-1 was over-expressed (fold difference = 2.2) in lithium responder patients compared with non-responder patients. In vitro evidence confirmed the putative role of IGF-1 on lithium mechanisms of action; indeed, IGF-1 increased lithium sensitivity selectively in LCLs from non-responder BD patients. In addition, serum IGF-1 levels are ele-vated in BD patients.[15] Changes in the expression of related genes were demonstrated to occur as an effect of lithium exposure (insulin-like growth factor 1 receptor alpha subunit (IGF-1-R alpha), insulin promoter factor 1 (IPF1), and insulin-like growth factor binding protein 5 precursor (IGF-binding protein 5 or IGFBP5)[16]).

The available evidence suggests that lithium restores the pro-inflammation status involved in BD pathogenesis modulating interleukin-signalling pathways. A growing number of studies demonstrated that inflammatory cytokines are closely associated with BD, especially during the acute phases of the disease. Plasma levels of several cytokines (TNF-α, TGF-β1, IL-23, and IL-17) were demonstrated to decrease after lithium treatment among BD patients who achieved response during a manic phase or euthymia.[17,18] However, confirmation of these findings is needed due to the paucity of available studies.

Other mood stabilizers

There is a paucity of pharmacogenetic studies investigating response to mood stabilizers other than lithium. Preliminary evidence of a possible effect of the functional—116C/G polymorphism in the XBP1 gene on valproate prophylactic efficacy was reported in Korean BD patients. The X-box binding protein 1 (XBP1) is an important molecule in the endoplasmic reticulum (ER)-stress response and it has been identified as a genetic risk factor for BD.[19]

Clinically relevant findings were instead reported for side effects that can be induced by some mood stabilizers. The most interesting pharmacogenetic findings regard valproate-induced hyperammonaemia, hepatic dysfunction, and immune-mediated cutaneous hypersensitivity reactions. The latter adverse drug reactions (ADRs) can be induced by carbamazepine and lamotrigine and they include a risk of potentially life-threatening Stevens–Johnson syndrome (SJS), toxic epidermal necrolysis (TEN), and drug-related rash with eosinophilia and systemic symptoms (DRESS).

Regarding valproate-induced hyperammonaemia, a missense polymorphism in the carbamoyl phosphate synthase 1 (CPS1) gene (4217C>A or rs1047891) was suggested to increase the risk and severity of hyperammonaemia in Caucasians, even if drug-plasmatic levels are within the therapeutic range.[20] The genotyping of this CPS1 SNP may be indicated in patients with suspected urea cycle disorder.

Valproate-induced liver impairment was related to mitochondrial DNA depletion and mutations in the POLG gene that codes for the mitochondrial DNA polymerase gamma in paediatric patients. Thus, POLG gene testing has been recommended in children/adolescents since they are particularly at risk of developing valproate-induced liver toxicity.[21]

Severe hypersensitivity reactions (cutaneous or systemic) to carbamazepine and lamotrigine have a frequency with a range of 1–10 per 10,000 new users. A 100% prevalence of carbamazepine-induced SJS was reported among Han Chinese carriers of the human leukocyte antigen HLA-B*1502 allele, compared with a frequency of this allele of only 3% among carbamazapine-tolerant patients.[22] Further case–control studies in Hong Kong Chinese and Thai populations confirmed the strong association of HLA-B*1502 with carbamazepine-induced SJS or TEN, but not with carbamazepine-induced maculopapular rash or DRESS. Ethnicity appears to play an important role in the association, since studies in Caucasians and in Japanese failed to identify any relationship between HLA-B*1502 status and SJS or TEN.[23] On the basis of these data, the US Food and Drug Administration (FDA) recommended that patients with ancestry from areas in which HLA-B*1502 is present (China, Thailand, Malaysia, Indonesia, the Philippines, Taiwan, and Vietnam) should be screened for this allele before starting treatment with carbamazepine. Given that more than 90% of drug-induced SJS/TEN occur within two months of starting treatment, patients who have been taking carbamazepine for at least a few months without developing severe cutaneous reactions are at low risk of developing SJS or TEN during continuation of treatment, even if they carry the HLA-B*1502 allele.[24]

Antipsychotics

Relatively recent studies demonstrated the efficacy of several second-generation antipsychotics (SGAs), both as monotherapy and in combination with mood stabilizers, in the treatment of acute phases of BD as well as for prophylaxis.[2] While first-generation antipsychotics (FGAs) are effective for the treatment of manic phases, they entail a relevant risk of extrapyramidal side effects and switch to a depressive phase, thus SGAs, are usually preferred. On the other hand, SGAs are not without side-effect risk, since they can cause significant weight gain, metabolic dysregulation (dyslipidemia, hyperglycaemia, and diabetes), sedation/somnolence and akathisia among those observed most frequently. As it was underlined in the Introduction of this chapter, side effects are one of the main factors responsible for poor treatment adherence, but metabolic side effects can also contribute to the development of severe medical conditions and increased mortality for cardiovascular diseases.[25] Further, clozapine is sometimes prescribed to treatment-resistant BD patients and agranulocytosis induced by this drug is a rare but life-threatening side effect. Thus, the identification of biomarkers of antipsychotic side effects is a milestone for providing tailored treatments able to improve BD prognosis. Despite the greatest part of studies were performed on samples with a diagnosis of schizophrenia, the biological mechanisms underlying side effects are supposed to overlap across different disorders. On the other hand, the same cannot be stated for treatment efficacy and very few pharmacogenetic data are available regarding antipsychotic response in BD. Thus, only the pharmacogenetics of antipsychotic side effects is discussed in the present chapter.

Metabolic side effects

Genetic factors play an important role in controlling weight gain that has been estimated to be around 60–80% through twin and family studies.[26] Given that cardiovascular disease is the primary cause of excess of mortality among severe psychiatric diseases,[25] the identification of genetic predictors of antipsychotic-induced metabolic side effects could be a turning point in the treatment of BD.

Several pharmacogenetic studies have investigated the genes that could influence antipsychotic-induced weight gain (AIWG), with focus mainly on homeostatic regulators expressed in hypothalamic areas that belong to the complex network that regulates appetite and satiety.

The most replicated pharmacogenetic association is with the serotonergic receptor 5-HTC2 (HTR2C) gene. The 5-HTC2 receptor is responsible for the serotonin-mediated anorexigenic action on the hypothalamic nuclei. Consistently, antagonists of 5-HTC2 receptors, such as clozapine and olanzapine, promote appetite increase. Carriers of the recessive T allele of the promoter polymorphism—759C/T—were demonstrated to be protected from substantial weight gain.[27]

Leptin and melanocortin receptor 4 (MC4R) are other essential components of one of the most important hypothalamic satiety signals. Leptin is mainly synthesized in the adipocytes of white adipose tissue and activates leptin receptors in the arcuate nucleus of the hypothalamus, resulting in a feeling of satiety. The leptin-2548A/G polymorphism may interact with the HTR2C–759C/T variant in affecting AIWG.[28] Neurons of the arcuate nucleus also express MC4R, activation of which decreases food intake while elevating energy utilization. This gene has been consistently associated with AIWG by four independent studies.[27]

The cannabinoid receptor 1 (CNR1) gene and the fatty acid amide hydrolase (FAAH gene) have been suggested as promising genetic factors involved in AIWG,[27] consistently with the observation that they play an important role in the mediation of leptin anorexigenic action.

A GWAS was aimed to identify genetic risk factors for metabolic side effects in patients treated with psychopharmacological medications.[29] The SNP rs7838490 (8q21.3 region) was associated with body mass index (BMI) alterations, while the rs11615724 (12q21) was associated with the effect of medications on decreasing HDL-C levels. Both markers are in intergenic regions. rs7838490 is located upstream of the gene matrix metalloproteinase 16 (MMP16), and it may regulate the expression of MMP16 and affect tumour necrosis factor receptor superfamily, member 1A (sTNFRSF1A), which may be involved in lipid regulation.

Extrapyramidal side effects

Pharmacogenetic data are mainly focused on antipsychotic-induced tardive dyskinesia that is the most severe among extrapyramidal side effects (EPS) due to its tendency to persist over time, its treatment-resistance, and its high frequency (around 20% of patients after prolonged treatment, but BD patients are more vulnerable to this EPS[30]).

Genes are hypothesized to play a relevant role in the risk of tardive dyskinesia, as suggested by increased risk of tardive dyskinesia in affected families.[31] In particular, the gene coding for the dopamine receptor 2 (DRD2), one of main target of antipsychotics (especially for those drugs with a higher risk of inducing this EPS), was suggested to be involved by a number of independent studies (especially the Taq1A polymorphism or rs1800497). The minor (T) Taq1A allele has been associated with a 40% reduction in striatal D2 receptor density (according to in vitro assays and in vivo imaging studies). This allele appears to be protective against tardive dyskinesia.[32] A functional missense mutation in the dopamine 3 receptor (DRD3, another target of antipsychotics) gene (ser9gly or rs6280) has been suggested to modulate the risk of tardive dyskinesia, but meta-analytic results did not support this hypothesis.[33] The 5-HT2A receptor (HTR2A gene) is a target of SGAs and it has been implicated in their reduced extrapyramidal side-effect profile. The HTR2A gene has also been associated with tardive dyskinesia susceptibility by several candidate gene studies in different ethnic groups.[34] Another relevant gene for the risk of tardive dyskinesia is CYP2D6 (member of the cytochrome P450 enzyme family) that is involved in the hepatic metabolism of several antipsychotics. CYP2D6 poor metabolizer status (homozygosity for null alleles) or intermediate metabolizer status (null allele heterozygosity) were associated with 1.64 and 1.43-fold greater odds of developing tardive dyskinesia.[35]

GWAS suggested the potential contribution of other genes to tardive dyskinesia. In particular, the gamma-aminobutyric acid (GABA) receptor signalling pathway (especially SLC6A11, GABRB2, and GABRG3 genes) may be involved in genetic susceptibility to treatment-resistant tardive dyskinesia in Asian populations.[36] A more interesting finding was the HSPG2 gene (coding for the heparan sulfate proteoglycan 2) since its replication by two independent GWAS on both Asian[37] and Caucasian[38] populations. This pharmacogenomic finding was supported by an increase in HSPG2 expression in subjects with lower risk of developing tardive dyskinesia, which may exert a protective effect via a cholinergic or basic fibroblast growth factor (FGF2) mediated neuroprotective mechanism.

Some data are available also for other types of EPS. A GWAS investigating antipsychotic-induced parkinsonism[39] has been replicated[38] supporting a role of the rs12678719 SNP in the zinc finger protein multitype 2 (ZFPM2) gene, especially in patients of African ancestry. The risk allele G was associated with a higher degree of nigrostriatal terminal degeneration in Parkinson disease.[38] Interestingly, another gene coding for a zinc finger protein (ZNF202) was associated with the development of abnormal movements during antipsychotic treatment. The association may be explained by the regulatory effect of ZNF202 on the expression of PLP1 (proteolipid protein 1) which mutations can determine the development of parkinsonism.[40]

Clozapine-induced agranulocytosis (CIA)

CIA is a rare (incidence 0.8%) but potentially fatal side effect of clozapine. Several pharmacogenetic case–control studies focused on CIA have produced inconsistent findings, mainly regarding the major histocompatibility complex (MHC) region (including human leukocyte antigen (HLA) class I, II, and III loci and some non-HLA genes), as well as a few non-MHC genes. HLA-DQB1 polymorphisms have been the ones most consistently associated with CIA.[41,42] Among them, an SNP (6672G>C) was found to confer a 16.9 times increased risk of CIA. A commercial test using this variant was marketed in 2007 but its clinical application is limited by its low sensitivity and low predictive validity.[41]

Antidepressants

The majority of patients with BD spend much more time in depressive episodes, including subsyndromal depressive symptoms, and bipolar depression accounts for the largest part of the morbidity and mortality of the illness. The pharmacological treatment of bipolar depression mostly consists of combinations of at least two drugs, and antidepressants are the most commonly prescribed drugs despite recommendations from evidence-based guidelines do not overtly support their use. Among antidepressants, best evidence exists for fluoxetine, but in combination with olanzapine. Although some guidelines recommend the use of selective serotonin reuptake inhibitors (SSRIs) or bupropion in combination with antimanic agents as first-choice treatment, others do not, based on the available evidence.[43] The current evidence mainly suggests that antidepressants may be effective in the brief-term treatment of bipolar depression but with the possibility of a mood switch towards (hypo)mania. The risk of mood switch should be taken into account particularly when prescribing tricyclic antidepressants (TCAs) or venlafaxine.[43] Few data exist in regard to the pharmacogenetics of antidepressant response in BD since studies were mainly focused on major depressive disorder or mixed samples including both unipolar and bipolar depression, resulting in non-specific information. On the other hand, the specific clinical issue of antidepressant-induced mania was investigated under the genetic perspective, thus it is discussed in the present chapter.

Antidepressant-induced mania (AIM)

Polymorphisms in the serotonin transporter (SLC6A4) were the mostly investigated variants in regard to AIM. Three previous meta-analyses were performed to clarify the role of the SLC6A4 5-HTTLPR polymorphism in AIM. The cumulative evidence suggests that S allele carriers may have an increased risk of AIM but probably with a small effect size while carriers of the L-A-10 haplotype (5-HTTLPR, rs25531, and the second intron variable number of tandem repeats (VNTR)) show a reduced risk.[44] The rs25531 and VNTR polymorphisms have functional effect as well as 5-HTTLPR. Particularly, the rs25531 affects the expression of the SLC6A4 gene in combination with 5-HTTLPR; indeed, the combination of the 5-HTTLPR L allele with the rs25531 A allele results in higher levels of expression, whereas the 5-HTTLPR L allele combined with the rs25531 G allele results in expression levels similar to those of the 5-HTTLPR S allele.[44] Thus, carriers of the 5-HTTLPR S allele and 5-HTTLPR-rs25531 LG haplotype may show higher synaptic serotonin levels after the administration of an antidepressant blocking the serotonin transporter, since their lower expression levels of the protein, and this mechanism may be involved in the induction of AIM.

Polypharmacy

As stated in the Introduction, polypharmacy is a very common issue in the treatment of BD, since an average of 3.31±1.46 psychotropic medications and 5.94±3.78 total medications was reported in BD patients.[45] The most useful genetic polymorphisms to predict treatment outcomes in this context are those in cytochrome (CYP) P450 genes. The CYP P450 superfamily is a class of enzymes with a major role in the oxidation and reduction of both endogenous and xenobiotic substances. CYP P450 enzymes are highly involved in the metabolism of antipsychotics, antidepressants, benzodiazepines, and some mood stabilizers (eg carbamazepine). Anyway, they represent only a minor route in valproate metabolism (approximately 10%) involving CYP2C9 and CYP2A6,[46] while lamotrigine is metabolized through the UDP glucuronosyltransferase enzyme and lithium elimination route is urinary without any metabolism. Given that CYP P450 enzymes are involved in the metabolism of a number of non-psychotropic drugs, it is expected that the information provided by their genotyping could be used to predict the risk and efficacy profiles of different drug combinations in each individual.

The isoforms mainly involved in psychotropic drug metabolism are CYP2D6, CYP2C19, CYP2C9, CYP1A2, and CYP3A4. Each of these genes is highly polymorphic, alleles are classified according to their activity in wild type (normal activity), reduced, or null activity and they define some metabolic groups. Accordingly, the wild type genotype is defined as extensive metabolizer (EM), which is characterized by the presence of two active alleles, while intermediate metabolizers (IMs) are characterized by the presence of one wild type allele plus a partially or totally defective allele and they are expected to be between EM and the poor metabolizer (PM) groups. PM shows a combination of two partially or totally defective alleles. Finally, the ultrarapid metabolizer (UM) category exists only for CYP2D6 and it is usually linked to multiple copies of the *1 or *2A allele.[47] Of note, the distribution of metabolizer groups varies substantially among ethnic groups. For example, the prevalence of PMs is estimated to be 5–10% in Caucasian populations and only 1–2% in Asian populations, whereas UMs constitute only 1–2% in Caucasian populations, but up to 30–40% in some Northern African populations. In addition, CYP enzymes can be inhibited or induced by drugs and diet. For example, paroxetine acts as a potent CYP2D6 inhibitor, thus it can convert an EM into a PM.[48]

The CYP2D6 gene is the most investigated one and it plays a role in the metabolism of at least 30 psychotropic medications, among them several antidepressants and antipsychotics (haloperidol, thioridazine, perphenazine, chlorpromazine, risperidone, aripiprazole, and iloperidone).[48]

The cumulative evidence from literature supports the involvement of CYP2D6 metabolizing status or CYP2D6 genotype in psychotropic drug-induced side-effect risk, including tardive dyskinesia, extrapyramidal symptoms, weight gain, sexual dysfunction, and cardiovascular and gastrointestinal side effects. Several antipsychotic (aripiprazole, risperidone, clozapine) and antidepressant (eg citalopram, fluoxetine, fluvoxamine, paroxetine, amitriptyline, clomipramine, desipramine, nortriptyline, imipramine) drugs already included CYP2D6 pharmacogenetic indications in their labelling (in the precautions, dosage and administration, warnings, clinical pharmacology, or drug interaction sections, for detailed information see[49]). Poorer evidence indicates that CYP2D6 is involved in the modulation of response to antipsychotic and antidepressant drugs.[50]

CYP2C19 mainly affects the metabolism of antidepressant drugs, but it shows minor influences on some antipsychotic medications. Particularly, it was demonstrated that clozapine concentration may be affected by CYP2C19 genotype resulting in a higher clozapine concentration in PMs compared with EMs.[48] The metabolism of quetiapine is also probably affected by polymorphisms in this gene, since it may influence prolactin levels during the administration of this drug.[51] Similarly, the CYP2C9 gene was mainly studied in regard to antidepressant pharmacokinetics and pharmacodynamics, but it was shown to potentially affect some of the olanzapine-induced side effects.[52]

CYP3A4 is the most abundant CYP3A enzyme in the human small intestine and liver, it metabolizes more than half of all human medications and an even higher percentage of psychotropic drugs than CYP2D6 but fewer studies are available. The *1G allele was associated with risperidone response,[50] but further studies are needed.

CYP1A2 is considered a low-affinity, high-capacity enzyme, and a significant metabolic clearance pathway for chlorpromazine, clozapine, olanzapine, and several antidepressants. The CYP1A2 UM genotype was associated with the greatest circulating clozapine to N-desmethylclozapine ratio and circulating olanzapine levels were associated with the CYP1A2 *1F/*1F genotype.[50]

Further research effort is needed to clarify the role of CYP genes other than CYP2D6 in affecting psychotropic efficacy and tolerability profiles, but the available data support the relevance of these genes.

Conclusion

Some genetic markers of treatment efficacy and side effects in BD are promising, but none is currently recommended for use in the clinical practice, some exceptions apart (see section on 'Other mood stabilizers'). The clinical applicability of personalized medicine based on pharmacogenetics has been demonstrated in other field

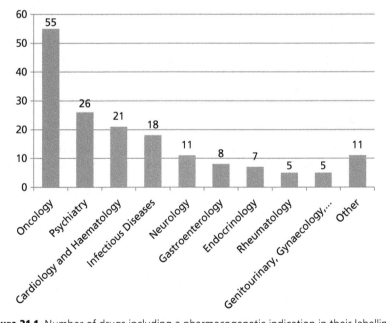

Figure 31.1 Number of drugs including a pharmacogenetic indication in their labelling according to the Food and Drug Administration (FDA) split by therapeutic area (updated to 20 May 2015). The 'Other' category includes: Analgesic and Anaesthesiology (n = 2), Dental (n = 1), Inborn Errors of Metabolism (n = 2), Pulmonary (n = 4), Toxicology (n = 1), and Transplantation (n = 1).

of medicine, such as for warfarin dosing, thiopurine myelosuppression in leukae-
mia, and abacavir hypersensitivity in HIV. However, these fields are experiencing
similar inertia, even in cases where the supporting evidence is strong[9] and psychiatry is actually the second field of medicine after oncology in terms of number of
drugs with a pharmacogenetic indication in their labelling according to the FDA
(Figure 31.1).

A promise for better elucidating the genetics of lithium response has been created
by the formation of the Consortium on Lithium Genetics (ConLiGen) to establish
the largest sample, to date, for the GWAS of lithium response in BD. The sample
currently comprises more than 1,200 patients, characterized by their response to
lithium. Preliminary results from this international study suggest a possible involvement of the sodium bicarbonate transporter (SLC4A10) gene in lithium response.[7]

A barrier to the implementation of pharmacogenetics in clinical practice is the
need for adequate educational training for clinicians. A recent study performed
at the Duke University reported discouraging data about clinicians' knowledge of
pharmacogenetic indications. Indeed, more than 50% of respondent clinicians were
not aware about any drug with a pharmacogenetic indication in the labelling, while
at the time of the survey there were more than 130 drugs reviewed by FDA with
pharmacogenetic labelling information. On the other hand, strong support for the
return of genetic research results to participants was found,[53] suggesting that educational programmes focused on the delivery of pharmacogenetic findings to clinicians would receive approval. The growing use of electronic medical records (EMRs)
may provide a route for introducing pharmacogenetics tests and decision support
to clinicians. By supplying clinical decision support derived from expert consensus
or FDA recommendations, model programmes for EMR-based pharmacogenetics
implementation may contribute to patient care.

References

1. Whiteford HA, Degenhardt L, Rehm J, Baxter AJ, Ferrari AJ, Erskine HE, et al. Global
   burden of disease attributable to mental and substance use disorders: findings from the
   Global Burden of Disease Study 2010, Lancet 2013;**382**:1575–86.

2. Jann MW. Diagnosis and treatment of bipolar disorders in adults: a review of the
   evidence on pharmacologic treatments, Am Health Drug Benefits 2014;7:489–99.

3. McGuffin P, Rijsdijk F, Andrew M, Sham P, Katz R, and Cardno A. The heritability of
   bipolar affective disorder and the genetic relationship to unipolar depression, Arch Gen
   Psychiatry 2003;**60**:497–502.

4. Cacabelos R, Martinez-Bouza R, Carril JC, Fernandez-Novoa L, Lombardi V,
   Carrera I, et al. Genomics and pharmacogenomics of brain disorders, Curr Pharm
   Biotechnol 2012;**13**:674–725.

5. Holmans P. Statistical methods for pathway analysis of genome-wide data for association
   with complex genetic traits, Adv Genet 2010;**72**:141–79.

6. Chang JS, Ha KS, Young Lee K, Sik Kim Y, and Min Ahn Y. The effects of long-term
   clozapine add-on therapy on the rehospitalization rate and the mood polarity patterns in
   bipolar disorders, J Clin Psychiatry 2006;**67**:461–7.

7. **Rybakowski JK.** Genetic influences on response to mood stabilizers in bipolar disorder: current status of knowledge, CNS Drugs 2013;**27**:165–73.

8. **Fabbri C, Di Girolamo G,** and **Serretti A.** Pharmacogenetics of antidepressant drugs: an update after almost 20 years of research, Am J Med Genet B Neuropsychiatr Genet 2013;**162B**:487–520.

9. **Salloum NC, McCarthy MJ, Leckband SG,** and **Kelsoe JR.** Towards the clinical implementation of pharmacogenetics in bipolar disorder, BMC Med 2014;**12**:90.

10. **Perlis RH, Smoller JW, Ferreira MA, McQuillin A, Bass N, Lawrence J,** et al. A genome-wide association study of response to lithium for prevention of recurrence in bipolar disorder, Am J Psychiatry 2009;**166**:718–25.

11. **Squassina A, Manchia M, Borg J, Congiu D, Costa M, Georgitsi M,** et al. Evidence for association of an ACCN1 gene variant with response to lithium treatment in Sardinian patients with bipolar disorder, *Pharmacogenomics* 2011;**12**:1559–69.

12. **Chen CH, Lee CS, Lee MT, Ouyang WC, Chen CC, Chong MY,** et al. Variant GADL1 and response to lithium therapy in bipolar I disorder, N Engl J Med 2014;**370**:119–28.

13. **Vlachadis N, Vrachnis N,** and **Economou E.** Variant GADL1 and response to lithium in bipolar I disorder, N Engl J Med 2014;**370**:1856.

14. **McCarthy MJ, Nievergelt CM, Kelsoe JR,** and **Welsh DK.** A survey of genomic studies supports association of circadian clock genes with bipolar disorder spectrum illnesses and lithium response, PLoS One 2012;**7**:e32091.

15. **Milanesi E, Hadar A, Maffioletti E, Werner H, Shomron N, Gennarelli M,** et al. Insulin-like growth factor 1 differentially affects lithium sensitivity of lymphoblastoid cell lines from lithium responder and non-responder bipolar disorder patients, J Mol Neurosci 2015;**56**:681–7.

16. **Farah R, Khamisy-Farah R, Amit T, Youdim MB,** and **Arraf Z.** Lithium's gene expression profile, relevance to neuroprotection A cDNA microarray study, Cell Mol Neurobiol 2013;**33**:411–20.

17. **Guloksuz S, Altinbas K, Aktas Cetin E, Kenis G, Bilgic Gazioglu S, Deniz G,** et al. Evidence for an association between tumor necrosis factor-alpha levels and lithium response, J Affect Disord 2012;**143**:148–52.

18. **Li H, Hong W, Zhang C, Wu Z, Wang Z, Yuan C,** et al. IL-23 and TGF-beta1 levels as potential predictive biomarkers in treatment of bipolar I disorder with acute manic episode, J Affect Disord 2015;**174**:361–6.

19. **Kim B, Kim CY, Lee MJ,** and **Joo YH.** Preliminary evidence on the association between XBP1-116C/G polymorphism and response to prophylactic treatment with valproate in bipolar disorders, Psychiatry Res 2009;**168**:209–12.

20. **Janicki PK, Bezinover D, Postula M, Thompson RS, Acharya J, Acharya V,** et al. Increased occurrence of valproic acid-induced hyperammonemia in carriers of T1405N polymorphism in carbamoyl phosphate synthetase 1 gene, ISRN Neurol 2013;**2013**:261497.

21. **FDA** (2013). 'FDA label for valproic acid and OTC, POLG' Retrieved 27 July 2015, from https://www.pharmgkb.org/label/PA166104825.

22. **Chung WH, Hung SI, Hong HS, Hsih MS, Yang LC, Ho HC,** et al. Medical genetics: a marker for Stevens–Johnson syndrome, *Nature* 2004;**428**:486.

23. **Franciotta D, Kwan P,** and **Perucca E.** Genetic basis for idiosyncratic reactions to antiepileptic drugs, Curr Opin Neurol 2009;**22**:144–9.

24. FDA (2013). 'Information for healthcare professionals: dangerous or even fatal skin reactions—carbamazepine (marketed as carbatrol, equetro, tegretol, and generics)'. Retrieved 27 July 2015, from http://www.fda.gov/Drugs/DrugSafety/PostmarketDrugSafetyInformationforPatientsandProviders/ucm124718.htm.

25. Osborn DP, Levy G, Nazareth I, Petersen I, Islam A, and King MB. Relative risk of cardiovascular and cancer mortality in people with severe mental illness from the United Kingdom's General Practice Research Database, Arch Gen Psychiatry 2007;**64**:242–9.

26. Gebhardt S, Theisen FM, Haberhausen M, Heinzel-Gutenbrunner M, Wehmeier PM, Krieg JC, et al. Body weight gain induced by atypical antipsychotics: an extension of the monozygotic twin and sib pair study, J Clin Pharm Ther 2010;**35**:207–11.

27. Shams TA and Muller DJ. Antipsychotic induced weight gain: genetics, epigenetics, and biomarkers reviewed, Curr Psychiatry Rep 2014;**16**:473.

28. Reynolds GP. Pharmacogenetic aspects of antipsychotic drug-induced weight gain—a critical review, Clin Psychopharmacol Neurosci 2012;**10**:71–7.

29. Athanasiu L, Brown AA, Birkenaes AB, Mattingsdal M, Agartz I, Melle I, et al. Genome-wide association study identifies genetic loci associated with body mass index and high density lipoprotein-cholesterol levels during psychopharmacological treatment—a cross-sectional naturalistic study, Psychiatry Res 2012;**197**:327–36.

30. Singh J, Chen G, and Canuso CM. Antipsychotics in the treatment of bipolar disorder, Handb Exp Pharmacol 2012;**187**-12.

31. Muller DJ, Chowdhury NI, and Zai CC. The pharmacogenetics of antipsychotic-induced adverse events, Curr Opin Psychiatry 2013;**26**:144–50.

32. Lencz T and Malhotra AK. Pharmacogenetics of antipsychotic-induced side effects, Dialogues Clin Neurosci 2009;**11**:405–15.

33. Tsai HT, North KE, West SL, and Poole C. The DRD3 rs6280 polymorphism and prevalence of tardive dyskinesia: a meta-analysis, Am J Med Genet B Neuropsychiatr Genet 2010;**153B**:57–66.

34. Lee HJ and Kang SG. Genetics of tardive dyskinesia, Int Rev Neurobiol 2011;**98**:231–64.

35. Patsopoulos NA, Ntzani EE, Zintzaras E, and Ioannidis JP. CYP2D6 polymorphisms and the risk of tardive dyskinesia in schizophrenia: a meta-analysis, Pharmacogenet Genomics 2005;**15**:151–8.

36. Inada T, Koga M, Ishiguro H, Horiuchi Y, Syu A, Yoshio T, et al. Pathway-based association analysis of genome-wide screening data suggest that genes associated with the gamma-aminobutyric acid receptor signaling pathway are involved in neuroleptic-induced, treatment-resistant tardive dyskinesia, Pharmacogenet Genomics 2008;**18**:317–23.

37. Syu A, Ishiguro H, Inada T, Horiuchi Y, Tanaka S, Ishikawa M, et al. Association of the HSPG2 gene with neuroleptic-induced tardive dyskinesia, *Neuropsychopharmacology* 2010;**35**:1155–64.

38. Greenbaum L, Smith RC, Lorberboym M, Alkelai A, Zozulinsky P, Lifschytz T, et al. Association of the ZFPM2 gene with antipsychotic-induced parkinsonism in schizophrenia patients, Psychopharmacology (Berl) 2012;**220**:519–28.

39. Alkelai A, Greenbaum L, Rigbi A, Kanyas K, and Lerer B. Genome-wide association study of antipsychotic-induced parkinsonism severity among schizophrenia patients, Psychopharmacology (Berl) 2009;**206**:491–9.

40. Aberg K, Adkins DE, Bukszar J, Webb BT, Caroff SN, Miller DD, et al. Genome-wide association study of movement-related adverse antipsychotic effects, Biol Psychiatry 2010;**67**:279–82.

41. **Ferentinos P** and **Dikeos D**. Genetic correlates of medical comorbidity associated with schizophrenia and treatment with antipsychotics, Curr Opin Psychiatry 2012;25:381–90.

42. **Goldstein JI, Jarskog LF, Hilliard C, Alfirevic A, Duncan L, Fourches D**, et al. Clozapine-induced agranulocytosis is associated with rare HLA-DQB1 and HLA-B alleles, Nat Commun 2014;5:4757.

43. **Vieta E** and **Valenti M**. Pharmacological management of bipolar depression: acute treatment, maintenance, and prophylaxis, CNS Drugs 2013;27:515–29.

44. **Frye MA, McElroy SL, Prieto ML, Harper KL, Walker DL, Kung S**, et al. Clinical risk factors and serotonin transporter gene variants associated with antidepressant-induced mania, J Clin Psychiatry 2015;76:174–80.

45. **Weinstock LM, Gaudiano BA, Epstein-Lubow G, Tezanos K, Celis-Dehoyos CE** and **Miller IW**. Medication burden in bipolar disorder: a chart review of patients at psychiatric hospital admission, Psychiatry Res 2014;216:24–30.

46. **Argikar UA** and **Remmel RP**. Effect of aging on glucuronidation of valproic acid in human liver microsomes and the role of UDP-glucuronosyltransferase UGT1A4, UGT1A8, and UGT1A10, Drug Metab Dispos 2009;37:229–36.

47. **Porcelli S, Fabbri C, Spina E, Serretti A**, and **De Ronchi D**. Genetic polymorphisms of cytochrome P450 enzymes and antidepressant metabolism, Expert Opin Drug Metab Toxicol 2011;7:1101–15.

48. **Muller DJ, Kekin I, Kao AC**, and **Brandl EJ**. Towards the implementation of CYP2D6 and CYP2C19 genotypes in clinical practice: update and report from a pharmacogenetic service clinic, Int Rev Psychiatry 2013;25:554–71.

49. **FDA** (2015). 'Table of pharmacogenomic biomarkers in drug labeling'. Retrieved 23 September 2015, from http://www.fda.gov/drugs/scienceresearch/researchareas/pharmacogenetics/ucm083378.htm.

50. **Altar CA, Hornberger J, Shewade A, Cruz V, Garrison J**, and **Mrazek D**. Clinical validity of cytochrome P450 metabolism and serotonin gene variants in psychiatric pharmacotherapy, Int Rev Psychiatry 2013;25:509–33.

51. **Cabaleiro T, Lopez-Rodriguez R, Roman M, Ochoa D, Novalbos J, Borobia A,** et al. Pharmacogenetics of quetiapine in healthy volunteers: association with pharmacokinetics, pharmacodynamics, and adverse effects, Int Clin Psychopharmacol 2015;30:82–8.

52. **Cabaleiro T, Lopez-Rodriguez R, Ochoa D, Roman M, Novalbos J**, and **Abad-Santos F**. Polymorphisms influencing olanzapine metabolism and adverse effects in healthy subjects, Hum Psychopharmacol 2013;28:205–14.

53. **Katsanis SH, Minear MA, Vorderstrasse A, Yang N, Reeves JW, Rakhra-Burris T**, et al. Perspectives on genetic and genomic technologies in an academic medical center: the duke experience, J Pers Med 2015;5:67–82.

Index